Reducing the Health Consequences of Smoking

25 YEARS OF PROGRESS

a report of the Surgeon General

1989

Executive Summary

U.S. DEPARTMENT OF HEALTH AND HUMAN SERVICES
Public Health Service
Centers for Disease Control
Center for Chronic Disease Prevention and Health Promotion
Office on Smoking and Health
Rockville, Maryland 20857

THE SECRETARY OF HEALTH AND HUMAN SERVICES
WASHINGTON, D.C. 20201

DEC 29 1988

The Honorable Jim Wright
Speaker of the House
of Representatives
Washington, D.C. 20515

Dear Mr. Speaker:

It is my pleasure to transmit to the Congress the 1989 Surgeon General's Report on the health consequences of smoking, as mandated by Section 8(a) of the Public Health Cigarette Smoking Act of 1969. The report was prepared by the Centers for Disease Control's Office on Smoking and Health.

This report, entitled Reducing the Health Consequences of Smoking: 25 Years of Progress, examines the fundamental developments over the past quarter century in smoking prevalence and in mortality caused by smoking. It highlights important gains in preventing smoking and smoking-related disease, reviews changes in programs and policies designed to reduce smoking, and emphasizes sources of continuing concern and remaining challenges.

During the past 25 years, smoking behavior has changed dramatically. Nearly half of all living adults who ever smoked have quit. The prevalence of smoking has declined steadily, with a particularly impressive decline among men. Smoking prevalence among men decreased from 50 percent in 1965 to 32 percent in 1987. As a result, lung cancer mortality rates among men are now leveling off after many decades of consistent increase. Despite this progress, the prevalence of smoking remains higher among blacks, blue-collar workers, and less-educated persons, than in the overall population. Smoking among high school seniors leveled off from 1981 through 1987 after previous years of decline.

In 1985, the last year for which estimates are available, approximately 390,000 Americans died as the result of past and current smoking. This represents more than one of every six deaths in the United States. Smoking remains the single most important preventable cause of death in our society.

To maintain our momentum toward a smoke-free society, we must focus our efforts on preventing smoking initiation and encouraging smoking cessation among high-risk populations. Increased public information activities, smoking prevention and cessation programs, and policies that encourage nonsmoking behavior should be pursued. Unless we meet this challenge successfully, smoking-related mortality will remain high well into the 21st Century.

Sincerely,

Otis R. Bowen, M.D.
Secretary

Enclosure

THE SECRETARY OF HEALTH AND HUMAN SERVICES
WASHINGTON, D.C. 20201

DEC 29 1988

The Honorable George Bush
President of the Senate
Washington, D.C. 20515

Dear Mr. President:

It is my pleasure to transmit to the Congress the 1989 Surgeon General's Report on the health consequences of smoking, as mandated by Section 8(a) of the Public Health Cigarette Smoking Act of 1969. The report was prepared by the Centers for Disease Control's Office on Smoking and Health.

This report, entitled Reducing the Health Consequences of Smoking: 25 Years of Progress, examines the fundamental developments over the past quarter century in smoking prevalence and in mortality caused by smoking. It highlights important gains in preventing smoking and smoking-related disease, reviews changes in programs and policies designed to reduce smoking, and emphasizes sources of continuing concern and remaining challenges.

During the past 25 years, smoking behavior has changed dramatically. Nearly half of all living adults who ever smoked have quit. The prevalence of smoking has declined steadily, with a particularly impressive decline among men. Smoking prevalence among men decreased from 50 percent in 1965 to 32 percent in 1987. As a result, lung cancer mortality rates among men are now leveling off after many decades of consistent increase. Despite this progress, the prevalence of smoking remains higher among blacks, blue-collar workers, and less-educated persons, than in the overall population. Smoking among high school seniors leveled off from 1981 through 1987 after previous years of decline.

In 1985, the last year for which estimates are available, approximately 390,000 Americans died as the result of past and current smoking. This represents more than one of every six deaths in the United States. Smoking remains the single most important preventable cause of death in our society.

To maintain our momentum toward a smoke-free society, we must focus our efforts on preventing smoking initiation and encouraging smoking cessation among high-risk populations. Increased public information activities, smoking prevention and cessation programs, and policies that encourage nonsmoking behavior should be pursued. Unless we meet this challenge successfully, smoking-related mortality will remain high well into the 21st Century.

Sincerely,

Otis R. Bowen, M.D.
Secretary

Enclosure

FOREWORD

Twenty-five years have elapsed since publication of the landmark report of the Surgeon General's Advisory Committee on Smoking and Health. By any measure, these 25 years have witnessed dramatic changes in attitudes toward and use of tobacco in the United States. The health consequences of tobacco use will be with us for many years to come, but those consequences have been greatly reduced by the social revolution that has occurred during this period with regard to smoking.

Since 1964, substantial changes have occurred in scientific knowledge of the health hazards of smoking, in the impact of smoking on mortality, in public knowledge of the dangers of smoking, in the prevalence of smoking and using other forms of tobacco, in the availability of programs to help smokers quit, and in the number of policies that encourage nonsmoking behavior and protect nonsmokers from exposure to environmental tobacco smoke. These changes and other significant developments, as well as the overall impact of the Nation's antismoking activities, are reviewed in detail in the individual chapters of this Report. Based on this review, five major conclusions of the entire Report were reached. The first two conclusions highlight important gains in preventing smoking and smoking-related disease in the United States. The last three conclusions emphasize sources of continuing concern and remaining challenges. The conclusions are:

1. **The prevalence of smoking among adults decreased from 40 percent in 1965 to 29 percent in 1987. Nearly half of all living adults who ever smoked have quit.**
2. **Between 1964 and 1985, approximately three-quarters of a million smoking-related deaths were avoided or postponed as a result of decisions to quit smoking or not to start. Each of these avoided or postponed deaths represented an average gain in life expectancy of two decades.**
3. **The prevalence of smoking remains higher among blacks, blue-collar workers, and less educated persons than in the overall population. The decline in smoking has been substantially slower among women than among men.**
4. **Smoking begins primarily during childhood and adolescence. The age of initiation has fallen over time, particularly among females. Smoking among high school seniors leveled off from 1980 through 1987 after previous years of decline.**
5. **Smoking is responsible for more than one of every six deaths in the United States. Smoking remains the single most important preventable cause of death in our society.**

The last 25 years have witnessed phenomenal changes in the way Americans think about tobacco use. More people now than ever before consider smoking to be outside the social norm. Antismoking programs and policies have contributed to this change. This shift in societal attitudes is almost certain to generate additional efforts to further limit the use of tobacco.

Almost half of all living Americans who ever smoked have quit. This is especially remarkable when one takes into account the powerful media images enticing people to smoke and the powerfully addictive nature of nicotine. As the downward trends in smoking behavior continue, we can expect to see a decline in the number of premature deaths and avoidable morbidity due to smoking.

For now, however, we must recognize that continued tobacco exposure in the population will cause a great deal of human suffering for many decades. Thus, we must not rest upon the laurels of the past quarter century. As long as children and adolescents continue to find reasons to use tobacco, replacements will be recruited for at least some of the smokers who quit or who die prematurely. If current trends continue, these replacements will be found disproportionately among minority groups, among the less educated, among the most economically disadvantaged, and among women.

We must look back on the last 25 years of change in order to look forward to our tasks for the future. Surely those tasks include expanding educational efforts for the young and old alike, restrictions against minors' access to tobacco, support for cessation activities, and restrictions against smoking in worksites, restaurants, transportation vehicles, and other public places.

The Public Health Service is dedicated to continuing the legacy of the 1964 Report. We hope this 25th Anniversary Report will stimulate new commitment to action by public health officials, civic leaders, educators, scientists, and the public at large on the problem of tobacco use, especially among children, adolescents, and high-risk groups.

Robert E. Windom, M.D.
Assistant Secretary for Health
Public Health Service

James O. Mason, M.D., Dr.P.H.
Director
Centers for Disease Control

PREFACE

Exactly 25 years ago, on January 11, 1964, Luther L. Terry, M.D., Surgeon General of the U.S. Public Health Service, released the report of the Surgeon General's Advisory Committee on Smoking and Health. That landmark document, now referred to as the first Surgeon General's Report on Smoking and Health, was America's first widely publicized official recognition that cigarette smoking is a cause of cancer and other serious diseases.

On the basis of more than 7,000 articles relating to smoking and disease already available at that time in the biomedical literature, the Advisory Committee concluded that cigarette smoking is a cause of lung cancer and laryngeal cancer in men, a probable cause of lung cancer in women, and the most important cause of chronic bronchitis. The Committee stated that "Cigarette smoking is a health hazard of sufficient importance in the United States to warrant appropriate remedial action."

What would constitute "appropriate remedial action" was left unspecified. But the release of the report was the first in a series of steps, still being taken 25 years later, to diminish the impact of tobacco use on the health of the American people.

This 1989 Report, the 20th in a series of Surgeon General's Reports on the Health Consequences of Smoking, spells out the dramatic progress that has been achieved in the past quarter century against one of our deadliest risks.

The circumstances surrounding the release of the first report in 1964 are worth remembering. The date chosen was a Saturday morning, to guard against a precipitous reaction on Wall Street. An auditorium in the State Department was selected because its security could be assured—it had been the site for press conferences of the late President John F. Kennedy, whose assassination had occurred less than 2 months earlier.

The first two copies of the 387-page, brown-covered Report were hand delivered to the West Wing of the White House at 7:30 on that Saturday morning. At 9:00, accredited press representatives were admitted to the auditorium and "locked in," without access to telephones. Surgeon General Terry and his Advisory Committee took their seats on the platform. The Report was distributed and reporters were allowed 90 minutes to read it. Questions were answered by Dr. Terry and his Committee members. Finally, the doors were opened and the news was spread. For several days, the Report furnished newspaper headlines across the country and lead stories on television newscasts. Later it was ranked among the top news stories of 1964.

During the quarter century that has elapsed since that Report, individual citizens, private organizations, public agencies, and elected officials have tirelessly pursued the Advisory Committee's call for "appropriate remedial action." Early on, the U.S. Congress adopted the Federal Cigarette Labeling and Advertising Act of 1965 and the

Public Health Cigarette Smoking Act of 1969. These laws required a health warning on cigarette packages, banned cigarette advertising in the broadcast media, and called for an annual report on the health consequences of smoking.

In 1964, the Public Health Service established a small unit called the National Clearinghouse for Smoking and Health (NCSH). Through the years, the Clearinghouse and its successor organization, the Office on Smoking and Health, have been responsible for the 20 reports on the health consequences of smoking previously mentioned, eight of which have been issued during my tenure as Surgeon General. In close cooperation with voluntary health organizations, the Public Health Service has supported highly successful school and community programs on smoking and health, has disseminated research findings related to tobacco use, and has ensured the continued public visibility of antismoking messages.

Throughout this period, tremendous changes have occurred. As detailed in this Report, we have witnessed expansion in scientific knowledge of the health hazards of smoking, growing public knowledge of the dangers of smoking, increased availability of programs to prevent young people from starting to smoke and to help smokers quit, and widespread adoption of policies that discourage the use of tobacco.

Most important, these developments have changed the way in which our society views smoking. In the 1940s and 1950s, smoking was chic; now, increasingly, it is shunned. Movie stars, sports heroes, and other celebrities used to appear in cigarette advertisements. Today, actors, athletes, public figures, and political candidates are rarely seen smoking. The ashtray is following the spittoon into oblivion.

Within this evolving social milieu, the population has been giving up smoking in increasing numbers. Nearly half of all living adults who ever smoked have quit. The most impressive decline in smoking has occurred among men. Smoking prevalence among men has fallen from 50 percent in 1965 to 32 percent in 1987. These changes represent nothing less than a revolution in behavior.

The antismoking campaign has been a major public health success. Those who have participated in this campaign can take tremendous pride in the progress that has been made.

The analysis in this Report shows that in the absence of the campaign, there would have been 91 million American smokers (15 to 84 years of age) in 1985 instead of 56 million. As a result of decisions to quit smoking or not to start, an estimated 789,000 smoking-related deaths were avoided or postponed between 1964 and 1985. Furthermore, these decisions will result in the avoidance or postponement of an estimated 2.1 million smoking-related deaths between 1986 and the year 2000.

This achievement has few parallels in the history of public health. It was accomplished despite the addictive nature of tobacco and the powerful economic forces promoting its use.

The Remaining Challenges

Despite this achievement, smoking will continue as the leading cause of preventable, premature death for many years to come, even if all smokers were to quit today. Smoking cessation is clearly beneficial in reducing the risk of dying from smoking-related diseases. However, for some diseases, such as lung cancer and emphysema, quitting may not reduce the risk to the level of a lifetime nonsmoker even after many years of abstinence. This residual health risk is one reason why approximately 390,000 Americans died in 1985 as the result of smoking, even after two decades of declining smoking rates.

The critical message here is that progress in curtailing smoking must continue, and ideally accelerate, to enable us to turn smoking-related mortality around. Otherwise, the disease impact of smoking will remain high well into the 21st century.

Just maintaining the current rate of progress is a challenge. Compared with nonsmokers, smokers are disproportionately found in groups that are harder to reach, and this disparity may increase over time. Greater effort and resources will need to be devoted to achieve equivalent reductions in smoking among those whose behavior has survived strong, countervailing social pressures.

Today, thanks to the remarkable progress of the past 25 years, we can dare to envision a smoke-free society. Indeed it can be said that the social tide is flowing toward that bold objective. To maintain momentum, we need to direct special attention to the following groups within our society:

Children and Adolescents

As a pediatric surgeon, and now as Surgeon General, I have dedicated my career to protecting the health of children. In the case of smoking, children and adolescents hold the key to progress toward curbing tobacco use in future generations.

If the adult rate of smoking were to continue at the present level, the impact of smoking on the future health and welfare of today's children would be enormous. Research has shown that one-fourth or more of all regular cigarette smokers die of smoking-related diseases. If 20 million of the 70 million children now living in the United States smoke cigarettes as adults (about 29 percent), then at least 5 million of them will die of smoking-related diseases. This figure should alarm anyone who is concerned with the future health of today's children.

Two additional factors make smoking among young people a preeminent public health concern: (1) the age of initiation of smoking, and (2) nicotine addiction. As this Report shows, four-fifths of smokers born since 1935 started smoking before age 21. The proportion of smokers who begin smoking during adolescence has been increasing over time, particularly among women.

In the Teenage Smoking Survey conducted by the Department of Health, Education, and Welfare in 1979, respondents were asked, "What would you say is the possibility that five years from now you will be a cigarette smoker?" Among smokers, half answered "definitely not" or "probably not." This response suggests that many children and adolescents are unaware of, or underestimate, the addictive nature of smoking. The predecessor to this volume, *The Health Consequences of Smoking: Nicotine Addiction*, provided a comprehensive review of the evidence that cigarettes and other forms of tobacco are addicting and that nicotine is the drug in tobacco that causes addiction.

These two factors refute the argument that smoking is a matter of free choice. Most smokers start smoking as teenagers and then become addicted. By the time smokers become adults, when they would be expected to have greater appreciation of the health effects of smoking, many have difficulty quitting. Today, 80 percent of smokers say they would like to quit; two thirds of smokers have made at least one serious attempt to quit. Characteristically, people quit smoking several times before becoming permanent ex-smokers.

The prevalence of daily smoking among high school seniors leveled off from 1981 through 1987, at about 20 percent, after previous years of decline. Each day, more than 3,000 American teenagers start smoking. If we can substantially reduce this number, we will soon achieve a major impact on smoking prevalence among adults. Although research efforts in prevention are increasing, prevention programs are not yet reaching large numbers of young people. The public health community should pay at least as much attention to the prevention of smoking among teenagers as it now pays to smoking cessation among adults. Comprehensive school health education, incorporating tobacco use prevention, should be provided in every school throughout the country.

Women

Since release of the first Surgeon General's Report, the prevalence of smoking among women has declined much more slowly than among men. If current trends continue, smoking rates will be about equal among men and women in the mid-1990s, after which women may smoke at a higher rate than men.

The public health impact of this trend is already being seen. Lung cancer mortality rates are increasing steadily among women, and estimates by the American Cancer Society indicate that this disease has now overtaken breast cancer as the number one cause of cancer death among women. Smoking during pregnancy poses special risks to the developing fetus and is an important cause of low birthweight and infant mortality. Smoking and oral contraceptive use interact to increase dramatically the risk of cardiovascular disease. Women's organizations and women's magazines have paid scant attention to these issues.

The key to addressing this problem is the prevention of smoking among female adolescents. The disparity in smoking prevalence between men and women is primarily a reflection of differences in smoking initiation. Smoking initiation has declined much more slowly among females than among males. This difference is due, in large part, to increasing initiation rates among less educated young women. Among high school seniors, the prevalence of daily smoking has been higher among females than among males each year since 1977.

In summary, women, and especially female adolescents not planning higher education, are an important target group for prevention activities.

Minorities

Smoking rates are higher in certain racial and ethnic minority groups, many of which already suffer from a disproportionate share of risk factors and illness. In particular, smoking prevalence has been consistently higher among black men than among white men (41 and 31 percent, respectively, in 1987). In addition, the limited data available show higher rates of smoking among Hispanic men than among white men.

Trends in smoking initiation, prevalence, and quitting among blacks and whites show similar rates of change from 1974 to 1985. Thus, the gap in smoking prevalence between blacks and whites is not widening. However, to reduce the gap in smoking between blacks and whites, prevention efforts must focus on blacks more successfully. The public health community is only now beginning to address this problem. The urgency of the situation is greater because cigarette companies are increasingly targeting their marketing efforts at blacks and Hispanics.

Blue-Collar Workers

The prevalence of smoking has been consistently higher among blue-collar workers than among white-collar workers. In 1985, 40 percent of blue-collar workers smoked compared with 28 percent of white-collar workers. Again, blue-collar workers are a major target of cigarette company advertising and promotional campaigns. Worksite smoking cessation programs, employee incentive programs, and policies banning or restricting smoking at the workplace are effective strategies to reach this group.

Toward a Smoke-Free Future

Because the general health risks of smoking are well known, because smoking is banned or restricted in a growing number of public places and worksites, and because smoking is losing its social acceptability, the overall prevalence of smoking in our society is likely to continue to decline. The progress we have achieved during the past quarter century is impressive.

Equally impressive, however, are the challenges we face. During the next quarter century and beyond, progress will be slow, and smoking-related mortality will remain high, unless the health community more effectively reaches children and adolescents, women, minorities, and blue-collar workers. Organizations that represent these groups can contribute substantially to the antismoking movement. In large part, the future health of these populations will depend on the degree to which schools, educators, parents' organizations, women's groups, minority organizations, employers, and employee unions join the campaign for a smoke-free society. Here in the United States, such a society is an attainable long-term goal.

Unfortunately, the looming epidemic of smoking and smoking-related disease in developing countries does not encourage similar optimism. According to the World Health Organization, increases in cigarette consumption between 1971 and 1981 exceeded population growth in all developing regions: by 77 percent in Africa, and by 30 percent in Asia and Latin America.

The topic of tobacco and health internationally, although critically important, especially for developing nations, is beyond the scope of this Report. I can only hope that the lessons we have learned in the United States, as detailed in this Report, will help other countries take the necessary steps to avoid the devastation caused by use of tobacco.

C. Everett Koop, M.D., Sc.D.
Surgeon General

ACKNOWLEDGMENTS

This Report was prepared by the Department of Health and Human Services under the general editorship of the Office on Smoking and Health, Ronald M. Davis, M.D., Director. The Managing Editors were Susan A. Hawk, Ed.M., M.S., and Thomas E. Novotny, M.D., Office on Smoking and Health.

The scientific editors of the Report were:

Kenneth E. Warner, Ph.D. (Senior Scientific Editor), Professor, Department of Public Health Policy and Administration, School of Public Health, University of Michigan, Ann Arbor, Michigan

Ronald M. Davis, M.D., Director, Office on Smoking and Health, Center for Chronic Disease Prevention and Health Promotion, Centers for Disease Control, Rockville, Maryland

John H. Holbrook, M.D., Professor of Internal Medicine, Department of Internal Medicine, University Hospital, Salt Lake City, Utah

Thomas E. Novotny, M.D., Medical Epidemiologist, Office on Smoking and Health, Center for Chronic Disease Prevention and Health Promotion, Centers for Disease Control, Rockville, Maryland

Judith K. Ockene, Ph.D., Associate Professor of Medicine, and Director, Division of Preventive and Behavioral Medicine, Department of Medicine, University of Massachusetts Medical School, Worcester, Massachusetts

Nancy A. Rigotti, M.D., Associate Director, Institute for the Study of Smoking Behavior and Policy, John F. Kennedy School of Government, Harvard University, Cambridge, Massachusetts, Instructor in Medicine, Harvard Medical School, Boston, Massachusetts

The following individuals prepared draft chapters or portions of the Report.

Elvin E. Adams, M.D., M.P.H., Associate Director, Health Department, General Conference of Seventh-Day Adventists, Washington, D.C.

Gregory N. Connolly, D.M.D., M.P.H., Director, Office for Nonsmoking and Health, Massachusetts Department of Public Health, Boston, Massachusetts

K. Michael Cummings, Ph.D., M.P.H., Director, Smoking Control Program, Roswell Park Memorial Institute, Buffalo, New York

Ronald M. Davis, M.D., Director, Office on Smoking and Health, Center for Chronic Disease Prevention and Health Promotion, Centers for Disease Control, Rockville, Maryland

Joseph R. DiFranza, M.D., Director of Research, Fitchburg Family Practice Residency Program, University of Massachusetts Medical Center, Fitchburg, Massachusetts

Michael P. Eriksen, Sc.D., Director, Behavioral Research Program, Department of Cancer Prevention and Control, The University of Texas M.D. Anderson Cancer Center, Houston, Texas

David P. Fan, Ph.D., Professor of Genetics and Cell Biology, University of Minnesota, St. Paul, Minnesota

Michael C. Fiore, M.D., M.P.H., Assistant Professor, Department of Medicine, Center for Health Sciences, University of Wisconsin, Madison, Wisconsin

Edwin B. Fisher, Jr., Ph.D., Associate Professor of Psychology, Director, Center for Health Behavior Research, Washington University, St. Louis, Missouri

Jeffrey E. Harris, M.D., Ph.D., Visiting Associate Professor, Department of Biostatistics, Harvard School of Public Health, Boston, Massachusetts; Clinical Associate, Medical Services, Massachusetts General Hospital, Boston, Massachusetts; Associate Professor of Economics, Massachusetts Institute of Technology, Cambridge, Massachusetts

Jan L. Hitchcock, Ph.D., Associate Director, Institute for the Study of Smoking Behavior and Policy, John F. Kennedy School of Government, Harvard University, Cambridge, Massachusetts

Thomas A. Hodgson, Ph.D., Chief Economist, Office of Analysis and Epidemiology, National Center for Health Statistics, Hyattsville, Maryland

Dietrich Hoffmann, Ph.D., Associate Director, Naylor Dana Institute for Disease Prevention, American Health Foundation, Valhalla, New York

Ilse Hoffmann, Research Coordinator, Naylor Dana Institute for Disease Prevention, American Health Foundation, Valhalla, New York

Juliette S. Kendrick, M.D., Deputy Chief, Pregnancy Epidemiology Branch, Division of Reproductive Health, Center for Chronic Disease Prevention and Health Promotion, Centers for Disease Control, Atlanta, Georgia

Lewis H. Kuller, M.D., Dr.P.H., Professor and Chairperson, Department of Epidemiology, Graduate School of Public Health, University of Pittsburgh, Pittsburgh, Pennsylvania

Eugene M. Lewit, Ph.D., Associate Professor, Departments of Medicine and Preventive Medicine and Community Health, Office of Primary Health Care Education, UMDNJ—New Jersey Medical School, Newark, New Jersey

Edward Lichtenstein, Ph.D., Research Scientist, Oregon Research Institute; Professor of Psychology, University of Oregon, Eugene, Oregon

Thomas E. Novotny, M.D., Medical Epidemiologist, Office on Smoking and Health, Center for Chronic Disease Prevention and Health Promotion, Centers for Disease Control, Rockville, Maryland

Judith K. Ockene, Ph.D., Associate Professor of Medicine, and Director, Division of Preventive and Behavioral Medicine, Department of Medicine, University of Massachusetts Medical School, Worcester, Massachusetts

Chris Leo Pashos, M.P.P., Project Coordinator, Institute for the Study of Smoking Behavior and Policy, John F. Kennedy School of Government, Harvard University, Cambridge, Massachusetts

Richard Peto, M.A., M.Sc., ICRF Cancer Studies Unit, Radcliffe Infirmary, Oxford, England

John P. Pierce, M.Sc., Ph.D., Chief, Epidemiology Branch, Office on Smoking and Health, Center for Chronic Disease Prevention and Health Promotion, Centers for Disease Control, Rockville, Maryland

John M. Pinney, Executive Director, Institute for the Study of Smoking Behavior and Policy, John F. Kennedy School of Government, Harvard University, Cambridge, Massachusetts

Edward T. Popper, M.B.A., D.B.A., Associate Professor of Marketing, Bryant College, Smithfield, Rhode Island

Patrick L. Remington, M.D., M.P.H., Medical Epidemiologist, Bureau of Community Health and Prevention, Wisconsin Division of Health, Madison, Wisconsin

Nancy A. Rigotti, M.D., Associate Director, Institute for the Study of Smoking Behavior and Policy, John F. Kennedy School of Government, Harvard University, Cambridge, Massachusetts, and Instructor in Medicine, Harvard Medical School, Boston, Massachusetts

Jonathan M. Samet, M.D., Professor of Medicine, Department of Medicine, Chief, Pulmonary Division, University of New Mexico, Albuquerque, New Mexico

Russell C. Sciandra, M.A., Associate Director, Smoking Control Program, Roswell Park Memorial Institute, Buffalo, New York

Carol Anne Soltanek, M.D., Resident, Southwestern Michigan Area Health Education Center, Kalamazoo, Michigan

Michael A. Stoto, Ph.D., Senior Staff Officer, Institute of Medicine, National Academy of Sciences, Washington, D.C.

Owen T. Thornberry, Ph.D., Director, Division of Health Interview Statistics, National Center for Health Statistics, Centers for Disease Control, Hyattsville, Maryland

Kenneth E. Warner, Ph.D., Professor, Department of Public Health Policy and Administration, School of Public Health, University of Michigan, Ann Arbor, Michigan

The editors acknowledge with gratitude the following distinguished scientists, physicians, and others who lent their support in the development of this Report by coordinating manuscript preparation, contributing critical reviews, or assisting in other ways.

Elvin E. Adams, M.D., M.P.H., Associate Director, Health Department, General Conference of Seventh-Day Adventists, Washington, D.C.

Charles Althafer, M.P.H., Assistant Director for Health Promotion and Risk Appraisal, Office of Program Planning and Evaluation, National Institute for Occupational Safety and Health, Centers for Disease Control, Atlanta, Georgia

Lynn M. Artz, M.D., M.P.H., Senior Policy Advisor, Office of Disease Prevention and Health Promotion, Office of the Assistant Secretary for Health, Washington, D.C.

Donald A. Berreth, Director, Office of Public Affairs, Centers for Disease Control, Atlanta, Georgia

Gayle M. Boyd, Ph.D., Program Director, Smoking, Tobacco and Cancer Program, Division of Cancer Prevention and Control, National Cancer Institute, Bethesda, Maryland

Allan Brandt, Ph.D., Department of Social Medicine and Health Policy, Harvard Medical School, Boston, Massachusetts

Lester Breslow, M.D., M.P.H., Professor, School of Public Health, and Director, Health Services Research, Jonsson Comprehensive Cancer Center, University of California, Los Angeles, Los Angeles, California

Clarice Brown, M.S., Data Analyst, Office of Prevention, Education, and Control, National Heart, Lung, and Blood Institute, Bethesda, Maryland

David P. Brown, M.D., Deputy Director, Division of Surveillance, Hazard Evaluations, and Field Studies, National Institute for Occupational Safety and Health, Centers for Disease Control, Atlanta, Georgia

Martin Brown, Ph.D., Surveillance and Operations Research Branch, Division of Cancer Prevention and Control, National Cancer Institute, Bethesda, Maryland

David M. Burns, M.D., Associate Professor of Medicine, Division of Pulmonary and Critical Care Medicine, University of California, San Diego Medical Center, San Diego, California

Dee Burton, Ph.D., Assistant Professor, Prevention Research Center, School of Public Health, University of Illinois at Chicago, Chicago, Illinois

Frank J. Chaloupka, Ph.D., Assistant Professor, Department of Economics, College of Business Administration, University of Illinois at Chicago, Chicago, Illinois

Paul D. Cleary, Ph.D., Department of Health Care Policy and The Division on Aging, Harvard Medical School, Boston, Massachusetts

Alexander Cohen, Ph.D., Deputy Director, Division of Biomedical and Behavioral Science, National Institute for Occupational Safety and Health, Centers for Disease Control, Atlanta, Georgia

Joel B. Cohen, Ph.D., Distinguished Service Professor and Director, Center for Consumer Research, University of Florida, Gainesville, Florida

Michael J. Cowell, F.S.A., Vice President and Corporate Actuary, UNUM Life Insurance Company, Portland, Maine

Joseph W. Cullen, Ph.D., Deputy Director, Division of Cancer Prevention and Control, National Cancer Institute, Coordinator for the National Cancer Institute's Smoking, Tobacco and Cancer Program, Bethesda, Maryland

Sir Richard Doll, Emeritus Professor of Medicine, University of Oxford, Acting Director, Imperial Cancer Research Fund, Cancer Epidemiology and Clinical Trials Unit, Oxford, England

J. David Erickson, D.D.S., Ph.D., Chief, Birth Defects and Genetic Diseases Branch, Division of Birth Defects and Developmental Disabilities, Center for Environmental Health and Injury Control, Centers for Disease Control, Atlanta, Georgia

Michael P. Eriksen, Sc.D., Director, Behavioral Research Program, Department of Cancer Prevention and Control, University of Texas M.D. Anderson Cancer Center, Houston, Texas

Virginia L. Ernster, Ph.D., Professor of Epidemiology, Department of Epidemiology and International Health, School of Medicine, University of California, San Francisco, California

Roberta G. Ferrence, Ph.D., Prevention Studies Department, Addiction Research Foundation, Toronto, Ontario, Canada

Jonathan E. Fielding, M.D., M.P.H., Professor of Public Health and Pediatrics, University of California at Los Angeles, Los Angeles, California, Vice President and Health Director, Johnson and Johnson Health Management, Inc., Santa Monica, California

John R. Finnegan, Jr., Ph.D., Assistant Professor, School of Public Health, University of Minnesota, Minneapolis, Minnesota

Martin Fishbein, Ph.D., Professor of Psychology and Research Professor, Institute of Communications Research, University of Illinois, Champaign–Urbana, Illinois

Brian R. Flay, D.Phil., Associate Professor and Director, Prevention Research Center, School of Public Health, University of Illinois at Chicago, Chicago, Illinois

William H. Foege, M.D., M.P.H., Executive Director, The Carter Center, Emory University, Atlanta, Georgia

Peter L. Frommer, M.D., Deputy Director, National Heart, Lung, and Blood Institute, National Institutes of Health, Bethesda, Maryland

Lawrence Garfinkel, M.A., Vice President for Epidemiology and Statistics, Director, Cancer Prevention, American Cancer Society, New York, New York

Donald W. Garner, J.D., Professor of Law, Southern Illinois University School of Law, Carbondale, Illinois

Russell E. Glasgow, Ph.D., Research Scientist, Oregon Research Institute, Eugene, Oregon

Thomas J. Glynn, Ph.D., Program Director for Smoking Research, Smoking, Tobacco, and Cancer Program, National Cancer Institute, Bethesda, Maryland

Frederick K. Goodwin, M.D., Administrator, Alcohol, Drug Abuse, and Mental Health Administration, Rockville, Maryland

Nancy P. Gordon, Sc.D., Behavioral Scientist, Division of Research, Northern California Kaiser Permanente Medical Care Program

Leonard Green, Ph.D., Professor of Psychology, Department of Psychology, Washington University, St. Louis, Missouri

Ellen R. Gritz, Ph.D., Director, Division of Cancer Control, Jonsson Comprehensive Cancer Center, University of California, Los Angeles, Los Angeles, California

Neil E. Grunberg, Ph.D., Associate Professor, Department of Medical Psychology, Uniformed Services University of the Health Sciences, Bethesda, Maryland

Dudley H. Hafner, Executive Vice President, American Heart Association, Dallas, Texas

James A. Harrell, M.A., Acting Director, Office of Disease Prevention and Health Promotion, Office of the Assistant Secretary for Health, Washington, D.C.

Jeffrey E. Harris, M.D., Ph.D., Visiting Associate Professor, Department of Biostatistics, Harvard School of Public Health, Boston, Massachusetts; Clinical Associate, Medical Services, Massachusetts General Hospital, Boston, Massachusetts; Associate Professor of Economics, Massachusetts Institute of Technology, Cambridge, Massachusetts

Jack E. Henningfield, Ph.D., Chief, Biology of Dependence and Abuse Potential Assessment Laboratory, Addiction Research Center, National Institute on Drug Abuse, Baltimore, Maryland

Carol J. Hogue, Ph.D., Director, Division of Reproductive Health, Center for Chronic Disease Prevention and Health Promotion, Centers for Disease Control, Atlanta, Georgia

Elvin Hilyer, Associate Director for Policy Coordination, Centers for Disease Control, Atlanta, Georgia

Richard Jessor, Ph.D., Professor of Psychology, Director of the Institute of Behavioral Science, University of Colorado at Boulder, Boulder, Colorado

Lloyd D. Johnston, Ph.D., Program Director, Institute for Social Research, University of Michigan, Ann Arbor, Michigan

John T. Kalberer, Jr., Ph.D., Deputy Director, Division of Disease Prevention, Office of Disease Prevention, Office of the Director, National Institutes of Health, Bethesda, Maryland

Martha F. Katz, M.P.A., Director, Office of Program Planning and Evaluation, Centers for Disease Control, Atlanta, Georgia

John H. Kelso, Acting Administrator, Health Resources and Services Administration, Rockville, Maryland

Larry Kessler, Sc.D., Surveillance and Operations Research Branch, National Cancer Institute, Bethesda, Maryland

A. Joan Klebba, M.A., Statistician, Division of Vital Statistics, National Center for Health Statistics, Centers for Disease Control, Hyattsville, Maryland

Lloyd J. Kolbe, Ph.D., Acting Director, Division of Adolescent and School Health, Center for Chronic Disease Prevention and Health Promotion, Centers for Disease Control, Atlanta, Georgia

Jeffrey P. Koplan, M.D., M.P.H., Director, Center for Chronic Disease Prevention and Health Promotion, Centers for Disease Control, Atlanta, Georgia

Lynn T. Kozlowski, Ph.D., Head, Behavioral Research on Tobacco Use, Addiction Research Foundation, Toronto, Ontario, Canada

Marshall W. Kreuter, Ph.D., Director, Division of Chronic Disease Control and Community Intervention, Center for Chronic Disease Prevention and Health Promotion, Centers for Disease Control, Atlanta, Georgia

Harry A. Lando, Ph.D., Associate Professor, Division of Epidemiology, School of Public Health, University of Minnesota, Minneapolis, Minnesota

Charles A. LeMaistre, M.D., President, University of Texas M.D. Anderson Cancer Center, Houston, Texas

Claude Lenfant, M.D., Director, National Heart, Lung, and Blood Institute, National Institutes of Health, Bethesda, Maryland

Eugene M. Lewit, Ph.D., Associate Professor, Departments of Medicine and Preventive Medicine and Community Health, Office of Primary Health Care Education, UMDNJ—New Jersey Medical School, Newark, New Jersey

Bryan R. Luce, M.B.A., Ph.D., Battelle Human Affairs Research Center, Washington, D.C.

Dolores M. Malvitz, Dr.P.H., Dental Disease Prevention Activity, Center for Prevention Services, Centers for Disease Control, Atlanta, Georgia

Alfred C. Marcus, Ph.D., Associate Director, Division of Cancer Control, Jonsson Comprehensive Cancer Center, University of California at Los Angeles, Los Angeles, California

James S. Marks, M.D., M.P.H., Deputy Director for Public Health Practice, Center for Chronic Disease Prevention and Health Promotion, Centers for Disease Control, Atlanta, Georgia

James O. Mason, M.D., Dr.P.H., Director, Centers for Disease Control, Atlanta, Georgia

Robin J. Mermelstein, Ph.D., Assistant Professor, Prevention Research Center, School of Public Health, University of Illinois at Chicago, Chicago, Illinois

Dannie C. Middleton, M.D., Medical Officer, Document Development Branch, Division of Standards Development and Technology Transfer, National Institute for Occupational Safety and Health, Centers for Disease Control, Atlanta, Georgia

Gregory J. Morosco, Ph.D., M.P.H., Coordinator, National Heart, Lung, and Blood Institute's Smoking Education Program, National Institutes of Health, Bethesda, Maryland

Joseph P. Mulholland, Ph.D., Bureau of Economics, Federal Trade Commission, Washington, D.C.

Hillary Murt, M.P.H., Research Associate, Department of Health Services Management and Policy, School of Public Health, University of Michigan, Ann Arbor, Michigan

Herbert W. Nickens, M.D., M.A., Director, Office of Minority Health, Public Health Service, Washington, D.C.

Richard W. Niemeier, Ph.D., Acting Director, Division of Standards Development and Technology Transfer, National Institute for Occupational Safety and Health, Centers for Disease Control, Atlanta, Georgia

Stuart L. Nightingale, M.D., Associate Commissioner for Health Affairs, Food and Drug Administration, Rockville, Maryland

Ira S. Ockene, M.D., Professor of Medicine; Director, Preventive Cardiology, Division of Cardiovascular Medicine, University of Massachusetts Medical School, Worcester, Massachusetts

Horace G. Ogden, Consultant, Gaithersburg, Maryland

Patrick M. O'Malley, Ph.D., Associate Research Scientist, Institute for Social Research, University of Michigan, Ann Arbor, Michigan

Mario A. Orlandi, Ph.D., M.P.H., Chief, Division of Health Promotion Research, American Health Foundation, New York, New York

Carole Tracy Orleans, Ph.D., Senior Investigator, Behavioral Medicine and Director of Smoking Cessation Services, Fox Chase Cancer Center, Philadelphia, Pennsylvania

Gerry Oster, Ph.D., Vice President, Policy Analysis, Inc., Brookline, Massachusetts

Clifford H. Patrick, Ph.D., Senior Public Health Advisor, Office of Minority Health, Washington, D.C.

Cheryl L. Perry, Ph.D., Associate Professor, Division of Epidemiology, School of Public Health, University of Minnesota, Minneapolis, Minnesota

Michael Pertschuck, J.D., Co-director, Advocacy Institute, Washington, D.C.

Edward L. Petsonk, M.D., Senior Medical Officer, Clinical Investigations Branch, Division of Respiratory Disease Studies, National Institute for Occupational Safety and Health, Centers for Disease Control, Atlanta, Georgia

John P. Pierce, M.Sc., Ph.D., Chief, Epidemiology Branch, Office on Smoking and Health, Center for Chronic Disease Prevention and Health Promotion, Centers for Disease Control, Rockville, Maryland

John M. Pinney, Executive Director, Institute for the Study of Smoking Behavior and Policy, John F. Kennedy School of Government, Harvard University, Cambridge, Massachusetts

Edward T. Popper, M.B.A., D.B.A., Associate Professor of Marketing, Bryant College, Smithfield, Rhode Island

William F. Raub, M.D., Deputy Director, National Institutes of Health, Bethesda, Maryland

Dorothy P. Rice, B.A., Sc.D.(Hon.), Professor in Residence, Department of Social and Behavioral Sciences, School of Nursing, University of California, San Francisco, San Francisco, California

Lynn Gloeckler Ries, M.S., Division of Cancer Prevention and Control, Surveillance and Operations Research Branch, National Cancer Institute, Bethesda, Maryland

Ruth Roemer, J.D., Adjunct Professor of Health Law, School of Public Health, University of California at Los Angeles, Los Angeles, California; Past President, American Public Health Association

Kenneth J. Rothman, Dr.P.H., Professor of Family and Community Health, University of Massachusetts Medical School, Worcester, Massachusetts

Jonathan M. Samet, M.D., Professor of Medicine, Department of Medicine; Chief, Pulmonary Division, University of New Mexico, Albuquerque, New Mexico

Thomas C. Schelling, Ph.D., Lucius N. Littauer Professor of Political Economy, Director, Institute for the Study of Smoking Behavior and Policy, John F. Kennedy School of Government, Harvard University, Cambridge, Massachusetts

Marvin A. Schneiderman, Ph.D., National Academy of Sciences, National Research Council, Board on Environmental Studies and Toxicology, Washington, D.C.

David Schottenfeld, M.D., M.Sc., John G. Searle Professor and Chairman, Department of Epidemiology, School of Public Health, Professor of Internal Medicine, School of Medicine, University of Michigan, Ann Arbor, Michigan

Lowell E. Sever, Ph.D., Assistant Director for Science, Division of Birth Defects and Developmental Disabilities, Center for Environmental Health and Injury Control, Centers for Disease Control, Atlanta, Georgia

Saul Shiffman, Ph.D., Associate Professor, Department of Psychology; Director, Psychology Clinic, University of Pittsburgh, Pittsburgh, Pennsylvania

Donald R. Shopland, Public Health Advisor, Smoking, Tobacco, and Cancer Program, Office of the Director, Division of Cancer Prevention and Control, National Cancer Institute, Bethesda, Maryland

John Slade, M.D., Department of Medicine, University of Medicine and Dentistry of New Jersey, New Brunswick, New Jersey

Jesse L. Steinfeld, M.D., former Surgeon General, Public Health Service, San Diego, California

Steven D. Stellman, Ph.D., Assistant Commissioner for Biostatistics and Epidemiologic Research, New York City Department of Health, New York, New York
Michael A. Stoto, Ph.D., Senior Staff Officer, Institute of Medicine, National Academy of Sciences, Washington, D.C.
James A. Swomley, Managing Director, American Lung Association, New York, New York
Owen T. Thornberry, Ph.D., Director, Division of Health Interview Statistics, National Center for Health Statistics, Centers for Disease Control, Hyattsville, Maryland
William M. Tipping, Executive Vice President and Chief Executive Officer, American Cancer Society, Atlanta, Georgia
Dennis D. Tolsma, M.P.H., Assistant Director for Public Health Practice, Centers for Disease Control, Atlanta, Georgia
Frederick L. Trowbridge, M.D., Director, Division of Nutrition, Center for Chronic Disease Prevention and Health Promotion, Centers for Disease Control, Atlanta, Georgia
Diana Chapman Walsh, Ph.D., University Professor, Professor of Public Health and Associate Director of the Health Policy Institute, Boston University, Boston, Massachusetts
Judith P. Wilkenfeld, J.D., Program Advisor, Cigarette Advertising and Testing, Federal Trade Commission, Washington, D.C.
Ronald W. Wilson, M.A., Director, Division of Epidemiology and Health Promotion, National Center for Health Statistics, Centers for Disease Control, Hyattsville, Maryland
Deborah M. Winn, Ph.D., Deputy Director, Division of Health Interview Statistics, National Center for Health Statistics, Hyattsville, Maryland
Ernst L. Wynder, M.D., President, American Health Foundation, New York, New York
James B. Wyngaarden, M.D., Director, National Institutes of Health, Bethesda, Maryland

The editors also acknowledge the contributions of the following staff members and others who assisted in the preparation of this Report.

Margaret Anglin, Secretary, Office on Smoking and Health, Rockville, Maryland
Charles Appiah, Project Clerk, The Circle, Inc., McLean, Virginia
John Artis, Courier, The Circle, Inc., McLean, Virginia
John L. Bagrosky, Associate Director for Program Operations, Office on Smoking and Health, Rockville, Maryland
Sonia Balakirsky, Secretary, Office on Smoking and Health, Rockville, Maryland
Carol A. Bean, Ph.D., Project Director, The Circle, Inc., McLean, Virginia
Marissa Bernstein, Editorial Assistant, The Circle, Inc., McLean, Virginia
Doreen M. Bonnett, Senior Editor, The Circle, Inc., McLean, Virginia
Catherine E. Burckhardt, Editorial Assistant, Office on Smoking and Health, Rockville, Maryland
Gayle A. Christman, Administrative Assistant, The Circle, Inc., McLean, Virginia
Carol K. Cummings, Secretary, Office on Smoking and Health, Rockville, Maryland

Karen M. Deasy, Assistant to the Director for Special Projects, Office on Smoking and Health, Rockville, Maryland

Joanna Ebling, Word Processing Specialist, The Circle, Inc., McLean, Virginia

David Fry, Editor, The Circle, Inc., McLean, Virginia

Lynn Funkhauser, Word Processing Specialist, The Circle, Inc., McLean, Virginia

Amy Garson, Student Intern, Office on Smoking and Health, Rockville, Maryland

Gary A. Giovino, Ph.D., Epidemiologist, Office on Smoking and Health, Rockville, Maryland

Arnetta G. Glover, Secretary, Office on Smoking and Health, Rockville, Maryland

Victoria M. Grier, Conference Coordinator, The Circle, Inc., McLean, Virginia

Andree C. Harris, Program Analyst, Center for Chronic Disease Prevention and Health Promotion, Centers for Disease Control, Atlanta, Georgia

Evridiki Hatziandreu, M.D., Dr.P.H., Epidemic Intelligence Service Officer, Office on Smoking and Health, Rockville, Maryland

Patricia E. Healy, Technical Information Specialist, Office on Smoking and Health, Rockville, Maryland

Timothy K. Hensley, Technical Publications Writer, Office on Smoking and Health, Rockville, Maryland

Robert S. Hutchings, Associate Director for Information and Program Development, Office on Smoking and Health, Rockville, Maryland

Karen Jacob, Senior Editor, The Circle, Inc., McLean, Virginia

Beth Jacobsen, Student Intern, Office on Smoking and Health, Rockville, Maryland

Sheila M. Jones, Word Processing Specialist, The Circle, Inc., McLean, Virginia

Kathleen M. Keever, Secretary, Department of Public Health Policy and Administration, School of Public Health, University of Michigan, Ann Arbor, Michigan

Rick Keir, Senior Editor, The Circle, Inc., McLean, Virginia

Jennifer L. Kirscht, M.P.H., Statistics Consultant, Department of Public Health Policy and Administration, School of Public Health, University of Michigan, Ann Arbor, Michigan

Laura Y. Martin, Program Analyst, Office of Program Planning and Evaluation, Centers for Disease Control, Atlanta, Georgia

Daniel F. McLaughlin, Editor, The Circle, Inc., McLean, Virginia

Sherry L. Mills, M.D., M.P.H., Epidemic Intelligence Service Officer, Office on Smoking and Health, Rockville, Maryland

Nancy A. Miltenberger, M.A., Senior Editor, The Circle, Inc., McLean, Virginia

Elizabeth Mugge, Special Assistant, Office of the Deputy Director, Division of Cancer Prevention and Control, National Cancer Institute, Bethesda, Maryland

Millie R. Naquin, M.Ed., Research Assistant, Office on Smoking and Health, Rockville, Maryland

Regina Nwankwo, Editor, The Circle, Inc., McLean, Virginia

Ruth C. Palmer, Secretary, Office on Smoking and Health, Rockville, Maryland

Lida Peterson, Computer Systems Manager, The Circle, Inc., McLean, Virginia

Renate Phillips, Desktop Publishing/Graphic Artist, The Circle, Inc., McLean, Virginia

Margaret E. Pickerel, Public Information and Publications Specialist, Office on Smoking and Health, Rockville, Maryland

Rose Mary Romano, Chief, Public Information Branch, Office on Smoking and Health, Rockville, Maryland

Tamara Shipp, Publications Assistant, The Circle, Inc., McLean, Virginia

Edwin Silverberg, Supervisor, Statistical Information Service, American Cancer Society

Linda R. Spiegelman, Administrative Officer, Office on Smoking and Health, Rockville, Maryland

Traion Stallings, Word Processing Specialist, The Circle, Inc., McLean, Virginia

Daniel R. Tisch, Senior Project Manager, The Circle, Inc., McLean, Virginia

Pamela Wilson, Editor, The Circle, Inc., McLean, Virginia

Louise G. Wiseman, Technical Information Specialist, Office on Smoking and Health, Rockville, Maryland

TABLE OF CONTENTS

CHAPTER 1

HISTORICAL PERSPECTIVE, OVERVIEW, AND CONCLUSIONS

CONTENTS

Historical Perspective

Each of the last five Surgeons General of the U.S. Public Health Service (PHS) has identified cigarette smoking as one of this Nation's most significant sources of death and disease. Today, more than one of every six American deaths is the result of cigarette smoking. Smoking is responsible for an estimated 30 percent of all cancer deaths, including 87 percent of lung cancer, the leading cause of cancer mortality; 21 percent of deaths from coronary heart disease; 18 percent of stroke deaths; and 82 percent of deaths from chronic obstructive pulmonary disease. Other forms of tobacco use, including pipe and cigar smoking and use of smokeless tobacco, are also associated with significantly elevated risks of disease and death (US DHEW 1979a; US DHHS 1986b).

Although the health hazards of tobacco use have been suspected for almost 400 years, the first reported clinical impressions of a relationship between tobacco and disease date from the 18th century, when tobacco use was associated with lip cancer (US DHEW 1979a) and nasal cancer (US DHHS 1986b). However, true scientific understanding of the health effects of tobacco has been achieved only in the present century. Broders (1920) published an article in the *Journal of the American Medical Association* linking tobacco use to lip cancer, and 8 years later, Lombard and Doering (1928) published an article in the *New England Journal of Medicine* noting that heavy smoking was more common among cancer patients than among control groups. Later, Pearl (1938) observed in the journal *Science* that heavy smokers had a shorter life expectancy than nonsmokers.

During the 1930s, the Nation's increasing rate of lung cancer and other diseases prompted the initiation of epidemiologic and laboratory studies of the relationship between tobacco use and disease. In the late 1940s and early 1950s, a number of retrospective epidemiologic studies, published by Wynder and Graham (1950) and by other investigators, provided scientific evidence strongly linking smoking to lung cancer. This association was soon thereafter supported by the emerging early findings of major prospective (cohort) mortality studies, including the work of Doll and Hill (1954, 1956) in Great Britain and Hammond and Horn (1958a, 1958b) in the United States. The strength and consistency of these results, combined with evidence from laboratory and autopsy studies, led a national scientific study group to conclude in 1957 that the relationship between smoking and lung cancer was causal (Study Group on Smoking and Health 1957).

On July 12 of that year, U.S. Surgeon General Leroy Burney issued a statement declaring that "The Public Health Service feels the weight of the evidence is increasingly pointing in one direction; that excessive smoking is one of the causative factors in lung cancer" (US PHS 1964). Two years later, in 1959, Surgeon General Burney said that "The weight of evidence at present implicates smoking as the principal factor in the increased incidence of lung cancer" (Burney 1959).

Increases in chronic diseases in other parts of the world led health authorities in other countries to examine the relationship between tobacco and disease, particularly in Europe and Scandinavia. In 1957, the British Medical Research Council reported that a major part of the increase in lung cancer was attributable to smoking (British Medical Research Council 1957). Later, the Royal College of Physicians (1962) issued a landmark document on smoking and health that concluded that "Cigarette smoking is the most likely cause of the recent world-wide increase in deaths from lung cancer . . . is an important predisposing cause of the development of chronic bronchitis . . . probably increases the risk of dying from coronary heart disease...has an adverse effect on healing of [gastric and duodenal] ulcers . . . [and] may be a contributing factor in cancer of the mouth, pharynx, oesophagus, and bladder."

On June 1, 1961, the presidents of the American Cancer Society, the American Public Health Association, the American Heart Association, and the National Tuberculosis Association (now the American Lung Association) urged President John F. Kennedy to establish a commission to study the health consequences of smoking. Representatives of these organizations met with Surgeon General Luther L. Terry in January 1962 to reiterate their call for action. In April, the Surgeon General presented a detailed proposal for an advisory group to reevaluate the position adopted by the Public Health Service in 1959. In calling for the advisory group, Dr. Terry cited new research on the adverse health effects of tobacco, a request from the Federal Trade Commission for guidance on policy regarding the labeling and advertising of tobacco products, and the findings in the new report of the Royal College of Physicians.

On July 27, 1962, following consultations between the White House and the Public Health Service, the Surgeon General held a meeting to define the work of an expert advisory group and to identify candidates for the committee. Meeting with the Surgeon General were representatives of the American Cancer Society, the American College of Chest Physicians, the American Heart Association, the American Medical Association, the Tobacco Institute, the Food and Drug Administration, the National Tuberculosis Association, the Federal Trade Commission, and the President's Office of Science and Technology. The group agreed on a list of more than 150 scientists and physicians. Each of the organizations had the right to veto any of the names on the list for any reason. Persons who had taken a public position on smoking and health were not considered for inclusion on the advisory committee.

Dr. Terry selected 10 individuals from the list to serve on the Surgeon General's Advisory Committee on Smoking and Health: Stanhope Bayne-Jones, M.D., LL.D., former Dean, Yale School of Medicine; Walter J. Burdette, M.D., Ph.D., University of Utah; William G. Cochrane, M.A., Harvard University; Emmanuel Farber, M.D., Ph.D., University of Pittsburgh; Louis F. Fieser, Ph.D., Harvard University; Jacob Furth, M.D., Columbia University; John B. Hickam, M.D., Indiana University; Charles LeMaistre, M.D., University of Texas; Leonard M. Schuman, M.D., University of Minnesota; and Maurice H. Seevers, M.D., Ph.D., University of Michigan.

The Advisory Committee held nine meetings from November 1962 through December 1963, during which they reviewed all the available data from animal laboratory experiments, clinical and autopsy studies, and retrospective and prospective epidemiologic studies. The Committee had access to over 7,000 publications pertaining to smoking and health, including more than 3,000 articles reporting research findings published after 1950. In evaluating evidence linking smoking to disease, the Committee restricted judgments of a causal relationship to those associations for which the evidence was (1) consistent, (2) strong, (3) specific, (4) supportive of appropriate temporal relationships, and (5) coherent (US PHS 1964).

The final Report of the Advisory Committee was released on January 11, 1964 (US PHS 1964). It concluded that "Cigarette smoking is causally related to lung cancer in men; the magnitude of the effect of cigarette smoking far outweighs all other factors. The data for women, though less extensive, point in the same direction . . . . The risk of developing lung cancer increases with duration of smoking and the number of cigarettes smoked per day, and is diminished by discontinuing smoking."

The Report also concluded that pipe smoking is causally related to lip cancer, that cigarette smoking is causally related to laryngeal cancer in men, and that "Cigarette smoking is the most important of the causes of chronic bronchitis." The Advisory Committee identified significant associations between smoking and cancer of the esophagus, cancer of the urinary bladder, coronary artery disease, emphysema, peptic ulcer disease, and low-birthweight babies, but it did not consider the available data to be sufficient to label these associations causal.

The Committee found that male cigarette smokers had a 70-percent excess mortality rate over men who had never smoked and that female smokers also had an elevated mortality rate, although less than that of males. The Advisory Committee concluded that "Cigarette smoking is a health hazard of sufficient importance in the United States to warrant appropriate remedial action."

"Remedial action" was initiated immediately after publication of the Advisory Committee's Report, when the Federal Trade Commission (FTC) proposed that cigarette packs and advertisements bear warning labels and that strict limitations be placed on the content of cigarette advertising. With passage of the Federal Cigarette Labeling and Advertising Act of 1965 (Public Law 89-92; amended in April 1970 by Public Law 91-222), Congress preempted the FTC's recommendation: beginning in 1966, a congressionally mandated health warning appeared on all cigarette packs but not on advertisements.

The Act also required the Secretary of Health, Education, and Welfare to submit annual reports to Congress on the health consequences of smoking, together with legislative recommendations, beginning no later than mid-1967. New reports of the Surgeon General on smoking and health were issued in each calendar year beginning in 1967, except for 1970, 1976, 1977, and 1987. (In 1976, a volume of selected chapters from the 1971–75 Reports was published. The report issued in 1978 was a joint Report for the years 1977 and 1978.) Thus, the present volume, commemorating the 25th anniversary of the 1964 Report, is the 20th Report in the series. In addition, in 1986, PHS issued a report on the health consequences of using smokeless tobacco (US DHHS 1986b). Table 1 identifies the previous reports and highlights their coverage.

The reports published since the 1964 Report have confirmed the scientific judgment of the Advisory Committee and have extended its findings. The evidence available today has reinforced the Advisory Committee's judgments of causality; converted most of its "significant associations" into causal relationships, adhering to the strict criteria described in the first Report; confirmed causal associations for relationships not contemplated in the 1964 Report (e.g., the health hazards of involuntary smoking (US DHHS 1986a)); and identified additional disease associations.

Accompanying the growth and dissemination of scientific knowledge has been increased public understanding of the hazards of smoking, reflected in decreases in smok-

TABLE 1.—Surgeon General's Reports on smoking and health, 1964–88

Year	Subject/Highlights
1964	First official report of the Federal Government on smoking and health. Concluded that "Cigarette smoking is a health hazard of sufficient importance in the United States to warrant appropriate remedial action." Concluded that cigarette smoking is a cause of lung cancer in men and a suspected cause of lung cancer in women. Identified many other causal relationships and smoking–disease associations (US PHS 1964).
1967	Confirmed and strengthened conclusions of 1964 Report. Stated that "The case for cigarette smoking as the principal cause of lung cancer is overwhelming." Found that evidence "strongly suggests that cigarette smoking can cause death from coronary heart disease." 1964 Report had described this relationship as an "association." Also concluded that "Cigarette smoking is the most important of the causes of chronic non-neoplastic bronchiopulmonary diseases in the United States." Identified measures of morbidity associated with smoking (US PHS 1968a).
1968	Updated information presented in 1967 Report. Estimated smoking-related loss of life expectancy among young men as 8 years for "heavy" smokers (over 2 packs per day) and 4 years for "light" smokers (less than 1/2 pack per day) (US PHS 1968b).
1969	Also supplemented 1967 Report. Confirmed association between maternal smoking and infant low birthweight. Identified evidence of increased incidence of prematurity, spontaneous abortion, stillbirth, and neonatal death (US PHS 1969).
1971	Reviewed entire field of smoking and health, with emphasis on most recent literature. Discussed new data indicating associations between smoking and peripheral vascular disease, atherosclerosis of the aorta and coronary arteries, increased incidence and severity of respiratory infections, and increased mortality from cerebrovascular disease and nonsyphilitic aortic aneurysm. Concluded that smoking is associated with cancers of the oral cavity and esophagus. Found that "Maternal smoking during pregnancy exerts a retarding influence on fetal growth" (US DHEW 1971).
1972	Examined evidence on immunological effects of tobacco and tobacco smoke, harmful constituents of tobacco smoke, and "public exposure to air pollution from tobacco smoke." Found tobacco and tobacco smoke antigenic in humans and animals; tobacco may impair protective mechanisms of immune system; nonsmokers' exposure to tobacco smoke may exacerbate allergic symptoms; carbon monoxide in smoke-filled rooms may harm health of persons with chronic lung or heart disease; tobacco smoke contains hundreds of compounds, several of which have been shown to act as carcinogens, tumor initiators, and tumor promoters. Identified carbon monoxide, nicotine, and tar as smoke constituents most likely to produce health hazards of smoking (US DHEW 1972).
1973	Presented evidence on health effects of smoking pipes, cigars, and "little cigars." Found mortality rates of pipe and cigar smokers higher than those of nonsmokers but lower than those of cigarette smokers. Found that cigarette smoking impairs exercise performance in healthy young men. Presented additional evidence on smoking as risk factor in peripheral vascular disease and problems of pregnancy (US DHEW 1973).

TABLE 1.—Continued

Year	Subject/Highlights
1974	Tenth Anniversary Report. Reviewed and strengthened evidence on major hazards of smoking. Reviewed evidence on association between smoking and atherosclerotic brain infarction and on synergistic effect of smoking and asbestos exposure in causing lung cancer (US DHEW 1974).
1975	Updated information on health effects of involuntary (passive) smoking. Noted evidence linking parental smoking to bronchitis and pneumonia in children during the first year of life (US DHEW 1975).
1976[a]	Compiled selected chapters from 1971–75 Reports (US DHEW 1976).
1977–78	Combined 2-year Report focused on smoking-related health problems unique to women. Cited studies showing that use of oral contraceptives potentiates harmful effects of smoking on the cardiovascular system (US DHEW 1978).
1979	Fifteenth Anniversary Report. Presented most comprehensive review of health effects of smoking ever published, and first Surgeon General's Report to carefully examine behavioral, pharmacologic, and social factors influencing smoking. Also first Report to consider role of adult and youth education in promoting nonsmoking. First Report to review health consequences of smokeless tobacco. Many new sections, including one identifying smoking as "one of the primary causes of drug interactions in humans" (US DHEW 1979a).
1980	Devoted to health consequences of smoking for women. Reviewed evidence that strengthened previous findings and permitted new ones. Noted projections that lung cancer would surpass breast cancer as leading cause of cancer mortality in women. Identified trend toward increased smoking by adolescent females (US DHHS 1980a).
1981	Examined health consequences of "the changing cigarette," i.e., lower tar and nicotine cigarettes. Concluded that lower yield cigarettes reduced risk of lung cancer but found no conclusive evidence that they reduced risk of cardiovascular disease, chronic obstructive pulmonary disease, and fetal damage. Noted possible risks from additives and their products of combustion. Discussed compensatory smoking behaviors that might reduce potential risk reductions of lower yield cigarettes. Emphasized that there is no safe cigarette and that any risk reduction associated with lower yield cigarettes would be small compared with benefits of quitting smoking (US DHHS 1981).
1982	Reviewed and extended understanding of the health consequences of smoking as a cause or contributory factor of numerous cancers. Included first Surgeon General's Report consideration of emerging epidemiologic evidence of increased lung cancer risk in nonsmoking wives of smoking husbands. Did not find evidence at that time sufficient to conclude that relationship was causal, but labeled it "a possible serious public health problem." Discussed potential for low-cost smoking cessation interventions (US DHHS 1982).
1983	Examined health consequences of smoking for cardiovascular disease. Concluded that cigarette smoking is one of three major independent causes of coronary heart disease (CHD) and, given its prevalence, "should be considered the most important of the known modifiable risk factors for CHD." Discussed relationships between smoking and other forms of cardiovascular disease (US DHHS 1983).

TABLE 1.—Continued

Year	Subject/Highlights
1984	Reviewed evidence on smoking and chronic obstructive lung disease (COLD). Concluded that smoking is the major cause of COLD, accounting for 80 to 90 percent of COLD deaths in the United States. Noted that COLD morbidity has greater social impact than COLD mortality because of extended disability periods of COLD victims (US DHHS 1984).
1985	Examined relationship between smoking and hazardous substances in the workplace. Found that for the majority of smokers, smoking is a greater cause of death and disability than their workplace environment. Risk of lung cancer from asbestos exposure characterized as multiplicative with smoking exposure. Observed special importance of smoking prevention among blue-collar workers because of their greater exposure to workplace hazards and their higher prevalence of smoking (US DHHS 1985).
1986	Focused on involuntary smoking, concluding that "Involuntary smoking is a cause of disease, including lung cancer, in healthy nonsmokers." Also found that, compared with children of nonsmokers, children of smokers have higher incidence of respiratory infections and symptoms and reduced rates of increase in lung function. Presented detailed examination of growth in restrictions on smoking in public places and workplaces. Concluded that simple separation of smokers and nonsmokers within same airspace reduces but does not eliminate exposure to environmental tobacco smoke (US DHHS 1986a).
1986[b]	Special Report of advisory committee appointed by the Surgeon General to study the health consequences of smokeless tobacco. Concluded that use of smokeless tobacco can cause cancer in humans and can lead to nicotine addiction (US DHHS 1986b).
1988	Established nicotine as a highly addictive substance, comparable in its physiological and psychological properties to other addictive substances of abuse (US DHHS 1988).

[a]Excluded from count of series volumes in text because no new evidence was reviewed.

[b]Excluded from count of series volumes in text because it was a Special Report, not in the series of reports on smoking and health.

ing prevalence and, in recent years, the intensification of public and private measures to discourage smoking. A quarter century after publication of the first Report, smoking remains the leading cause of preventable premature death in our society, but per capita cigarette consumption is declining annually, and analyses of consumption and disease trends augur eventual decreases in smoking's toll.

Given these changes, the remaining toll of tobacco-related disease, and the Surgeon General's objective of a smoke-free society by the year 2000 (Koop 1984), Surgeon General C. Everett Koop devotes this 25th anniversary edition of the Surgeon General's Report to an assessment of progress against smoking in the quarter century since the first Report was published.

Highlights of Conclusions and Findings

Major Conclusions

As the present Report documents, knowledge of the health consequences of smoking has expanded dramatically since 1964, and programs and policies to combat the hazards of smoking have proliferated. The essential chapter-specific conclusions relating to these and other topics of this Report are presented at the end of each chapter and are reproduced in the final Section of this introductory Chapter. The major conclusions of the entire Report, immediately following, address fundamental developments over the past quarter century in smoking prevalence and in mortality caused by smoking. The first two conclusions highlight important gains in preventing smoking and smoking-related disease in the United States. The last three conclusions emphasize sources of continuing concern and remaining challenges.

1. **The prevalence of smoking among adults decreased from 40 percent in 1965 to 29 percent in 1987. Nearly half of all living adults who ever smoked have quit.**

2. **Between 1964 and 1985, approximately three-quarters of a million smoking-related deaths were avoided or postponed as a result of decisions to quit smoking or not to start. Each of these avoided or postponed deaths represented an average gain in life expectancy of two decades.**

3. **The prevalence of smoking remains higher among blacks, blue-collar workers, and less educated persons than in the overall population. The decline in smoking has been substantially slower among women than among men.**

4. **Smoking begins primarily during childhood and adolescence. The age of initiation has fallen over time, particularly among females. Smoking among high school seniors leveled off from 1980 through 1987 after previous years of decline.**

5. **Smoking is responsible for more than one of every six deaths in the United States. Smoking remains the single most important preventable cause of death in our society.**

Key New Findings

While this Report is designed to provide a retrospective view of smoking and health over the past 25 years, several findings never previously documented in a report of the Surgeon General emerged during the process of reviewing and analyzing the voluminous materials consulted for the study. Discussed in detail throughout the Report, key new findings include the following:

- Cigarette smoking is a major cause of cerebrovascular disease (stroke), the third leading cause of death in the United States.

- By 1986, lung cancer caught up with breast cancer as the leading cause of cancer death in women. Women smokers' relative risk of lung cancer has increased by a factor of more than four since the early 1960s and is now comparable to the relative risk identified for men in that earlier period. Gender differences in smoking behavior are disappearing; consistent with this, gender differences in the relative risks of and mortality from smoking-related diseases are narrowing.

- Cigarette smoking is associated with cancer of the uterine cervix.

- To date, 43 chemicals in tobacco smoke have been determined to be carcinogenic.

- In 1985, approximately 390,000 deaths were attributable to cigarette smoking. This figure is greater than other recent estimates of smoking-attributable mortality, reflecting the use of higher relative risks of smoking-related diseases for women and, especially in the case of lung cancer, for men. These higher relative risks were derived from the largest and most recent prospective study of smoking and disease, conducted by the American Cancer Society.

- Disparities in smoking prevalence, quitting, and initiation between groups with the highest and lowest levels of educational attainment are substantial and have been increasing. Educational attainment appears to be the best single sociodemographic predictor of smoking.

- There is growing recognition that prevention and cessation interventions need to target specific populations with a high smoking prevalence or at high risk of smoking-related disease. These populations include minority groups, pregnant women, military personnel, high school dropouts, blue-collar workers, unemployed persons, and heavy smokers.

- One-quarter of high school seniors who have ever smoked had their first cigarette by sixth grade, one-half by eighth grade. Associated with knowledge of this fact is a growing consensus that smoking prevention education needs to begin in elementary school.

- Whereas past smoking control efforts targeting children and adolescents focused exclusively on prevention of smoking, the smoking control community has identified the need to develop cessation programs for children and adolescents addicted to nicotine.

- As of mid-1988, more than 320 local communities had adopted laws or regulations restricting smoking in public places. This compares with a total of about 90 as of the end of 1985, a more than threefold increase in 3 years. The number of new State laws restricting smoking in public places in 1987 exceeded the number passed in any preceding year.

- A growing body of evidence on the role of economic incentives in influencing health behavior has contributed to increased interest in and use of such incentives to discourage use of tobacco products. These include excise taxation of tobacco products, workplace financial incentives, and insurance premium differentials for smokers and nonsmokers.

- In marked contrast to the trends in virtually all other areas of smoking control policy, the number of legal restrictions on children's access to tobacco products has decreased over the past quarter century. Studies indicate that vendor compliance with minimum-age-of-purchase laws is the exception rather than the rule.

- The marketing of a variety of alternative nicotine delivery systems has heightened concern within the public health community about the future of nicotine addiction. The most prominent development in this regard was the 1988 test marketing by a major cigarette producer of a nicotine delivery device having the external appearance of a cigarette and being promoted as "the cleaner smoke."

- While over 50 million Americans continue to smoke, more than 90 million would be smoking in the absence of the changes in the smoking-and-health environment that have occurred since 1964.

- Quitting and noninitiation of smoking between 1964 and 1985, encouraged by changes in that environment, have been or will be associated with the postponement or avoidance of almost 3 million smoking-related deaths. That figure reflects the three-quarters of a million deaths noted in conclusion 2 above, and an additional 2.1 million deaths estimated to be postponed or avoided between 1986 and the year 2000.

Overview

Coverage of the Report

As the major conclusions and new findings suggest, progress against smoking is necessarily measured in several dimensions. Ultimately, the most important measure is the burden of mortality, morbidity, and disability associated with smoking. Secondarily, changes in the prevalence of smoking and its distribution among sociodemographic groups foretell the future course of smoking-related disease. Behavioral changes in turn reflect a myriad of social and psychological influences that have evolved over the past 25 years. These include public knowledge of smoking hazards and attitudes toward the behavior; availability and effectiveness of smoking prevention and cessation programs; and adoption of smoking-related social policies, often reflections of public attitudes and opinions. At the heart of all these phenomena is the substantial and expanding body of scientific knowledge about the health consequences of smoking.

The 1989 Report examines changes in each of these dimensions over the past quarter century. The Report includes a Foreword by the Assistant Secretary for Health and the Director of the Centers for Disease Control, a Preface by the Surgeon General of the U.S. Public Health Service, and the following chapters.

Chapter 1. Historical Perspective, Overview, and Conclusions

Chapter 2. Advances in Knowledge of the Health Consequences of Smoking

Chapter 3. Changes in Smoking-Attributable Mortality

Chapter 4. Trends in Public Beliefs, Attitudes, and Opinions About Smoking

Chapter 5. Changes in Smoking Behavior and Knowledge About Determinants

Chapter 6. Smoking Prevention, Cessation, and Advocacy Activities

Chapter 7. Smoking Control Policies

Chapter 8. Changes in the Smoking-and-Health Environment: Behavioral and Health Consequences

A key to abbreviations used throughout the Report is found at the end of the volume.

Analysis of changes in scientific–medical understanding follows the core tradition of the Surgeon General's Report series. Chapter 2 summarizes current knowledge of the health consequences of smoking and examines how it has advanced, both qualitatively and quantitatively, beyond that reflected in the original Surgeon General's Report. The Chapter also summarizes knowledge of the physicochemical nature of tobacco smoke.

Chapter 3 examines the ultimate population impact of smoking-disease relationships in its review of changes in smoking-attributable mortality. The patterns of mortality have changed in predictable ways, reflecting variations in the rates and sociodemographic distribution of smoking prevalence (the subject of much of Chapter 5). In particular, smoking-attributable mortality in women has increased dramatically, the predictable consequence of the rapid growth in smoking by women in the middle decades of the century. Shifts in sociodemographic patterns of smoking, with greater prevalence now found among blue-collar workers and some minorities than among the white-collar population, presage a continuing disproportionate burden of illness for the Nation's poor and minority populations.

One element of the decision of whether or not to smoke is personal understanding of the dangers involved. Chapter 4 reviews changes in public knowledge since 1964. The most basic findings from scientific research on the health consequences of smoking have been conveyed to and accepted by the American public, at least at a generalized level. Nevertheless, survey research reveals important gaps in public understanding of the hazards of smoking. Smokers report less understanding of the basic consequences of smoking than do nonsmokers; furthermore, smokers often do not internalize, or personalize, the hazards they acknowledge as applying to smokers in general. In addition, knowledge of smoking-and-health facts beyond the most basic information is not possessed by significant numbers of Americans. Thus, a substantial educational task remains.

Although significant gaps remain, it is also clear that the public has a much better appreciation of the hazards of smoking than it did 25 years ago. Associated with the growing acceptance of smoking as a health hazard for the smoker, and more recently as a hazard for nonsmokers, is a growing public desire to restrict smoking in public places to protect the rights of nonsmokers to breathe clean air. Opinions about smoking and the appropriate role of smoking control are also considered in Chapter 4.

The relationship between knowledge and opinion change, on the one hand, and subsequent behavior change, on the other, is quite complex. Nevertheless, substantial smoking behavior change has occurred since issuance of the first Surgeon General's Report and has often followed shifts in beliefs and opinions about smoking. The many dimensions of such behavior change are explored in Chapter 5. Part I of the Chapter examines empirical evidence on behavior change across a number of smoking behaviors and across the major sociodemographic groups. Several previous reports of the Surgeon General have included consideration of these trends (US DHEW1979a;US DHHS 1980a,1983, 1985, 1988). Part II of Chapter 5 reviews the evolution of understanding of smoking behaviors and their determinants. The 1979 Surgeon General's Report devoted several chapters to the psychological and social determinants of smoking (US DHEW 1979a). Most recently, the phenomenon of nicotine addiction was reviewed thoroughly by the Surgeon General (US DHHS 1988).

Changes in public attitudes toward smoking and in the prevalence of smoking are reflected in the rapid expansion in the 1980s of State and local laws and workplace policies restricting smoking. The Nation's growing nonsmoking ethos is also reflected in more attention to both voluntary and regulatory measures intended to prevent the initiation of tobacco use or to assist smokers to quit. The number of smoking-cessation techniques and programs has expanded. Smoking policy discussions today concern such diverse activities as excise taxation, restriction of advertising and promotion of tobacco products, limitation of children's access to tobacco products, and regulation of the newly emerging nicotine-based products collectively referred to as "alternative nicotine delivery systems."

Chapters 6 and 7 examine developments over the past quarter century in voluntary programmatic efforts and public policies directed at smoking control, respectively. Chapter 6 describes separately programs directed at smoking prevention and cessation, and highlights the work of the major voluntary health associations. The Chapter reviews such diverse efforts as comprehensive school health education curricula and antismoking public service announcements on the broadcast media. Chapter 6 concludes with a brief overview of advocacy and lobbying activities related to smoking and health. Advocacy activities are purely voluntary in nature, yet most have been directed at promoting smoking control policies, particularly in recent years. As such, a discussion of advocacy serves as a logical transition between the focus of Chapter 6 on voluntary efforts to combat smoking and concentration in Chapter 7 on policy measures.

Coverage of developments in smoking control policies in Chapter 7 has few precedents in prior reports of the Surgeon General, despite the first Report's call for "appropriate remedial action" a quarter of a century ago (US PHS 1964). The major exception was the substantial attention accorded workplace and Government smoking restriction policies in the 1986 Report (US DHHS 1986a). Otherwise, the report series' principal references to policy have come in the form of legislative recommendations to the Congress. Yet, as noted above, policies intended to diminish smoking and its disease burden have become increasingly common in both the public and private sectors. Thus, as part of the history of smoking and health, and as a determinant of progress against smoking, smoking-related policy is examined in detail in this 25th anniversary Report. Coverage of policy in Chapter 7 includes documentation of trends in specific policies, analogous to the coverage afforded smoking restrictions in the 1986 Report. Policies are grouped into three categories: policies pertaining to information and education (Part I), economic incentives (Part II), and direct restrictions (Part III). Where possible, discussion includes examination of scientific understanding of specific policy effects. Such understanding derives from a growing and increasingly sophisticated body of empirical social science research.

Collectively, the program and policy efforts discussed in Chapters 6 and 7, combined with changing public knowledge and social norms, have encouraged tens of millions of Americans not to smoke. As examined in Chapter 8, this behavioral change can be credited with the avoidance of many hundreds of thousands of premature deaths and the associated saving of millions of life-years. Chapter 8 reviews these and other findings on the behavioral and health consequences of changes in the Nation's smoking-and-health environment.

Conclusions pertaining to the findings of each of the Report's chapters are reviewed in the final Section of this introductory Chapter.

By all accounts, the 1964 Report of the Surgeon General's Advisory Committee is a landmark document in the history of public health and a seminal contribution to the Nation's efforts to understand and combat tobacco-related morbidity and mortality. The present Report chronicles progress against smoking in the intervening 25 years, demonstrating an extraordinary array of advances in knowledge, changes in norms and behavior, and effects on the health of the American people. By any reasonable measure, the burden of smoking remains enormous; but the legacy of the 1964 Report is a society that has made impressive strides toward ridding itself of this most preventable source of disease, disability, and death.

1990 Health Objectives for the Nation

In 1979, PHS released the first Surgeon General's Report on Health Promotion and Disease Prevention (US DHEW 1979b). The Report identified 15 priority areas, including smoking, in which significant health gains could be expected in the 1980s, with appropriate actions. Subsequently, working with health experts from both the private and public sectors, the PHS established 226 specific health objectives for the Nation (US DHHS 1980b). Seventeen of these pertain directly to cigarette smoking (Table 2). Many others relate to smoking as well, because they address the prevention of heart disease, cancer, burn injuries, and other smoking-related disease problems. In 1986, the PHS published a midcourse assessment of progress toward achieving the 226 objectives (US DHHS 1986c). One of the goals of the present Report is to offer additional insight in this assessment as it relates to the 17 smoking objectives. This is discussed in the relevant chapters.

PHS is currently developing national health goals for the year 2000, again working with organizations and individuals in the private and public sectors. The reduction of

TABLE 2.—1990 health objectives for the nation pertaining to smoking

Reduced risk factors	1. By 1990, the proportion of adults who smoke should be reduced to below 25 percent. 2. By 1990, the proportion of women who smoke during pregnancy should be no greater than one-half the proportion of women overall who smoke.	3. By 1990, the proportion of children and youth aged 12 to 18 years who smoke should be reduced to below 6 percent. 4. By 1990, the sales-weighted average tar yield of cigarettes should be reduced to below 10 mg. The other components of cigarette smoke known to cause disease should also be reduced proportionately.
Increased public/professional awareness	5. By 1990, the share of the adult population aware that smoking is one of the major risk factors for heart disease should be increased to at least 85 percent. 6. By 1990, at least 90 percent of the adult population should be aware that smoking is a major cause of lung cancer, as well as multiple other cancers including laryngeal, esophageal, bladder, and other types. 7. By 1990, at least 85 percent of the adult population should be aware of the special risk of developing and worsening chronic obstructive pulmonary disease, including bronchitis and emphysema, among smokers.	8. By 1990, at least 85 percent of women should be aware of the special health risks for women who smoke, including the effect on outcomes of pregnancy and the excess risk of cardiovascular disease with oral contraceptive use. 9. By 1990, at least 65 percent of 12-year-olds should be able to identify smoking cigarettes with increased risk of serious disease of the heart and lungs.

TABLE 2.—Continued

Improved services/protection	10. By 1990, at least 35 percent of all workers should be offered employer/employee-sponsored or -supported smoking cessation programs either at the worksite or in the community. 11. By 1985, tar, nicotine, and carbon monoxide yields should be prominently displayed on each cigarette package and promotional material. 12. By 1985, the present cigarette warning should be strengthened to increase its visibility and impact, and to give the consumer additional needed information on the specific multiple health risks of smoking. Special consideration should be given to rotational warnings and to identification of special vulnerable groups.	13. By 1990, laws should exist in all 50 States and all jurisdictions prohibiting smoking in enclosed public places, and establishing separate smoking areas at work and in dining establishments. 14. By 1990, major health and life insurers should be offering differential insurance premiums to smokers and nonsmokers.
Improved surveillance/evaluation	15. By 1985, insurance companies should have collected, reviewed, and made public their actuarial experience on the differential life experience and hospital utilization by specific cause among smokers and nonsmokers, by sex. 16. By 1990, continuing epidemiologic research should have delineated the unanswered research questions regarding low-yield cigarettes, and preliminary partial answers to these should have been generated by research efforts.	17. By 1990, in addition to biomedical hazard surveillance, continuing examination of the changing tobacco product and the sociological phenomena resulting from those changes should have been accomplished.

SOURCE: US DHHS (1980b).

tobacco use is one of 21 priority areas in which objectives are being formulated. PHS intends to publish the objectives in 1990.

Limitations of Coverage

Despite the broad scope of this Report, certain limitations have had to be placed on coverage. Two in particular are worthy of mention here:

(1) The Report focuses primarily, but not exclusively, on cigarette smoking, reflecting its dominance among forms of tobacco use, in terms of both prevalence and disease impact. This focus also reflects the desire to represent the principal interest of the 1964 Advisory Committee in this 25th anniversary Report. Pipe and cigar smoking are much less prevalent than cigarette smoking but also carry significant health risks (US DHEW 1979a). Growing use of smokeless tobacco products (snuff and chewing tobacco), primarily by adolescent males, has focused national attention on the prevalence and health consequences of using these tobacco products (Connolly et al. 1986). This subject was recently reviewed thoroughly by an advisory committee to the Surgeon General (US DHHS 1986b) and in a National Cancer Institute monograph (Boyd and Darbey, in press).

(2) The Report concentrates on smoking in the United States. Both within the United States and around the world, there is growing concern about the spread of smoking, particularly in the world's poorer countries. While per capita cigarette consumption is stable or falling in most developed nations, it is rising in Third World countries. Rates of smoking-related chronic diseases are also increasing rapidly, to the point that tobacco is expected to soon become the leading cause of premature, preventable mortality in the Third World, as it is at present in the developed world (Aoki, Hisamichi, Tominaga 1988).

Concentration of this Report on smoking in the United States is no reflection on the relative importance of the international situation. Rather, it results from the principal objective of reviewing where this Nation has come in its efforts to control smoking-related disease since the 1964 report of the Surgeon General's Advisory Committee. The Public Health Service hopes that this review, like its predecessors, will prove to be of value to scientists, health professionals, and public health officials in countries throughout the world.

Development of the Report

This Report was developed by the Office on Smoking and Health (OSH), Center for Chronic Disease Prevention and Health Promotion, Centers for Disease Control, Public Health Service of the U.S. Department of Health and Human Services, as part of the Department's responsibility, under Public Law 91-222, to report new and current information on smoking and health to the U.S. Congress.

The scientific content of this Report was produced through the efforts of more than 130 scientists in the fields of medicine, the biological and social sciences, public health, and policy analysis. Manuscripts for the Report, constituting drafts of chapters or sections of chapters, were prepared by 33 scientists selected for their expertise in the specific content areas. An editorial team including the Director of OSH, a medical epidemiologist from OSH, and four non-Federal experts edited and consolidated the individual manuscripts into chapters. These draft chapters were subjected to an intensive outside peer review, with each chapter reviewed by 5 to 12 individuals knowledgeable about the chapter's subject matter. Incorporating the reviewers' comments, the editors revised the chapters and assembled a draft of the complete Report. The draft Report was then submitted to 25 distinguished scientists for their review and comment on the entirety of its contents. Simultaneously, the draft Report was submitted to 9 institutes and agencies within the U.S. Public Health Service for their review. Comments from the senior scientific reviewers and the agencies were then used to prepare the final draft of the Report, which was then reviewed by the Offices of the Assistant Secretary for Health and the Secretary, Department of Health and Human Services.

Chapter Conclusions

Chapter 2: Advances in Knowledge of the Health Consequences of Smoking

Part I. Health Consequences

1. The 1964 Surgeon General's Report concluded that cigarette smoking increases overall mortality in men, causes lung and laryngeal cancer in men, and causes chronic bronchitis. The Report also found significant associations between smoking and numerous other diseases.
2. Reports of the Surgeon General since 1964 have concluded that smoking increases mortality and morbidity in both men and women. Disease associations identified as causal since 1964 include coronary heart disease, atherosclerotic peripheral vascular disease, lung and laryngeal cancer in women, oral cancer, esophageal cancer, chronic obstructive pulmonary disease, intrauterine growth retardation, and low-birthweight babies.
3. Cigarette smoking is now considered to be a probable cause of unsuccessful pregnancies, increased infant mortality, and peptic ulcer disease; to be a contributing factor for cancer of the bladder, pancreas, and kidney; and to be associated with cancer of the stomach.
4. Accumulating research has elucidated the interaction effects of cigarette smoking with certain occupational exposures to increase the risk of cancer, with alcohol ingestion to increase the risk of cancer, and with selected medications to produce adverse effects.
5. A decade ago, the 1979 Report of the Surgeon General found smokeless tobacco to be associated with oral cancer. In 1986, the Surgeon General concluded that smokeless tobacco was a cause of this disease.
6. Research in the present decade has established that involuntary smoking is a cause of disease, including lung cancer, in healthy nonsmokers, and that the children of parents who smoke have an increased frequency of respiratory infections and symptoms.

7. In 1964, tobacco use was considered habituating. A substantial body of evidence accumulated since then, and summarized in the 1988 Surgeon General's Report, has established that cigarettes and other forms of tobacco are addicting. Given the prevalence of smoking, tobacco use is the Nation's most widespread form of drug dependency.
8. Studies dating from the 1950s have consistently documented the benefits of smoking cessation for smokers in all age groups.
9. Recent evidence, including that presented in this 1989 Report of the Surgeon General, documents that cigarette smoking is a cause of cerebrovascular disease (stroke) and is associated with cancer of the uterine cervix.

Part II. The Physicochemical Nature of Tobacco

1. The estimated number of compounds in tobacco smoke exceeds 4,000, including many that are pharmacologically active, toxic, mutagenic, and carcinogenic.
2. Forty-three carcinogens have been identified in tobacco smoke.
3. Carcinogenic tobacco-specific nitrosamines are found in high concentrations in smokeless tobacco.

Chapter 3: Changes in Smoking-Attributable Mortality

1. Lung cancer death rates increased two- to fourfold among older male smokers over the two decades between the American Cancer Society's two Cancer Prevention Studies (CPS-I, 1959–65, and CPS-II, 1982–86). Lung cancer death rates for younger male smokers fell about 30 to 40 percent during this period.
2. Lung cancer death rates increased four- to sevenfold among female smokers aged 45 years or older in CPS-II compared with CPS-I, while lung cancer death rates among younger women declined 35 to 55 percent.
3. The two-decade interval witnessed a two- to threefold increase in death rates from chronic obstructive pulmonary disease (COPD) in female smokers aged 55 years or older.
4. There was no change in the age-adjusted death rates for lung cancer and COPD between CPS-I and CPS-II among men and women who never smoked regularly.
5. Overall death rates from coronary heart disease (CHD) declined substantially between CPS-I and CPS-II. The decline in CHD mortality among nonsmokers, however, was notably greater than among current cigarette smokers.
6. In CPS-II, the relative risks of death from cerebrovascular lesions were 3.7 and 4.8 for men and women smokers under age 65. Increased risks of stroke were also observed among older smokers and former smokers. Along with the recently reported results of other studies, these findings strongly support a causal role for cigarette smoking in thromboembolic and hemorrhagic stroke.
7. In 1985, smoking accounted for 87 percent of lung cancer deaths, 82 percent of COPD deaths, 21 percent of CHD deaths, and 18 percent of stroke deaths. Among men and women less than 65 years of age, smoking accounted for more than 40 percent of CHD deaths.

8. The large increase in smoking-attributable mortality among American women between 1965 and 1985 was a direct consequence of their adoption of lifelong cigarette smoking, especially from their teenage years onward.
9. In 1985, 99 percent of smoking-attributable deaths occurred among people who started smoking before the 1964 Surgeon General's Report. For this group, the annual smoking-attributable fatality rate is about 7,000 deaths per 1 million persons at risk.
10. For 10 causes of death, a total of 337,000 deaths were attributable to smoking in 1985. These represented 22 percent of all deaths among men and 11 percent among women. If other cardiovascular, neoplastic, and respiratory causes of death were included—as well as deaths among newborns and infants resulting from maternal smoking, deaths from cigarette-caused residential fires, and lung cancer deaths among nonsmokers due to environmental tobacco smoke—the total smoking-attributable mortality was about 390,000 in 1985.

Chapter 4: Trends in Public Beliefs, Attitudes, and Opinions About Smoking

1. In the 1950s, 40 to 50 percent of adults believed that cigarette smoking is a cause of lung cancer. By 1986, this proportion had increased to 92 percent (including 85 percent of current smokers).
2. Between 1964 and 1986, the proportion of adults who believed that cigarette smoking increases the risk of heart disease rose from 40 to 78 percent. A similar increase occurred among smokers, from 32 to 71 percent.
3. The proportion of adults who believed that cigarette smoking increases the risk of emphysema and chronic bronchitis rose from 50 percent in 1964 to 81 percent (chronic bronchitis) and 89 percent (emphysema) in 1986. These proportions increased among current smokers from 42 percent in 1964 to 73 percent (chronic bronchitis) and 85 percent (emphysema) in 1986.
4. Despite these impressive gains in public knowledge, substantial numbers of smokers are still unaware of or do not accept important health risks of smoking. For example, the proportions of smokers in 1986 who did not believe that smoking increases the risk of developing lung cancer, heart disease, chronic bronchitis, and emphysema were 15 percent, 29 percent, 27 percent, and 15 percent, respectively. These percentages correspond to between 8 and 15 million adult smokers in the United States.
5. In 1985, substantial percentages of women of childbearing age did not believe that smoking during pregnancy increases the risk of stillbirth (32 percent), miscarriage (25 percent), premature birth (24 percent), and having a low-birthweight baby (15 percent). Of women in this age group, 28 percent did not believe that women taking birth control pills have a higher risk of stroke if they smoke.
6. Some smokers today do not recognize their own personal risk from smoking or they minimize it. In 1986, only 18 percent of smokers were "very concerned" about the effects of smoking on their health, and 24 percent were not at all concerned.

7. In 1986, about half of current smokers and 40 percent of never smokers incorrectly believed that a person would have to smoke 10 or more cigarettes per day before it would affect his or her health.
8. A national survey conducted in 1983 by Louis Harris and Associates found that the public underestimates the health risks of smoking compared with many other health risks.
9. Many smokers underestimate the population impact of smoking. In 1987, 28 percent of smokers (and 16 percent of the general population) disagreed with the statement, "Most deaths from lung cancer are caused by cigarette smoking."
10. The proportion of high school seniors who believe that smoking a pack or more of cigarettes per day causes great risk of harm increased from 51 percent in 1975 to 66 percent in 1986.
11. In 1986, about three-quarters of adults believed that using chewing tobacco or snuff is harmful to health.
12. The social acceptability of smoking in public is declining, as measured by the proportion of adults who find it annoying to be near a person smoking cigarettes. This proportion increased from 46 percent in 1964 to 69 percent in 1986.
13. A majority of the public favors policies restricting smoking in public places and worksites, prohibiting the sale of cigarettes to minors, and increasing the cigarette tax to fund the medicare program. Recent surveys indicate that about half the public supports a ban on cigarette advertising.

Chapter 5: Changes in Smoking Behavior and Knowledge About Determinants

Part I. Changes in Smoking Behavior

1. Prevalence of cigarette smoking has declined substantially among men, slightly among women, and hardly at all among those without a high school diploma. From 1965–87, the prevalence of smoking among men 20 years of age and older decreased from 50.2 to 31.7 percent. Among women, the prevalence of smoking decreased from 31.9 to 26.8 percent. Smoking prevalence among whites fell steadily. Among blacks, the prevalence of smoking changed very little between 1965 and 1974; subsequently, prevalence declined at a rate similar to that of whites during the same period. Smoking prevalence has consistently been higher among blue-collar workers than among white-collar workers.
2. Annual per capita (18 years of age and older) sales of manufactured cigarettes decreased from 4,345 cigarettes in 1963 to 3,196 in 1987, a 26-percent reduction. Total cigarette sales increased gradually to 640 billion cigarettes in 1981 and then fell to 574 billion in 1987.
3. In 1965, 29.6 percent of adults who had ever smoked cigarettes had quit. This proportion (quit ratio) increased to 44.8 percent in 1987. The rate of increase in the quit ratio from 1965–85 was similar for men and women. The rate of change in quitting activity in recent years is similar for whites and blacks. From 1965–85, the quit ratio increased more rapidly among college graduates than among adults without a high school diploma.

4. Of all adults who smoked at any time during the year 1985–86, 70 percent had made at least one serious attempt to quit during their lifetime and one-third stopped smoking for at least 1 day during that year.
5. The age of initiation of smoking has declined over time, particularly among females. Among smokers born since 1935, more than four-fifths started smoking before the age of 21.
6. Trends in prevalence of cigarette smoking among those aged 20 to 24 years are an indicator of trends in initiation. By this measure, initiation has declined between 1965 and 1987 from 47.8 to 29.5 percent. Initiation has fallen four times more rapidly among males than among females. The rate of decline has been similar among whites and blacks. Initiation has decreased three times more rapidly among those with 13 or more years of education than among those with less education.
7. The prevalence of daily cigarette smoking among high school seniors decreased from 29 percent in 1976 to 21 percent in 1980, after which prevalence leveled off at 18 to 21 percent. Prevalence among females has consistently exceeded that among males since 1977. Prevalence was lower for students with plans to pursue higher education than for those without such plans. The difference in prevalence by educational plans widened throughout this period; in 1987, smoking rates were 14 percent and 30 percent in these two groups, respectively.
8. The best sociodemographic predictor of smoking patterns appears to be level of educational attainment. Marked differences in smoking prevalence, quitting, and initiation have occurred and have increased over time between more and less educated people.
9. The domestic market share of filtered cigarettes increased from 1 percent in 1952 to 94 percent in 1986. The market share of low-tar cigarettes (15 mg or less) increased from 2 percent in 1967 to 56 percent in 1981, after which this proportion fell slightly and then stabilized at 51 to 53 percent. The market share of longer cigarettes (94 to 121 mm) increased from 9 percent in 1967 to 40 percent in 1986.
10. Between 1964 and 1986, use of smokeless tobacco (snuff and chewing tobacco) declined among men and women 21 years of age and older. However, among males aged 17 to 19, snuff use increased fifteenfold and use of chewing tobacco increased more than fourfold from 1970–86.
11. Differences in prevalence of cigarette smoking and smokeless tobacco use between young males and young females suggest that the prevalence of any tobacco use is similar in these two groups.
12. From 1964 to 1986, the prevalence of pipe and cigar smoking declined by 80 percent among men.

Part II. Changes in Knowledge About the Determinants of Smoking Behavior

1. Smoking was viewed as a habit in 1964 and is now understood to be an addiction influenced by a wide range of interacting factors, including pharmacologic effects of nicotine; conditioning of those effects to numerous activities, emotions, and settings; socioeconomic factors; personal factors such as coping resources; and social influence factors.

2. Since 1964, there has been a gradual evolution of understanding of the progression of smoking behavior through the broad stages of development, regular use, and cessation. Each of these stages is differentially affected by multiple and interacting determinants.
3. Views of determinants of smoking are affected by the predominating theoretical and methodological perspectives. In smoking, the earlier focus on broad, dispositional variables (e.g., extraversion) has given way to an emphasis on situation-specific and interactional variables; a focus on a search for a single cause has given way to a focus on multiple and interacting causes.

Chapter 6: Smoking Prevention, Cessation, and Advocacy Activities

Part I. Smoking Prevention Activities

1. Diverse program approaches to the prevention of smoking among youth grew out of antismoking education efforts in the 1960s. These approaches include media-based programs and resources; smoking prevention as part of multicomponent school health education; psychosocial prevention curricula; and a variety of other resources developed and sponsored by professional and voluntary health organizations, Federal and State agencies, and schools and community groups.
2. Psychosocial curricula addressing youths' motivations for smoking and the skills they need to resist influences to smoke have emerged as the program approach with the most positive outcomes. Evolution in program content has been accompanied by a shift since the 1960s in prevention program focus from youths in high school and college to adolescents in grades 6 through 8.
3. Existing prevention programs vary greatly in the extent to which they have been evaluated and used. Psychosocial prevention curricula have been intensively developed over the last decade and have been the most thoroughly evaluated and best documented; however, they are generally not part of a dissemination system. More widely disseminated smoking prevention materials and programs, such as those using mass media and brochures, have not always been as thoroughly evaluated; however, they have achieved wider use in the field.
4. The model of stages of smoking behavior acquisition underlies current smoking prevention programs and suggests new intervention opportunities, ranging from prevention activities aimed at young children to cessation programs for adolescent smokers.
5. There has been and continues to be a lack of smoking prevention programs that target youth at higher risk for smoking, such as those from lower socioeconomic backgrounds or school dropouts.

Part II. Smoking Education and Cessation Activities

1. During the past 25 years, national voluntary health agencies, especially the American Cancer Society, the American Heart Association, and the American

Lung Association, have played a significant role in educating the public about the hazards of tobacco use.

2. Individual and group smoking cessation programs evolved from an emphasis on conditioning-based approaches in the 1960s, to the cognitively based self-management procedures of the 1970s, to the relapse prevention and pharmacologically based components of the 1980s.
3. There has recently been an increased emphasis on targeting specific groups of smokers for cessation activities (e.g., pregnant women, Hispanics, blacks).
4. Packaging and marketing of self-help smoking cessation materials have become more sophisticated and there is more of an emphasis on relapse prevention, while much of the content has changed relatively little over the years.
5. Mass-mediated quit-smoking programs have become an increasingly popular strategy for influencing the smoking behavior of a large number of smokers.
6. The 1980s have seen an increase in the promotion of smoking control efforts in the workplace in response to increasing demand and opportunity for worksite wellness programs and smoking control policies.
7. In the last decade there has been an increasing interest in involving physicians and other health care professionals in smoking control efforts. Medical organizations have played a more prominent role in smoking and health during the 1980s than they had in the past.

Part III. Antismoking Advocacy and Lobbying

1. Lobbying and advocacy efforts have expanded through the increasing commitment of the national voluntary health agencies to political action and the formation of coalitions at the local, State, and national levels.
2. Antismoking advocacy and lobbying have evolved over the past 25 years and now focus on a growing number of local, State, and national legislative and regulatory initiatives designed to reduce smoking, regulate the cigarette product, and prevent the uptake of smoking by children and adolescents.

Chapter 7: Smoking Control Policies

Part I. Policies Pertaining to Information and Education

1. The Federal Government's efforts to reduce the health consequences of cigarette smoking have consisted primarily of providing the public with information and education about the hazards of tobacco use. Two of the most well-known mechanisms are the publication of Surgeon General's Reports and the requirement of warning labels on cigarette packages. A system of rotating health warning labels is now required for all cigarette and smokeless tobacco packaging and advertisements.
2. Current laws do not require health warning labels on all tobacco products and do not require monitoring of the communications effectiveness of the warnings. Furthermore, existing laws do not provide administrative mechanisms to update the

contents of labels to prevent the overexposure of current messages or to reflect advances in scientific knowledge, such as new information about the addictive nature of tobacco use.

3. There is insufficient evidence to determine the independent effect of cigarette warning labels, particularly the rotating warning labels required since 1985, on public knowledge about the health effects of smoking or on smoking behavior.
4. Information about tar and nicotine yields appears on all cigarette advertisements but not on all cigarette packages. Levels of other hazardous constituents of tobacco smoke, such as carbon monoxide, hydrogen cyanide, and ammonia, are not disclosed on packages or advertisements. Little information is available to the public about the identity or health consequences of the additives in tobacco products.
5. Declines in adult per capita cigarette consumption have occurred in years of major dissemination of information on the health hazards of smoking. These include 1964, the year of the first Surgeon General's Report on smoking and health, and 1967–70, when antismoking public service announcements were widely broadcast on radio and television, as mandated by the Federal Communications Commission's Fairness Doctrine.
6. In 1985, when cigarette advertising and promotion totaled 2.5 billion dollars, cigarettes were the most heavily advertised product category in the outdoor media (e.g., billboards), second in magazines, and third in newspapers. Over the past decade, the majority of cigarette marketing expenditures has shifted from traditional print advertising to promotional activities (e.g., free samples, coupons, sponsorship of sporting events).
7. An estimated 1 percent of the budget allocated to disease prevention by the U.S. Department of Health and Human Services is devoted specifically to tobacco control. These expenditures totaled 39.5 million dollars in 1986.

Part II. Economic Incentives

1. Cigarette excise taxes are imposed by the Federal Government (16 cents per pack), all State governments, and nearly 400 cities and counties. On average, Federal and State excise taxes add 34 cents per pack to the price of cigarettes. Cigarette excise tax rates have fallen since 1964 in real terms because the rate and magnitude of periodic tax increases have not kept pace with inflation.
2. Studies demonstrate that increases in the price of cigarettes decrease smoking, particularly by adolescents. It has been estimated that an additional 100,000 or more persons will live to age 65 as a result of the price increases induced by the 1983 doubling of the Federal excise tax on cigarettes.
3. In 1964, smoking status was not considered in the determination of insurance premiums. Currently, nearly all life insurers but only a few health, disability, and property and casualty insurers offer premium discounts for nonsmokers. Few health insurers reimburse for the costs of smoking cessation programs or treatment.

Part III. Direct Restrictions on Smoking

1. Restrictions on smoking in public places and at work are growing in number and comprehensiveness, as a result of both Government actions and private initiatives. Forty-two States and more than 320 communities have passed laws restricting smoking in public, and an estimated one-half of large businesses have a smoking policy for their employees.
2. The goal of these smoking restrictions is to protect individuals from the consequences of involuntary tobacco smoke exposure, but they may also contribute to reductions in smoking prevalence by changing the attitudes and behavior of current and potential smokers. Insufficient research has been undertaken to determine the extent, if any, of these effects.
3. There are fewer legal restrictions on children's access to tobacco products now than in 1964, despite what has been learned since then about the dangers of tobacco use, its addictive nature, and the early age of initiation of smoking.
4. As of January 1, 1988, laws in 43 States and the District of Columbia restricted the sale of cigarettes to minors. Nevertheless, tobacco products are relatively easy for children to obtain through vending machines and over-the-counter purchases because of low levels of compliance with and enforcement of current laws.
5. Tobacco products have been exempted by law or administrative decision from the jurisdiction of Federal regulatory agencies under whose authority they might otherwise fall.

Chapter 8: Changes in the Smoking-and-Health Environment: Behavioral and Health Consequences

1. All birth cohorts born between 1901 and 1960 experienced reductions in the prevalence of smoking relative to the rates that would have been expected in the absence of the antismoking campaign. By 1985, the gap between actual (reported) prevalence and that which would have been expected ranged from 6 percentage points for the eldest female cohort to 28 percentage points for the youngest male cohort.
2. In 1985, an estimated 56 million Americans 15 to 84 years of age were smokers. In the absence of the antismoking campaign, an estimated 91 million would have been smokers.
3. Adult per capita cigarette consumption has fallen 3 to 8 percent in years of major smoking-and-health events, such as publication of the first Surgeon General's Report on smoking and health in 1964. Per capita consumption fell each of the years the Fairness Doctrine antismoking messages were presented on television and radio (1967–70).
4. By 1987, adult per capita cigarette consumption would have exceeded its actual level by an estimated 79 to 89 percent had the antismoking campaign never occurred.
5. One of the most substantial behavioral responses to concerns about smoking and health has been the shift toward filtered cigarettes in the 1950s and low-tar and

low-nicotine cigarettes in the 1970s. The net health impact of these product changes is unknown.

6. As a result of the antismoking campaign, an estimated 789,000 deaths were postponed during the period 1964 through 1985, 112,000 in 1985 alone. The average life expectancy gained per postponed death was 21 years.
7. The avoidance of smoking-related mortality associated with the antismoking campaign will represent a growing percentage of smoking-related mortality over time, as the principal beneficiaries of the campaign, younger men and women, reach the ages at which smoking-related disease is most common. Campaign-induced quitting and noninitiation through 1985 will result in the postponement or avoidance of an estimated 2.1 million smoking-related deaths between 1986 and the year 2000.

References

AOKI, M., HISAMICHI, S., TOMINAGA, S. (eds.) *Smoking and Health 1987*. Proceedings of the 6th World Conference on Smoking and Health, Tokyo, November, 9–12, 1987. Amsterdam: Excerpta Medica, 1988.

BOYD, G., DARBEY, C.M. (eds.) *Smokeless Tobacco Use in the United States*, NCI Monograph. National Cancer Institute, in press.

BRITISH MEDICAL RESEARCH COUNCIL. Tobacco smoking and cancer of the lung. Statement by the Medical Research Council. *British Medical Journal* 1:1523–1524, 1957.

BRODERS, A.C. Squamous-cell epithelioma of the lip. A study of five hundred and thirty-seven cases. *Journal of the American Medical Association* 74(10):656–664, March 6, 1920.

BURNEY, L.E. Smoking and lung cancer. A statement of the Public Health Service. *Journal of the American Medical Association* 171(13):1829–1837, November 28, 1959.

CONNOLLY, G.N., WINN, D.M., HECHT, S.S., HENNINGFIELD, J.E., WALKER, B. JR., HOFFMANN, D. The reemergence of smokeless tobacco. *New England Journal of Medicine* 314(16):1020–1027, April 17, 1986.

DOLL, R., HILL, A.B. The mortality of doctors in relation to their smoking habits. A preliminary report. *British Medical Journal* 1(4877):1451–1455, June 26, 1954.

DOLL, R., HILL, A.B. Lung cancer and other causes of death in relation to smoking. A second report on the mortality of British doctors. *British Medical Journal* 2:1071–1081, November 10, 1956.

HAMMOND, E.C., HORN, D. Smoking and death rates—Report on forty-four months of follow-up on 187,783 men. I. Total mortality. *Journal of the American Medical Association* 166(10):1159–1172, March 8, 1958a.

HAMMOND, E.C., HORN, D. Smoking and death rates—Report on forty-four months of follow-up of 187,783 men. II. Death rates by cause. *Journal of the American Medical Association* 166(11):1294–1308, March 15, 1958b.

KOOP, C.E. *A Smoke-Free Society by the Year 2000*. Julia M. Jones Lecture, presented at the annual meeting of the American Lung Association, Miami Beach, Florida, May 20, 1984.

LOMBARD, H.L., DOERING, C.R. Cancer studies in Massachusetts. 2. Habits, characteristics and environment of individuals with and without cancer. *New England Journal of Medicine* 198(10):481–487, April 26, 1928.

PEARL, R. Tobacco smoking and longevity. *Science* 87(2253):216–217, March 4, 1938.

ROYAL COLLEGE OF PHYSICIANS. *Smoking and Health. Summary and Report of the Royal College of Physicians of London on Smoking in Relation to Cancer of the Lung and Other Diseases*. New York: Pitman Publishing, 1962.

STUDY GROUP ON SMOKING AND HEALTH. Smoking and health. Joint report of the Study Group on Smoking and Health. *Science* 125(3258):1129–1133, June 7, 1957.

U.S. DEPARTMENT OF HEALTH AND HUMAN SERVICES. *The Health Consequences of Smoking for Women. A Report of the Surgeon General*. U.S. Department of Health and Human Services, Public Health Service, Office of the Assistant Secretary for Health, Office on Smoking and Health, 1980a.

U.S. DEPARTMENT OF HEALTH AND HUMAN SERVICES. *Promoting Health/Preventing Disease: Objectives for the Nation*. U.S. Department of Health and Human Services, Public Health Service, 1980b.

U.S. DEPARTMENT OF HEALTH AND HUMAN SERVICES. *The Health Consequences of Smoking. The Changing Cigarette: A Report of the Surgeon General*. U.S. Department of Health and Human Services, Public Health Service, Office of the Assistant Secretary for Health, Office on Smoking and Health. DHHS Publication No. (PHS) 81-50156, 1981.

U.S. DEPARTMENT OF HEALTH AND HUMAN SERVICES. *The Health Consequences of Smoking: Cancer. A Report of the Surgeon General.* U.S. Department of Health and Human Services, Public Health Service, Office on Smoking and Health. DHHS Publication No. (PHS) 82-50179, 1982.

U.S. DEPARTMENT OF HEALTH AND HUMAN SERVICES. *The Health Consequences of Smoking: Cardiovascular Disease. A Report of the Surgeon General.* U.S. Department of Health and Human Services, Public Health Service, Office on Smoking and Health. DHHS Publication No. (PHS) 84-50204, 1983.

U.S. DEPARTMENT OF HEALTH AND HUMAN SERVICES. *The Health Consequences of Smoking: Chronic Obstructive Lung Disease. A Report of the Surgeon General.* U.S. Department of Health and Human Services, Public Health Service, Office on Smoking and Health. DHHS Publication No. (PHS) 84-50205, 1984.

U.S. DEPARTMENT OF HEALTH AND HUMAN SERVICES. *The Health Consequences of Smoking: Cancer and Chronic Lung Disease in the Workplace. A Report of the Surgeon General.* U.S. Department of Health and Human Services, Public Health Service, Office on Smoking and Health. DHHS Publication No. (PHS) 85-50207, 1985.

U.S. DEPARTMENT OF HEALTH AND HUMAN SERVICES. *The Health Consequences of Involuntary Smoking. A Report of the Surgeon General.* U.S. Department of Health and Human Services, Public Health Service, Centers for Disease Control. DHHS Publication No. (CDC) 87-8398, 1986a.

U.S. DEPARTMENT OF HEALTH AND HUMAN SERVICES. *The Health Consequences of Using Smokeless Tobacco. A Report of the Advisory Committee to the Surgeon General, 1986.* U.S. Department of Health and Human Services, Public Health Service. NIH Publication No. 86-2874, April 1986b.

U.S. DEPARTMENT OF HEALTH AND HUMAN SERVICES. *The 1990 Health Objectives for the Nation: A Midcourse Review.* U.S. Department of Health and Human Services, Public Health Service, Office of Disease Prevention and Health Promotion, November 1986c.

U.S. DEPARTMENT OF HEALTH AND HUMAN SERVICES. *The Health Consequences of Smoking: Nicotine Addiction. A Report of the Surgeon General, 1988.* U.S. Department of Health and Human Services, Public Health Service, Centers for Disease Control, Center for Health Promotion and Education, Office on Smoking and Health. DHHS Publication No. (CDC) 88-8406, 1988.

U.S. DEPARTMENT OF HEALTH, EDUCATION, AND WELFARE. *The Health Consequences of Smoking. A Report of the Surgeon General: 1971.* U.S. Department of Health, Education, and Welfare, Public Health Service, Health Services and Mental Health Administration. DHEW Publication No. (HSM) 71-7513, 1971.

U.S. DEPARTMENT OF HEALTH, EDUCATION, AND WELFARE. *The Health Consequences of Smoking. A Report of the Surgeon General: 1972.* U.S. Department of Health, Education, and Welfare, Public Health Service, Health Services and Mental Health Administration. DHEW Publication No. (HSM) 72-7516, 1972.

U.S. DEPARTMENT OF HEALTH, EDUCATION, AND WELFARE. *The Health Consequences of Smoking.* U.S. Department of Health, Education, and Welfare, Public Health Service, Health Services and Mental Health Administration. DHEW Publication No. (HSM) 73-8704, 1973.

U.S. DEPARTMENT OF HEALTH, EDUCATION, AND WELFARE. *The Health Consequences of Smoking. 1974.* U.S. Department of Health, Education, and Welfare, Public Health Service, Center for Disease Control. DHEW Publication No. (CDC) 74-8704, 1974.

U.S. DEPARTMENT OF HEALTH, EDUCATION, AND WELFARE. *The Health Consequences of Smoking. 1975.* U.S. Department of Health, Education, and Welfare, Public Health Service, Center for Disease Control. HEW Publication No. (CDC) 77-8704, 1975.

U.S. DEPARTMENT OF HEALTH, EDUCATION, AND WELFARE. *San Diego Smoking Research Project. Five Year Status*. U.S. Department of Health, Education, and Welfare, Center for Disease Control. DHEW Project No. 200-75-0516:1–7, 1976.

U.S. DEPARTMENT OF HEALTH, EDUCATION, AND WELFARE. *The Health Consequences of Smoking, 1977–1978*. U.S. Department of Health, Education, and Welfare, Public Health Service, Office of the Assistant Secretary for Health, Office on Smoking and Health. DHEW Publication No. (PHS) 79-50065, 1978.

U.S. DEPARTMENT OF HEALTH, EDUCATION, AND WELFARE. *Smoking and Health. A Report of the Surgeon General*. U.S. Department of Health, Education, and Welfare, Public Health Service, Office of the Assistant Secretary for Health, Office on Smoking and Health. DHEW Publication No. (PHS) 79-50066, 1979a.

U.S DEPARTMENT OF HEALTH, EDUCATION, AND WELFARE. *Healthy People. The Surgeon General's Report on Health Promotion and Disease Prevention*. U.S. Department of Health, Education, and Welfare, Public Health Service, Office of the Assistant Secretary for Health. DHEW Publication No. 79-55071, 1979b.

U.S. PUBLIC HEALTH SERVICE. *Smoking and Health. Report of the Advisory Committee to the Surgeon General of the Public Health Service*. U.S. Department of Health, Education, and Welfare, Public Health Service, Center for Disease Control. PHS Publication No. 1103, 1964.

U.S. PUBLIC HEALTH SERVICE. *The Health Consequences of Smoking. A Public Health Service Review: 1967*. U.S. Department of Health, Education, and Welfare, Public Health Service, Health Services and Mental Health Administration. PHS Publication No. 1696, revised 1968a.

U.S. PUBLIC HEALTH SERVICE. *The Health Consequences of Smoking. 1968 Supplement to the 1967 Public Health Service Review*. U.S. Department of Health, Education, and Welfare, Public Health Service, Health Services and Mental Health Administration. DHEW Publication No. 1696, 1968b.

U.S. PUBLIC HEALTH SERVICE. *The Health Consequences of Smoking. 1969 Supplement to the 1967 Public Health Service Review*. U.S. Department of Health, Education, and Welfare, Public Health Service. DHEW Publication No. 1969-2 (Supplement), 1969.

WYNDER, E.L., GRAHAM, E.A. Tobacco smoking as a possible etiologic factor in bronchiogenic carcinoma: A study of 684 proved cases. *Journal of the American Medical Association* 143:329–396, May 27, 1950.

CHAPTER 2

ADVANCES IN KNOWLEDGE OF THE HEALTH CONSEQUENCES OF SMOKING

CONTENTS

INTRODUCTION

The purpose of this Chapter is to summarize and compare the state of biomedical knowledge concerning tobacco and health in 1989 with that presented in the 1964 Surgeon General's Report (see Table 13). The Chapter addresses major tobacco-related disorders that are well documented in the medical literature; it does not consider many areas of current research that may prove to be important but are in an early or provisional state of investigation.

The 1964 Surgeon General's Report was a landmark publication that included a survey of more than 7,000 available scientific articles on smoking and health. The Advisory Committee that prepared the 1964 Report reviewed and assessed epidemiologic, clinical, pathological, and experimental data for evidence linking smoking to disease. To reach conclusions concerning the causality of associations between smoking and disease, the Committee constructed a framework for evaluating the evidence. With regard to causality, the Committee concluded:

> The causal significance of an association is a matter of judgment which goes beyond any statement of statistical probability. To judge or evaluate the causal significance of the association between attribute or agent and the disease, or effect upon health, a number of criteria must be utilized, no one of which is an all-sufficient basis for judgment. These criteria include:
>
> a) the consistency of the association
>
> b) the strength of the association
>
> c) the specificity of the association
>
> d) the temporal relationships of the association
>
> e) the coherence of the association (US PHS 1964).

These criteria were applied throughout the 1964 Report. When the word "cause" was used in the 1964 Report, it was felt to convey "the notion of a significant, effectual relationship between an agent and an associated disorder or disease in the host." Use of the word "cause" in relation to cigarette smoking did not exclude other agents as causes; rather, the members of the Advisory Committee shared "a common conception of the multiple etiology of biological processes."

The principal findings on the health effects of smoking were summarized in the Surgeon General's 1964 Report as follows:

1. Cigarette smoking is associated with a 70-percent increase in the age-specific death rates of men.
2. Cigarette smoking is causally related to lung cancer in men; the magnitude of the effect of cigarette smoking far outweighs all other factors. The data for women, though less extensive, point in the same direction.
3. Cigarette smoking is the most important of the causes of chronic bronchitis in the United States and increases the risk of dying from chronic bronchitis and

emphysema. A relationship exists between cigarette smoking and emphysema, but it has not been established that the relationship is causal.

4. It is established that male cigarette smokers have a higher death rate from coronary artery disease than nonsmoking males. Although the causative role of cigarette smoking in deaths from coronary disease is not proven, the Committee considers it more prudent from the public health viewpoint to assume that the established association has causative meaning than to suspend judgment until no uncertainty remains.
5. Pipe smoking appears to be causally related to lip cancer. Cigarette smoking is a significant factor in the causation of cancer of the larynx in men. The evidence supports the belief that an association exists between tobacco use and cancer of the esophagus, and between cigarette smoking and cancer of the urinary bladder in men, but the data are not adequate to decide whether these relationships are causal.
6. Women who smoke cigarettes during pregnancy tend to have babies of lower birthweight. It is not known whether this decrease in birthweight has any influence on the biological fitness of the newborn.
7. Epidemiologic studies indicate an association between cigarette smoking and peptic ulcer that is greater for gastric than for duodenal ulcer.
8. The habitual use of tobacco is related primarily to psychological and social drives, reinforced and perpetuated by the pharmacologic actions of nicotine.

Since 1967, the U.S. Department of Health and Human Services has transmitted to the U.S. Congress mandated reports on the health consequences of smoking. Some of the reports have been encyclopedic reviews similar to the 1964 Report, whereas others have focused on the relationship between smoking and a specific topic. The Federal unit charged with preparing these annual reports, the Office on Smoking and Health, now has more than 57,000 documents on smoking and health in its Technical Information Center database.

Research performed during the subsequent 25 years has substantiated and strengthened the conclusions of the 1964 Advisory Committee. Studies published since 1964 have also established associations between smoking and disease in areas for which data did not exist in 1964, shed light on pathogenetic mechanisms of tobacco-related disease, and added scientific depth to areas mentioned only briefly in the 1964 Report.

PART I: HEALTH CONSEQUENCES

Smoking and Overall Mortality [See Chapter 3 for more detailed discussion]

The major prospective studies of the disease risks associated with smoking completed in the 1960s and 1970s contributed substantially to an understanding of the relationship between smoking and disease (US DHEW 1979). These studies provided estimates of both the relative and attributable risks related to cigarette and other types of smoking (Table 1) (US DHEW 1979). Male cigarette smokers had approximately 70 percent higher overall death rates than nonsmokers; the excess mortality of female

TABLE 1.—Mortality ratios of current cigarette-only smokers, by cause of death in eight prospective epidemiologic studies

Cause of death	British doctors[1]	Males in 25 States[2]		U.S. veterans[3]	Japanese study[4]	Canadian veterans[5]	Males in 9 States[6]	Swedish[7]		California occupations[8]
		45–64	65–79					Males	Females	
All cancers[a] (140–205)		2.14	1.76	2.21	1.62		1.97			
Cancer of lung and bronchus (162–163)	14.0	7.84	11.59	12.14	3.64	14.2	10.73	7.0	4.5	15.9
Cancer of larynx (161)		6.09	8.99	9.96	13.59		13.10			
Cancer of buccal cavity (140–141)	13.0[b]			4.09	7.04	3.9[b]	2.80			
Cancer of pharynx (145–148)		9.90[c]	2.93[c]	12.54	2.81					1.0
Cancer of esophagus (150)	4.7	4.17	1.74	6.17	2.57	3.3	6.60			
Cancer of bladder and other (181)	2.1	2.20	2.96	2.15	0.98	1.3	2.40	1.8	1.6	0.7
Cancer of pancreas (157)	1.6	2.69	2.17	1.84	1.83	2.1		3.1	2.5	6.0
Cancer of kidney (180)		1.42	1.57	1.45	1.11	1.4	1.50			
Cancer of stomach (151)		1.42	1.26	1.60	1.51	1.9	2.30	0.9	2.3	
Cancer of intestines (152–153)				1.27	1.27	1.4	0.50			0.8
Cancer of rectum (154)	2.7	1.01[d]	1.17[d]	0.98	0.91	0.6	0.80			0.9
All cardiovascular disease (330–334, 400–468)		1.90	1.31	1.75			1.57			
CHD (420)	1.6	2.08	1.36	1.74	1.96	1.6	1.70	1.7	1.3	2.0
Cerebrovascular lesions (330–334)	1.3	1.38	1.06	1.52	1.14	0.9	1.30	1.0	1.1	1.8
Aortic aneurysm (nonsyphilitic) (451)	6.6	2.62	4.92	5.24		1.8		1.6		
Hypertension (440–447)		1.40	1.42	1.67	2.51	1.6	1.20	1.3	1.4	1.0
General arteriosclerosis (450)	1.4			1.86		3.3	2.00	2.0	2.0	

TABLE 1.—Continued

Cause of death	British doctors[1]	Males in 25 States[2]		U.S. veterans[3]	Japanese study[4]	Canadian veterans[5]	Males in 9 States[6]	Swedish[7]		California occupations[8]
		45–64	65–79					Males	Females	
All respiratory disease (nonneoplastic)							2.85			
Emphysema and/or bronchitis	24.7			10.08			2.30	1.6	2.2[f]	4.3
Emphysema without bronchitis (527.1)		6.55	11.41	14.17		7.7				
Bronchitis (500–502)				4.49		11.3				
Respiratory tuberculosis (001–008)	5.0			2.12	1.27					
Asthma (241)				3.47						
Influenza and pneumonia (480–498)	1.4	1.86	1.72	1.87		1.4	2.60			2.4
Certain other conditions										
Stomach ulcer (540)	2.5[e]	4.06	4.13	4.13	2.06[e]					
Duodenal ulcer (541)		2.86	1.50	2.98		6.9	2.16			0.5
Cirrhosis (581)	3.0	2.06	1.97	3.38	1.35	2.3	1.93	2.4	0.8	4.0
Parkinsonism (350)	0.4			0.26						
All causes	1.64	1.88	1.43	1.84	1.22	1.52	1.70	1.4	1.2	1.78

[a]Numbers in parentheses represent International Classification of Diseases (ICD) codes.
[b]Includes cancers of larynx, buccal cavity, and pharynx.
[c]Includes cancers of buccal cavity and pharynx.
[d]Includes cancers of intestines and rectum.
[e]Includes stomach ulcer and duodenal ulcer.
[f]Includes emphysema, bronchitis, and asthma.
SOURCE: Studies cited are as follows: [1]Doll and Hill (1956); [2]Hammond (1966); [3]Kahn (1966); [4]Hirayama (1967); [5]Best, Josie, Walker (1961); [6] Hammond and Horn (1958); [7]Cederlof et.al. (1975); [8]Dunn, Linden, Breslow (1960). US DHEW (1979).

cigarette smokers was somewhat less than that of men, but it increased over the followup intervals. A strong dose–response relationship was found between exposure to cigarette smoke and excess mortality; cessation of cigarette smoking was associated with a decrease in this excess mortality. The relative risks were greater for smoking-related cancers and chronic obstructive pulmonary disease (COPD) than for coronary heart disease (CHD); however, because of the higher mortality rates for CHD the smoking-attributable mortality associated with CHD accounted for over one-third of the excess mortality due to smoking-related diseases.

There have been relatively few long-term longitudinal studies that have measured the overall effects of cigarette smoking since these earlier reports. Results from a new American Cancer Society (ACS) prospective study (Cancer Prevention Study II, CPS-II) and a detailed discussion of total smoking-related mortality are presented in Chapter 3. Based on this study, cigarette smoking is currently estimated to account for 21 percent of all CHD deaths, 30 percent of all cancer deaths, and 82 percent of all COPD deaths.

The Multiple Risk Factor Intervention Trial (MRFIT) is a recent prospective study that screened 361,662 men aged 35 to 57 years between 1972 and 1974 and has been following them since then, both through the Social Security Administration and the National Death Index files. To gauge smoking status, only the number of cigarettes smoked per day at enrollment was reported. Because former smokers were included in the nonsmoker category, the risk comparisons in this study between nonsmokers and smokers are conservative in estimating the effects of smoking. Findings for the 6 years of followup for the MRFIT enrollees screened from 1972–73 are consistent with the studies reported in the 1960s, despite changes in the type of cigarettes in terms of tar and nicotine yield and the increased use of filters (see later section of this Chapter and Chapter 5). The MRFIT study shows that smoking status and number of cigarettes smoked per day have remained powerful predictors for total mortality and the development of CHD, stroke, cancer, and COPD. In the study population, there were an estimated 2,249 (29 percent) excess deaths due to smoking, of which 35 percent were from CHD and 21 percent from lung cancer. The nonsmoker–former smoker group had 30 percent fewer total cancers than the smoking group over the 6-year followup.

A study of a random sample of 25,129 Swedish men between 1964 and 1979 evaluated the relationship between cigarette smoking (prevalence of 32 percent), pipe smoking (27 percent), cigar smoking (5 percent), and subsequent mortality (Table 2; Carstensen, Pershagen, Eklund 1987). The all-cause relative death rate was 1.7-fold higher for those smoking greater than 15 g of tobacco per day (estimated as 16 to 25 cigarettes equaling 20 g or a package of pipe tobacco lasting 1 to 4 days equaling 16 g). The relative risks associated with cigarette smoking were consistent both with those of the current MRFIT sample and the earlier cohorts from the 1950s and 1960s. The risks were also increased for pipe and cigar smokers for many of the causes of death.

Epidemiologic studies have shown that cigarette smoking exerts an adverse effect on mortality in older as well as younger age groups. The 17-year followup of the Alameda County Study (Kaplan et al. 1987) demonstrates an increased risk of death even among older cigarette smokers. The adjusted relative risk of death among smokers at entry was 1.46 (age 60 to 69) and 1.43 at age 70 or more. Smoking remained the strongest predictor of mortality even in this older age group. Other studies have also substantiated that smoking remains an important risk factor in the older age groups (Jajich, Ostfeld, Freeman 1984).

TABLE 2.—Mortality ratios for selected causes in Swedish males, 1964–1979, by type of smoking

	Type of smoking[a]		
Cause of death	Cigarettes only	Pipe only	Cigars only
Cancer of oral cavity and larynx (140–146, 148, 161)[b]	2.9 (8)	1.4 (3)	0.6 (1)
Cancer of esophagus (150)	3.7 (9)	3.6 (6)	6.5 (2)
Cancer of liver and biliary passages (155–156)	3.0 (13)	1.7 (5)	7.2 (4)
Cancer of pancreas (157)	3.3 (28)	2.8 (19)	1.0 (1)
Cancer of trachea, bronchus, and lung (162)	7.4 (77)	7.2 (59)	7.6 (11)
Cancer of bladder (188)	4.2 (17)	4.0 (16)	1.9 (1)
Ischemic heart disease (410–414)	1.48 (399)	1.39 (366)	1.16 (42)
Aortic aneurysm (nonsyphilitic) (441)	2.1 (11)	2.1 (11)	5.1 (4)
Bronchitis and emphysema (490–492)	3.3 (18)	3.6 (16)	1.3 (1)
Peptic ulcer (531–534)	2.0 (11)	2.8 (13)	4.0 (3)
Cirrhosis of liver (571)	1.8 (21)	0.7 (4)	2.7 (3)
Suicide, accidents, and violence (E800–E999)	1.7 (90)	0.9 (35)	2.5 (10)
All causes	1.45 (1,063)	1.29 (866)	1.39 (131)

NOTE: Death rates standardized for age and residence. Never smokers constitute the reference group. Number of deaths are given in parentheses.

[a]The mean grams of tobacco smoked per day in 1963, standardized for age and residence, was estimated to be 10.7 in cigarette smokers, 8.4 in pipe smokers, and 13.5 in cigar smokers.

[b]Numbers in parentheses are ICD-8 codes.

SOURCE: Carstensen, Pershagen, Eklund (1987).

Lung Cancer

Introduction

One of the most prominent conclusions of the 1964 Report was the determination that "Cigarette smoking is causally related to lung cancer in men; the magnitude of the effect far outweighs all other factors. The data for women, though less extensive, point in the same direction." The epidemiologic evidence available in 1964 on smoking and lung cancer was already extensive. Sharply increasing lung cancer mortality rates in the United States across the 20th century provided indisputable documentation of a new epidemic. Clinical observations and early epidemiologic findings suggested that tobacco smoking was associated with lung cancer, but hypotheses related to air pollution, occupation, and other factors were also extant. By 1964, however, the epidemiologic data, derived from 29 retrospective and 7 prospective studies, were conclusive: smoking was causally related to cancer of the lung. Further support for this conclusion was obtained from animal studies showing that condensates of tobacco smoke were carcinogenic and from the demonstration that tobacco smoke contained carcinogens (US DHHS 1982). The evidence compiled through 1964 also provided additional insight into quantitative aspects of respiratory carcinogenesis by tobacco smoke. The risk of lung cancer was shown to increase with the amount and duration of smoking and to decline with cessation of smoking.

In the 25 years since the 1964 Report, voluminous evidence has continued to support the causal relationship between smoking and lung cancer. The new evidence has been sufficient to establish that smoking also causes lung cancer in women; more comprehensive epidemiologic data have provided expanded descriptions of dose–response relationships between smoking and lung cancer risk. Research has also been directed at environmental and host factors determining susceptibility to tobacco smoke. New investigative techniques in molecular and cellular biology are now providing insight into the molecular mechanisms of carcinogenesis by tobacco smoke.

Dose–Response Relationships

The 1964 Report reviewed evidence from retrospective and prospective epidemiologic investigations that documented dose–response relationships between lung cancer risk and measures of exposure to tobacco smoke. This evidence was cited by the 1964 Report in relation to the criterion of strength of association for determining causality. Investigation of dose–response relationships for lung cancer has subsequently been extended. Mathematical models have been applied to the epidemiologic data to gain biological insight into respiratory carcinogenesis. The cigarette has evolved substantially since 1964 with modifications designed to reduce tar and nicotine yields. Recent research has addressed the risks of smoking the newer products. Studies of lung cancer and involuntary smoking have examined lung cancer risks at low dose levels (US DHHS 1986a).

Abundant epidemiologic evidence has shown dose–response relationships of lung cancer risk with cigarettes smoked per day, degree of inhalation, and age at initiation of regular smoking. For the purpose of illustration, selected examples of dose–response relationships from two of the early, large prospective epidemiologic studies are reviewed here. Figure 1 shows lung cancer mortality ratios for males by the number of cigarettes smoked per day. For those who smoked more than 40 cigarettes per day, the risk of dying of lung cancer was 23 times greater than the risk experienced by nonsmokers.

Figure 2 illustrates the lung cancer mortality ratios for males by self-reported degree of inhalation of cigarette smoke. These data confirm that even those who reported "just puffing" on cigarettes still had a significantly increased risk of lung cancer. Those who reported inhaling "none" or "slightly" experienced a risk of developing lung cancer that was eight times greater than that of nonsmokers. The relative risk increased to 17 for those who inhaled deeply.

Figure 3 shows lung cancer mortality ratios for males by the age they began smoking. The risk of developing lung cancer was greatest for those who began smoking at an early age.

Mathematical modeling of dose–response relationships, in the biological framework of a multistage model of carcinogenesis, has provided further insight into the nature of dose–response relationships for smoking and lung cancer. Using data from the prospective study of British doctors, Doll and Peto (1978) have performed the most widely cited analysis. They compared regular smokers and lifelong nonsmokers and showed that lung cancer incidence increased with the square of the amount smoked daily, but with the duration of smoking raised to a power of 4 to 5. This finding implies that duration of smoking is the stronger determinant of lung cancer risk and that initiation of smoking during the teenage years will have serious consequences for lung cancer risk (Peto 1986).

Commercial cigarettes have continuously evolved through the addition of filters and other modifications designed to reduce tar and nicotine yields (US DHHS 1981). Since extensive modification of the cigarette began in the 1950s, it has only recently become possible to investigate smokers with predominant use of the newer products. Evidence from prospective and case–control studies and assessment of temporal trends of lung cancer mortality indicate somewhat lower risks for cigarettes with reduced tar and nicotine yield, although the risks remain markedly higher than for nonsmokers (US DHHS 1982).

Doll and Peto (1981) examined trends of lung cancer mortality in males in the United States, Britain, and other European countries. They concluded that the international differences and the temporal trends were generally consistent with the tar yields and tar intakes across time and across countries.

Relevant information is also available from case–control and prospective studies. In the United States, investigations spanning the 1960s and 1970s have shown somewhat reduced lung cancer risks in smokers who switched from nonfilter to filter cigarettes (Bross and Gibson 1968; Wynder, Mabuchi, Beattie 1970; Hammond et al. 1976; Wynder and Stellman 1979). More recent studies continue to document lower risks in smokers of filter cigarettes compared with smokers of nonfilter cigarettes. In a case–control study conducted in Western Europe, the relative risk for lifelong nonfilter cigarette smokers was approximately twice that for smokers of filter cigarettes alone

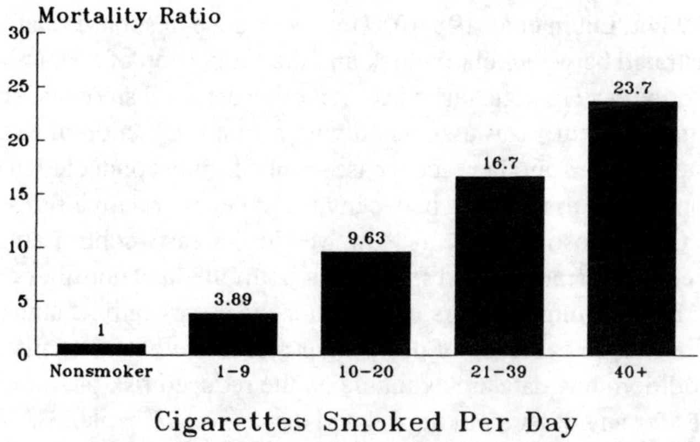

FIGURE 1.—Lung cancer mortality ratio for males by cigarettes smoked per day
SOURCE: U.S. Veterans (Kahn 1966).

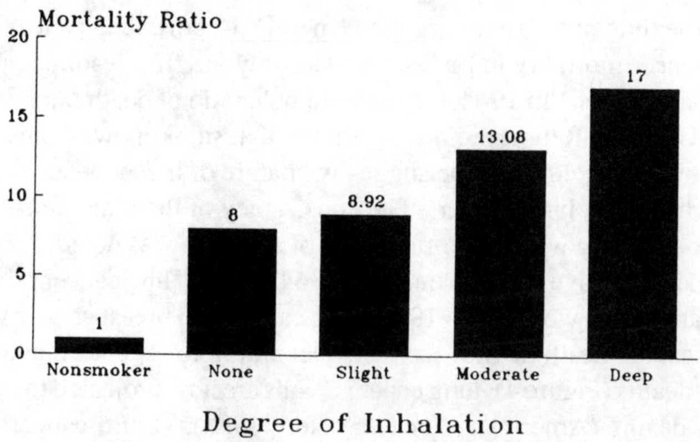

FIGURE 2.—Lung cancer mortality ratio for males by degree of inhalation
SOURCE: CPS-I (Hammond 1966).

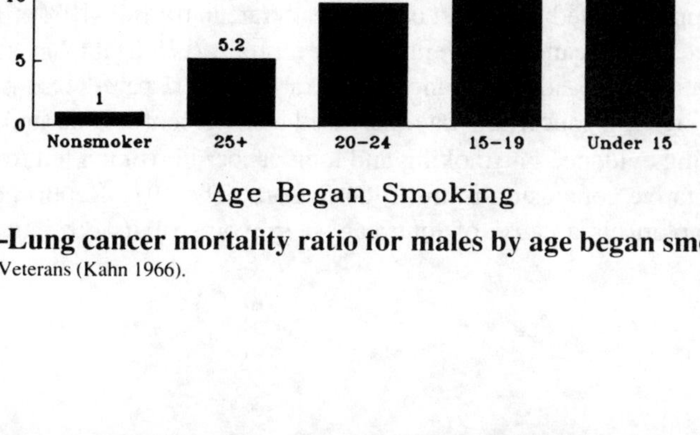

FIGURE 3.—Lung cancer mortality ratio for males by age began smoking
SOURCE: U.S. Veterans (Kahn 1966).

(Lubin et al. 1984a; Lubin et al. 1984b). However, dose–response relationships could not be demonstrated between relative risk and the proportion of years nonfilter brands were smoked or with a cigarette tar index. Among sustained smokers, switching from nonfilter to filter cigarettes was associated with a small reduction in risk (Lubin et al. 1984a). The results from another recent case–control study conducted in Cuba also did not show a convincing association between tar intake and relative risk of lung cancer (Joly, Lubin, Caraballoso 1983). In New Mexico, a case–control study found that lifelong filter cigarette smokers and smokers of both filter and nonfilter cigarettes were at lower risk than lifelong smokers of nonfilter cigarettes only (Pathak et al. 1986). However, there was no evidence of decreasing risk as the extent of filter smoking increased. In addition, few data are available on the reduced risk of smoking low-tar or filter cigarettes for any other smoking-related disease (see Chapter 3).

Women and Lung Cancer

In 1964, at the time of the first Surgeon General's Report, lung cancer was the leading cause of cancer mortality in males, but was only the fifth leading cause of cancer mortality among women. In 1964, the male–female ratio of death rates from lung cancer was 6.7. The 1964 Report did not determine that smoking was causally related to lung cancer in women, although the suggestive nature of the evidence was cited in the Report's conclusion on lung cancer. The consistency of the male–female differences in lung cancer mortality with temporal trends of smoking was noted.

In the 25 years that have elapsed since the 1964 Report, lung cancer mortality has increased dramatically in women. In 1986, lung cancer and breast cancer were the leading causes of cancer death in U.S. women, accounting for approximately equal numbers of cancer deaths (Figure 4); lung cancer deaths are now projected to have surpassed breast cancer deaths (American Cancer Society 1988). Lung cancer mortality for women now equals that observed for men three decades earlier and the male–female ratio of death rates has now fallen to 2.0.

Since the late 1970s, the rise in the age-adjusted death rates of lung cancer among men began to level off (Horm and Kessler 1986). In contrast, lung cancer death rates among women continue to climb (Figure 4). As Figures 4 and 5 demonstrate, lung cancer is the only major cancer whose death rates have increased substantially and steadily since the 1930s. The dramatic increase among women began approximately 30 years after the increase for men, consistent with the later adoption of smoking by women; the slope of the curve for women appears to be nearly identical to that of men 30 years earlier. Figure 4 also demonstrates that among women, the lung cancer death rate closely approximated the breast cancer death rate in the mid-1980s. Illustrative of the importance of lung cancer in overall cancer mortality is the fact that, excluding lung cancer, the Nation's age-adjusted cancer death rate fell by 13 percent from 1950 through 1982. Including lung cancer, the rate increased by 8 percent (Bailar and Smith 1986).

The mounting evidence on smoking and lung cancer in women led to a strengthening of the tentative conclusion in the 1964 Report. The 1971 Report concluded that "Cigarette smoking is a cause of lung cancer in women but accounts for a smaller

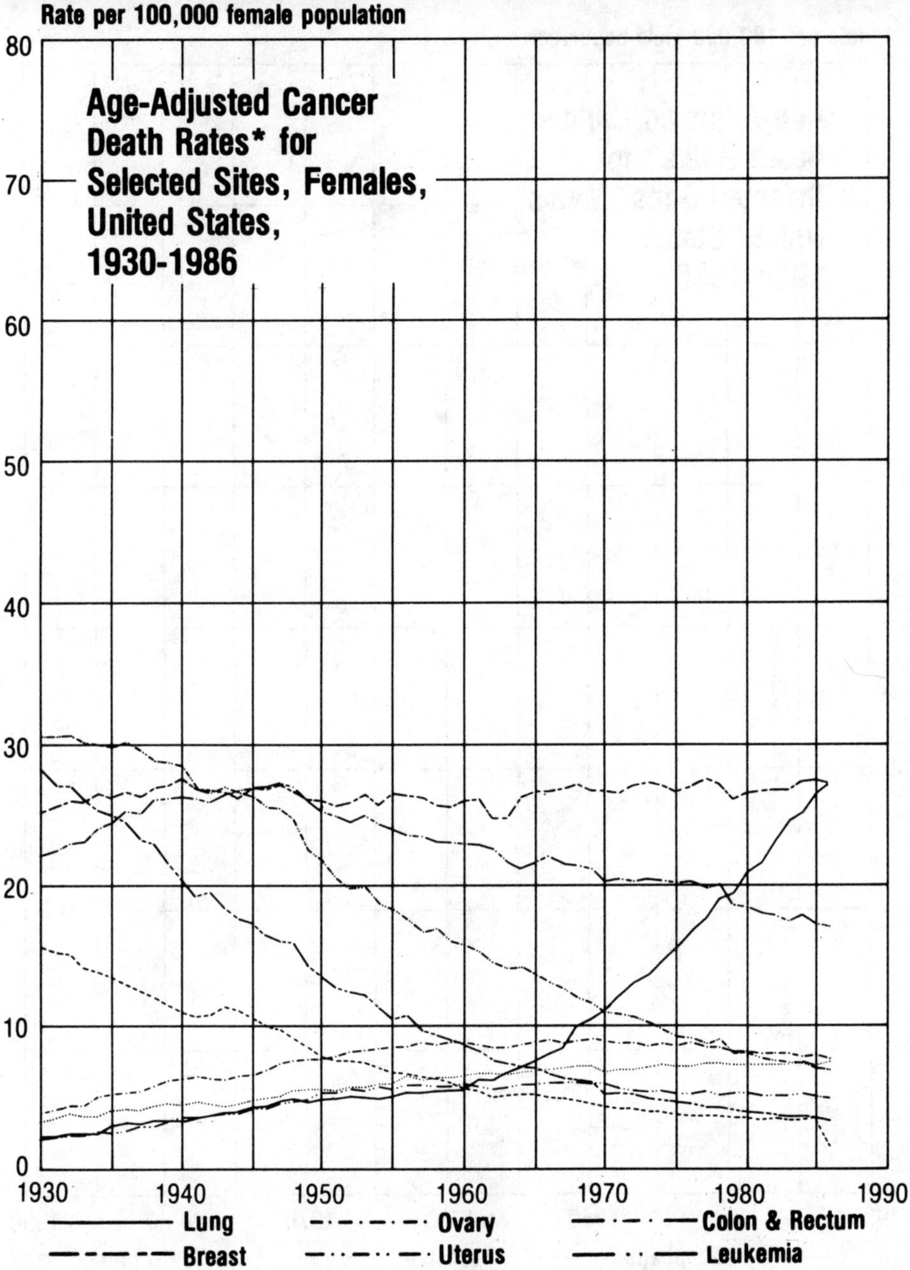

FIGURE 4.—Age-adjusted cancer death rates* for selected sites, females, United States, 1930–86

*Adjusted to the age distribution of the 1970 U.S. Census population.

SOURCES OF DATA: National Center for Health Statistics; U.S. Bureau of the Census.

proportion of cases than in men" (US DHEW 1971). The conclusion of the 1979 Report was similar (US DHEW 1979). The 1980 Report (US DHHS 1980), concerned with smoking and women, and the 1982 Report (US DHHS 1982), concerned with smoking and cancer, comprehensively reviewed the epidemiologic data and reaffirmed the earlier conclusions concerning the causal association of smoking and lung cancer in

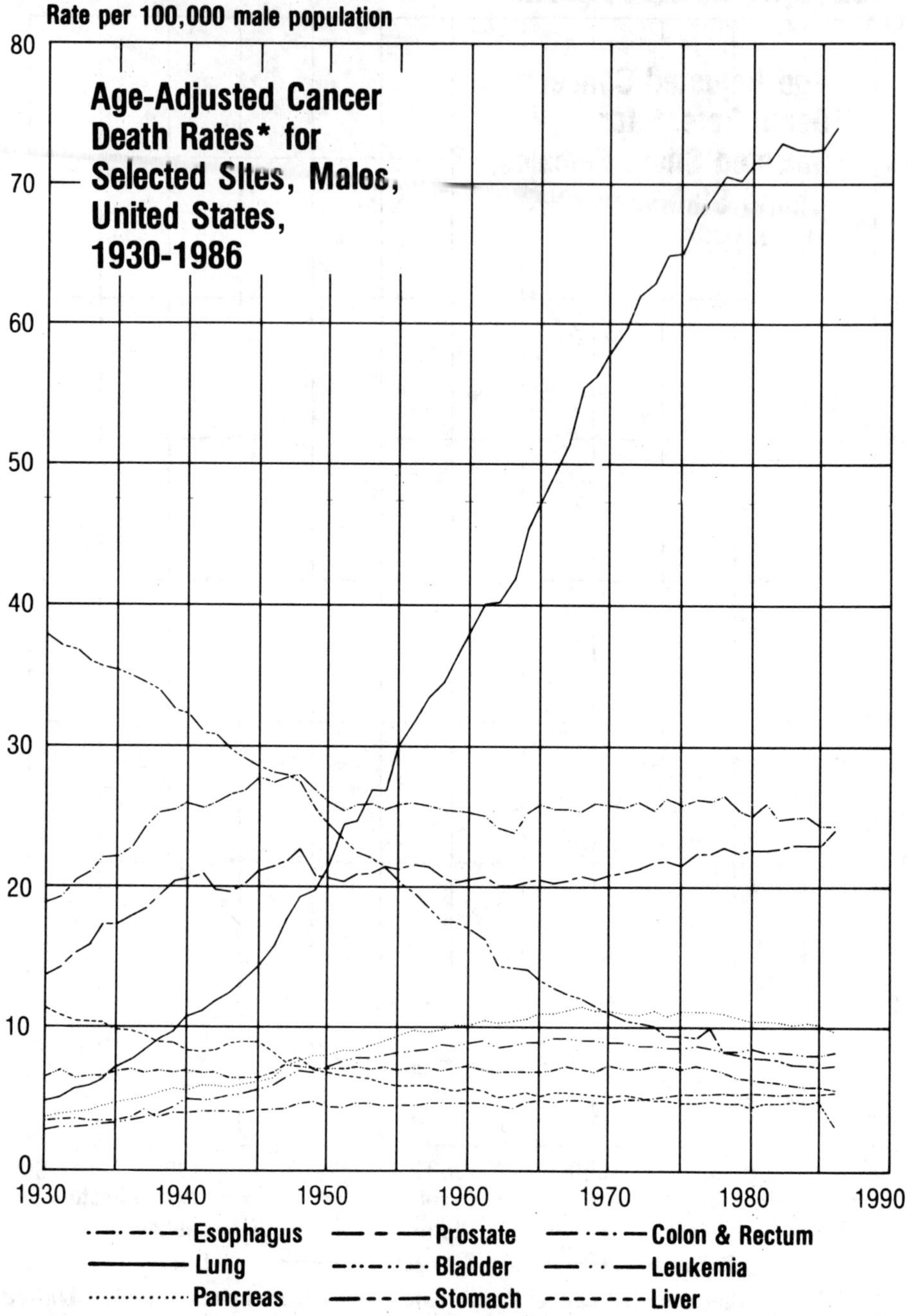

FIGURE 5.—Age-adjusted cancer death rates* for selected sites, males, United States, 1930–86

*Adjusted to the age distribution of the 1970 U.S. Census population.

SOURCES OF DATA: National Center for Health Statistics; U.S. Bureau of the Census.

women; the evidence also provided comprehensive descriptions of dose–response relationships with findings similar to those reported previously for men. Recently reported dose–response relationships from the American Cancer Society Cancer Prevention Study II for lung cancer and women extend these observations (Figure 6).

These data also dramatically illustrate that the current lung cancer epidemic in women is confined to those who smoke cigarettes (Figure 7).

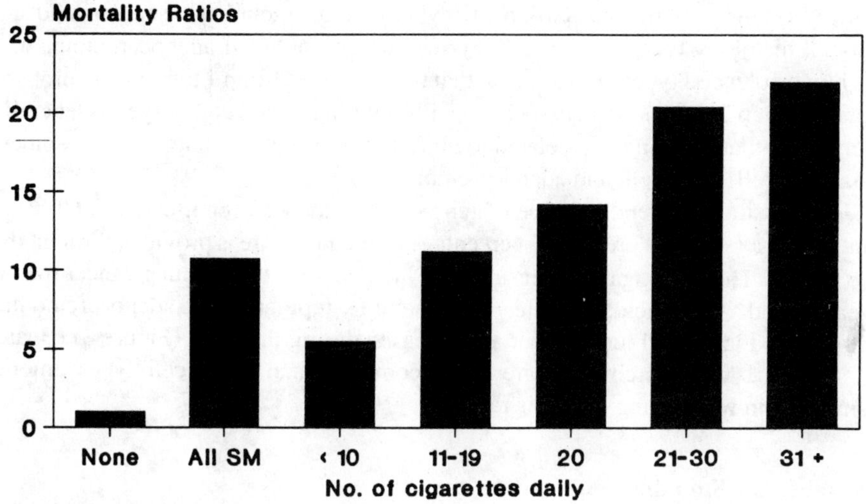

FIGURE 6.—Lung cancer mortality ratios of female cigarette smokers, compared to never smokers, by daily cigarette consumption

SOURCE: CPS-II 1982–86, ACS.

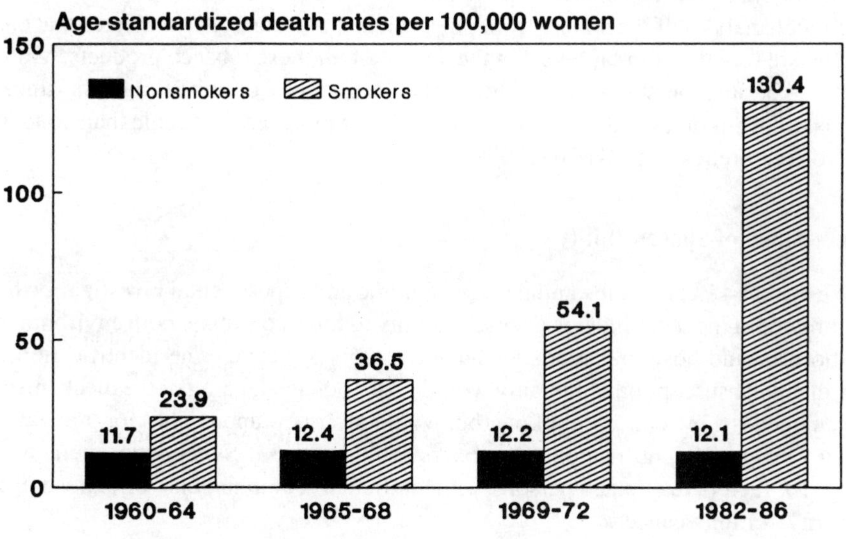

FIGURE 7.—Lung cancer death rates among females over time

SOURCE: CPS-I and CPS-II, ACS.

Type of Lung Cancer and Smoking

At the time of the 1964 Surgeon General's Report, the Kreyberg classification of lung tumors was being investigated. Group 1 Kreyberg tumors included the epidermoid and small-cell histology types; Group 2 Kreyberg tumors included adenocarcinoma and bronchioalveolar cell types. It was felt at that time that the Group 1 tumors, but probably not the Group 2 tumors, were associated with smoking. The 1982 Surgeon General's Report noted that smoking was related to all four major types of lung cancer: epidermoid, small cell, large cell, and adenocarcinoma.

A detailed study of trends in type of lung cancer has been reported from Olmsted County, MN, a region where a large percentage of medical care is provided through the Mayo Clinic. The investigators measured the incidence by type of lung cancer over a 45-year period. The incidence rates for squamous (epidermoid), adenocarcinoma, small-cell, and large-cell lung cancer all increased during this time (Figure 8) (Beard et al. 1985). Adenocarcinomas are more common than other cell types among nonsmokers, in whom lung cancer is rare.

Pipe and Cigar Smoking

Mortality ratios for lung cancer in those who have always smoked only cigars or pipes are significantly higher than in nonsmokers (US DHHS 1982). The mortality ratios are lower, however, than among those who have always smoked cigarettes. The risk of lung cancer increases in relation to the number of cigars smoked per day, the number of pipesful smoked per day, and the degree of smoke inhalation. The lower risk of lung cancer among pipe and cigar smokers compared with cigarette smokers is due to the lesser amount of tobacco smoked and the lower degree of inhalation.

Chemical analysis of the smoke from pipes, cigars, and cigarettes indicates that carcinogens are found in similar levels in the smoke of all these tobacco products. Additionally, experimental studies have shown that in a variety of animal models, smoke condensates from pipes and cigars are equally, if not more, carcinogenic than condensates from cigarettes (US DHEW 1979).

Determinants of Susceptibility

Since the 1964 Report, substantial epidemiologic and experimental investigation has been directed at the determinants of susceptibility to tobacco smoke; both environmental exposures and host characteristics have been investigated. The identification of determinants of susceptibility not only would further understanding of the mechanisms of carcinogenesis by tobacco smoking, but would offer new approaches for prevention of lung cancer by identification of smokers at higher risk. Synergistic interactions among risk factors may place persons with particular combinations of exposures at higher risk for lung cancer.

Interactions among risk factors, such as cigarette smoking and occupational exposures, may be either synergistic or antagonistic; synergism refers to an increased effect of the independent exposures when both are present, whereas antagonism refers to

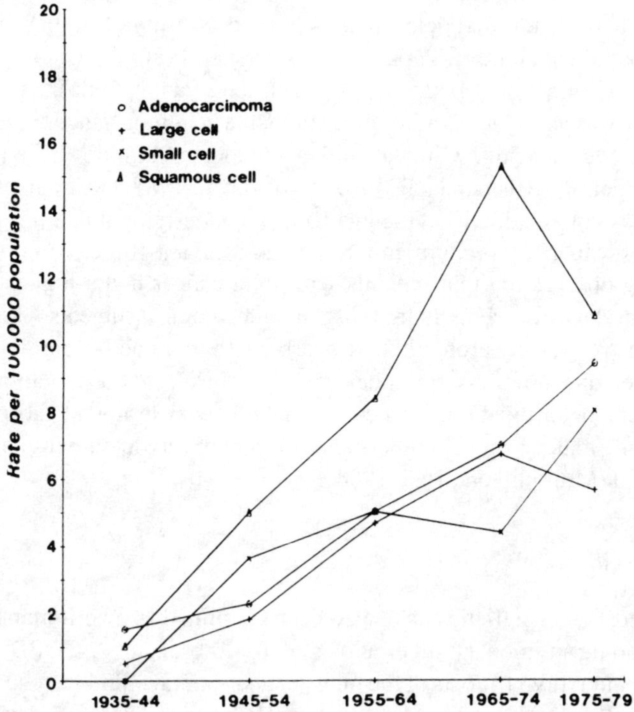

FIGURE 8.—Mean annual incidence rates per 100,000 population for males of bronchogenic carcinoma by cell type, Olmsted County, MN, 1935–79, by decade

SOURCE: Beard et al. (1985).

a reduced effect. Statistical methods are used with epidemiologic data to describe interactions. Either an additive or a multiplicative scale may be used to measure interaction statistically (Saracci 1987). For two exposures, on an additive scale, the sum of the two independent relative risks reduced by one is compared with the relative risk observed when both exposures are present. On a multiplicative scale, the comparison relative risk value is the product of the two independent relative risks. For public health purposes, a positive departure from additivity is considered to represent synergism (Saracci 1987). As the extent of interaction increases, the proportion of the excess cases attributable to the interaction also increases (Saracci 1987).

This Section briefly reviews the current evidence on host characteristics and environmental agents that may modify the risk of cigarette smoking.

Familial Factors

The 1964 Report considered and dismissed the "constitutional hypothesis" that predilections to cigarette smoking and to lung cancer share a common genetic origin. The Report did consider that genetic factors might determine susceptibility for a minority of cases. Subsequent epidemiologic studies have provided empirical evidence of possible genetic or familial determinants of susceptibility (Tokuhata and Lilienfeld 1963a, 1963b; Samet, Humble, Pathak 1986; Ooi et al. 1986). For example, in a recent case–control study in New Mexico (Samet, Humble, Pathak 1986), a parental history of lung cancer was associated with a fivefold increase in lung cancer risk, after adjustment for cigarette smoking. Clinical studies of selected families have also indicated familial aggregation (Brisman et al. 1967; Lynch et al. 1982; Goffman et al. 1982).

Research has not yet identified the mechanisms underlying the familial aggregation of lung cancer. In 1973, Kellermann, Shaw, and Luyten-Kellerman (1973) reported the promising observation that patients with lung cancer had a higher degree of inducibility of aryl hydrocarbon hydroxylase than did control subjects. Because this enzyme converts polycyclic aromatic hydrocarbons to more active carcinogens and because enzyme concentrations are under genetic control, this observation suggested a possible genetic determinant of lung cancer risk. However, not all subsequent studies have been confirmatory, and the inheritance of inducibility in humans has not yet been fully described (Mulvihill and Bale 1984).

Other Host Factors

Acquired host characteristics have also been examined as determinants of lung cancer risk including pulmonary tuberculosis, chronic bronchitis, COPD, disorders associated with interstitial fibrosis of the lung, and peripheral pulmonary scars. However, the evidence related to these disorders is incomplete and frequently is derived from case series rather than from epidemiologic investigations. Recent epidemiologic evidence, however, has indicated increased lung cancer risk for smokers with COPD compared with unaffected smokers (Peto et al. 1983; Samet, Humble, Pathak 1986; Skillrud, Offord, Miller 1986).

Occupational Exposures

Diverse agents inhaled in the workplace have been shown to cause lung cancer. Interaction between occupational exposures and smoking was the focus of the 1985 Report of the Surgeon General (US DHHS 1985). That Report concluded that "For the majority of American workers who smoke, cigarette smoking represents a greater cause of death and disability than their workplace environment." The Report also highlighted the limitations of the evidence on interactions between smoking and occupational exposures.

Little new information has become available since the 1985 Report. The evidence remains strongest for interactions of smoking with exposure to radon decay products and with exposure to asbestos (Saracci 1987). For both exposures, the preponderance of the evidence indicates synergism (Doll and Peto 1985; National Research Council 1988), although the results of some individual investigations are inconsistent with synergism.

Ambient Air Pollution

The 1964 Report noted that lung cancer mortality rates tended to be higher in urban than in rural locations. Air pollution was considered a plausible explanation for these differences. The association of lung cancer with atmospheric pollution derives biological plausibility from the presence of carcinogens in polluted air and has some support from epidemiologic data. However, epidemiologic investigation of ambient air pollution as a risk factor for lung cancer has been hampered by methodological problems, including the necessity of considering cigarette smoking and the difficulty of assessing pollution exposure (NIH 1986). Recent epidemiologic investigations have not shown strong effects of air pollution (Samet et al. 1987; Buffler et al. 1988); and Doll and Peto (1981), in their review of the causes of cancer, estimated that only 1 to 2 percent of lung cancer was related to air pollution.

Indoor Air Pollution

As the hazards posed by ambient air pollution from conventional fossil fuels have diminished in some countries, the relevance of indoor air quality for health has become increasingly apparent. Studies of time–activity patterns demonstrate that residents of more developed countries, including the United States, spend on average little time outdoors (Spengler and Sexton 1983; Samet, Marbury, Spengler 1987). Indoor spaces may be polluted by entry of contaminants from outdoor air and by indoor sources including those related to human activity, such as tobacco smoking, building materials, combustion devices, personal care and other household products, and other sources. A trend of reduced building ventilation in the aftermath of the energy problems of the 1970s may have worsened indoor air quality.

Two pollutants in indoor air have been causally linked to lung cancer: environmental tobacco smoke (ETS) (US DHHS 1986a) and radon (National Research Council 1988). The evidence on ETS and cancer was comprehensively reviewed in the 1986 Report (see Section on Involuntary Smoking in this Chapter).

Radon is an inert gas that is formed from radium during the natural decay of uranium. The predominant source of radon in indoor air is the soil beneath structures. Radon diffuses through the ground into basement and crawl spaces, and then throughout the air in a home, or crosses cracks and other penetrations in homes on concrete slabs to enter the indoor environment. Radon daughters are invariably present in indoor air and a wide range of concentrations has been observed in homes (Samet et al. 1988). Some homes have levels comparable to those measured in uranium mines, but the majority of homes probably have levels that are currently considered acceptable.

Radon decays into short-lived particulate decay products. Two of the decay products emit alpha particles, which are highly effective in damaging cells because of their high energy and high mass. When these alpha emissions take place within the lung, the epithelial lining of the tracheobronchial tree may be damaged and lung cancer may ultimately result. Extensive epidemiologic data from studies of uranium and other underground miners have established a causal association between exposure to radon daughters and lung cancer (National Research Council 1988). The committee on the Biological Effects of Ionizing Radiation (BEIR) IV concluded that the studies of miners indicated synergism between cigarette smoking and radon decay products (National Research Council 1988). The evidence, however, was not considered adequate to determine if the interaction was multiplicative or submultiplicative.

To date, epidemiologic investigations of domestic radon daughters as a risk factor for lung cancer have been limited and preliminary (Samet et al. 1988). However, it is assumed that radon decay products are carcinogenic in the indoor environment as they are in the mining environment. Dosimetric analyses indicate equivalent carcinogenicity in the domestic and mining environments (National Research Council 1988). Thus, radon must be considered one of the most important factors interacting with cigarette smoking. All smokers are exposed to radon, some at unacceptable levels. Quantitative estimates of the contribution of radon to lung cancer are variable. The estimates vary with the underlying assumptions and the risk model employed (Samet et al. 1988).

Although cigarette smoking is by far the major cause of lung cancer, radon must also be considered a cause of the disease. The public health burden of radon-related lung cancer is substantially increased by the synergism between cigarette smoking and radon exposure.

Diet

Diet has recently been considered as potentially influencing the risk of lung cancer in smokers. Nutrients of particular interest include preformed vitamin A, carotene, vitamin E, and vitamin C (Colditz, Stampfer, Willett 1987).

An enlarging body of experimental and epidemiologic evidence supports the hypothesis that the risk for certain cancers varies inversely with consumption of preformed vitamin A or beta-carotene, its precursor (Peto et al. 1981; National Academy of Sciences 1982; Colditz, Stampfer, Willett 1987). The biological plausibility of this hypothesis derives from the known effects of vitamin A deficiency on the differentiation of epithelial surfaces, from in vitro and in vivo models, which show that retinoids can suppress the development of malignancy, and from possible anticarcinogenic activity of beta-carotene, the principal dietary precursor of vitamin A (Peto et al. 1981; National Academy of Sciences 1982). The epidemiologic evidence indicates a protective effect of dietary vitamin A intake from vegetable sources, but not of preformed vitamin A, which is derived from meat and dairy sources, and vitamin supplements. Clinical trials on vitamin A and lung cancer risk are in progress.

Vitamins E and C are antioxidants, which might have anticancer effects. To date, the epidemiologic data on these vitamins are sparse and inconclusive (Colditz, Stampfer, Willett 1987).

Smoking Cessation

Cessation of cigarette smoking results in a gradual decrease in lung cancer risk. Several of the prospective and retrospective epidemiologic studies have demonstrated a reduction in lung cancer risk over time following smoking cessation. One example is provided from the U.S. Veterans study (Kahn 1966) (Figure 9).

Other recent studies have continued to confirm the benefit of smoking cessation for lung cancer risk (Lubin et al. 1984b; Alderson, Lee, Wang 1985; Pathak et al. 1986; Higgins, Mahan, Wynder 1988). For example, Lubin and colleagues (1984b) described the pattern of reduction in risk following smoking cessation in a case–control study that

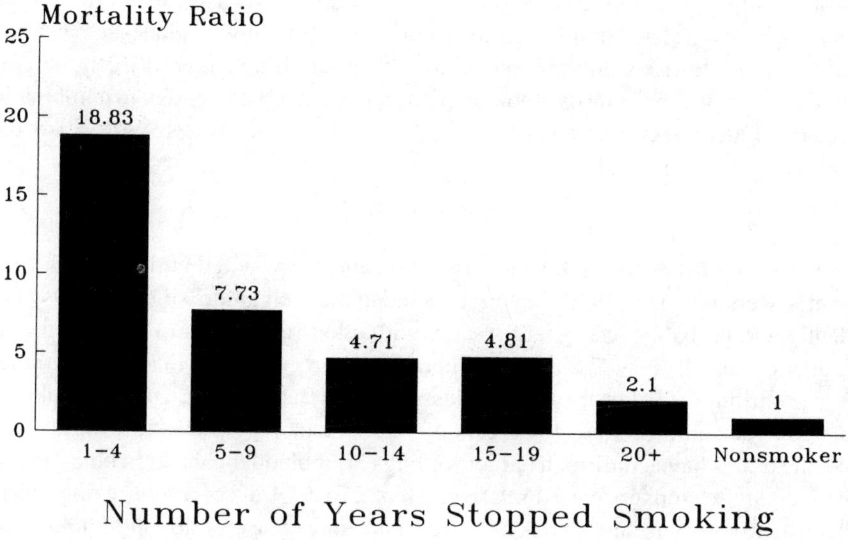

FIGURE 9.—Lung cancer mortality ratio for male former smokers
SOURCE: U.S. Veterans (Kahn 1966).

involved 7,181 lung cancer patients and 11,006 controls. For men and women in this study who had smoked for less than 20 years and had not smoked for 10 years, the risks of lung cancer were approximately the same as those of lifelong nonsmokers. On the basis of the study of British physicians, Peto and Doll (1984) have suggested that the effect of cigarette smoking cessation is to fix the age-specific risk of lung cancer at the rate achieved at the time of cessation, based on the smoking history up to that time. According to this analysis, the former smoker's relative risk of lung cancer declines as the background rate for lung cancer rises with age.

Therefore, smoking cessation is clearly beneficial in reducing the risk of lung cancer compared with continued smoking; but cessation may not reduce the risk to the levels of a lifetime nonsmoker even after many years of cessation. (See Table 2, Chapter 3.)

Laryngeal, Oral, and Esophageal Cancer

The 1964 Surgeon General's Report concluded that cigarette smoking was causally related to laryngeal cancer in men and that pipe smoking was causally related to lip cancer (US PHS 1964). Subsequent reports reviewed the accumulating epidemiologic evidence that established that cancers of the larynx, oral cavity, and esophagus are caused by smoking in both men and women. The mortality ratios for these cancers are similar for smokers whether they smoke cigars, pipes, or cigarettes. A strong dose–response relationship exists, and the risk decreases with cessation, compared with continued smoking. Recent studies have confirmed these findings (Blot et al. 1988; Elwood et al. 1984; Schottenfeld 1984). (See Chapter 3.)

Alcohol consumption is also a risk factor for oral, pharyngeal, laryngeal, and esophageal cancer. The combination of alcohol and smoking produces a synergistic increase in risk. In one study (Schottenfeld 1984), for all upper airway cancers combined, the risk was 8.6 for those smoking 30 or more cigarettes per day in combination with 20 oz of alcohol consumed per week.

Bladder and Kidney Cancer

A relationship between smoking and bladder cancer was noted in the 1964 Surgeon General's Report. The 1979 Report concluded that cigarette smoking acts independently and probably acts synergistically with other risk factors to increase the risk of bladder cancer. The 1982 Surgeon General's Report concluded that cigarette smoking is a contributory factor for both bladder and kidney cancer. Cigarette smoking is estimated to account for 30 to 40 percent of bladder cancer (US DHHS 1982).

Recent studies have confirmed earlier findings. For bladder cancer, in both men and women, cigarette smokers have a relative risk of 2 to 3. A dose–response relationship has been demonstrated, and the risk of bladder cancer decreases following smoking cessation (McLaughlin et al. 1984; Hartge et al. 1987; Zahm, Hartge, Hoover 1987).

There is a positive association between smoking and kidney cancer, with relative risks ranging from 1 to more than 5. The increased risk of kidney cancer due to cigarette smoking is found for both males and females, and there is a dose–response relationship, as measured by the number of cigarettes smoked per day.

Pancreatic Cancer

The first Surgeon General's Report did not examine the relationship between smoking and cancer of the pancreas. Several subsequent reports of the Surgeon General have noted that cigarette smoking is a contributory factor for pancreatic cancer.

The major prospective epidemiologic studies have consistently shown an increased risk of pancreatic cancer among both male and female cigarette smokers. The mortality ratio for cigarette smokers compared with nonsmokers is generally in the range of 2 to

3. A detailed review of the epidemiology of pancreatic cancer was written by Gordis and Gold (1984).

For those in the MRFIT Study who smoked 40 or more cigarettes a day, the mortality ratio for pancreatic cancer was 2.3 compared with nonsmokers. Other recent studies (Mack et al. 1986; Whittemore et al. 1985) report that cigarette smoking is strongly and consistently related to pancreatic cancer. Most epidemiologic studies show a dose–response relationship between cigarette smoking and pancreatic cancer for both men and women and a gradual decline in the risk of developing pancreatic cancer following smoking cessation (US DHHS 1982; Mack et al. 1986).

Autopsy studies report hyperplastic changes in the pancreatic duct cells and atypical changes in their nuclei among cigarette smokers compared with nonsmokers. The pancreas is probably exposed to tobacco carcinogens or carcinogenic metabolites present in bile or blood (US DHHS 1982).

Stomach Cancer

The 1964 Surgeon General's Report reviewed smoking and stomach cancer and, on the basis of the limited evidence available at that time, concluded that there was no relationship between smoking and stomach cancer. Evidence from prospective and retrospective studies available more recently has shown a small but consistent increase in mortality ratios, averaging approximately 1.5 for smokers compared with nonsmokers. Dose–response relationships have been demonstrated for the number of cigarettes smoked per day. The 1982 Surgeon General's Report concluded that cancer of the stomach is associated with cigarette smoking.

Cervical Cancer

Cancer of the uterine cervix was not reviewed in the 1964 Surgeon General's Report. The 1982 Report of the Surgeon General reviewed the studies published up to that time and concluded that further research was necessary to define whether there was an association between cigarette smoking and cervical cancer.

There are several risk factors for cervical cancer including early and frequent coitus, multiple sexual partners, pregnancy at an early age, and the presence of sexually transmitted diseases. Some of these risk factors may also be associated with smoking.

Winkelstein and coworkers (1984) reviewed 12 studies dealing with smoking and cervical cancer, and in most studies there was a positive relationship that could not be explained by other risk factors. Two studies published in 1985 confirmed these findings (Clarke et al. 1985; Greenberg et al. 1985).

Baron and coworkers (1986) reported on a case–control study of 1,174 patients with cervical cancer. Cigarette smoking was associated with a statistically significant increase in risk for cervical cancer. LaVecchia and associates (1986) in Italy studied the relationship between cigarette smoking and the risk of cervical neoplasia in a case–control study of 183 women with intraepithelial neoplasia. Cigarette smoking was associated with an increased risk of intraepithelial neoplasia and invasive cancer. This association could not be totally explained by potential confounding factors. In a case–

control study of 480 patients with cervical cancer, there was a 50-percent excess risk of cancer among cigarette smokers (Brinton et al. 1986). This excess risk persisted after adjustment for sexual practices associated with smoking such as age at first intercourse and number of sexual partners. There was a twofold excess risk of cervical cancer for women who smoked more than 40 cigarettes per day. The dose–response relationship persisted after adjusting for several variables. There was no increased risk of cervical cancer among former smokers.

The finding of nicotine and cotinine in the cervical secretions of cigarette smokers (Sasson et al. 1985) and of mutagenic mucus in the cervix of smokers (Holly et al. 1986) complements the epidemiologic findings.

In summary, more than 15 epidemiologic studies have consistently shown an increased risk for cervical carcinoma in cigarette smokers compared with nonsmokers. Supportive clinical studies provide a plausible biological basis for the relationship. The available data confirm an association between cigarette smoking and carcinoma of the uterine cervix.

Endometrial Cancer

Several studies have reported that endometrial cancer is less frequent among women who smoke cigarettes than among nonsmokers (Baron et al. 1986). Cigarette smoking exerts an antiestrogenic effect that may explain this inverse association. The public health significance of this association is limited because of the overall adverse impact of cigarette smoking on morbidity and mortality.

Coronary Heart Disease

The 1964 Surgeon General's Report (US PHS 1964) noted that male cigarette smokers have higher death rates from CHD than nonsmokers. Subsequent reports concluded that cigarette smoking can cause death from CHD and that smoking is one of the major independent risk factors for heart attack, manifested as fatal and nonfatal myocardial infarction and sudden cardiac death. Smoking also increases the risk of heart attack recurrence among survivors of a myocardial infarction (US DHEW 1979). The 1980 Report (US DHHS 1980) noted the increased risk of CHD among women who smoke. It also described the synergistic interaction between smoking and oral contraceptive use that substantially increases CHD risk. The 1983 Report (US DHHS 1983) stated that cigarette smoking is a major cause of CHD and noted the decreased risk of CHD among former smokers compared with current smokers.

Epidemiology

The findings from several prospective studies involving more than 20 million person-years of observation in North America, Northern Europe, and Japan have been remarkably similar: cigarette smokers are at increased risk for fatal and nonfatal myocardial infarction and for sudden death. Overall, smokers have a 70 percent greater

CHD death rate, a two- to fourfold greater incidence of CHD, and a two- to fourfold greater risk for sudden death than nonsmokers (US DHHS 1983).

Although women experience lower CHD rates than men, cigarette smoking is a major determinant of CHD in women. In a recent prospective study of 119,404 female nurses, smoking accounted for approximately one-half of the coronary events (Willett et al. 1987). Cigarette smoking produces a greater relative CHD risk in men and women under 50 years of age than in those over 50 years of age (Glover, Kuber et al. 1982; Rosenberg, Miller et al. 1983).

Dose–response relationships between cigarette smoking and CHD mortality have been demonstrated for several measures of exposure to cigarettes, including the number of cigarettes smoked per day, the depth of inhalation, the age at which smoking began, and the number of years of smoking (US DHHS 1983). Smoking cigarettes with reduced yields of tar and nicotine has not been found to reduce CHD risk (Kaufman et al. 1983).

Coronary Heart Disease Risk Factors

The risk of experiencing a heart attack is multifactorial (US DHHS 1983). The presence of one or more of the major CHD risk factors, cigarette smoking, hypercholesterolemia, and hypertension, identifies individuals at high or very high risk. These risk factors interact synergistically to greatly increase CHD risk (Figure 10). The risk of CHD associated with cigarette smoking is comparable to that associated with the other major CHD risk factors.

The risk of CHD is greatly increased among diabetic men and women who smoke cigarettes (Suarez and Barrett-Connor 1984; Stamler, Wentworth, Neaton 1986), and the sex differences in CHD are substantially reduced among diabetics. Among the MRFIT screenees free of a history of heart attack, there were 5,245 diabetics and 350,977 nondiabetic men aged 35 to 57 years at the time of enrollment (Suarez and Barrett-Connor 1984). The CHD death rate was much higher among diabetics than among nondiabetics. Smokers had higher CHD death rates than nonsmokers among both diabetics and nondiabetics. Six-year CHD mortality was 4.0/1,000 for nonsmokers who were nondiabetic and 23.2/1,000 for diabetics who smoked at least 36 cigarettes per day.

Hyperlipoproteinemia is a primary cause of premature coronary atherosclerosis and heart attacks. Cigarette smoking substantially increases the risk of CHD among individuals with genetic familial hyperlipidemias. Williams and coworkers (Williams et al. 1986; Hopkins, Williams, Hunt 1984) studied four large Utah pedigrees with familial hypercholesterolemia. They noted a substantially increased risk of CHD within the high-risk pedigrees in relation to cigarette smoking.

Miettinen and Gylling (1988) have recently completed a long-term followup of 96 patients with familial hypercholesterolemia. Cigarette smoking was a significant predictor of coronary mortality after adjustment for disease history, sex, and various metabolic parameters.

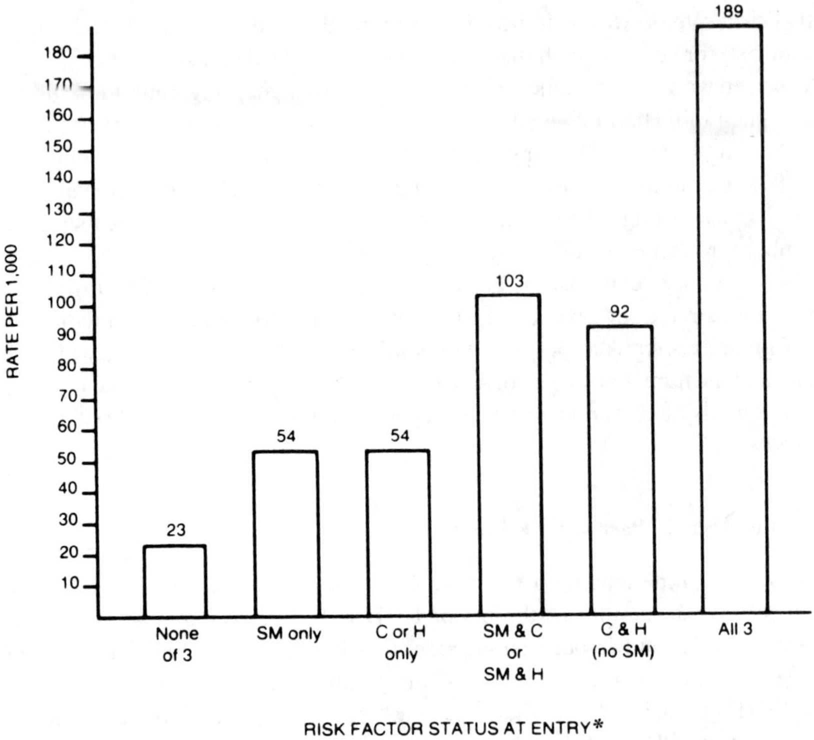

FIGURE 10.—Major risk factor combinations, 10-year incidence of first major coronary events, males aged 30 to 59 years at entry, Pooling Project

*Definitions of the three major risk factors and their symbols: hypercholesterolemia (C), ≥250 mg/dh; elevated blood pressure (H), diastolic pressure ≥90 mm Hg; cigarette smoking (SM), any current use of cigarettes at entry.

NOTE: All rates were age-adjusted by 10-year age groups to the U.S. white male population, 1980.

SOURCE: Pooling Project Research Group (1978).

Pathophysiological Mechanisms

Autopsy studies indicate that cigarette smoking has a significant positive association with atherosclerosis (US DHHS 1983). Studies have noted the strongest relationship of cigarette smoking with aortic atherosclerosis, but smokers also show increased coronary atherosclerosis compared with nonsmokers (US DHHS 1983). Smokers undergoing coronary angiography have more coronary artery disease than nonsmokers (Pearson 1984). Cigarette smokers who continue to smoke following transluminal coronary angioplasty may be more likely to require repeat angioplasty than nonsmokers (Galan et al. 1988)

Cigarette smoking exerts both acute and chronic adverse coronary effects (US DHHS 1983; Holbrook et al. 1984). It contributes to acute ischemic and occlusive events through several possible mechanisms: an imbalance between myocardial oxygen supply and demand, coronary artery spasm, a hypercoagulable state, increased platelet adhesiveness and aggregation, and a decreased ventricular fibrillation threshold (US

DHHS 1983; Martin et al. 1984; Fitzgerald, Oates, Nowak 1988). Cigarette smoking also contributes to the development of coronary atherosclerosis. Possible mechanisms for this chronic effect include: repetitive endothelial injury, a decreased high-density lipoprotein (HDL)/low-density lipoprotein (LDL) cholesterol ratio, abnormalities in the synthesis of thromboxane A2 and prostacyclin, and increased neutrophil elastase activity (Holbrook, in press; Nowak et al. 1987; Weitz et al. 1987).

Clinical Correlations

Cigarette smoking has an adverse effect on individuals with symptomatic or asymptomatic CHD. Compared with nonsmokers, smokers having a positive exercise test (Rautaharju et al. 1986; Gordon et al. 1986) or a history of coronary bypass surgery (Vlietstra et al. 1986; Kemp et al. 1986) face a worse prognosis. Smokers who have angina pectoris have a higher risk of death than nonsmokers (Hubert, Holford, Kannel 1982) and have a poorer long-term prognosis after a myocardial infarction (Ronnevik, Gundersen, Abrahamsen 1985; Kuller et al. 1982). Continuing to smoke increases the likelihood of recurrent acute myocardial infarction and sudden death (Hallstrom, Cobb, Ray 1986). Smoking may also cause silent ischemic disturbances in patients with stable angina pectoris (Deanfield et al. 1986).

Cigarette smoking interferes with the efficacy of medication used to treat CHD such as propranolol, atenolol, and nifedipine (Deanfield et al. 1984).

Smoking Cessation

Prospective epidemiologic studies have documented a substantial reduction in CHD death rates following smoking cessation (US DHHS 1983). While some studies have shown a benefit within 2 years after quitting, other studies have suggested that the former smoker's CHD risk gradually decreases over a period of several years (Cook et al. 1986). For heavier smokers, the residual CHD risk is proportional to the total lifetime exposure to cigarettes.

Cerebrovascular Disease (Stroke)

In the United States stroke is the third leading cause of death. It is also a major cause of morbidity, with more than 400,000 Americans suffering nonfatal strokes each year (Harrison's Principles of Internal Medicine 1987).

There are two major types of cerebrovascular disease: (1) cerebral infarction due to occlusion of a vessel by an embolus or thrombosis, and (2) cerebral hemorrhage, including subarachnoid and parenchymal. The terms cerebrovascular accident and stroke are nonspecific and usually refer to clinical syndromes.

A stroke may be caused by disease of the extra- or intracranial blood vessels. Embolization from the heart or extracranial arteries is also an important cause of stroke. The stroke can result from hemorrhage from a blood vessel or from occlusion of an artery because of atherosclerosis, thrombosis, or embolization. In the Framingham study, atherothrombotic brain infarction accounted for the majority of strokes (Wolf,

Dawber et al. 1978). Improved diagnostic methods have provided a better categorization of the causes of stroke. Epidemiologic studies have shown that hypertension is the most important risk factor for stroke (US DHHS 1983).

The 1964 Report of the Surgeon General stated that the large epidemiologic studies of Hammond and Horn (1958) and Dorn (1958) had found a moderate increase in the mortality rate from cerebrovascular disease in cigarette smokers compared with nonsmokers.

The 1971 Report (US DHEW 1971) reviewed six major prospective epidemiologic studies. Cigarette smokers in these studies experienced increased stroke mortality compared with nonsmokers. The 1980 Report (US DHHS 1980) noted that women who smoke have an increased risk of subarachnoid hemorrhage. The 1983 Report (US DHHS 1983) reviewed the data associating cigarette smoking with stroke and found an increased risk for stroke among smokers that was most evident in younger age groups. It also noted that women cigarette smokers experience an increased risk for subarachnoid hemorrhage and that the concurrent use of both cigarettes and oral contraceptives greatly increased this risk.

Since the release of the 1983 Surgeon General's Report the relationship between cigarette smoking and stroke has been clarified in several large studies involving men and women.

The risk of stroke was evaluated in a prospective study of 8,006 Japanese-American men living in Hawaii (Abbott et al. 1986). After 12 years of followup, cigarette smokers had two to three times the risk of thromboembolic or hemorrhagic stroke compared with nonsmokers. The increased risk was independent of other risk factors such as hypertension and CHD. Those smokers who stopped smoking during the course of the study experienced more than a 50-percent reduction in the risk of stroke compared with continuing smokers.

The impact of cigarette smoking on stroke incidence was assessed prospectively in the Framingham Study of 4,255 men and women (Wolf et al. 1988). This cohort was followed for 26 years, and the diagnoses were confirmed by clinical examination. Cigarette smoking made a significant, independent contribution to the risk of stroke. The risk increased as the number of cigarettes smoked increased. Smoking cessation resulted in a significant decrease in stroke risk so that 5 years after stopping smoking the risk was at the level of nonsmokers.

The relationship between cigarette smoking and the risk of stroke was evaluated in a prospective study of 118,539 middle-aged women who were followed for 8 years (Colditz, Bonita, Stampfer 1988). Compared with nonsmoking women, those who smoked 1 to 14 cigarettes per day had a relative risk of fatal and nonfatal stroke of 2.2. Those who smoked 25 or more cigarettes per day had a relative risk of fatal and nonfatal stroke of 3.7. In this latter group of women, the relative risk of subarachnoid hemorrhage was 9.8. The contribution of cigarette smoking to increased stroke risk was independent of other risk factors. Smoking cessation resulted in a prompt decrease in stroke risk; the relative risk of stroke in women who had stopped smoking for 2 years was 1.4, compared with women who had never smoked. The authors of this study also reviewed eight prospective cohort studies and seven case–control studies involving women, and concluded that most of these studies had shown a positive association between cigarette smoking and stroke (Table 3).

In the ongoing study of approximately 1.2 million persons (CPS-II), cigarette smokers under the age of 65 years experienced increased risks of death from stroke. For men and women (current smokers), the relative risks of death from stroke were 3.7 and 4.9, respectively. The relative risks for those over age 65 years were 1.9 and 1.5 for men and women, respectively (Chapter 3).

Cigarette smoking was associated with decreased cerebral blood flow in a recent clinical study involving 192 normal volunteers (Rogers, Meyer et al. 1983). In a subsequent study of 268 normal volunteers, abstention from cigarette smoking improved cerebral perfusion (Rogers, Meyer et al. 1985).

As already noted in this Chapter, cigarette smoking increases the risk for CHD, and consequently for congestive heart failure, both of which increase the risk for stroke. Data from the Medical Research Council study on the treatment of mild hypertension illustrate the impact of cigarette smoking on the efficacy of drug therapy and stroke incidence (Medical Research Council Working Party 1985). Nonsmokers receiving propranolol to control hypertension experienced a reduction in stroke incidence, while cigarette smokers did not.

Wolf and coworkers (1988) recently reviewed the association between cigarette smoking and stroke and concluded that it is causal. These investigators noted that the causal connection is supported by all of the traditional epidemiologic criteria; these include an increased risk for stroke among smokers compared with nonsmokers that is independent of other risk factors, a dose–response relationship, and a decrease in stroke risk with smoking cessation (Abbott et al. 1986; Wolf et al. 1988; Colditz, Bonita, Stampfer 1988). The aforementioned recent clinical studies also confirm that cigarette smoking increases the risk for stroke. Thus, current evidence indicates that cigarette smoking is a cause of stroke and that smoking cessation reduces the risk for stroke.

Atherosclerotic Peripheral Vascular Disease

Lower extremity arterial vascular disease causes substantial mortality and morbidity; the complications may include intermittent claudication, tissue ischemia and gangrene, and ultimately, loss of the limb.

The 1964 Surgeon General's Report commented that little is known about the relationship of smoking to peripheral arteriosclerosis. Subsequent reports have described the evidence establishing that cigarette smoking is a cause of and the most powerful risk factor for atherosclerotic peripheral vascular disease and that smoking cessation is the most important intervention in the management of this problem (US DHEW 1971, 1979; US DHHS 1983).

Cigarette smoking is directly related to the extent of atherosclerotic disease involving large and small arteries in the lower extremity (Criqui et al. 1985). Cigarette smoking also causes peripheral vasoconstriction. Epidemiologic and clinical studies have clearly demonstrated that cigarette smokers have a higher prevalence than nonsmokers

TABLE 3.—Summary of studies of cigarette smoking and stroke in women

First author	Cohort size	Type of stroke	No. of cases	Relative risk	Comments
		Prospective cohort studies			
Colditz	118,539	All	274	2.2 (95% CI, 1.5–3.3) 2.7 (95% CI, 1.9–3.7) 3.7 (95% CI, 2.7–5.1)	1–14 cigarettes/day 15–24 cigarettes/day ≥25 cigarettes/day
Salonen	4,334	Infarction Other	21 38	1.4 (90% CI, 0.4–5.0) 0.8 (90% CI, 0.3–2.2)	
Tanaka	1,681	Hemorrhage Infarction	30 81	2.1 (NS) 1.0 (NS)	Included 780 men
Sacco	2,421	Subarachnoid hemorrhage	22	1.6	Relative risk was 2.9 for heavy smokers
Vessey	17,000	Subarachnoid hemorrhage Nonhemorrhagic	13 33	3.0 1.4	
Doll	6,194	Cerebral thrombosis	68	0.5 for 15–24 cigarettes/day	Risk tended to decrease with amount smoked
Layde	46,000	Subarachnoid hemorrhage	20		Smokers had higher risk of fatal subarachnoid hemorrhage
Petitti	16,759	Subarachnoid hemorrhage Other	11 23	5.7 (90% CI, 1.8–17.8) 4.8 (90% CI, 2.3–9.8)	
Wolf	2,421	All	238	1.6 (p<0.025)	
		Case–control studies			
Taha		Subarachnoid hemorrhage	124	2.6 for aneurysm	Based on 68 female cases
Bell		Subarachnoid hemorrhage	134	3.7(90% CI, 2.3–5.9)	
Collaborative study		Hemorrhage Thrombosis	192 140		Smoking doubled risk No increased risk
Abu-Zeid		Hemorrhage Thrombosis	137 410	1.4 (NS) 2.4 (p<0.001)	Included men
Bonita		Subarachnoid hemorrhage	70	4.7 (95% CI, 2.9–7.6)	Dose–response relationship not significant
Bonita		Not subarachnoid hemorrhage	53	2.6 (95% CI, 1.4–4.6)	
Herman		Stroke	125	1.2 (95% CI, 0.7–2.3)	Included 78 men

NOTE: CI, confidence interval; NS, not significant.

SOURCE: Colditz, Bonita, Stampfer (1988).

of both symptomatic and asymptomatic lower extremity arterial disease (US DHHS 1983).

In the Lipid Research Clinic prevalence study (Pomrehn et al. 1986), 48 percent of individuals with claudication were current cigarette smokers compared with 30 percent of the controls. Smoking was twice as frequent among individuals developing leg pain, compared with those not developing leg pain, during the exercise test. In the Framingham Study, the risk of developing intermittent claudication was directly and strongly related to cigarette smoking (Kannel and Shurtleff 1973).

Diabetes mellitus and cigarette smoking are the key risk factors for lower extremity arterial disease and subsequent amputation. Peripheral neuropathy and lower extremity arterial disease and infection predispose individuals with diabetes to gangrene and amputation (Herman, Teutsch, Geiss 1987). Diabetics have a sixteenfold increased risk of lower extremity amputation compared with nondiabetics; about 50 percent of the lower extremity amputations in the United States are performed on diabetics. Approximately 31,000 American diabetics undergo such surgery each year. The disease tends to be more progressive and occurs at younger ages in diabetic smokers than in nonsmokers.

In a study in Sweden, practically all diabetic patients under the age of 60 years with gangrene were cigarette smokers (Lithner 1983). The prevalence of lower extremity arterial disease was evaluated for diabetic subjects. One-third of the smokers had evidence of peripheral vascular disease compared with only 16 percent of the nonsmokers. Diabetics who stopped smoking for at least 2 years had a 30 percent lower prevalence of lower extremity arterial disease than those who continued to smoke.

Epidemiologic studies in a Rochester, MN, population (Zimmerman et al. 1981) demonstrated that for 1,073 residents over the age of 30 who were diagnosed with diabetes mellitus between 1945 and 1969, about 8 percent of men and 7 percent of women had clinical evidence of peripheral vascular disease at the time that diabetes was diagnosed. The annual incidence of lower extremity arterial disease among the diabetics was 21/1,000 for men and 17.6/1,000 for women; about 20 percent had gangrene and 36 percent had intermittent claudication. Among diabetics with lower extremity arterial disease, 77 percent of men and 43 percent of women had been cigarette smokers compared with 55 percent of normal control men and 36 percent of normal control women.

Effective treatment of diabetes mellitus and smoking cessation are the two most important interventions to prevent the development of atherosclerotic peripheral vascular disease.

Atherosclerotic Aortic Aneurysm

The 1964 Report of the Surgeon General commented on the increased mortality rates for aortic aneurysm in cigarette smokers compared with nonsmokers. The 1969 Report concluded that there is a close association between cigarette smoking and death caused by aortic aneurysm. The 1983 Report summarized the epidemiologic data and noted that the mortality rate for abdominal aortic aneurysm was 2 to 8 times greater in cigarette smokers than in nonsmokers. As already noted, pathology studies have shown a significant association between cigarette smoking and atherosclerosis that is most striking in the aorta (US DHHS 1983).

Chronic Obstructive Pulmonary Disease

In the 1950s, increasing morbidity and mortality from chronic respiratory conditions prompted clinical and epidemiologic investigations of the etiology of chronic bronchitis, emphysema, and related disorders. A variety of terms have subsequently been applied to permanent airflow obstruction in cigarette smokers. In the 1984 Surgeon General's Report, chronic obstructive lung disease (COLD) referred to chronic mucus hypersecretion, airways abnormalities, and emphysema. In this Report, the term COPD is used for the permanent airflow obstruction that develops in cigarette smokers. Thirty years ago, the most widely advanced hypothesis on the etiology of COPD linked progressive lung damage to recurrent respiratory infection and atmospheric pollution (Stuart-Harris 1954). However, epidemiologic investigations, largely carried out in the United Kingdom, quickly indicated the predominant role of cigarette smoking in causing COPD (Stuart-Harris 1968a,b).

By 1964, the evidence was sufficiently compelling to support the conclusion by the Advisory Committee to the Surgeon General that "Cigarette smoking is the most important of the causes of chronic bronchitis in the United States, and increases the risk of dying from chronic bronchitis and emphysema" (US PHS 1964). The Report stopped short of classifying the relationship between cigarette smoking and emphysema as causal, however. The Report also noted the increased prevalence of respiratory symptoms and the reduction of lung function in smokers. The epidemiologic data cited in support of these conclusions were drawn from seven prospective studies of mortality in relation to cigarette smoking and about a dozen surveys of respiratory morbidity; only one prospective study on lung function had been reported at that time.

In the 25 years that have elapsed since the release of the 1964 Surgeon General's Report, the findings of numerous laboratory, clinical, and epidemiologic studies have continued to reaffirm the predominant role of cigarette smoking in causing COPD and have extended understanding of the pathogenesis, pathophysiology, and natural history of this disorder. As the evidence has accumulated, the conclusions of the Surgeon General's Reports on cigarette smoking and COPD have been strengthened. The 1967 Surgeon General's Report labeled cigarette smoking as the most important of the causes of COPD (US PHS 1968). In the 1971 and 1979 Reports, the conclusions of the 1964 and 1967 Reports were strengthened (US DHEW 1979). Increased morbidity and mortality from chronic bronchitis and emphysema were documented in cigarette smokers compared with nonsmokers. Additionally, autopsy evidence confirmed that the lungs of smokers were widely damaged, and the evolving protease–antiprotease hypothesis provided a framework for understanding mechanisms through which cigarette smoke causes emphysema.

The 1984 Surgeon General's Report focused on COLD (US DHHS 1984). The overall conclusion of the Report was: "Cigarette smoking is the major cause of chronic obstructive lung disease in the United States for both men and women. The contribution of cigarette smoking to chronic obstructive lung disease morbidity and mortality far outweighs all other factors." In contrast to the sparse evidence in the 1964 Report, the 1984 Report reviewed numerous cross-sectional and longitudinal studies of morbidity and mortality. The longitudinal studies described the evolution of the cigarette-related decline in lung function that leads to impairment sufficient to result in a clinical diagnosis of COPD.

This Section provides an overview of the evidence on COPD that has accumulated since the 1964 Report in the areas of pathogenesis, pathophysiology, and natural history of COPD and the role of cigarette smoking.

Pathogenesis

The 1964 Report described the deposition of cigarette-smoke particles and gases in the lungs and the effects of cigarette smoke on lung defenses but did not address the mechanisms by which cigarette smoking causes COPD (US PHS 1964). Much of the subsequent investigation of the mechanism of lung injury by cigarette smoke was sparked by the observation that homozygous deficiency of alpha$_1$-antitrypsin, the major protease inhibitor, is associated with familial panlobular emphysema (Laurell and Eriksson 1963; Eriksson 1964). This observation led to the hypothesis, generally referred to as the protease–antiprotease hypothesis, that the development of emphysema results from an imbalance between proteolytic enzymes and their inhibitors (Janoff 1985; Niewoehner 1988). Cigarette smoking is postulated to produce unchecked proteolytic activity by increasing proteolytic enzyme activity in the lung while decreasing antiprotease activity.

Experimental and clinical observations have been consistent with the protease–antiprotease hypothesis (US DHHS 1984). Observations that smokers, compared with nonsmokers, have an increased number of neutrophils in peripheral blood (Yeung and dy Buncio 1984), in bronchoalveolar lavage fluid, and in lung biopsy specimens (Hunninghake and Crystal 1983) provide indirect evidence for an increased elastase burden in smokers' lungs, since neutrophils are the primary source of elastase (Janoff 1985). Furthermore, elastase levels are elevated in bronchial lavage fluid immediately after smoking cigarettes (Fera et al. 1986). Cigarette smoking has also been shown to decrease the levels and activity of antiproteases, an effect attributed to oxidants in cigarette smoke and the pulmonary macrophages of smokers (Janoff 1985; US DHHS 1984). Animal models confirm that unchecked proteolytic activity can cause emphysema (US DHHS 1984).

The lungs of patients with COPD generally display both emphysema and abnormalities of the small airways. Mechanisms by which cigarette smoke damages small airways have not been so extensively investigated as the factors determining the development of emphysema.

Pathophysiology

The lungs of smokers with COPD generally have both thickening and narrowing of airways and emphysema, although the extent of these two processes is variable (US DHHS 1984). Both the airways changes and emphysema produce airflow obstruction.

The 1964 Report noted that smokers' lungs displayed airways changes and emphysema; however, the pathophysiological correlates of these changes were not explored.

Subsequent investigations, correlating structural changes with function, have described the relationship between smoking-caused changes in lung structure and airflow obstruction. Emphysema and small-airway injury contribute to the physiological impairment found in COPD; in individuals with symptomatic airflow obstruction, either type of injury may be predominant, but both are probably important (US DHHS 1984). While the 1964 Report described effects of cigarette smoking on the airways, the importance of the small airways as a site of airflow obstruction was not recognized until the late 1960s (Hogg, Macklem, Thurlbeck 1968). More recent investigations have confirmed that measures of small-airway injury are correlated with the degree of airflow obstruction (US DHHS 1984; Hale et al. 1984; Nagai, West, Thurlbeck 1985). Autopsy studies have shown that changes in the small airways develop in the lungs of young smokers and antedate the development of symptomatic airflow obstruction (Niewoehner, Kleinerman, Rice 1974).

The importance of emphysema in producing chronic airflow obstruction has also been amply documented since the 1964 Report. Emphysema reduces the driving pressure for expiratory flow and contributes to increased airways resistance by reducing tethering of small airways. In patients with symptomatic airflow obstruction, the extent of anatomic emphysema is correlated with the severity of airflow obstruction, as are small-airway abnormalities (US DHHS 1984; Hale et al. 1984; Nagai, West, Thurlbeck 1985). Thus, the smoking-caused lung changes in the airways and parenchyma have both been unequivocally linked to airflow obstruction.

Natural History of COPD and the Role of Cigarette Smoking

Nearly all the epidemiologic evidence reviewed in the 1964 Report was cross-sectional in nature. These data established that cigarette smoking increased respiratory symptoms and reduced the level of ventilatory function, but they did not provide insight into the temporal evolution of COPD. Subsequent cross-sectional studies have provided more complete quantitative descriptions of the effects of cigarette smoking on lung function, and new longitudinal studies have partially described the evolution of lung function changes in smokers and the factors determining the rate of change over time.

The numerous cross-sectional studies published since the 1964 Surgeon General's Report have shown that cigarette smoking is a strong determinant of the level of ventilatory function, which is most often assessed by the measurement of the 1-sec forced expiratory volume (FEV_1). The level of FEV_1 declines as the amount of smoking increases (US DHHS 1984). Multiple regression techniques have been applied to data from several different populations to describe the quantitative relationship between the amount smoked and loss of ventilatory function. These analyses indicate that ventilatory function declines in a linear fashion with cumulative consumption of cigarettes, usually expressed as pack-years (Burrows et al. 1977; Dockery et al. 1988). For example, based on analysis of data from 8,191 men and women from six U.S. cities, Dockery and others (1988) reported that male smokers of average height lose 7.4 mL of FEV_1

on average for each pack-year and that women lose 4.4 mL per pack-year. Although the decline in mean level of FEV_1 appears small, the distributions of lung function level in smokers and in nonsmokers are different; the distribution for smokers is skewed toward lower levels so that a much greater proportion of smokers than nonsmokers have levels below the usual limit of normal (Figure 11) (US DHHS 1984; Burrows et al. 1977; Dockery et al. 1988).

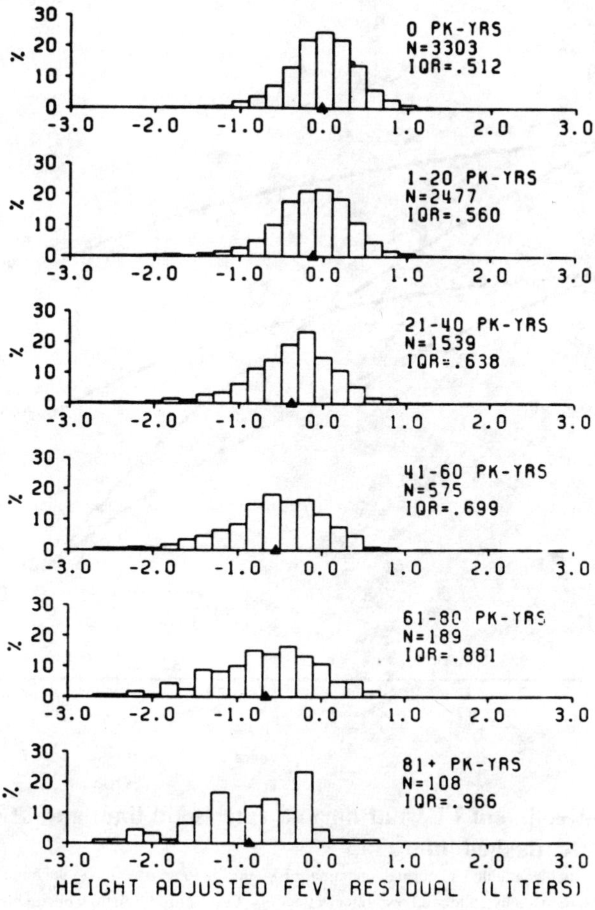

FIGURE 11.—Percent distribution of predicted values of forced expiratory volume in 1-sec (FEV_1) in subjects with varying pack-years of smoking.

NOTE: Triangle indicates mean. IQR is interquartile range.

SOURCE: Dockery et al. (1988).

The longitudinal studies published since the 1964 Report have partially described the natural history of lung function changes in COPD (Fletcher et al. 1976; US DHHS 1984). Ventilatory function, as measured by FEV_1, for example, increases during childhood and reaches a peak level during early adulthood (Figure 12). From the peak level, ventilatory function declines with increasing age. In cigarette smokers who develop symptomatic airflow obstruction, a similar loss of function takes place, but at a more rapid rate than in nonsmokers and in smokers who do not develop disease. A physician is likely to diagnose COPD when continued excessive loss of ventilatory function results in sufficient impairment to cause dyspnea and limitation of activity.

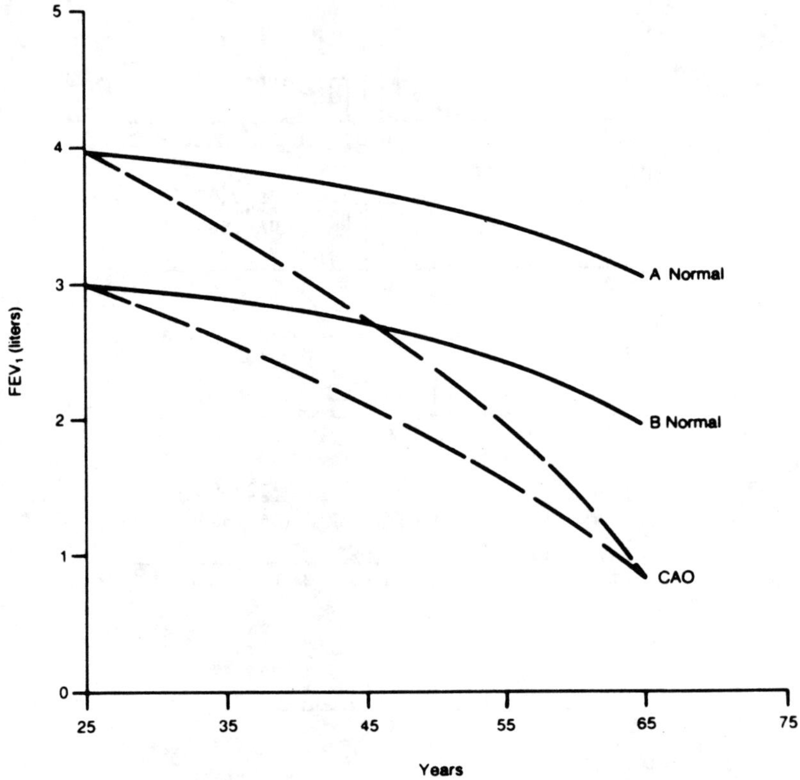

FIGURE 12.—Decline of FEV$_1$ at normal rate (solid line) and at an accelerated rate (dashed line)

NOTE: A, person who has attained a "normal" maximal FEV$_1$ during lung growth and development; B, person whose maximal FEV$_1$ has been reduced by childhood respiratory infection. CAO, chronic airflow obstruction.

SOURCE: Samet et al. (1983).

The factors influencing rate of lung function decline in cigarette smokers have not yet been fully characterized. The rate of decline tends to increase with the amount smoked, and former smokers generally revert to the rate of loss of nonsmokers. In fact, the excessive decline observed in some smokers may represent a common physiological consequence of different pathophysiological mechanisms. Habib and coworkers (1987) carefully characterized 13 subjects from a longitudinal study in Tucson with a mean annual decline in FEV$_1$ greater than 60 mL per year. Clinically, these subjects were not unique and none had alpha$_1$-antitrypsin deficiency. Physiological assessment suggested that some were developing emphysema, whereas others appeared to have disease of the large and/or small airways.

The studies of longitudinal change in lung function have spanned only segments of the full natural history of COPD, and many questions remain unanswered. It is unclear, for example, whether the excessive decline takes place at a constant rate in continuous smokers, as suggested by much of the epidemiologic evidence, or whether the excessive decline occurs intermittently after some triggering event. The factors determining the susceptibility of individuals to cigarette smoking are also unclear. Current hypotheses emphasize determinants of protease–antiprotease imbalance, level of nonspecific airways reactivity, and severe respiratory illness during early childhood.

Since the release of the 1964 Surgeon General's Report, abundant evidence has indicated the overwhelming importance of cigarette smoking in causing COPD; in fact, COPD would be an uncommon condition in the United States without cigarette smoking. Unfortunately, death rates due to COPD have paralleled those for lung cancer and have increased progressively over the last 25 years (National Center for Health Statistics 1986). The trends are consistent with cohort changes in smoking; in this regard, while age-specific rates for males have been increasing at older ages, a recent decline in COPD mortality has been observed at younger ages (US DHHS 1984). While important scientific questions remain unanswered concerning the pathogenesis of COPD, the available evidence provides sufficient rationale for preventing COPD through smoking prevention and cessation.

Pregnancy and Infant Health

Several endpoints have been studied to evaluate the adverse effects of smoking on pregnancy, including (1) infant birthweight; (2) fetal and infant mortality; (3) congenital malformations; (4) fertility; and (5) long-term effects on the child.

The 1964 Report indicated an association between smoking and low-birthweight babies (US PHS 1964), but it did not consider the evidence sufficient to establish a causal relationship.

The 1969 Report (US PHS 1969) confirmed the association between maternal smoking and low-birthweight babies, an increased incidence of prematurity, spontaneous abortions, stillbirths, and neonatal deaths. The 1971 Report (US DHEW 1971) concluded that maternal smoking during pregnancy exerts a retarding influence on fetal growth. The 1973 Report (US DHEW 1973) noted that cigarette smoking is a probable cause of increased late fetal mortality and infant mortality. The 1977–78 Report (US DHEW 1978) noted a dose–response relationship between smoking and abruptio placentae, placenta previa, bleeding during pregnancy, and prolonged premature rupture of membranes, as well as the association of smoking during pregnancy with impaired physical and intellectual development of the offspring. The 1979 Report (US DHEW 1979) linked smoking with sudden infant death syndrome. The 1980 Report (US DHHS 1980) noted that up to 14 percent of preterm deliveries in the United States may be attributed to maternal smoking. It also surveyed studies of men and women suggesting that cigarette smoking may impair fertility.

In 1985, the Center for Health Promotion and Education of the Centers for Disease Control, Atlanta, GA, defined the fetal tobacco syndrome as follows. (1) The mother smoked 5 or more cigarettes a day throughout the pregnancy. (2) The mother had no evidence of hypertension during pregnancy, specifically no preeclampsia and documentation of normal blood pressure at least once after the first trimester. (3) The newborn has symmetrical growth retardation at term, 37 weeks, defined as birthweight less than 2,500 g, and a ponderal index (weight in grams divided by length) greater than 2.32. (4) There is no obvious cause of intrauterine growth retardation, that is, congenital malformation or infection (Nieburg et al. 1985).

Infant Birthweight

A clear dose–response relationship exists between the number of cigarettes smoked during pregnancy and the birthweight deficit (US DHHS 1980; Committee to Study the Prevention of Low Birthweight 1985). Compared with nonsmokers, light and heavy smokers have a 54- and 130-percent increase, respectively, in the prevalence of newborns weighing less than 2,500 g. A review of five studies including 113,000 births in the United States, Canada, and Wales found that from 21 to 39 percent of the incidence of low birthweight was attributed to maternal cigarette smoking (Committee to Study the Prevention of Low Birthweight 1985). Also, cigarette smoking seems to be a more significant determinant of birthweight than the mother's prepregnancy height, weight, parity, payment status, or history of previous pregnancy outcome, or the infant's sex. The reduction in birthweight associated with maternal tobacco use seems to be a direct effect of smoking on fetal growth.

Mothers who smoke also have increased rates of premature delivery. The newborns are also smaller at every gestational age. The infants display symmetrical fetal growth retardation with deficits in measurements of crown–heel length, chest and head circumferences, and birthweight.

A recent study in Boston (Lieberman et al. 1985) attempted to evaluate the reasons for differences in rates of prematurity between blacks and whites. Of the 1,365 black women, 34.7 percent were cigarette smokers compared with only 23.4 percent of the white women. Cigarette smoking and low hematocrit levels were two of the most important risk factors accounting for the differences in prematurity rates between blacks and whites.

Finally, a number of careful studies have found that the effect of cigarette smoking on birthweight is not mediated through decreased maternal appetite or weight gain (US DHHS 1980).

The most widely accepted hypothesis relating maternal smoking and the effects on the fetus and newborn is intrauterine hypoxia (Rush and Cassano 1983). The hypoxia could occur as a result of factors associated with smoking, such as increased levels of carbon monoxide (CO) in the blood, reduction of blood flow, or inhibition of respiratory enzymes. There is strong experimental evidence that maternal smoking causes fetal hypoxia.

Several studies have demonstrated that smoking cessation prior to or during pregnancy can partly reverse the reduction in the child's birthweight (Rush and Cassano 1983; Hebel, Fox, Sexton 1988). In a large study using the 1970 British Birth Cohort (Lieberman et al. 1987), an inverse relationship between measures of social class and the prevalence of smoking was demonstrated that was similar to that seen in the United States. In all social class groups, babies of the nonsmokers weighed more than those whose mothers had smoked during pregnancy, and the women who had stopped smoking either before or during pregnancy had babies with higher birthweights than women who continued to smoke throughout pregnancy.

Fetal and Perinatal Mortality

Kleinman and colleagues (1988) from the National Center for Health Statistics used Missouri birth records from 1979–83 (Table 4) to study the relationship between cigarette smoking in mothers and infant mortality. Among the 134,429 primiparas, the infant mortality rates (adjusted for age, parity, education, and marital status) were (per 1,000 subjects) 15.1 for white nonsmokers, 18.8 for whites who smoked less than 1 pack of cigarettes per day, and 23.3 for whites who smoked more than 1 pack of cigarettes per day. For black nonsmoking women, the infant mortality rate (per 1,000 women) was 26.0; for blacks who smoked less than 1 pack per day, 32.4; and for blacks who smoked greater than 1 pack per day, 39.9. Mortality was increased during the fetal, neonatal, and postneonatal periods. It was estimated that if all pregnant women stopped smoking, the number of fetal and infant deaths would be reduced by approximately 10 percent. In the United States this would result in about 4,000 fewer infant deaths each year. A study conducted by the Office on Smoking and Health attributed approximately 2,500 infant deaths to maternal smoking in 1984 (CDC 1987).

Stein and associates (1981) have studied the causes of spontaneous abortion in three New York City hospitals. They compared women with spontaneous abortion to controls (women who carried their pregnancy to 28 weeks or more). Within the spontaneous abortion groups, they then compared those with evidence of chromosomal abnormalities and those with apparently normal chromosomes. The odds of a spontaneous abortion increased by 46 percent for the first 10 cigarettes smoked per day and by 61 percent for the first 20 cigarettes smoked. Smoking was not associated with the spontaneous abortion of chromosomally abnormal conceptions, but only with those in which the chromosomes were normal. These results were not confounded by such factors as maternal age or race.

Congenital Malformations

Evidence that exposure to tobacco and cigarette smoking could be related to congenital malformations is less clear. About 3 percent of all live births have major congenital malformations (Behrman and Vaughn 1987). Maternal smoking has not been demonstrated to be a major risk factor for the induction of congenital malformations, although elevated risks have been reported in some studies. Kelsey and coworkers (1978) reported an increased risk of 1.6 for congenital malformations among the

TABLE 4.—Infant mortality rates and odds ratios (95% confidence intervals), by maternal race, among 134,429 primiparas, based on multiple logistic regression, Missouri, 1979–83

	Crude rates (per 1,000)		Adjusted rates (per 1,000)		Adjusted odds ratios	
	Whites	Blacks	Whites	Blacks	Whites	Blacks
Marital status						
Married	14.5	25.4	15.9	29.5	1.00	1.00
Unmarried	24.0	28.6	21.0	27.2	1.33 (1.18–1.50)	0.92 (0.73–1.16)
Education (years)						
<12	22.9	33.2	19.8	34.1	1.36 (1.16–1.59)	
12	15.2	25.9	16.7	28.8	1.14 (1.02–1.28)	
>12	12.8	21.5	14.6	25.3	1.00	
Age (years)						
<18	24.0	33.7	18.8	32.2	1.24 (1.06–1.45)	
18–19	18.2	26.0	16.3	27.9	1.08 (0.95–1.22)	
20–24	14.2	23.4	15.2	26.0	1.00	
25–29	13.2	27.1	16.1	27.6	1.06 (0.94–1.20)	
30–34	16.1	19.9	18.6	31.9	1.23 (1.01–1.50)	
≥35	25.4	69.3	31.1	52.9	2.09 (1.49–2.93)	
Smoking						
0	13.9	25.3	15.1	26.0	1.00	
<1 pack/day	19.1	33.7	18.8	32.4	1.25 (1.13–1.39)	
≥1 pack/day	24.3	41.5	23.3	39.9	1.56 (1.37–1.77)	

SOURCE: Kleinman et al. (1988).

offspring of women smoking more than 1 pack of cigarettes per day compared with women reporting no smoking during pregnancy. Similarly, Himmelberger, Brown, and Cohen (1978) reported a 2.3-fold higher risk of congenital abnormalities for smoking mothers than for nonsmokers.

One study has also reported an increased frequency of congenital malformations based on the smoking habits of the father (Schardein 1985). The trends with paternal smoking were independent of maternal smoking level, maternal and paternal age, and social class.

The relatively low incidence of congenital malformations, the different types of malformations, and the various possible biological mechanisms have made the study of the relationship between environmental factors and congenital malformations extremely difficult. New techniques to monitor pregnancy outcomes may enhance our understanding of the interrelationship between cigarette smoking, other environmental factors, and congenital malformations.

Fertility

A recent study has substantiated previous reports that suggested that women who smoke may have reduced fertility (Baird and Wilcox 1985). Data on smoking history and number of noncontraceptive cycles until conception were collected from 678 pregnant women. Of nonsmokers, 38 percent conceived in their first cycle compared with 28 percent of smokers. Smokers were 3.4 times more likely than nonsmokers to have taken greater than 1 year to conceive. After adjustment for other risk factors, it was estimated that the fertility of smokers was 72 percent of that of nonsmokers. Heavy smokers experienced lower fertility than light smokers. Fertility was not affected by the husbands' smoking.

The effects of cigarette smoking on sperm quality in men (Ablin 1986) were also evaluated in relation to density, motility, and morphological abnormalities in 238 age-related smokers and 135 nonsmokers. Spermatozoa from smokers possessed significantly decreased density and motility compared with those from nonsmokers. Morphological abnormalities of the sperm were also noted more frequently among smokers than among nonsmokers (Ablin 1986).

Long-Term Effects on the Child

Relatively few studies have evaluated the long-term consequences of smoking during pregnancy on the child. One of the larger recent studies looked at neurological handicaps among children up to 14 years of age whose mothers had smoked during pregnancy and among control children born in northern Finland in 1966 (Rantakallio and Koiranen 1987). Seventy-eight children of smokers and 62 controls had mental retardation (IQs less than 85), cerebral palsy, or epilepsy. The incidence of mental retardation alone was 15.9/1,000 among the children of the mothers who smoked and 13.9 among the controls. For any combination of mental retardation, cerebral palsy, and epilepsy, the rates were 42.8/1,000 for children of smoking mothers and 34/1,000 for the controls, a relative risk of 1.27 with confidence limits of 0.90 to 1.79.

Naeye and Peters (1984) investigated the mental development of smokers' children by comparing siblings whose mothers smoked in one but not in subsequent pregnancies and found that hyperactivity, short attention span, and lower scores on spelling and reading tests were more frequent for the children whose mother had smoked during pregnancy, but the differences were relatively small, the test scores being only 2 to 4 percent lower. Dunn also studied neurological and electroencephalographic abnormalities among 6-year-old children of smokers and found these conditions to be slightly more common in the children of mothers who had smoked during pregnancy, but again the differences were not statistically significant. Small sample sizes in many of these studies and the relative infrequency of the events of interest limit interpretation of the studies (Dunn et al. 1977).

Peptic Ulcer

The 1964 Surgeon General's Report noted an association between peptic ulcer and cigarette smoking. The 1979 Report stated that the relationship between cigarette smoking and peptic ulcer is significant enough to suggest a causal relationship. Peptic ulcer disease is more likely to occur, less likely to heal, and more likely to cause death in smokers than in nonsmokers.

Cigarette smoking retards the healing of peptic ulcer (Sontag et al. 1984; Lane and Lee 1988; Korman et al. 1983). A large trial of cimetidine, a drug used in the treatment of peptic ulcer, was reported in 1984 by Sontag and associates. Ulcer recurrence was much more frequent among smokers compared with nonsmokers for both the placebo- and the cimetidine-treated groups.

Nicotine decreases pyloric sphincter pressure and therefore permits increased reflux of duodenal contents into the stomach. Nicotine also decreases pancreatic bicarbonate secretion. This may impair neutralization of gastric acid in the duodenum, contributing to the formation and persistence of duodenal ulcers. Smoking cessation probably reduces the incidence of peptic ulcer and is an important component of peptic ulcer treatment even with the available effective drug therapy.

Osteoporosis

The 1964 Report did not discuss osteoporosis. The interest in osteoporosis is fairly recent because of the increasing number of older individuals, especially women, at risk of fracture; the better methods of measuring bone mineral mass; and the understanding of osteoporosis pathophysiology and risk factors.

Osteoporosis leading to fractures, especially of the hip, wrist, and spine, is an important cause of disability and death, predominantly among postmenopausal women. About 15 to 20 million persons in the United States have osteoporosis. Each year about 1.3 million fractures are attributed to this disease (Journal of the American Medical Association 1984).

Smoking may be a risk factor for osteoporosis (Willett et al. 1983). Women smokers have an earlier age of menopause, an important risk factor for osteoporosis (Willett et al. 1983). Smokers may have a lower intake of calcium during adolescence and young adult life when maximum bone mineral mass is reached (Sandler et al. 1985). Smokers also weigh less than nonsmokers (US DHHS 1988). Obesity substantially reduces the risk of hip fracture (Kiel et al. 1987). Overweight women have higher endogenous estrogen levels and greater bone mass (Cauley et al. 1986). Exogenous estrogen intake among postmenopausal women results in a decreased risk of fracture (Ernster et al. 1988). Women who smoke and are on estrogen therapy may have reduced levels of estrogens in their blood compared with levels for nonsmoking women. Among women who smoked and were given high doses of estradiol, blood levels of estrone and estradiol were only one-half of those among nonsmokers (Jensen, Christiansen, Rodbro 1985). Increased hepatic metabolism of exogenous oral estrogen may result in lower estrogen levels among postmenopausal cigarette smokers.

Several case–control studies have evaluated the relationship between osteoporosis and cigarette smoking. Most find an increased risk of fractures among smokers. However, problems with study design, especially the potential effects of confounders such as obesity and age, have limited the interpretation of these studies, as have contradictory findings. For example, a large study of hip fractures among postmenopausal women in four Connecticut hospitals did not find any differences in risk between smokers and nonsmokers (Kreiger et al. 1982). A study in Iowa by Sowers (Sowers, Wallace, Lemke 1985) of 86 women aged 20 to 35 years did not find any relationship between forearm bone mineral mass and smoking during maximal bone mineralization. A study in Denmark (Jensen 1986) compared bone mineral content among 77 long-term smokers and 103 nonsmokers. Bone mineral content correlated with fat mass. For the same degrees of obesity, smokers did not have any lower level of bone mineral content than nonsmokers. The results of these studies suggest that the effect of smoking as a risk factor for osteoporosis and fracture among postmenopausal women may be primarily determined by the inverse relationship between smoking and obesity. It is possible that the early age of menopause among smokers may also contribute to the risk of osteoporosis.

Involuntary Smoking

The issue of involuntary smoking was not raised in the 1964 Surgeon General's Report. The first report of the Surgeon General to address the possible health effects of involuntary smoking was published in 1972 (US DHEW 1972). Over the ensuing 15 years, evidence on the adverse consequences of involuntary smoking began to amass, with several hundred papers being published. In 1986, the Surgeon General's Report (US DHHS 1986a) focused exclusively on this subject.

Nonsmoking adults exposed to ETS have a higher frequency of symptomology, such as eye irritation and upper respiratory symptoms (US DHHS 1986a). The relationship between lung cancer among nonsmokers and ETS has been documented in both case–control and longitudinal studies. Most of these studies have measured the increased risk of lung cancer among nonsmoking women, usually wives exposed to their husbands' tobacco smoke. A 1.3-fold increased risk of lung cancer has been estimated from these studies and is consistent with the amount of exposure to carcinogens from

ETS (US DHHS 1986a), the duration of exposure, and the differences in the distribution of potential carcinogens between sidestream and mainstream smoke.

The 1986 Surgeon General's Report on involuntary smoking concluded (US DHHS 1986a):

1. Involuntary smoking is a cause of disease, including lung cancer, in healthy nonsmokers.
2. The children of parents who smoke compared with the children of nonsmoking parents have an increased frequency of respiratory infections, increased respiratory symptoms, and slightly smaller rates of increase in lung function as the lung matures.
3. The simple separation of smokers and nonsmokers within the same airspace may reduce, but does not eliminate, the exposure of nonsmokers to ETS.

Another major review on involuntary smoking was released in 1986 by the National Research Council (NRC). This report concluded that the risk of lung cancer is approximately 30 percent higher for nonsmoking spouses of smokers than it is for nonsmoking spouses of nonsmokers (NRC 1986).

Since release of the 1986 Surgeon General's Report, five additional studies examining ETS exposure and lung cancer in nonsmokers have been published (Brownson et al. 1987; Dalager et al. 1986; Humble, Samet, Pathak 1987; Gao et al. 1987; Pershagen, Hrubec, Svensson 1987). All five noted a correlation between ETS exposure and lung cancer among nonsmokers. Thus, of the 16 epidemiologic studies in the scientific literature, 14 have noted a positive association.

Smokeless Tobacco

In 1979 the Surgeon General's Report included, for the first time, a review of the health consequences of using smokeless tobacco (snuff and chewing tobacco) (US DHEW 1979). In 1986, a special Surgeon General's Report, *The Health Consequences of Using Smokeless Tobacco* (US DHHS 1986b), reviewed smokeless tobacco in depth and concluded that it can cause cancer in humans. The relationship between smokeless tobacco use and cancer is strongest for the use of snuff and for cancer of the oral cavity. Smokeless tobacco can also cause oral leukoplakia, which may progress to neoplastic transformation with continued use of smokeless tobacco.

Addiction to Smoking

The 1964 Surgeon General's Report referred to tobacco use as habituating. Fifteen years later, the 1979 Report concluded that smoking was "the prototypical substance abuse dependency" (US DHEW 1979). The entire 1988 Report (US DHHS 1988) was dedicated to an exhaustive review of tobacco use as an addiction. The 1988 Report concluded:

1. Cigarettes and other forms of tobacco are addicting.
2. Nicotine is the drug in tobacco that causes addiction.
3. The pharmacologic and behavioral processes that determine tobacco addiction are similar to those that determine addiction to drugs such as heroin or cocaine.

These findings are discussed in greater detail in Part II of Chapter 5 on determinants of smoking behavior.

PART II. THE PHYSICOCHEMICAL NATURE OF TOBACCO

The 1964 Surgeon General's Report on Smoking and Health (US PHS 1964) gave impetus to intensified investigations on the physicochemical nature and composition of tobacco smoke and the identification of biologically active agents in tobacco and tobacco smoke and their modes of action.

In 1936 Brückner listed 120 known components in tobacco smoke. This number grew to about 450 in 1959 (Johnstone and Plimmer 1959), to about 950 in 1968 (Stedman 1968), to 3,875 in 1982 (Dube and Green 1982), and to 3,996 in 1988 (Roberts 1988). Today, the estimated number of known compounds in tobacco smoke exceeds 4,000, including some that are pharmacologically active, toxic, mutagenic, or carcinogenic (US DHEW 1979; US DHHS 1983). Such diverse biological effects of cigarette smoke constituents provide a framework for understanding the multiple adverse consequences of smoking.

Since about 1960, both the composition of cigarette tobacco and the components and shape of the cigarette itself have undergone significant changes that effected reductions in standardized measurements of tar, nicotine, and other toxic agents in the smoke (Norman 1982). Perhaps the greatest advances have been made in understanding the pharmacology and toxicology of nicotine (Benowitz 1986; US DHHS 1988) and in delineating the nature and mode of action of the major carcinogens in tobacco smoke (US DHHS 1982; Hoffmann and Hecht, 1989).

Processed, unadulterated tobacco contains at least 2,550 known compounds (Dube and Green 1982). The bulk of the dried tobacco consists of carbohydrates and proteins. Other important constituents are alkaloids (0.5 to 5 percent), with nicotine as the predominant compound (90 to 95 percent of total alkaloids), and terpenes (0.1 to 3 percent), polyphenols (0.5 to 4.5 percent), phytosterols (0.1 to 2.5 percent), carboxylic acids (0.1 to 0.7 percent), alkanes (0.1 to 0.4 percent), and alkali nitrates (0.01 to 5 percent). In addition, tobacco contains traces of aromatic hydrocarbons, aldehydes, ketones, amines, nitriles, N- and O-heterocyclic compounds, pesticides, and more than 30 metallic compounds (Wynder and Hoffmann 1967; US DHEW 1979).

The composition of the processed tobacco in cigarettes influences the chemistry and toxicity of the smoke. Cigarettes manufactured in the United States are made with blends of bright, burley, and oriental tobaccos that generate weakly acidic mainstream smoke (pH 5.5 to 6.2) in which nicotine occurs in protonated form in the particulate matter. The sidestream smoke (SS) of these cigarettes is neutral to alkaline (pH 6.5 to 8.0), and part of the nicotine in SS is present in unprotonated form in the vapor phase (Brunnemann and Hoffmann 1974). These observations are important because unprotonated nicotine is readily absorbed through the buccal mucosa (US DHHS 1988).

The 400 to 500 mg of mainstream smoke (MS) freshly emerging from the mouthpiece of a cigarette is an aerosol containing about 10^{10} particles per mL; these range in diameter from 0.1 to 1.0 μm (mean diameter 0.2 μm) and are dispersed in a vapor phase (Ingebrethsen 1986). About 95 percent of the MS effluents of a nonfilter cigarette are composed of 400 to 500 individual gaseous compounds with nitrogen, oxygen, and

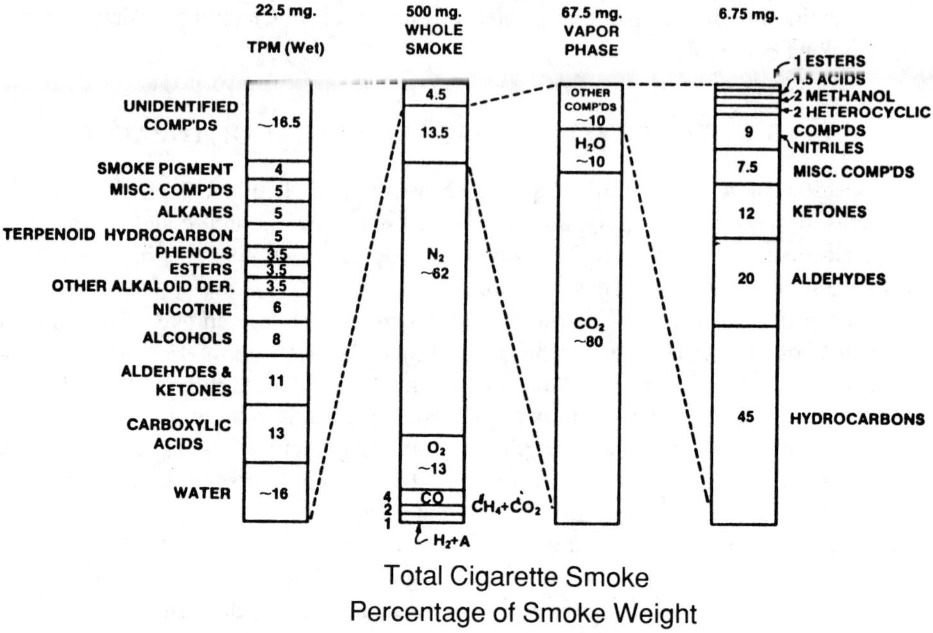

FIGURE 13.—Composition of cigarette mainstream smoke
SOURCE: Dube and Green (1982).

carbon dioxide as major constituents; the particulate matter of MS contains at least 3,500 individual compounds (Figure 13; Dube and Green 1982).

Like all organic combustion products, tobacco smoke contains free radicals, highly reactive oxygen- and carbon-centered types in the vapor phase, and relatively stable radicals in the particulate phase. The principal of the latter appears to be a quinone/hydroquinone complex capable of reducing molecular oxygen to superoxide, and, eventually, to hydrogen peroxide and hydroxyl radicals (Nakayama, Kodama, Nagata 1984; Church and Pryor 1985).

For chemical analysis, the smoke is arbitrarily separated into vapor and particulate phases. Those smoke components of which more than 50 percent appear in the vapor phase of fresh MS are considered volatile smoke constituents; all others are particulate phase components (Figure 13). Tables 5 and 6 list the major types of components identified and their estimated concentration in the smoke of one cigarette (US DHHS 1982; Hoffmann and Hecht 1989). The quantitative data presented here were obtained by machine smoking of cigarettes under standardized laboratory conditions using the method of the Federal Trade Commission (Pillsbury et al. 1969); therefore, the data do not fully reflect the human setting. This applies especially to smokers of low-yield cigarettes who tend to compensate for the low nicotine delivery by drawing smoke more intensely and inhaling more deeply (US DHHS 1988).

Table 6 does not contain information about the nature and concentration of at least 30 metals in the smoke. These compounds are not listed because less than 1 percent of the metals in tobacco are transferred into the smoke and constitute together only ≤80 μg/g(Jenkins, Goldey, Williamson 1985). Tables 5 and 6 also lack descriptions of the

TABLE 5.—Major constituents of the vapor phase of the mainstream smoke of nonfilter cigarettes

Compound[a]	Concentration/cigarette
Nitrogen	280–320 mg (56–64%[b])
Oxygen	50–70 mg (11–14%[b])
Carbon dioxide	45–65 mg (9–13%[b])
Carbon monoxide	14–23 mg (2.8–4.6%[b])
Water	7–12 mg (1.4–2.4%[b])
Argon	5 mg (1.0%[b])
Hydrogen	0.5–1.0 mg
Ammonia	10–130 μg
Nitrogen oxides (NO_x)	100–600 μg
Hydrogen cyanide	400–500 μg
Hydrogen sulfide	20–90 μg
Methane	1.0–2.0 mg
Other volatile alkanes (20)	1.0–1.6 mg[c]
Volatile alkenes (16)	0.4–0.5 mg
Isoprene	0.2–0.4 mg
Butadiene	25–40 μg
Acetylene	20–35 μg
Benzene	12–50 μg
Toluene	20–60 μg
Styrene	10 μg
Other volatile aromatic hydrocarbons (29)	15–30 μg
Formic acid	200–600 μg
Acetic acid	300–1,700 μg
Propionic acid	100–300 μg
Methyl formate	20–30 μg
Other volatile acids (6)	5–10 μg[c]
Formaldehyde	20–100 μg
Acetaldehyde	400–1,400 μg
Acrolein	60–140 μg

TABLE 5.—Continued

Compound[a]	Concentration/cigarette
Other volatile aldehydes (6)	80–140 μg
Acetone	100–650 μg
Other volatile ketones (3)	50–100 μg
Methanol	80–180 μg
Other volatile alcohols (7)	10–30 μg[c]
Acetonitrile	100–150 μg
Other volatile nitriles (10)	50–80 μg[c]
Furan	20–40 μg
Other volatile furans (4)	45–125 μg[c]
Pyridine	20–200 μg
Picolines (3)	15–80 μg
3-Vinylpyridine	10–30 μg
Other volatile pyridines (25)	20–50 μg[c]
Pyrrole	0.1–10 μg
Pyrrolidine	10–18 μg
N-Methylpyrrolidine	2.0–3.0 μg
Volatile pyrazines (18)	3.0–8.0 μg
Methylamine	4–10 μg
Other aliphatic amines (32)	3–10 μg

[a]Numbers in parentheses represent individual compounds identified in a given group.
[b]Percent of total effluent.
[c]Estimate.
SOURCE: Hoffmann and Hecht (1989).

chemical nature and concentrations in cigarette smoke of agricultural chemicals and pesticides, which originate from the residues of such compounds in tobacco. There are many variations in the qualitative and quantitative aspects relative to such agents in tobacco from region to region and from year to year. Overall, the use of agricultural chemicals has also been greatly reduced (Wittekindt 1985). Nevertheless, it is fairly certain that commercial tobaccos contain up to a few parts per million of DDT, DDD,

TABLE 6.—Major constituents of the particulate matter of the mainstream smoke of nonfilter cigarettes

Compound[a]	μg/cigarette
Nicotine	1,000–3,000
Nornicotine	50–150
Anatabine	5–15
Anabasine	5–12
Other tobacco alkaloids (17)	NA
Bipyridyls (4)	10–30
n-Hentriacontane (n-$C_{31}H_{64}$)	100
Total nonvolatile hydrocarbons (45)[b]	300–400[b]
Naphthalene	2–4
Other naphthalenes (23)	3–6[b]
Phenanthrenes (7)	0.2–0.4[b]
Anthracenes (5)	0.05–0.1[b]
Fluorenes (7)	0.6–1.0[b]
Pyrenes (6)	0.3–0.5[b]
Fluoranthenes (5)	0.3–0.45[b]
Carcinogenic polynuclear aromatic hydrocarbons (11)[c]	0.1–0.25
Phenol	80–160
Other phenols (45)[b]	60–180[b]
Catechol	200–400
Other catechols (4)	100–200[b]
Other dihydroxybenzenes (10)	200–400[b]
Scopoletin	15–30
Other polyphenols (8)[b]	NA
Cyclotenes (10)[b]	40–70[b]
Quinones (7)	0.5
Solanesol	600–1,000

TABLE 6.—Continued

Compound[a]	μg/cigarette
Neophytadienes (4)	200–350
Limonene	30–60
Other terpenes (200–250)[b]	NA
Palmitic acid	100–150
Stearic acid	50–75
Oleic acid	40–110
Linoleic acid	60–150
Linolenic acid	150–250
Lactic acid	60–80
Indole	10–15
Skatole	12–16
Other indoles (13)	NA
Quinolines (7)	2–4
Other N-heterocyclic hydrocarbons (55)	NA
Benzofurans (4)	200–300
Other O-heterocyclic hydrocarbons (42)	NA
Stigmasterol	40–70
Sitosterol	30–40
Campesterol	20–30
Cholesterol	10–20
Aniline	0.36
Toluidines	0.23
Other aromatic amines (12)	0.25
Tobacco-specific N-nitrosamines (4)[c]	0.34–2.7
Glycerol	120

NOTE: NA, not available.
[a]Numbers in parentheses represent individual compounds identified in a given group.
[b]Estimate.
[c]See Table 7 for details.
SOURCE: Hoffmann and Hecht (1989).

and maleic hydrazide; fewer than 20 percent of these contaminants are transferred into the smoke stream.

The 1964 Surgeon General's Report listed five polynuclear aromatic hydrocarbons (PAHs) and three N-heterocyclic hydrocarbons as known carcinogenic smoke constituents (US PHS 1964). By the criteria for carcinogenicity of chemicals as set by the International Agency for Research on Cancer (1986), the carcinogens identified to date in tobacco smoke include 11 PAHs, 4 N-heterocyclic hydrocarbons, 9 N-nitrosamines, 3 aromatic amines, 3 aldehydes, 6 volatile carcinogens, 6 inorganic compounds, and the radioelement polonium-210 (Table 7; Hoffmann and Hecht 1989).

The Changing Cigarette

As discussed in Part I, epidemiologic studies have documented a dose–response relationship between the number of cigarettes smoked and the development of cancer of the lung, larynx, oral cavity, esophagus, pancreas, bladder, and kidney (US DHHS 1982; IARC 1986). Bioassays for tumorigenicity with whole smoke and with tar have also demonstrated a dose–response relationship (US DHHS 1982). As tar and nicotine yields in cigarette smoke gradually declined, other toxic and tumorigenic agents, such as CO, volatile N-nitrosamines, and carcinogenic PAHs, were also successfully reduced (Hoffmann, Tso, Gori 1980; Hoffmann et al. 1984; US DHHS 1981). However, it was soon realized that the smoker of low-yield cigarettes tended to compensate for reduced nicotine delivery by intensified smoking (US DHHS 1988), and therefore exposure may not actually have been lowered. Based on values generated by smoking machines under standardized conditions, Figure 14 shows the reduction in sales-weighted tar and nicotine delivery of the average U.S. cigarette. Arrows in the graph point to the introduction of technical changes in the manufacture of cigarettes at various times. These changes have influenced the machine-measured sales-weighted average nicotine and tar deliveries (Norman 1982). Technical issues in the machine measurements of delivered tar and nicotine yields also arose during 1982; modifications of the testing procedure were suggested (Federal Trade Commission 1984). The data shown in Figure 14 are based on the consistent testing procedures. Since 1981, the tar delivery of U.S. cigarettes has averaged between 13.0 and 12.7 mg, while nicotine delivery has remained stable at 0.9 mg per cigarette. (See Chapter 5, Table 26.) In the smoke of popular U.S. low-yield cigarettes, the reduction of nicotine, the primary pharmacologic factor in tobacco addiction (US DHHS 1988), has not occurred to the same extent as has the reduction of tar. The same development has been observed with cigarettes in the United Kingdom (Jarvis and Russell 1985).

Some modifications in the makeup of commercial cigarettes have led to a selective reduction of toxic and tumorigenic agents. Filter tips of cellulose acetate, the most common cigarette filter material, can selectively remove phenols and volatile N-nitrosamines from the smoke stream. Perforated filter tips selectively reduce CO and hydrogen cyanide (HCN) levels, and charcoal filters may selectively reduce volatile aldehydes and HCN. The incorporation into the tobacco blend of reconstituted tobacco sheets, expanded tobacco, and tobacco ribs has also contributed to a selective reduction of PAHs in cigarette smoke. The incorporation of ribs and stems and the utiliza-

TABLE 7.—Tumorigenic agents in tobacco and tobacco smoke

Compounds	Processed tobacco (per gram)	Mainstream smoke (per cigarette)	Evidence for IARC evaluation of carcinogenicity	
			In lab animals	In humans
PAH				
Benz(a)anthracene		20–70 ng	Sufficient	NA
Benzo(b)fluoranthene		4–22 ng	Sufficient	NA
Benzo(j)fluoranthene		6–21 ng	Sufficient	NA
Benzo(k)fluoranthene		6–12 ng	Sufficient	NA
Benzo(a)pyrene	0.1–90 ng	20–40 ng	Sufficient	Probable
Chrysene		40–60 ng	Sufficient	NA
Dibenz(a,h)anthracene		4 ng	Sufficient	NA
Dibenzo(a,i)pyrene		1.7–3.2 ng	Sufficient	NA
Dibenzo(a,l)pyrene		Present	Sufficient	NA
Indeno(1,2,3-c,d)pyrene		4–20 ng	Sufficient	NA
5-Methylchrysene		0.6 ng	Sufficient	NA
Aza-arenes				
Quinoline		1–2 µg	NA	NA
Dibenz(a,h)acridine		0.1 ng	Sufficient	NA
Dibenz(a,j)acridine		3–10 ng	Sufficient	NA
7H-Dibenzo(c,g)carbazole		0.7 ng	Sufficient	NA
N-Nitrosamines				
N-Nitrosodimethylamine	ND–215 ng	0.1–180 ng	Sufficient	NA
N-Nitrosoethyl methylamine		3–13 ng	Sufficient	NA
N-Nitrosodiethylamine		ND–25 ng	Sufficient	NA
N-Nitrosopyrrolidine	ND–360 ng	1.5–110 ng	Sufficient	NA
N-Nitrosodiethanolamine	ND–6,900 ng	ND–36 ng	Sufficient	NA
N′-Nitrosonornicotine	0.3–89 µg	0.12–3.7 µg	Sufficient	NA
4-(Methylnitrosamino)-1-(3-pyridyl)-1-butanone	0.2–7 µg	0.08–0.77 µg	Sufficient	NA
N′-Nitrosoanabasine	0.01–1.9 µg	0.14–4.6 µg	Limited	NA
N-Nitrosomorpholine	ND–690 ng		Sufficient	NA

TABLE 7.—Continued

Compounds	Processed tobacco (per gram)	Mainstream smoke (per cigarette)	Evidence for IARC evaluation of carcinogenicity	
			In lab animals	In humans
Aromatic amines				
2-Toluidine		30–200 ng	Sufficient	Inadequate
2-Naphthylamine		1–22 ng	Sufficient	Sufficient
4-Aminobiphenyl		2–5 ng	Sufficient	Sufficient
Aldehydes				
Formaldehyde[a]	1.6–7.4 μg	70–100 μg[a]	Sufficient	NA
Acetaldehyde[a]	1.4–7.4 mg	18–1,400 mg[a]	Sufficient	NA
Crotonaldehyde	0.2–2.4 μg	10–20 μg	NA	NA
Miscellaneous organic compounds				
Benzene		12–48 μg	Sufficient	Sufficient
Acrylonitrile		3.2–15 μg	Sufficient	Limited
1, 1-Dimethylhydrazine	60–147 μg		Sufficient	NA
2-Nitropropane		0.73–1.21 μg	Sufficient	NA
Ethylcarbamate	310–375 ng	20–38 ng	Sufficient	NA
Vinyl chloride		1–16 ng	Sufficient	Sufficient
Inorganic compounds				
Hydrazine	14–51 ng	24–43 ng	Sufficient	Inadequate
Arsenic	500–900 ng	40–120 ng	Inadequate	Sufficient
Nickel	2,000–6,000 ng	0–600 ng	Sufficient	Limited
Chromium	1,000–2,000 ng	4–70 ng	Sufficient	Sufficient
Cadmium	1,300–1,600 ng	41–62 ng	Sufficient	Limited
Lead	8–10 μg		Sufficient	Inadequate
Polonium-210	0.2–1.2 pCi	0.03–1.0 pCi	NA	NA

NOTE: ND, no data; NA, evaluation has not been done by IARC.

[a]The Fourth Report of the Independent Scientific Committee on "Smoking and Health" (1988) published values for the 14 leading U.K. cigarettes in 1986 (51.4 percent of the market) of 20–105 μg/cigarette (mean, 59 μg) for formaldehyde and 550–1,150 μg/cigarette (mean, 910 μg) for acetaldehyde.

SOURCE: Hoffmann and Hecht (1989).

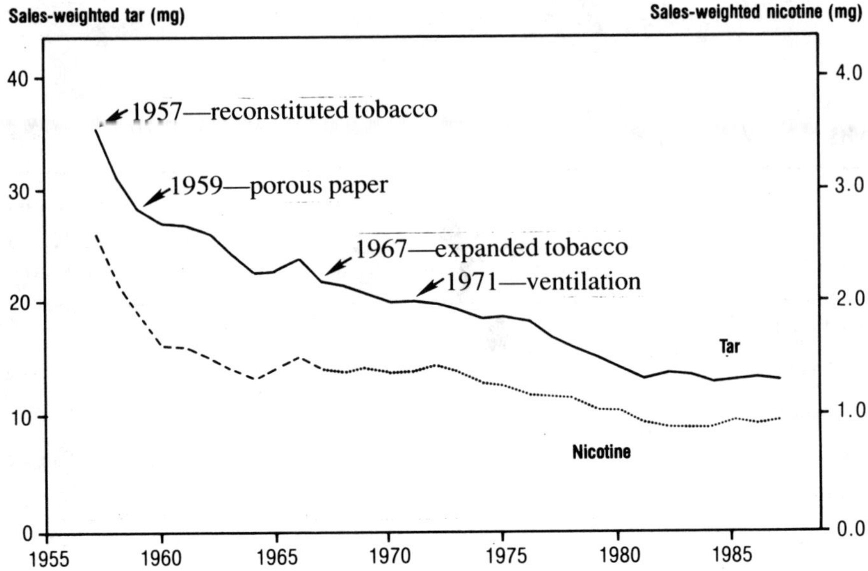

FIGURE 14.—"Tar" and nicotine content of U.S. cigarettes, sales-weighted average basis, 1957–87

NOTE: Nicotine values for 1957–67 are estimates.

SOURCE: 1957–67, Wakeham (1976), fourth-quarter estimates for each year; 1968–81, FTC (1984); 1982–87, derived from FTC data tape of annual cigarette company submissions to the FTC. This database is the same as that used for the ongoing FTC tobacco report series. Since 1981, these reports have not listed the sales-weighted tar average. Historical events are noted in R. J. Reynolds (1988).

tion of more burley varieties in the tobacco blend have led to an increase in the nitrate content of the U.S. blended cigarette from 0.5 percent to between 1.2 to 1.5 percent. This development brought about a reduction of the smoke yields of tar, phenols, and PAHs, but has caused an increase of the nitrogen oxides in the smoke and thus has increased the potential for N-nitrosamine formation (US DHHS 1981, 1982; Hoffmann et al. 1984). The development of the low-yield cigarette has also necessitated an enrichment of the flavor "bouquet" in the smoke either by tobacco selection or by addition of natural or synthetic flavor compounds. These facts and the practice of smoking low-yield cigarettes more intensely make it difficult to evaluate whether these new types of cigarettes are in fact less hazardous to the smoker (see Chapter 8). Changes in the market share of filtered cigarettes, lower yield cigarettes, mentholated cigarettes, and longer cigarettes are presented in Chapter 5.

Environmental Tobacco Smoke

SS is the smoke generated during smoldering of tobacco products between puffs. When it is obtained under standard laboratory conditions, undiluted SS contains far higher amounts of toxic and tumorigenic agents than MS, which is drawn puff by puff through the unlit end of the cigarette. Table 8 presents data for those toxic agents in SS that are known carcinogens, tumor promoters, and cocarcinogens. The release of volatile N-nitrosamines and aromatic amines into the SS is remarkably higher than that into MS (US DHHS 1988; Guerin 1987). Whereas filter tips, especially perforated

TABLE 8.—Some toxic and tumorigenic agents in undiluted cigarette sidestream smoke

Compound	Type of toxicity	Amount in sidestream smoke (per cigarette)	Amount in sidestream smoke/ amount in mainstream smoke
Vapor phase			
Carbon monoxide	T	26.8–61 mg	2.5–14.9
Carbonyl sulfide	T	2–3 μg	0.03–0.13
Benzene	C	400–400 μg	8–10
Formaldehyde	C	1,500 μg	50
3-Vinylpyridine	SC	300–450 μg	24–34
Hydrogen cyanide	T	14–110 μg	0.06–0.4
Hydrazine	C	90 ng	3
Nitrogen oxides (NO_x)	T	500–2,000 μg	3.7–12.8
N-Nitrosodimethylamine	C	200–1,040 ng	20–130
N-Nitrosopyrrolidine	C	30–390 ng	6–120
Particulate phase			
Tar	C	14–30 mg	1.1–15.7
Nicotine	T	2.1–46 mg	1.3–21
Phenol	TP	70–250 μg	1.3–3.0
Catechol	CoC	58–290 μg	0.67–12.8
o-Toluidine	C	3 μg	18.7
2-Naphtylamine	C	70 ng	39
4-Aminobiphenyl	C	140 ng	31
Benz(a)anthracene	C	40–200 ng	2–4
Benzo(a)pyrene	C	40–70 ng	2.5–20
Quinoline	C	15–20 μg	8–11
NNN	C	0.15–1.7 μg	0.5–5.0
NNK	C	0.2–1.4 μg	1.0–22
N-Nitrosodiethanolamine	C	43 ng	1.2
Cadmium	C	0.72 μg	7.2
Nickel	C	0.2–2.5 μg	13–30
Polonium-210	C	0.5–1.6 pCi	1.06–3.7

NOTE: C, carcinogenic; CoC, cocarcinogenic; SC, suspected carcinogen; T, toxic; TP, tumor promoter; NNN, N′-Nitrosonornicotine; NNK, 4-(methylnitrosamino)-(3-pyridyl)-1-butanone.
SOURCE: Hoffmann and Hecht (1989).

ones, can significantly reduce the concentration of toxic and tumorigenic agents in MS, they have no reducing effect on the agents emitted into the SS (Adams, O'Mara-Adams, Hoffmann 1987).

SS is the major source of ETS. The smoke diffusing through the cigarette paper, the smoke emerging from the burning cone during active smoking, and that portion of MS that is exhaled also contribute to ETS. Table 9 presents some data for toxic agents resulting from tobacco combustion in indoor environments (US DHHS 1988; Hoffmann and Hecht 1989). The concentrations of toxic agents in ETS appear low in comparison with their levels in undiluted cigarette MS. With regard to exposure factors, one needs to take into account the fact that the active inhalation of MS is limited to the time it takes to smoke each cigarette, whereas the inhalation of ETS is constant over several hours spent in the polluted environment. This is reflected in the results of measurements of the uptake of nicotine by active and passive smokers (US DHHS 1988).

Smokeless Tobacco

As noted above, the special Report of the Surgeon General, *The Health Consequences of Using Smokeless Tobacco*, has shown that tobacco chewers and snuff dippers face an increased risk for cancer of the oral cavity (US DHHS 1986b). In the United States the four primary smokeless tobacco types are plug tobacco, loose leaf tobacco, twist tobacco, and snuff.

The composition of processed, unadulterated tobacco has been discussed. Chewing tobacco and snuff are made with various flavor additives (LaVoie et al. 1989). It is of special significance that the preparation of smokeless tobacco products, which entails curing, fermentation, and aging, occurs under conditions favoring the formation of tobacco-specific N-nitrosamines (TSNAs) from nicotine and other tobacco alkaloids such as nornicotine, anatabine, and anabasine (Figure 15). Of the six identified TSNAs in smokeless tobacco, N′-nitrosonornicotine (NNN) and 4-(methylnitrosamino)-1-(3-pyridyl)-1-butanone (NNK) are strong carcinogens in mice, rats, and hamsters, inducing benign and malignant tumors of the oral cavity, nasal cavity, esophagus, lung, liver, and pancreas (Hecht and Hoffmann 1988; Rivenson et al. 1988). Table 10 presents chemical–analytical data for TSNAs in U.S. smokeless tobacco products (Hoffmann and Hecht 1988). The concentrations of carcinogenic nitrosamines in smokeless tobacco exceed those in other consumer products by at least 2 orders of magnitude (US DHHS 1986b). During tobacco chewing and snuff dipping, additional amounts of carcinogenic TSNAs are most likely also formed endogenously in the oral cavity (Hoffmann and Hecht 1988). Carcinogenic TSNAs have been regarded as a major factor for the association of snuff-dipping with oral cancer in humans (Craddock 1983).

Other carcinogens identified in smokeless tobacco are volatile nitrosamines (N-nitrosodimethylamine, ≤215 ppb), N-nitrosomorpholine (≤40 ppb), N-nitrosodiethylamine (≤6,800 ppb), formaldehyde (≤7,000 ppb), crotonaldehyde (≤2,400 ppb), and benzo(*a*)pyrene (≤90 ppb), as well as traces of the radioelement polonium-210 (≤0.6 pCi/g) (US DHHS 1986; Hoffmann et al. 1987; Chamberlain, Schlotzhauer, Chortyk 1988).

TABLE 9.—Some toxic and tumorigenic agents in indoor environments polluted by tobacco smoke

Pollutant	Location	Concentration/m^3
Nitric oxide	Workrooms	50–440 μg
	Restaurants	17–270 μg
	Bars	80–520 μg
	Cafeterias	2.5–48 μg
Nitrogen dioxide	Workrooms	68–410 μg
	Restaurants	40–190 μg
	Bars	2–116 μg
	Cafeterias	67–200 μg
Hydrogen cyanide	Living rooms	8–122 μg
Benzene	Public places	20–317 μg
Formaldehyde	Living rooms	23–50 μg
Acrolein	Public places	30–120 μg
Acetone	Public places	360–5,800 μg
Phenols (volatile)	Coffee houses	7.4–11.5 ng
N-Nitrosodimethylamine	Restaurants, public places	0–240 ng
N-Nitrosodiethylamine	Restaurants, public places	0–200 ng
Nicotine	Public places	1–6 μg
	Restaurants	3–10 μg
	Workrooms	1–13.8 μg
Benzo(a)pyrene	Restaurants, public places	3.3–23.4 ng

SOURCE: Hoffmann and Hecht (1989).

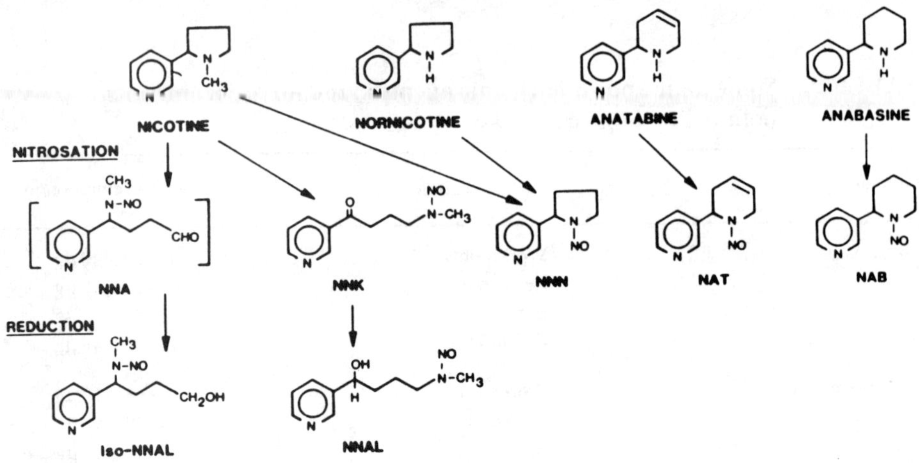

FIGURE 15.—Formation of tobacco-specific N-nitrosamines

TABLE 10.—Tobacco-specific N-nitrosamines in U.S. smokeless tobacco (ppb)

Product	NNN	NNK	NAT	NAB
Loose leaf tobacco	670–8,200 (6[a])	380 (1)	2,300 (1)	140 (1)
Plug tobacco	3,400–4,300 (3)			
Snuff—moist	3,120–135,000 (26)	100–13,600 (25)	1,340–339,000 (20)	10–6,700 (16)
Snuff—dry	9,000–52,000 (3)	1,800–13,000 (3)	18,000–38,000 (3)	60–60,000 (3)

NOTE: NNN, N′-Nitrosonornicotine; NNK, 4-(methylnitrosamino)-1-(3-pyridyl)-1-butanone; NAT, N′-nitrosoanatabine; NAB, N′-nitrosoanabasine.

[a]Number in parentheses is the number of samples analyzed.

SOURCE: Hoffmann and Hecht (1988).

Toxicity and Carcinogenicity of Tobacco Smoke

Undiluted tobacco smoke is too toxic to be tolerated by laboratory animals primarily because of the acute toxic effects of CO. CO in cigarette smoke increases with ascending puff number from 2 to 5 volume percent (the average CO content of cigarette smoke is 3.5 to 4.5 volume percent). The acute toxicity of tobacco smoke is also due to HCN, nicotine, and volatile aldehydes. In vitro short-term exposure to cigarette smoke causes ciliastasis, an effect primarily attributable to HCN (300 to 500 μg/cigarette) and volatile aldehydes (500 to 2,000 μg/cigarette). The long-term exposure of laboratory animals to diluted cigarette smoke causes impairment of mucociliary clearance, mucus hypersecretion, and epithelial lesions. Cigarette smoke constituents responsible for this effect are both the gas phase, primarily HCN and volatile aldehydes, and the particulate phase (US DHEW 1979; US DHHS 1984).

Long-term inhalation of diluted cigarette smoke by mice has resulted in adenomas and adenocarcinomas of the lung, whereas such inhalation in rats has only led to a few isolated tumors of the lung. In Syrian golden hamsters, long-term smoke inhalation studies have regularly induced benign and malignant tumors of the larynx and only a few lung tumors. These observations strongly suggest, and studies of particulate deposition and determination of carboxyhemoglobin (COHb) and nicotine–cotinine in the blood of the smoke-exposed animals have confirmed, that laboratory animals do not inhale the smoke deeply. Intratracheal instillation of cigarette tar and one of its fractions has resulted in lung tumors, including bronchogenic carcinomas (Mohr and Reznik 1978; Dalbey et al. 1980; US DHHS 1982).

The particulate matter (more often called "tar") suspended in organic solvents has induced carcinoma in the rat after subcutaneous injection and benign and malignant tumors in the skin of mice and rabbits after topical application. The major tumor initiators reside in the PAH-enriched neutral subfractions, whereas the tumor promoters and cocarcinogens are found in the weakly acidic fraction as well as in the polaric neutral subfraction (Wynder and Hoffmann 1967; Mohr and Reznik 1978; US DHHS 1982; Hoffmann and Hecht 1988).

As discussed earlier, combined chemical–analytical studies have led to the identification of several organ-specific carcinogens in cigarette smoke. The diversity of these carcinogens and those identified as contact carcinogens may cause ambiguity as to which among them are most important. Table 11, which is based on extensive laboratory studies, lists the likely causative agents associated with the increased risk of cigarette smokers for cancer of the various organs (Hoffmann and Hecht 1988).

Nicotine

It is generally held that nicotine is the active pharmacologic agent in tobacco that determines the addictive behavior of the tobacco smoker (US DHHS 1988). Nicotine, together with CO, is also regarded as a major contributor to cigarette smokers' increased risk of cardiovascular disease (US DHHS 1983, 1988). In addition to nicotine, tobacco contains various other alkaloids, most of which are 3-pyridyl derivatives. In the blended U.S. cigarette, nicotine constitutes 85 to 95 percent of the total alkaloids. During the smoking of a nonfilter cigarette, about 15 percent of the nicotine appears in the MS, 35 to 40 percent appears in the SS, 15 to 20 percent is deposited in the butt, and the remainder is broken down into pyrolysis products. The major pyrolysis products of nicotine are CO, carbon dioxide, 3-vinylpyridine, 3-methylpyridine, pyridine, myosmine, and 2,3′-dipyridyl (US DHHS 1982).

As discussed earlier, the absorption of nicotine from tobacco smoke is pH dependent. When tobacco smoke reaches the small airways and alveoli of the lung, nicotine is rapidly absorbed. In chewing tobacco and snuff with their alkaline pH, nicotine is primarily absorbed through the mucous membranes of the oral cavity. Nicotine enters the blood and is rapidly transported to the brain, which has specific receptor sites for

TABLE 11.—Likely causative agents for tobacco-related cancers

Organ	Initiator or carcinogen	Enhancing agents
Lung, larynx	PAH	Catechol (cocarcinogen) Weakly acidic tumor promoters
	NNK	Acrolein, crotonaldehyde (?)
	Polonium-210 (minor factor), acetaldehyde, formaldehyde	
Esophagus	NNN	
Pancreas	NNK(?)	
Bladder	4-Aminobiphenyl 2-Naphthylamine	
Oral cavity (smoking)	PAH NNK, NNN	Ethanol
Oral cavity (snuff dipping)	NNK, NNN	Irritation (?) Herpes simplex (?)
	Polonium-210	

NOTE: PAH, polynuclear aromatic hydrocarbons; NNK, 4-(methylnitrosoamino)-1-(3-pyridyl)-1-butanone; NNN, N′-Nitrosonornicotine.
SOURCE: Hoffmann and Hecht (1989).

the drug. The effects of nicotine on the central nervous system are associated with the development of tobacco dependence (US DHHS 1988).

Nicotine is metabolized primarily in the liver and, to a smaller extent, in the lung. About 10 to 15 percent of the absorbed nicotine is excreted unchanged in the urine. The primary metabolites of nicotine are cotinine and nicotine-N′-oxide. Cotinine is further metabolized extensively, with only 17 percent of it appearing unchanged in the urine (Benowitz 1986; Neurath et al. 1987; US DHHS 1988). Cotinine measurements in saliva, serum, or urine serve as an indicator for nicotine uptake by tobacco chewers, active smokers, and involuntary smokers. It takes 18 to 20 hr to eliminate one-half of the cotinine present in an active smoker through renal excretion; an involuntary smoker shows a considerably slower rate of elimination (Sepkovic, Haley, Hoffmann 1986; US DHHS 1988).

Biological Markers

Techniques for the determination of current and lifetime exposures to tobacco products include the examination of medical records and data from prospective and case–control studies as well as the utilization of biological markers. The development of highly sensitive and reproducible methods has led to increased use of biological markers for uptake of tobacco smoke constituents.

Table 12 lists those biochemical markers that are currently used to determine exposure to tobacco smoke components after active inhalation of MS and also after involuntary uptake of ETS. Some of these markers are also the basis for measuring the transfer of smoke constituents from the maternal bloodstream to a developing fetus.

The tobacco-specific alkaloid nicotine and its major metabolite, cotinine, are most frequently used as serum and urine indicators of the uptake of tobacco smoke by active smokers and also to indicate ETS exposure in nonsmokers. Unlike CO, nicotine is not

TABLE 12.—Biochemical markers for the uptake of tobacco smoke

Smoke constituent	Biochemical marker	Substrate	Method	Sensitivity	Critical value[a]
Nicotine	Nicotine	Serum Urine	GC	1 ng/mL	0
		Serum Urine	RIA	0.2 ng/mL	0
	Cotinine	Saliva Serum Urine	GC	5 ng/mL	0
		Saliva Serum Urine	RIA	1 ng/mL	0
Carbon monoxide (CO)	COHb	Blood	Oximeter	±0.1%	0.9 ±0.7%
	CO	Exhaled air	GC	±1 ppm	5.6 ±2.7 ppm
Hydrogen cyanide (HCN)	Thiocyanate (SCN^-)	Saliva Serum Urine	Autoanalyzer (color reaction)	±5 µmol/L	100 µmol/L
Nitrogen oxides (NO_x)	Nitrosoproline	Urine	GC/TEA	±0.4 µg/L	2.0 ±1.5 µg/24 hours
Ethylene (CH_2=CH_2)	Globin-adduct	Blood	GC	±5pmol/gHb	58 ±25 pmol/gHb
4-Aminobiphenyl	Globin-adduct	Blood	GC	?	<70 pg/gHb
Tobacco-specific nitrosamines	Globin-adduct	Blood	GC	?	Not established

[a]Critical values, values measured in nonsmokers.

SOURCE: International Agency for Research on Cancer (1987).

only taken up by inhalation but also is absorbed through the mucous membranes in the oral cavity. Therefore, it is possible to determine user uptake of hydrophilic agents from chewing tobacco and snuff by means of nicotine–cotinine measurements. The analytical assessment of nicotine and cotinine in physiological fluids is done primarily by gas chromatography and radioimmunoassay (IARC 1986). Both methods are highly sensitive (between 0.2 and 5 ng/mL), and there is little or no interference by other smoke components. After environmental exposure, the average nicotine and cotinine levels in saliva, plasma, and urine of nonsmokers vary from 0.5 to 4.0 µg/mL, whereas the average amount of nicotine in the serum of cigarette smokers ranges from 15 to 40 µg/mL and lies between 500 and 2,000 µg/mL in saliva and urine. Cotinine concentration varies from 150 to 350 µg/mL in plasma, from 150 to 400 µg/mL in saliva, and can go up to 2,000 µg/mL in urine (Jarvis et al. 1984; US DHHS 1988). In snuff dippers and tobacco chewers, plasma nicotine levels were found between 3 to 22 µg/mL and plasma cotinine was 200 to 400 µg/mL (US DHHS 1986).

One of the oldest methods for estimating the inhalation of tobacco smoke is the determination of COHb in blood. Since some CO is endogenously formed, the background values for COHb in the blood of nonsmokers without occupational exposure to CO range from 0.5 to 1.5 percent (National Research Council 1977). Smoking only a few cigarettes per day elevates COHb levels to 2.0 percent. In a study of men aged 34 to 64 years, cigarette smokers had average COHb concentrations of 4.7 percent; cigar smokers, 2.9 percent; and pipe smokers, 2.2 percent (Wald et al. 1981; Wald and Ritchie 1984). The COHb values of nonsmokers after ETS exposure do not markedly exceed 1.5 percent; thus, COHb cannot serve as an indicator of exposure to ETS (NRC 1986). Since CO is only slowly released from the blood in the process of exhaling, the smoking intensity of a cigarette smoker can also be assessed by the analysis of CO in the exhaled breath. The critical value for CO, the value above that of a nonsmoker, is 5.6±2.7 ppm in exhaled breath; again this method is not applicable to the dosimetry of nonsmoker ETS exposures.

HCN, a major tobacco smoke constituent (>100 µg/cigarette), is absorbed upon inhalation and is detoxified in the liver, yielding SCN^-. Since SCN^- can also originate from dietary intake, only values above 100 µmol of SCN^- per L of serum as measured for cigarette smokers are meaningful for dosimetry of uptake. In general, the average cigarette smoker has SCN^- levels between 100 and 250 µmol/L of serum (US DHHS 1987).

A number of studies have clearly demonstrated that the mutagenic activity of the urine of cigarette smokers is higher than that of nonsmokers (IARC 1986). The most widely applied method for determining mutagenic activity of urine samples was developed by Yamasaki and Ames (1977), using a resin to concentrate the body fluid and, upon metabolic activation, measuring the mutagenic activity on bacterial tester strains TA98 and TA1538. In general, the urine of cigarette smokers exhibits at least twice the mutagenic activity of that measured in nonsmokers' urine.

In summary, there are several biochemical indicators that enable investigators to assay the uptake of tobacco smoke by individuals or by groups of individuals. Whereas analyses of exhaled CO, of COHb, and of SCN^- and nicotine–cotinine in saliva, serum, and urine are well suited for determining the smoking intensity of an active smoker, only nicotine and cotinine determinations in serum and urine can also serve as indicators for the exposure of nonsmokers to ETS.

Summary

The 1964 Surgeon General's Report was a landmark study that reviewed and assessed the available epidemiologic, clinical, pathological, and experimental literature for evidence linking cigarette smoking to disease. The principal findings of that Report are summarized in Table 13. In men, cigarette smoking was found to increase overall mortality and to cause lung and laryngeal cancer. Several other important conclusions were also drawn (Table 13).

Since 1964, 20 reports of the Surgeon General (including this Report) have been released on tobacco and health that substantiate and strengthen the original conclusions of the 1964 Report. These reports have also established associations between smoking and disease in areas for which data did not exist, shed light on pathogenetic mechanisms of tobacco-related disease, and added scientific depth to areas mentioned only briefly in the 1964 Report.

A review of Table 13 allows the reader to survey quickly the state of knowledge on cigarette smoking and health in 1989 and to compare it with what was known in 1964. Of the 27 principal effects presented in Table 13, 13 were first noted in 1964; among those 13 effects, many have been strengthened since 1964. Recent reports of the Surgeon General have also covered important topics not even mentioned in the 1964 Report. For example, these reports have concluded that involuntary smoking can cause disease, including lung cancer, in healthy nonsmokers and that smokeless tobacco can cause oral cancer. The most recent Surgeon General's Report also concluded that the use of cigarettes and other forms of tobacco is addicting (US DHHS 1988).

Much progress has been made in understanding the physicochemical nature of tobacco smoke. Today, the estimated number of compounds in tobacco smoke exceeds 4,000, including some that are pharmacologically active, toxic, mutagenic, or carcinogenic. The diverse biological effects of tobacco smoke constituents provide a framework for understanding the multiple adverse consequences of smoking. For example, the identification of 43 different carcinogenic substances in tobacco smoke helps explain why cigarette smoking can cause cancer at different sites including the lung, larynx, oral cavity, and esophagus; why cigarette smoking is a contributory factor for the development of cancer at different sites including the bladder, kidney, and pancreas; and why cigarette smoking is associated with cancer of the stomach and uterine cervix.

The central role of cigarette smoking as a massive, preventable personal and public health problem can now be better appreciated. In the United States, it is a major cause of CHD, this country's most common cause of death; cigarette smoking is estimated to account for 21 percent of all CHD deaths. Cigarette smoking is the major cause of lung cancer, the most common cause of cancer death in the United States; smoking is estimated to account for 87 percent of lung cancer deaths and 30 percent of all cancer deaths. While lung cancer death rates for women who are nonsmokers have not increased since the early 1960s, comparable death rates for women who smoke cigarettes have increased more than fourfold. In 1986, lung cancer and breast cancer were the

TABLE 13.—Summary of the principal effects of cigarette smoking

Effect first discussed in Surgeon General's Reports	Year first discussed in a Surgeon General's Report	Current knowledge in 1989
Mortality and morbidity		
Overall mortality, increased in men	1964	Overall mortality increased in men and women
Overall morbidity, increased	1967	Overall morbidity increased
Cardiovascular		
CHD, mortality increased in men	1964	A major cause of coronary heart disease in men and women
Cerebrovascular disease (stroke), mortality increased	1964	A cause of cerebrovascular disease (stroke)
Atherosclerotic aortic aneurysm, mortality increased	1967	Increased mortality from atherosclerotic aortic aneurysm
Atherosclerotic peripheral vascular disease, risk factor	1971	A cause and most important risk factor for atherosclerotic peripheral vascular disease
Cancer		
Lung cancer, the major cause in men	1964	The major cause of lung cancer in men and women
Laryngeal cancer, a cause in men	1964	The major cause of laryngeal cancer in men and women
Oral cancer (lip), a cause (pipe smoking)	1964	A major cause of cancer of the oral cavity (lip, tongue, mouth, pharynx)
Esophageal cancer, associated with	1964	A major cause of esophageal cancer
Bladder cancer, associated with	1964	A contributory factor for bladder cancer
Pancreatic cancer, increased mortality	1967	A contributory factor for pancreatic cancer
Renal cancer, increased mortality	1968	A contributory factor for renal cancer
Gastric cancer, associated with	1982	An association with gastric cancer
Cervical cancer, possible association with	1982	An association with cervical cancer

TABLE 13.—Continued

Effect first discussed in Surgeon General's Reports	Year first discussed in a Surgeon General's Report	Current knowledge in 1989
Pulmonary		
Chronic bronchitis, the major cause	1964	The major cause of chronic bronchitis
Emphysema, increased mortality	1964	The major cause of emphysema
Women		
Low-birthweight babies, associated with	1964	A cause of intrauterine growth retardation
Unsuccessful pregnancy, associated with	1980	A probable cause of unsuccessful pregnancies
Other effects		
Tobacco habit, related to psychological and social drives	1964	Cigarette smoking and other forms of tobacco use are addicting
Involuntary smoking, irritant effect	1972	A cause of disease, including lung cancer, in healthy nonsmokers
Peptic ulcer disease, associated with	1964	A probable cause of peptic ulcer disease
Occupational interactions, adverse	1971	Adverse occupational interactions that increase the risk of cancer
Alcohol interactions, adverse	1971	Adverse interactions with alcohol that increase the risk of cancer
Drug interactions, adverse	1979	Adverse drug interactions
Nonmalignant oral disease, associated with	1969	An association with nonmalignant oral disease
Smokeless tobacco, associated with oral cancer	1979	Smokeless tobacco is a cause of oral cancer

leading causes of cancer death in U.S. women, accounting for approximately equal numbers of cancer deaths. Cigarette smoking is the major cause of COPD, an effect that far outweighs all other factors; smoking is estimated to account for 82 percent of COPD deaths. (See Chapter 3.)

The 1964 Report of the Surgeon General stated that death rates from cerebrovascular disease (stroke) were increased in cigarette smokers compared with nonsmokers, but it drew no conclusions concerning causality. In the current 1989 Report, for the first time, cigarette smoking is cited as a cause of stroke, the third most common cause of death in the United States. Stopping smoking reduces the risk of stroke.

The effect of smoking on pregnancy was briefly mentioned in the 1964 Report. Many studies have subsequently shown that cigarette smoking causes fetal growth retardation and is a probable cause of unsuccessful pregnancies.

Table 13 summarizes other important smoking associations with several diseases, including atherosclerotic aortic aneurysm, atherosclerotic peripheral vascular disease, and peptic ulcer disease; it also includes occupational and alcohol-related interactions with smoking that increase the risk of cancer.

Finally, the reports of the Surgeon General have emphasized the benefits of quitting for smokers of all ages.

CONCLUSIONS

Part I. Health Consequences

1. The 1964 Surgeon General's Report concluded that cigarette smoking increases overall mortality in men, causes lung and laryngeal cancer in men, and causes chronic bronchitis. The Report also found significant associations between smoking and numerous other diseases.
2. Reports of the Surgeon General since 1964 have concluded that smoking increases mortality and morbidity in both men and women. Disease associations identified as causal since 1964 include coronary heart disease, atherosclerotic peripheral vascular disease, lung and laryngeal cancer in women, oral cancer, esophageal cancer, chronic obstructive pulmonary disease, intrauterine growth retardation, and low-birthweight babies.
3. Cigarette smoking is now considered to be a probable cause of unsuccessful pregnancies, increased infant mortality, and peptic ulcer disease; to be a contributing factor for cancer of the bladder, pancreas, and kidney; and to be associated with cancer of the stomach.
4. Accumulating research has elucidated the interaction effects of cigarette smoking with certain occupational exposures to increase the risk of cancer, with alcohol ingestion to increase the risk of cancer, and with selected medications to produce adverse effects.
5. A decade ago, the 1979 Report of the Surgeon General found smokeless tobacco to be associated with oral cancer. In 1986, the Surgeon General concluded that smokeless tobacco was a cause of this disease.

6. Research in the present decade has established that involuntary smoking is a cause of disease, including lung cancer, in healthy nonsmokers, and that the children of parents who smoke have an increased frequency of respiratory infections and symptoms.
7. In 1964, tobacco use was considered habituating. A substantial body of evidence accumulated since then, and summarized in the 1988 Surgeon General's Report, has established that cigarettes and other forms of tobacco are addicting. Given the prevalence of smoking, tobacco use is the Nation's most widespread form of drug dependency.
8. Studies dating from the 1950s have consistently documented the benefits of smoking cessation for smokers in all age groups.
9. Recent evidence, including that presented in this 1989 Report of the Surgeon General, documents that cigarette smoking is a cause of cerebrovascular disease (stroke) and is associated with cancer of the uterine cervix.

Part II. The Physicochemical Nature of Tobacco

1. The estimated number of compounds in tobacco smoke exceeds 4,000, including many that are pharmacologically active, toxic, mutagenic, and carcinogenic.
2. Forty-three carcinogens have been identified in tobacco smoke.
3. Carcinogenic tobacco-specific nitrosamines are found in high concentrations in smokeless tobacco.

References

ABBOTT, R.D., YIN, Y., REED, D.M., YANO, K. Risk of stroke in male cigarette smokers. *New England Journal of Medicine* 315(12):717–720, September 18, 1986.

ABLIN, R.J. Cigarette smoking and quality of sperm. (Letter.) *New York State Journal of Medicine* 86(2):108, February 1986.

ABU-ZEID, H.A.H., CHOI, N.W., MAINI, K.K., HSU, P.-H., NELSON, N.A. Relative role of factors associated with cerebral infarction and cerebral hemorrhage. A matched pair case–control study. *Stroke* 8(1):106–112, January–February 1977.

ADAMS, J.D., O'MARA-ADAMS, K.J., HOFFMANN, D. Toxic and carcinogenic agents in undiluted mainstream smoke and sidestream smoke of different types of cigarettes. *Carcinogenesis* 8(5):729–731, 1987.

ALDERSON, M.R., LEE, P.N., WANG, R. Risks of lung cancer, chronic bronchitis, ischaemic heart disease, and stroke in relation to type of cigarette smoked. *Journal of Epidemiology and Community Health* 39(4):286–293, December 1985.

AMERICAN CANCER SOCIETY. *Cancer Facts and Figures—1988.* New York: American Cancer Society, 1988.

BAILAR, J.C. III., SMITH, E.M. Progress against cancer? *New England Journal of Medicine* 314(19):1226–1232, May 1986.

BAIRD, D.D., WILCOX, A.J. Cigarette smoking associated with delayed conception. *Journal of the American Medical Association* 253(20):2979–2983, 1985.

BARON, J.A., BYERS, T., GREENBERG, E.R., CUMMINGS, K.M., SWANSON, M. Cigarette smoking in women with cancers of the breast and reproductive organs. *Journal of National Cancer Institute* 77(3):677–680, September 1986.

BEARD, C.M., ANNEGERS, J.F., WOOLNER, L.B., KURLAND, L.T. Bronchogenic carcinoma in Olmsted County, 1935–1979. *Cancer* 55:2026–2030, 1985.

BEHRMAN, R.E., VAUGHN, V.C. (eds.) *Nelson's Textbook of Pediatrics*, Thirteenth Edition. Philadelphia: W.B. Saunders, 1987.

BELL, B.A., SYMON, L. Smoking and subarachnoid haemorrhage. *British Medical Journal* 1(6163):577–578, March 3, 1979.

BENOWITZ, N.L. Clinical pharmacology of nicotine. *Annual Review of Medicine* 37:21–22, 1986.

BEST, E.W.R., JOSIE, G.H., WALKER, C.B. A Canadian study of mortality in relation to smoking habits. A preliminary report. *Canadian Journal of Public Health* 52:99–106, March 1961.

BLOT, W.J., MCLAUGHLIN, J.K., WINN, D.M., AUSTIN, D.F., GREENBERG, R.S., PRESTON-MARTIN, S., BERNSTEIN, L., SCHOENBERG, J.B., STEMHAGEN, A., FRAUMENI, J.F. JR. Smoking and drinking in relation to oral pharyngeal cancer. *Cancer Research* 48:3282–3287, June 1, 1988.

BONITA, R. Cigarette smoking, hypertension and the risk of subarachnoid hemorrhage: A population-based case–control study. *Stroke* 17(5):831–835, September–October 1986.

BONITA, R., SCRAGG, R., STEWART, A., JACKSON, R., BEAGLEHOLE, R. Cigarette smoking and risk of premature stroke in men and women. *British Medical Journal* 293(6538):6–8, July 1986.

BRINTON, L.A., SCHAIRER, C., HAENSZEL, W., STOLLEY, P., LEHMAN, H.F., LEVINE, R., SAVITZ, D.A. Cigarette smoking and invasive cervical cancer. *Journal of the American Medical Association* 255(23):3265–3269, 1986.

BRISMAN, R., BAKER, R.R., ELKINS, R., HARTMANN, W.H. Carcinoma of lung in four siblings. *Cancer* 20(11):2048–2053, November 1967.

BROSS, I.D., GIBSON, R. Risks of lung cancer in smokers who switch to filter cigarettes. *American Journal of Public Health* 58(18):1396–1403, 1968.

BROWNSON, R.C., REIF, J.S., KEEFE, T.J., FERGUSON, S.W., PRITZL, J.A. Risk factors for adenocarcinoma of the lung. *American Journal of Epidemiology* 125(1):25–34, January 1987.

BRUNNEMANN, K.D., HOFFMANN, D. The pH of tobacco smoke. *Food and Cosmetics Toxicology* 12(1):115–124, February 1974.

BUFFLER, P.A., COOPER, S.P., STINNETT, S., CONTANT, C., SHIRTS, S., HARDY, R.J., AGU, V., GEHAN, B., BURAU, K. Air pollution and lung cancer mortality in Harris County, Texas, 1979–1981. *American Journal of Epidemiology* 128(4):683–699, October 1988.

BURROWS, B., KNUDSON, R.J., CLINE, M.G., LEBOWITZ, M.D. Quantitative relationships between cigarette smoking and ventilatory function. *American Review of Respiratory Disease* 115:195–205, 1977.

CARSTENSEN, J.M., PERSHAGEN, G., EKLUND, G. Mortality in relation to cigarette and pipe smoking: 16 years' observation of 25,000 Swedish men. *Journal of Epidemiology and Community Health* 41:166–172, 1987.

CAULEY, J.A., GUTAI, J.P., SANDLER, R.B., LAPORTE, R.E., KULLER, L., SASHIN, D. The relationship of endogenous estrogen to bone density and bone area in normal postmenopausal women. *American Journal of Epidemiology* 124(5):752–761, 1986.

CEDERLOF, R., FRIBERG, L., HRUBEC, Z., LORICH, U. *The Relationship of Smoking and Some Social Covariables to Mortality and Cancer Morbidity. A Ten Year Follow-up in a Probability Sample of 55,000 Swedish Subjects Age 18–69, Part 1/2*. Stockholm, Sweden: Karolinska Institute, Department of Environmental Hygiene, 1975.

CENTERS FOR DISEASE CONTROL. Smoking-attributable mortality and years of potential life lost—United States, 1984. *Morbidity and Mortality Weekly Report* 36(42):693–697, October 30, 1987.

CHAMBERLAIN, W.J., SCHLOTZHAUER, W.S., CHORTYK, O.T. Chemical composition of nonsmoking tobacco products. *Journal of Agricultural and Food Chemistry* 36(1):48–50, 1988.

CHURCH, D.F., PRYOR, W.A. Free-radical chemistry of cigarette smoke and its toxicological implications. *Environmental Health Perspectives* 64:111–126, December 1985.

CLARKE, E.A., HATCHER, J., MCKEOWN-EYSSEN, G.E., LICKRISH, G.M. Cervical dysplasia: Association with sexual behavior, smoking, and oral contraceptive use? *American Journal of Obstetrics and Gynecology* 151(5):612–616, March 1, 1985.

COLDITZ, G.A., BONITA, R., STAMPFER, M.J., WILLETT, W.C., ROSNER, B., SPEIZER, F.E., HENNEKENS, C.H. Cigarette smoking and risk of stroke in middle-aged women. *New England Journal of Medicine* 318(15):937–941, April 14, 1988.

COLDITZ, G.A., STAMPFER, M.J., WILLETT, W.C. Diet and lung cancer. A review of the epidemiologic evidence in humans. *Archives of Internal Medicine* 147:157–160, January 1987.

COMMITTEE TO STUDY THE PREVENTION OF LOW BIRTHWEIGHT. *Preventing Low Birthweight.* Washington, D.C.: National Academy Press, 1985.

COOK, D.G., POCOCK, S.J., SHAPER, A.G., KUSSICK, S.J. Giving up smoking and the risk of heart attacks. A report from The British Regional Heart Study. *Lancet* 2(8520):1376–1380, December 13, 1986.

CRADDOCK, V.M. Nitrosamines and human cancer: Proof of an association? *Nature* 306 (5944):638, December 15, 1983.

CRIQUI, M.H., FRONEK, A., KLAUBER, M.R., BARRETT-CONNOR, E., GABRIEL, S.W. Peripheral arterial disease in large vessels is epidemiologically distinct from small vessel disease. (Abstract.) *CVD Epidemiology Newsletter* 37:67, January 1985.

DALAGER, N.A, PICKLE, L.W., MASON, T.J., CORREA, P., FONTHAM, E., STEMHAGEN, A., BUFFLER, P.A., ZIEGLER, R.G., FRAUMENI, J.F. JR. The relation of passive smoking to lung cancer. *Cancer Research* 46(9):4808–4811, September 1986.

DALBEY, W.E., NETTESHEIM, D., GRIESEMER, R., CATON, J.E., GUERIN, M.R. Chronic inhalation of cigarette smoke by F344 rats. *Journal of the National Cancer Institute* 64(2):383–388, February 1980.

DEANFIELD, J.E., SHEA, M.J., WILSON, R.A., HORLOCK, P., DELANDSHERE, C.M., SELWYN, A.P. Direct effects of smoking on the heart: Silent ischemic disturbances of coronary flow. *American Journal of Cardiology* 57(13):1005–1009, May 1, 1986.

DEANFIELD, J., WRIGHT, C., KRIKLER, S., RIBEIRO, P., FOX, K. Cigarette smoking and the treatment of angina with propranolol, atenolol, and nifedipine. *New England Journal of Medicine* 310(15):951–954, April 12, 1984.

DOCKERY, D.W., SPEIZER, F.E., FERRIS, B.G. JR., WARE, J.H., LOUIS, T.A., SPIRO, A. III. Cumulative and reversible effects of lifetime smoking on simple tests of lung function in adults. *American Review of Respiratory Disease* 137:286–292, 1988.

DOLL, R., GRAY, R., HAFNER, B., PETO, R. Mortality in relation to smoking: 22 years' observations on female British doctors. *British Medical Journal* 280(6219):967–971, April 5, 1980.

DOLL, R., HILL, A.B. Lung cancer and other causes of death in relation to smoking. A second report on the mortality of British doctors. *British Medical Journal* 2:1071–1081, November 10, 1956.

DOLL, R., PETO, R. Cigarette smoking and bronchial carcinoma: Dose and time relationships among regular smokers and lifelong non-smokers. *Journal of Epidemiology and Community Health* 32(4):303–313, December 1978.

DOLL, R., PETO, R. The causes of cancer: Quantitative estimates of avoidable risks of cancer in the United States today. *Journal of the National Cancer Institute* 66(6):1191–1308, June 1981.

DOLL, R., PETO, R. *Effects on Health of Exposure to Asbestos*. London: Her Majesty's Stationery Office, 1985.

DORN, H.F. The mortality of smokers and nonsmokers. 1958.

DUBE, M.F., GREEN, C.R. Methods of collection of smoke for analytical purposes. *Recent Advances in Tobacco Science: Formation, Analysis, and Composition of Tobacco Smoke* 8:42–102, 1982.

DUNN, H.G., MCBURNEY, A.K., INGRAM, S., HUNTER, C.M. Maternal cigarette smoking during pregnancy and the child's subsequent development: II. Neurological and intellectual maturation to the age of 6 1/2 years. *Canadian Journal of Public Health* 68(1):43–50, January–February 1977.

DUNN, J.E. JR., LINDEN, G., BRESLOW, L. Lung cancer mortality experience of men in certain occupations in California. *American Journal of Public Health* 50(10):1475–1487, October 1960.

ELWOOD, J.M., PEARSON, J.C.G., SKIPPEN, D.H., JACKSON, S.M. Alcohol, smoking, social and occupational factors in the aetiology of cancer of the oral cavity, pharynx and larynx. *International Journal of Cancer* 34:603–612, 1984.

ERIKSSON, S. Pulmonary emphysema and alpha$_1$-antitrypsin deficiency. *Acta Medica Scandinavica* 175:197–205, 1964.

ERNSTER, V.L., BUSH, T.L., HUGGINS, G.R., HULKA, B.S., KELSEY, J.L., SCHOTTENFELD, D. Benefits and risks of menopausal estrogen and/or progestin hormone use. *Preventive Medicine* 17:201–223, 1988.

FEDERAL TRADE COMMISSION. *Report to Congress Pursuant to the Federal Cigarette Labeling and Advertising Act for the Year 1981*. Federal Trade Commission, July 1984.

FEDERAL TRADE COMMISSION. *"Tar," Nicotine and Carbon Monoxide of the Smoke of 207 Varieties of Domestic Cigarettes.* Federal Trade Commission, January 1985.

FERA, T., ABBOUD, R.T., RICHTER, A., JOHAL, S.S. Acute effect of smoking on elastase-like esterase activity and immunologic neutrophil elastase levels in bronchoalveolar lavage fluid. *American Review of Respiratory Disease* 133(4):568–573, April 1986.

FITZGERALD, G.A., OATES, J.A., NOWAK, J. Cigarette smoking and hemostatic function. *American Heart Journal* 115:267–271, 1988.

FLETCHER, C., PETO, R., TINKER, C., SPEIZER, F.E. *The Natural History of Chronic Bronchitis and Emphysema.* Oxford: Oxford University Press, 1976.

GALAN, K.M., DELIGONUL, U., KERN, M.J., CHAITMAN, B.R., VANDORMAEL, M.G. Increased frequency of restenosis in patients continuing to smoke cigarettes after percutaneous transluminal coronary angioplasty. *American Journal of Cardiology* 61:260–263, 1988.

GAO, Y.T., BLOT, W.J., ZHENG, W., ERSHOW, A.G., HSU, C.W., LEVIN, L., ZHANG, R., FRAUMENI, J.F. Lung cancer among Chinese women. *International Journal of Cancer* 40(5):604–609, November 15, 1987.

GLOVER, M.U., KUBER, M.T., WARREN, S.E., VIEWEG, W.V.R. Myocardial infarction before age 36: Risk factor and artiographic analysis. *American Journal of Cardiology* 49(7):1600–1603, May 1982.

GOFFMAN, T.E., HASSINGER, D.D., MULVIHILL, J.J. Familial respiratory tract cancer. Opportunities for research and prevention. *Journal of the American Medical Association* 247(7):1020–1023, February 19, 1982.

GORDIS, L., GOLD, E.B. Epidemiology of pancreatic cancer. *World Journal of Surgery* 8:808–821, 1984.

GORDON, D.J., EKELUND, L.-G., KARON, J.M., PROBSTFIELD, J.L., RUBENSTEIN, C., SHEFFIELD, T., WEISSFELD, L. Predictive value of the exercise tolerance test for mortality in North American men: The Lipid Research Clinics Mortality Follow-up Study. *Circulation* 74(2):252–261, 1986.

GREENBERG, E.R., VESSEY, M., MCPHERSON, K., YEATES, D. Cigarette smoking and cancer of the uterine cervix. *British Journal of Cancer* 51:139–141, January 1985.

GUERIN, M.R. Formation and physicochemical nature of sidestream smoke. In: O'Neill, I.K., Brunnemann, K.D., Dodet, B., Hoffmann, D. (eds.) *Environmental Carcinogens, Methods of Analysis and Exposure Measurements, Volume 9—Passive Smoking*, IARC Scientific Publications No. 81. Lyon, France: World Health Organization, International Agency for Research on Cancer, 1987, pp. 11–23.

HABIB, M.P., KLINK, M.E., KNUDSON, D.E., BLOOM, J.W., KALTENBORN, W.T., KNUDSON, R.J. Physiologic characteristics of subjects exhibiting accelerated deterioration of ventilatory function. *American Review of Respiratory Disease* 136:638–645, 1987.

HALE, K.A., EWING, S.L., GOSNELL, B.A., NIEWOEHNER, D.E. Lung disease in long-term cigarette smokers with and without chronic air-flow obstruction. *American Review of Respiratory Disease* 130(5):716–721, November 1984.

HALLSTROM, A.P., COBB, L.A., RAY, R. Smoking as a risk factor for recurrence of sudden cardiac arrest. *New England Journal of Medicine* 314(5):271–275, 1986.

HAMMOND, E.C. Smoking in relation to the death rates of one million men and women. In: Haenszel, W. (ed.) *Epidemiological Approaches to the Study of Cancer and Other Chronic Diseases*, National Cancer Institute Monograph 19. U.S. Department of Health, Education, and Welfare, Public Health Service, NCI, January 1966, pp. 127–204.

HAMMOND, E.C., HORN, D. Smoking and death rates—Report on forty-four months of follow-up on 187,783 men. I. Total mortality. *Journal of the American Medical Association* 166(10):1159–1172, March 8, 1958.

HAMMOND, E.C., GARFINKEL, L., SEIDMAN, H., LEW, E.A. "Tar" and nicotine content of cigarette smoke in relation to death rates. *Environmental Research* 12(3):263–274, December 1976.

HARRISON'S PRINCIPLES OF INTERNAL MEDICINE, Eleventh Edition. McGraw-Hill, 1987.

HARTGE, P., SILVERMAN, D., HOOVER, R., SCHAIRER, C., ALTMAN, R., AUSTIN, D., CANTOR, K., CHILD, M., KEY, C., MARRETT, L.D., MASON, T.J., MEIGS, J.W., MYERS, M.H., NARAYANA, A., SULLIVAN, J.W., SWANSON, G.M., THOMAS, D., WEST, D. Changing cigarette habits and bladder cancer risk: A case–control study. *Journal of the National Cancer Institute* 78(6):1119–1125, June 1987.

HEBEL, J.R., FOX, N.L., SEXTON, M. Dose–response of birth weight to various measures of maternal smoking during pregnancy. *Journal of Clinical Epidemiology* 41(5):483–489, 1988.

HECHT, S.S., HOFFMANN, D. Tobacco-specific nitrosamines, an important group of carcinogens in tobacco and tobacco smoke. *Carcinogenesis* 9(6):875–884, 1988.

HERMAN, B., LEYTEN, A.C.M., VAN LUIJK, J.H., FRENKEN, C.W.G.M., OP DE COUL, A.A.W., SCHULTE, B.P.M. An evaluation of risk factors for stroke in a Dutch community. *Stroke* 13(3):334–339, May–June 1982.

HERMAN, W.H., TEUTSCH, S.M., GEISS, L.S. Diabetes mellitus. In: Amler, R.W., Dull, H.B. (eds.) *Closing the Gap: The Burden of Unnecessary Illness.* New York: Oxford University Press, 1987, pp. 72–82.

HIGGINS, I.T.T., MAHAN, C.M., WYNDER, E.L. Lung cancer among cigar and pipe smokers. *Preventive Medicine* 17(1):116–128, January 1988.

HIMMELBERGER, D.U., BROWN, B.W. JR., COHEN, E.N. Cigarette smoking during pregnancy and the occurrence of spontaneous abortion and congenital abnormality. *American Journal of Epidemiology* 108(6):470–479, 1978.

HIRAYAMA, T. *Smoking in Relation to the Death Rates of 265,118 Men and Women in Japan.* Tokyo: National Cancer Center, September 1967.

HOFFMANN, D., BRUNNEMANN, K.D., ADAMS, J.D., HECHT, S.S. Formation and analysis of N-nitrosamines in tobacco products and their endogenous formation in consumers. In: O'Neill, J.K., Von Borstel, R.C., Miller, C.T., Long, J., Bartsch, H. (eds.) *N-Nitroso Compounds: Occurrence, Biological Effects and Relationship to Human Cancer*, IARC Scientific Publication No. 57. Geneva: International Agency for Research on Cancer, 1984, pp. 743–762.

HOFFMANN, D., HECHT, S.S. Smokeless tobacco and cancer. In: *ISI Atlas of Science: Pharmacology*, Volume 2, 1988, pp. 46–52.

HOFFMANN, D., HECHT, S.S. Advances in tobacco carcinogenesis. In: Grover, P. (ed.) *Handbook of Experimental Pharmacology, 1988*. Springer-Verlag, 1989.

HOFFMANN, D., TSO, T.C., GORI, G.B. The less harmful cigarette. *Preventive Medicine* 9(2):287–296, March 1980.

HOGG, J.C., MACKLEM, P.T., THURLBECK, W.M. Site and nature of airway obstruction in chronic obstructive lung disease. *New England Journal of Medicine* 278(25):1355–1360, June 20, 1968.

HOLBROOK, J.H. Cigarette smoking and coronary heart disease. *Eighth International Atherosclerosis Symposium Proceedings (Rome)*, Excerpta Medica International Congress Series. Elsevier Science Publishers, in press.

HOLBROOK, J.H., GRUNDY, S.M., HENNEKENS, C.H., KANNEL, W.B., STRONG, J.P. Cigarette smoking and cardiovascular diseases: A statement for health professionals by a task force appointed by the steering committee of the American Heart Association. *Circulation* 70(6):1114A–1117A, December 1984.

HOLLY, E.A., PETRAKIS, N.L., FRIEND, N.F., SARLES, D.L., LEE, R.E., FLANDER, L.B. Mutagenic mucus in the cervix of smokers. *Journal of the National Cancer Institute* 76(6): 983–986, June 1986.

HOPKINS, P.N., WILLIAMS, R.R., HUNT, S.C. Magnified risks from cigarette smoking for coronary prone families in Utah. *Western Journal of Medicine* 141:196–202, August 1984.

HORM, J.W., KESSLER, L.G. Falling rates of lung cancer in men in the United States. *Lancet* 1(8478):425–426, February 1986.

HUBERT, H.B., HOLFORD, T.R., KANNEL, W.B. Clinical characteristics and cigarette smoking in relation to prognosis of angina pectoris in Framingham. *American Journal of Epidemiology* 115(2):231–242, February 1982.

HUMBLE, C.G., SAMET, J.M., PATHAK, D.R. Marriage to a smoker and lung cancer risk. *American Journal of Public Health* 77(5):598–602, May 1987.

HUNNINGHAKE, G.W., CRYSTAL, R.G. Cigarette smoking and lung destruction. Accumulation of neutrophils in the lungs of cigarette smokers. *American Review of Respiratory Disease* 128(5):833–838, November 1983.

INGEBRETHSEN, B.J. Aerosol studies of cigarette smoke. *Recent Advances in Tobacco Science* 12:54–142, 1986.

INTERNATIONAL AGENCY FOR RESEARCH ON CANCER. *Tobacco Smoking*, IARC Monographs on the Evaluation of the Carcinogenic Risk of Chemicals to Humans, Volume 38. Lyon: International Agency for Research on Cancer, 1986.

INTERNATIONAL AGENCY FOR RESEARCH ON CANCER. *Environmental Carcinogens. Methods of Analysis and Exposure Measurement. Volume 9—Passive Smoking*, IARC Scientific Publications No. 81. Lyon: International Agency for Research on Cancer, 1987.

JAJICH, C.L., OSTFELD, A.M., FREEMAN, D.H. JR. Smoking and coronary heart disease mortality in the elderly. *Journal of the American Medical Association* 252(20):2831–2834, November 23–30, 1984.

JANOFF, A. Elastases and emphysema. Current assessment of the protease–antiprotease hypothesis. *American Review of Respiratory Disease* 132:417–433, 1985.

JARVIS, M.J., RUSSELL, M.A.H. Tar and nicotine yields of U.K. cigarettes 1972–1983: Sales-weighted estimates from non-industry sources. *British Journal of Addiction* 80:429–434, 1985.

JARVIS, M., TUNSTALL-PEDOE, H., FEYERABEND, C., VESEY, C., SALLOOJEE, Y. Biochemical markers of smoke absorption and self reported exposure to passive smoking. *Journal of Epidemiology and Community Health* 38(4):335–339, December 1984.

JENKINS, R.W. JR., GOLDEY, C., WILLIAMSON, T.G. Neutron activation analysis in tobacco and tobacco smoke studies: 2R1 cigarette composition smoke transference and butt filtration. *Beitrage zur Tabakforschung* 13(2):59–65, December 1985.

JENSEN, G.F. Osteoporosis of the slender smoker revisited by epidemiologic approach. *European Journal of Clinical Investigation* 16:239–242, 1986.

JENSEN, J., CHRISTIANSEN, C., RODBRO, P. Cigarette smoking, serum estrogens, and bone loss during hormone-replacement therapy early after menopause. *New England Journal of Medicine* 313:973–975, 1985.

JOHNSTONE, R.A.W., PLIMMER, J.R. The chemical constituents of tobacco and tobacco smoke. *Chemical Reviews* 59(5):885–936, 1959.

JOLY, O.G., LUBIN, J.H., CARABALLOSO, M. Dark tobacco and lung cancer in Cuba. *Journal of the National Cancer Institute* 70(6):1033–1039, June 1983.

JOURNAL OF THE AMERICAN MEDICAL ASSOCIATION. Osteoporosis—Consensus Conference. *Journal of the American Medical Association* 252(6):799–802, August 10, 1984.

KAHN, H.A. The Dorn study of smoking and mortality among U.S. veterans: Report on eight and one-half years of observation. In: Haenszel, W. (ed.) *Epidemiological Approaches to the Study of Cancer and Other Chronic Diseases*, NCI Monograph 19. U.S. Department of Health, Education, and Welfare, Public Health Service, National Cancer Institute, January 1966, pp. 1–125.

KANNEL, W.B., SHURTLEFF, D. The Framingham Study. Cigarettes and the development of intermittent claudication. *Geriatrics* 28(2):61–68, February 1973.

KAPLAN, G.A., SEEMAN, T.E., COHEN, R.D., KNUDSEN, L.P., GURALNIK, J. Mortality among the elderly in the Alameda County Study: Behavioral and demographic risk factors. *American Journal of Public Health* 77(3):307–312, March 1987.

KAUFMAN, D.W., HELMRICH, S.P., ROSENBERG, L., MIETTINEN, O.S., SHAPIRO, S. Nicotine and carbon monoxide content of cigarette smoke and the risk of myocardial infarction in young men. *New England Journal of Medicine* 308(8):409–413, February 24, 1983.

KELLERMANN, G., SHAW, C.R., LUYTEN-KELLERMAN, M. Aryl hydrocarbon hydroxylase inducibility and bronchogenic carcinoma. *New England Journal of Medicine* 289(18):934–937, 1973.

KELSEY, J.L., DWYER, T., HOLFORD, T.R., BRACKEN, M.B. Maternal smoking and congenital malformations: An epidemiological study. *Journal of Epidemiology and Community Health* 32:102–107, 1978.

KEMP, H.G., KRONMAL, R.A., VLIETSTRA, R.E., FRYE, R.L., PARTICIPANTS IN THE CORONARY ARTERY SURGERY STUDY. Seven year survival of patients with normal or near normal coronary arteriograms: A CASS Registry Study. *Journal of the American College of Cardiology* 7(3):479–483, March 1986.

KIEL, D.P., FELSON, D.T., ANDERSON, J.J., WILSON, P.W.F., MOSKOWITZ, M.A. Hip fracture and the use of estrogens in postmenopausal women. The Framingham Study. *New England Journal of Medicine* 317(19):1169–1174, November 5, 1987.

KLEINMAN, J.C., PIERRE, M.B. JR., MADANS, J.H., LAND, J.H., SCHRAMM, W.F. The effects of maternal smoking on fetal and infant mortality. *American Journal of Epidemiology* 127(2):274–282, 1988.

KORMAN, M.G., HANSKY, J., EAVES, E.R., SCHMIDT, G.T. Influence of cigarette smoking on healing and relapse in duodenal ulcer disease. *Gastroenterology* 85:871–874, 1983.

KREIGER, N., KELSEY, J., HOLFORD, T.R., O'CONNOR, T. An epidemiologic study of hip fracture in postmenopausal women. *American Journal of Epidemiology* 116(1):141–148, 1982.

KULLER, L., MEILAHN, E., TOWNSEND, M., WEINBERG, G. Control of cigarette smoking from a medical perspective. *Annual Review of Public Health* 3:153–178, 1982.

LANE, M.R., LEE, S.P. Recurrence of duodenal ulcer after medical treatment. *Lancet* 1:1147–1149, May 21, 1988.

LAURELL, C.-B., ERIKSSON, S. The electrophoretic α-globulin pattern of serum in α_1-antitrypsin deficiency. *Scandinavian Journal of Clinical Investigations* 15:132–140, 1963.

LAVECCHIA, C., FRANCESCHI, S., DECARLI, A., FASOLI, M., GENTILE, A., TOGNONI, G. Cigarette smoking and the risk of cervical neoplasia. *American Journal of Epidemiology* 123(1):22–29, January 1986.

LAVOIE, E.J., TUCCIARONE, P., KAGAN, M., ADAMS, J.D., HOFFMANN, D. Analyses of steam distillates and aqueous extracts of smokeless tobacco. *Journal of Agricultural and Food Chemistry* 37(1):154–157, January–February 1989.

LAYDE, P.M., BERAL, V., KAY, C.R. Further analyses of mortality in oral contraceptive users. Royal College of General Practitioners' Oral Contraceptives Study. *Lancet* 1(8219):541–546, March 7, 1981.

LIEBERMAN, E., RYAN, K.J., MONSON, R.R., SCHOENBAUM, S.C. Risk factors accounting for racial differences in the rate of premature birth. *New England Journal of Medicine* 317(12):743–748, 1987.

LITHNER, F. Is tobacco of importance for the development and progression of diabetic vascular complications? *Acta Medica Scandinavica* 687(Supplement):33–36, 1983.

LUBIN, J.H., BLOT, W.J., BERRINO, F., FLAMANT, R., GILLIS, C.R., KUNZE, M., SCHMAHL, D., VISCO, G. Patterns of lung cancer risk according to type of cigarette smoked. *International Journal of Cancer* 33(5):569–576, 1984a.

LUBIN, J.H., BLOT, W.J., BERRINO, F., FLAMANT, R., GILLIS, C.R., KUNZE, M., SCHMAHL, D., VISCO, G. Modifying risk of developing lung cancer by changing habits of cigarette smoking. *British Medical Journal* 288(6435):1953–1956, June 30, 1984b.

LYNCH, H.T., FAIR, P.R., ALBANO, W.A., RUMA, T.A., BLACK, L., LYNCH, J., SHONKA, M. Genetic/epidemiological findings in a study of smoking-associated tumors. *Cancer Genetics and Cytogenetics* 6(2):163–169, June 1982.

MACK, T.M., YU, M.C., HANISCH, R., HENDERSON, B.E. Pancreas cancer and smoking, beverage consumption, and past medical history. *Journal of the National Cancer Institute* 76(1):49–60, 1986.

MARTIN, J.L., WILSON, J.R., FERRARO, N., LASKEY, W.K., KLEAVELAND, J.P., HIRSHFELD, J.W. JR. Acute coronary vasoconstrictive effects of cigarette smoking in coronary heart disease. *American Journal of Cardiology* 54(1):56–60, July 1, 1984.

MCLAUGHLIN, J.K., MANDEL, J.S., BLOT, W.J., SCHUMAN, L.M., MEHL., E.S., FRAUMENI, J.F. JR. A population-based case–control study of renal cell carcinoma. *Journal of the National Cancer Institute* 72(2):275–284, February 1984.

MEDICAL RESEARCH COUNCIL WORKING PARTY. MRC trial of treatment of mild hypertension: Principal results. *British Medical Journal* 291(6488):97–104, July 13, 1985.

MIETTINEN, T.A., GYLLING, H. Mortality and cholesterol metabolism in familial hypercholesterolemia. Long-term follow-up of 96 patients. *Arteriosclerosis* 8:163–167, March–April 1988.

MOHR, U., REZNIK, G. Tobacco carcinogenesis. In: Harris, C.C. (ed.) *Pathogenesis and Therapy of Lung Cancer*. New York: Marcel Dekker, 1978, pp. 263–367.

MULVIHILL, J.J., BALE, A.E. Ecogenetics of lung cancer: Genetic susceptibility in the etiology of lung cancer. In: Mizell, C.M., Correa, P. (eds.) *Proceedings of the International Lung Cancer Update Conference*. Deerfield Beach, Florida: Verlag-Chemie International, 1984, pp. 141–152.

NAEYE, R.L., PETERS, E.C. Mental development of children whose mothers smoked during pregnancy. *Obstetrics and Gynecology* 64(5):601–607, November 1984.

NAGAI, A., WEST, W.W., THURLBECK, W.M. The National Institutes of Health Intermittent Positive-Pressure Breathing Trial: Pathology studies. II. Correlation between morphologic findings, clinical findings, and evidence of expiratory air-flow obstruction. *American Review of Respiratory Disease* 132:946–953, 1985.

NAKAYAMA, T., KODAMA, M., NAGATA, C. Generation of hydrogen peroxide and superoxide anion radical from cigarette smoke. *Gann: Japanese Journal of Cancer Research* 75(2):95–98, February 1984.

NATIONAL ACADEMY OF SCIENCES. *Diet, Nutrition, and Cancer*. Washington, D.C.: National Academy Press, 1982.

NATIONAL CENTER FOR HEALTH STATISTICS. *Health, United States, 1986*. U.S. Department of Health and Human Services, Public Health Service, National Center for Health Statistics. DHHS Publication No. (PHS) 87-1232, December 1986.

NATIONAL INSTITUTES OF HEALTH, NATIONAL INSTITUTE OF ENVIRONMENTAL HEALTH SCIENCES. Airborne pollutants and respiratory cancer reproductive and developmental toxicology. *Environmental Health Perspectives* 70, December 1986.

NATIONAL RESEARCH COUNCIL. *Carbon Monoxide.* National Research Council, Committee on Medical and Biologic Effects of Environmental Pollutants. Washington, D.C.: National Academy Press, 1977.

NATIONAL RESEARCH COUNCIL. *Environmental Tobacco Smoke. Measuring Exposures and Assessing Health Effects.* Washington, D.C.: National Academy Press, 1986.

NATIONAL RESEARCH COUNCIL. *Health Risks of Radon and Other Internally Deposited Alpha-Emitters. BEIR IV.* Washington, D.C.: National Academy Press, 1988.

NEURATH, G.B., DUNGER, M., ORTH, D., PEIN, F.G. Trans-3130-hydroxycotinine as a main metabolite in urine of smokers. *International Archives of Occupational and Environmental Health* 59:199–201, 1987.

NIEBURG, P., MARKS, J.S., MCLAREN, N.M., REMINGTON, P.L. The fetal tobacco syndrome. *Journal of the American Medical Association* 253(20):2998–2999, May 24–31, 1985.

NIEWOEHNER, D.E. Cigarette smoking, lung inflammation, and the development of emphysema. *Journal of Laboratory and Clinical Medicine* 111(1):15–27, January 1988.

NIEWOEHNER, D.E., KLEINERMAN, J., RICE, D.B. Pathologic changes in the peripheral airways of young cigarette smokers. *New England Journal of Medicine* 291(15):755–758, 1974.

NORMAN, V. Changes in smoke chemistry of modern day cigarettes. *Recent Advances in Tobacco Science* 8:141–177, 1982.

NOWAK, J., MURRAY, J.J., OATES, J.A., FITZGERALD, G.A. Biochemical evidence of a chronic abnormality in platelet and vascular function in healthy individuals who smoke cigarettes. *Circulation* 76(1):6–14, July 1987.

OOI, W.L., ELSTON, R.C., CHEN, V.W., BAILEY-WILSON, J.E., ROTHSCHILD, H. Increased familial risk for lung cancer. *Journal of the National Cancer Institute* 76(2):217–222, February 1986.

PATHAK, D.R., SAMET, J.M., HUMBLE, C.G., SKIPPER, B.J. Determinants of lung cancer risk in cigarette smokers in New Mexico. *Journal of the National Cancer Institute* 76(4):597–604, April 1986.

PEARSON, T.A. Coronary arteriography in the study of the epidemiology of coronary artery disease. *Epidemiologic Reviews* 6:140–166, 1984.

PERSHAGEN, G., HRUBEC, Z., SVENSSON, C. Passive smoking and lung cancer in Swedish women. *American Journal of Epidemiology* 125(1):17–24, January 1987.

PETITTI, D.B., WINGERD, J., PELLEGRIN, F., RAMCHARAN, S. Risk of vascular disease in women: Smoking, oral contraceptives, noncontraceptive estrogens, and other factors. *Journal of the American Medical Association* 242(11):1150–1154, September 14, 1979.

PETO, R. Overview of cancer time-trend studies in relation to changes in cigarette manufacture. In: Zaridze, D.G., Peto, R. (eds.) *Tobacco: A Major International Health Hazard*, IARC Scientific Publications No. 74. Lyon, France: International Agency for Research on Cancer, 1986, pp. 211–226.

PETO, R., DOLL, R. Keynote address: The control of lung cancer. In: Mizell, M., Correa, P. (eds.) *Lung Cancer: Causes and Prevention.* Deerfield Beach, Florida: Verlag Chemie International, 1984, pp. 1–19.

PETO, R., DOLL, R., BUCKLEY, J.D., SPORN, M.B. Can dietary beta-carotene materially reduce cancer rates? *Nature* 290:201–208, March 19, 1981.

PETO, R., SPEIZER, F.E., COCHRANE, A.L., MOORE, F., FLETCHER, C.M., TINKER, C.M., HIGGINS, I.T.T., GRAY, R.G., RICHARDS, S.M., GILLILAND, J., NORMAN-

SMITH, B. The relevance in adults of air-flow obstruction, but not of mucus hypersecretion, to mortality from chronic lung disease. Results from 20 years of prospective observation. *American Review of Respiratory Disease* 128(3):491–501, September 1983.

PILLSBURY, H.C., BRIGHT, C.C., O'CONNOR, K.J., IRISH, F.W. Tar and nicotine in cigarette smoke. *Journal of the Association of Official Analytical Chemists* 52(3):458–462, 1969.

POMREHN, P., DUNCAN, B., WEISSFELD, L., WALLACE, R.B., BARNES, R., HEISS, G., EKELUND, L.-G., CRIQUI, M.H., JOHNSON, N., CHAMBLESS, L.E. The association of dyslipoproteinemia with symptoms and signs of peripheral arterial disease: The Lipid Research Clinics Program Prevalence Study. *Circulation* 73(Supplement 1):1–100, 1986.

POOLING PROJECT RESEARCH GROUP. Relationship of blood pressure, serum cholesterol, smoking habit, relative weight and ECG abnormalities to incidence of major coronary events: Final report of the Pooling Project. *Journal of Chronic Diseases* 31(4):201–306, April 1978.

R.J. REYNOLDS TOBACCO COMPANY. *Chemical and Biological Studies on New Cigarette Prototypes That Heat Instead of Burn Tobacco.* Winston-Salem, North Carolina: R.J. Reynolds Tobacco Company, 1988.

RANTAKALLIO, P., KOIRANEN, M. Neurological handicaps among children whose mothers smoked during pregnancy. *Preventive Medicine* 16:597–606, 1987.

RAUTAHARJU, P.M., PRINEAS, R.J., EIFLER, W.J., FURBERG, C.D., NEATON, J.D., CROW, R.S., STAMLER, J., CUTLER, J.A. Prognostic value of exercise electrocardiogram in men at high risk of future coronary heart disease: Multiple Risk Factor Intervention Trial experience. *Journal of the American College of Cardiology* 8(1):1–10, July 1986.

RIVENSON, A., HOFFMANN, D., PROKOPCZYK, B., AMIN, S., HECHT, S.S. Induction of lung and exocrine pancreas tumors in F344 rats by tobacco-specific and *areca*-derived N-nitrosamines. *Cancer Research* 48(23):6912–6917, December 1, 1988.

ROBERTS, D.L. Natural tobacco flavor. *Recent Advances in Tobacco Science: Chemical and Sensory Aspects of Tobacco Flavor* 14:49–81, 1988.

ROGERS, R.L., MEYER, J.S., SHAW, T.G., MORTEL, K.F., HARDENBERG, J.P., ZAID, R.R. Cigarette smoking decreases cerebral blood flow suggesting increased risk for stroke. *Journal of the American Medical Association* 250(20):2796–2800, November 25, 1983.

ROGERS, R.L., MEYER, J.S., JUDD, B.W., MORTEL, K.F. Abstention from cigarette smoking improves cerebral perfusion among elderly chronic smokers. *Journal of the American Medical Association* 253(20):2970–2974, May 24–31, 1985.

RONNEVIK, P.K., GUNDERSEN, T., ABRAHAMSEN, A.M. Effect of smoking habits and timolol treatment on mortality and reinfarction in patients surviving acute myocardial infarction. *British Heart Journal* 54(2):134–139, August 1985.

ROSENBERG, L. Case–control studies of risk factors for myocardial infarction among women. In: Eaker, E.D., Packard, B., Wenger, N.K., Clarkson, T.B., Tyroler, H.A. (eds.) *Coronary Heart Disease in Women. Proceedings of an N.I.H. Workshop*, 1987, pp. 70–77.

ROSENBERG, L., MILLER, D.R., KAUFMAN, D.W., HELMRICH, S.P., VAN DE CARR, S., STOLLEY, P.D., SHAPIRO, S. Myocardial infarction in women under 50 years of age. *Journal of the American Medical Association* 250(20):2801–2806, November 25, 1983.

RUSH, D., CASSANO, P. Relationship of cigarette smoking and social class to birth weight and perinatal mortality among all births in Britain, April 5–11, 1970. *Journal of Epidemiology and Community Health* 37:249–255, 1983.

SACCO, R.L., WOLF, P.A., BHARUCHA, N.E., MEEKS, S.L., KANNEL, W.B., CHARETTE, J., MCNAMARA, P.M., PALMER, E.P., D'AGOSTINO, R. Subarachnoid and intracerebral hemorrhage: Natural history, prognosis, and precursive factors in the Framingham Study. *Neurology* 34:847–854, July 1984.

SALONEN, J.T., PUSKA, P., TUOMILEHTO, J., HOMAN, K. Relation of blood pressure, serum lipids, and smoking to the risk of cerebral stroke: A longitudinal study in eastern Finland. *Stroke* 13(3):327–333, May–June 1982.

SAMET, J.M., HUMBLE, C.G., PATHAK, D.R. Personal and family history of respiratory disease and lung cancer risk. *American Review of Respiratory Disease* 134(3):466–470, September 1986.

SAMET, J.M., HUMBLE, C.G., SKIPPER, B.E., PATHAK, D.R. History of residence and lung cancer risk in New Mexico. *American Journal of Epidemiology* 125(5):800–811, 1987.

SAMET, J.M., MARBURY, M.C., SPENGLER, J.D. Health effects and sources of indoor air pollution. Part I. *American Review of Respiratory Disease* 136:1486–1508, 1987.

SAMET, J.M., TAGER, I.B., SPEIZER, F.E. The relationship between respiratory illness in childhood and chronic air-flow obstruction in adulthood. *American Review of Respiratory Disease* 127(4):508–523, April 1983.

SAMET, J.M., WIGGINS, C.L., HUMBLE, C.G., PATHAK, D.R. Cigarette smoking and lung cancer in New Mexico. *American Review of Respiratory Disease* 137:1110–1113, 1988.

SANDLER, R.B., SLEMENDA, C.W., LAPORTE, R.E., CAULEY, J.A., SCHRAMM, M.M., BARRESI, M.L., KRISKA, A.M. Postmenopausal bone density and milk consumption in childhood and adolescence. *American Journal of Clinical Nutrition* 42:270–274, August 1985.

SARACCI, R. The interactions of tobacco smoking and other agents in cancer etiology. *Epidemiologic Reviews* 9:175–193, 1987.

SASSON, I.M., HALEY, N.J., HOFFMANN, D., WYNDER, E.L., HELLBERG, D., NILSSON, S. Cigarette smoking and neoplasia of the uterine cervix: Smoke constituents in cervical mucus. *New England Journal of Medicine* 312(5):315–316, January 31, 1985.

SCHARDEIN, J.L. *Chemically Induced Birth Defects.* New York: Marcel Dekker, 1985.

SCHOTTENFELD, D. Epidemiology of cancer of the esophagus. *Seminars in Oncology* 11(2):92–100, June 1984.

SEPKOVIC, D.W., HALEY, N.J., HOFFMANN, D. Elimination from the body of tobacco products by smokers and passive smokers. (Letter.) *Journal of the American Medical Association* 256(7):863, August 15, 1986.

SKILLRUD, D.M., OFFORD, K.P., MILLER, R.O. Higher risk of lung cancer in chronic obstructive pulmonary disease. A prospective, matched, controlled study. *Annals of Internal Medicine* 105(4):503–507, October 1986.

SLONE, D., SHAPIRO, S., KAUFMAN, D.W., ROSENBERG, L., MIETTINEN, O.S., STOLLEY, P.D. Risk of myocardial infarction in relation to current and discontinued use of oral contraceptives. *New England Journal of Medicine* 305:420–424, August 21, 1981.

SONTAG, S., GRAHAM, D.Y., BELSITO, A., WEISS, J., FARLEY, A., GRUNT, R., COHEN, N., KINNEAR, D., DAVIS, W., ARCHAMBAULT, A., ACHORD, J., THAYER, W., GILLIES, R., SIDIROV, J., SABESIN, S.M., DYCK, W., FLESHLER, B., CLEATOR, I., WENGER, J., OPEKUN, A. JR. Cimetidine, cigarette smoking, and recurrence of duodenal ulcer. *New England Journal of Medicine* 311(11):689–693, September 13, 1984.

SOWERS, M., WALLACE, R.B., LEMKE, J.H. Correlates of forearm bone mass among women during maximal bone mineralization. *Preventive Medicine* 14:585–596, 1985.

SPENGLER, J.D., SEXTON, K. Indoor air pollution: A public health perspective. *Science* 221(4605):9–17, July 1, 1983.

STAMLER, J., WENTWORTH, D.N., NEATON, J.D., MRFIT RESEARCH GROUP. Middle-aged American men at very low risk of coronary death: 6-year findings on the 356,222 screenees of the Multiple Risk Factor Intervention Trial (MRFIT). Paper presented at the Tenth World Congress of Cardiology, Washington, D.C., September 1986.

STEDMAN, R.L. The chemical composition of tobacco and tobacco smoke. *Chemical Reviews* 68(2):153–207, April 1968.

STEIN, Z., KLINE, J., LEVIN, B., SUSSER, M., WARBURTON, D. Epidemiologic studies of environmental exposures in human reproduction. In: Berg, G.G., Maillie, H.D. (eds.) *Measurement of Risks*. New York: Plenum Press, 1981, pp. 163–183.

STUART-HARRIS, C.H. The epidemiology and evolution of chronic bronchitis. *British Journal of Tuberculosis and Diseases of the Chest* 48(3):169–178, July 1954.

STUART-HARRIS, C.H. Chronic bronchitis. (Part I). *Abstracts of World Medicine* 42(9): 649–669, September 1968a.

STUART-HARRIS, C.H. Chronic bronchitis. (Part II). *Abstracts of World Medicine* 42(10): 737–751, 1968b.

SUAREZ, L., BARRETT-CONNOR, E. Interaction between cigarette smoking and diabetes mellitus in the prediction of death attributed to cardiovascular disease. *American Journal of Epidemiology* 120(5):670–675, 1984.

SULLIVAN, J.M., VANDER ZWAAG, R., LEMP, G.F., HUGHES, J.P., MADDOCK, V., KROETZ, F.W., RAMANATHAN, K.B., MIRVIS, D.M. Postmenopausal estrogen use and coronary atherosclerosis. *Annals of Internal Medicine* 108(3):358–363, March 1988.

TAHA, A., BALL, K.P., ILLINGWORTH, R.D. Smoking and subarachnoid haemorrhage. *Journal of the Royal Society of Medicine* 75(5):332–335, May 1982.

TANAKA, H., UEDA, Y., HAYASHI, M., DATE, C., BABA, T., YAMASHITA, H., SHOJI, H., TANAKA, Y., OWADA, K., DETELS, R. Risk factors for cerebral hemorrhage and cerebral infarction in a Japanese rural community. *Stroke* 13(1):62–73, 1982.

TOKUHATA, G.K., LILIENFELD, A.M. Familial aggregation of lung cancer in humans. *Journal of the National Cancer Institute* 30(2):289–312, February 1963a.

TOKUHATA, G.K., LILIENFELD, A.M. Familial aggregation of lung cancer among hospital patients. *Public Health Reports* 78(4):277–283, April 1963b.

U.S. DEPARTMENT OF HEALTH AND HUMAN SERVICES. *The Health Consequences of Smoking for Women. A Report of the Surgeon General.* U.S. Department of Health and Human Services, Public Health Service, Office of the Assistant Secretary for Health, Office on Smoking and Health, 1980.

U.S. DEPARTMENT OF HEALTH AND HUMAN SERVICES. *The Health Consequences of Smoking. The Changing Cigarette: A Report of the Surgeon General.* U.S. Department of Health and Human Services, Public Health Service, Office of the Assistant Secretary for Health, Office on Smoking and Health. DHHS Publication No. (PHS) 81-50156, 1981.

U.S. DEPARTMENT OF HEALTH AND HUMAN SERVICES. *The Health Consequences of Smoking: Cancer. A Report of the Surgeon General.* U.S. Department of Health and Human Services, Public Health Service, Office on Smoking and Health. DHHS Publication No. (PHS) 82-50179, 1982.

U.S. DEPARTMENT OF HEALTH AND HUMAN SERVICES. *The Health Consequences of Smoking: Cardiovascular Disease. A Report of the Surgeon General.* U.S. Department of Health and Human Services, Public Health Service, Office on Smoking and Health. DHHS Publication No. (PHS) 84-50204, 1983.

U.S. DEPARTMENT OF HEALTH AND HUMAN SERVICES. *The Health Consequences of Smoking: Chronic Obstructive Lung Disease. A Report of the Surgeon General.* U.S. Department of Health and Human Services, Public Health Service, Office on Smoking and Health. DHHS Publication No. (PHS) 84-50205, 1984.

U.S. DEPARTMENT OF HEALTH AND HUMAN SERVICES. *The Health Consequences of Smoking: Cancer and Chronic Lung Disease in the Workplace. A Report of the Surgeon General.* U.S. Department of Health and Human Services, Public Health Service, Office on Smoking and Health. DHHS Publication No. (PHS) 85-50207, 1985.

U.S. DEPARTMENT OF HEALTH AND HUMAN SERVICES. *The Health Consequences of Involuntary Smoking. A Report of the Surgeon General.* U.S. Department of Health and Human Services, Public Health Service, Centers for Disease Control. DHHS Publication No. (CDC) 87-8398, 1986a.

U.S. DEPARTMENT OF HEALTH AND HUMAN SERVICES. *The Health Consequences of Using Smokeless Tobacco. A Report of the Advisory Committee to the Surgeon General, 1986.* U.S. Department of Health and Human Services, Public Health Service. NIH Publication No. 86-2874, April 1986b.

U.S. DEPARTMENT OF HEALTH AND HUMAN SERVICES. *The Health Consequences of Smoking: Nicotine Addiction. A Report of the Surgeon General, 1988.* U.S. Department of Health and Human Services, Public Health Service, Centers for Disease Control, Center for Health Promotion and Education, Office on Smoking and Health. DHHS Publication No. (CDC) 88-8406, 1988.

U.S. DEPARTMENT OF HEALTH, EDUCATION, AND WELFARE. *The Health Consequences of Smoking. A Report to the Surgeon General: 1971.* U.S. Department of Health, Education, and Welfare, Public Health Service, Health Services and Mental Health Administration. DHEW Publication No. (HSM) 71-7513, 1971.

U.S. DEPARTMENT OF HEALTH, EDUCATION, AND WELFARE. *The Health Consequences of Smoking. A Report of the Surgeon General: 1972.* U.S. Department of Health, Education, and Welfare, Public Health Service, Health Services and Mental Health Administration. DHEW Publication No. (HSM) 72-7516, 1972.

U.S. DEPARTMENT OF HEALTH, EDUCATION, AND WELFARE. *The Health Consequences of Smoking.* U.S. Department of Health, Education, and Welfare, Public Health Service, Health Services and Mental Health Administration. DHEW Publication No. (HSM) 73-8704, 1973.

U.S. DEPARTMENT OF HEALTH, EDUCATION, AND WELFARE. *The Health Consequences of Smoking, 1977–1978.* U.S. Department of Health, Education, and Welfare, Public Health Service, Office of the Assistant Secretary for Health, Office on Smoking and Health. DHEW Publication No. (PHS) 79-50065, 1978.

U.S. DEPARTMENT OF HEALTH, EDUCATION, AND WELFARE. *Smoking and Health. A Report of the Surgeon General.* U.S. Department of Health, Education, and Welfare, Public Health Service, Office of the Assistant Secretary for Health, Office on Smoking and Health. DHEW Publication No. (PHS) 79-50066, 1979.

U.S. PUBLIC HEALTH SERVICE. *Smoking and Health. Report of the Advisory Committee to the Surgeon General of the Public Health Service.* U.S. Department of Health, Education, and Welfare, Public Health Service, Center for Disease Control. PHS Publication No. 1103, 1964.

U.S. PUBLIC HEALTH SERVICE. *The Health Consequences of Smoking. A Public Health Service Review: 1967.* U.S. Department of Health, Education, and Welfare, Public Health Service. PHS Publication No. 1696, revised 1968.

U.S. PUBLIC HEALTH SERVICE. *The Health Consequences of Smoking. 1969 Supplement to the 1967 Public Health Service Review.* U.S. Department of Health, Education, and Welfare, Public Health Service. PHS Publication No. 1696-2 (Supplement), 1969.

VESSEY, M.P., LAWLESS, M., YEATES, D. Oral contraceptives and stroke: Findings in a large prospective study. *British Medical Journal* 289(6444):530–531, September 1, 1984.

VLIETSTRA, R.E., KRONMAL, R.A., OBERMAN, A., FRYE, R.L., KILLIP, T. III. Effect of cigarette smoking on survival of patients with angiographically documented coronary artery disease: Report from the CASS Registry. *Journal of the American Medical Association* 255(8):1023–1027, February 28, 1986.

WAKEHAM, H. Sales weighted average "tar" and nicotine deliveries of U.S. cigarettes from 1957 to present. In: Wynder, E., Hecht, S. (eds.) *Lung Cancer*, UICC Technical Report Series, Volume 25. Geneva: International Union Against Cancer, 1976, pp. 151–152.

WALD, N.J., IDLE, M., BOREHAM, J., BAILEY, A., VANVUNAKIS, H. Serum cotinine levels in pipe smokers: Evidence against nicotine as cause of coronary heart disease. *Lancet* 2:775–777, October 10, 1981.

WALD, N.J., RITCHIE, C. Validation of studies on lung cancer in non-smokers married to smokers. (Letter.) *Lancet* 1(8385):1067, May 12, 1984.

WEITZ, J.I., CROWLEY, K.A., LANDMAN, S.L., LIPMAN, B., YU, J. Increased neutrophil elastase activity in cigarette smokers. *Annals of Internal Medicine* 107:680–682, 1987.

WHITTEMORE, A.S., PAFFENBERGER, R.S. JR., ANDERSON, K., LEE, J.E. Early precursors of site-specific cancers in college men and women. *Journal of the National Cancer Institute* 74:43–51, 1985.

WILLETT, W.C., GREEN, A., STAMPFER, M.J., SPEIZER, F.E., COLDITZ, G.A., ROSNER, B., MONSON, R.R., STASON, W., HENNEKENS, C.H. Relative and absolute excess risks of coronary heart disease among women who smoke cigarettes. *New England Journal of Medicine* 317(20):1303–1309, November 19, 1987.

WILLETT, W., STAMPFER, M.J., BAIN, C., LIPNICK, R., SPEIZER, F.E., ROSNER, B., CRAMER, D., HENNEKENS, C.H. Cigarette smoking, relative weight, and menopause. *American Journal of Epidemiology* 117(6):651–658, 1983.

WILLIAMS, R.R., HASSTEDT, S.J., WILSON, D.E., ASH, K.O., YANOWITZ, F.F., REIBER, G.E., KUIDA, H. Evidence that the men with familial hypercholesterolemia can avoid early coronary death: An analysis of 77 gene carriers in four Utah pedigrees. *Journal of the American Medical Association* 255(2):219–224, January 10, 1986.

WINKELSTEIN, W. JR., SHILLITOE, E.J., BRAND, R., JOHNSON, K.K. Further comments on cancer of the uterine cervix, smoking, and herpesvirus infection. *American Journal of Epidemiology* 119(1):1–8, January 1984.

WITTEKINDT, W. Changes in recommended plant protecting agents for tobacco. *Tabak Journal International* 5:390,392–394, October 1985.

WOLF, P.A., D'AGOSTINO, R.B., KANNEL, W.B., BONITA, R., BELANGER, A.J. Cigarette smoking as a risk factor for stroke. The Framingham Study. *Journal of the American Medical Association* 259(7):1025–1029, February 19, 1988.

WOLF, P.A., DAWBER, T.R., THOMAS, H.E. JR., KANNEL, W.B. Epidemiologic assessment of chronic atrial fibrillation and risk of stroke: The Framingham Study. *Neurology* 28:973–977, October 1978.

WYNDER, E.L., HOFFMANN, D. *Tobacco and Tobacco Smoke. Studies in Experimental Carcinogenesis.* New York: Academic Press, 1967.

WYNDER, E.L., MABUCHI, K., BEATTIE, E.F. JR. The epidemiology of lung cancer. *Journal of the American Medical Association* 213(13):2221–2228, September 28, 1970.

WYNDER, E.L., STELLMAN, S.D. Impact of long-term filter cigarette usage on lung and larynx cancer risk: A case–control study. *Journal of the National Cancer Institute* 62(3):471–477, March 1979.

YAMASAKI, E., AMES, B.N. Concentration of mutagens from urine by adsorption with the nonpolar resin XAD-2: Cigarette smokers have mutagenic urine. (Detecting Carcinogens in Urine or Aqueous Liquids/Salmonella Test). *Proceedings of the National Academy of Science* 74(8):3555–3559, August 1977.

YEUNG, M.C, DY BUNCIO, A. Leukocyte count, smoking, and lung function. *American Journal of Medicine* 76(1):31–37, January 1984.

ZAHM, S.H., HARTGE, P., HOOVER, R. The National Bladder Cancer Study: Employment in the chemical industry. *Journal of the National Cancer Institute* 79(2):217–222, August 1987.

ZIMMERMAN, B.R., PALUMBO, P.J., O'FALLON, W.M., OSMUNDSON, P.J., KAZIMER, F.J. A prospective study of peripheral occlusive arterial disease in diabetes. I. Clinical characteristics of the subjects. *Mayo Clinic Proceedings* 56:217–222, April 1981.

CHAPTER 3

CHANGES IN SMOKING-ATTRIBUTABLE MORTALITY

CONTENTS

Introduction

In 1938, Raymond Pearl reported elevated death rates among white males who smoked tobacco, especially those aged 30 to 60 years (Pearl 1938). Pearl's study of 6,800 subjects revealed the increase in mortality risk to be highest among heavy smokers. In 1954, Hammond and Horn reported on the 20-month followup of their prospective study of 188,000 white men, aged 50 to 69 years (Hammond and Horn 1954). Death rates were highest among men who smoked cigarettes but not other tobacco products, and increased with the amount of cigarette use. Overall, the number of deaths among cigarette smokers was 52 percent greater than would be expected from nonsmokers' mortality rates. Most of the increased mortality could be attributed to deaths from cancer and especially from coronary heart disease (CHD).

In 1964, the Advisory Committee to the Surgeon General reviewed seven prospective studies of smoking and mortality, encompassing over 1.7 million entrants. For the 1.1 million male enrollees, the overall mortality ratio, defined as the observed number of deaths in current cigarette smokers divided by the number expected from nonsmokers' rates, was 1.68. "For all seven studies," the Committee stated, "coronary artery disease is the chief contributor to the excess number of deaths of cigarette smokers over nonsmokers, with lung cancer uniformly in second place. For all seven studies combined, coronary artery disease (with a mortality ratio of 1.7) accounts for 45 percent of the excess deaths among cigarette smokers, whereas lung cancer (with a ratio of 10.8) accounts for 16 percent" (US PHS 1964, p. 30).

In 1979, the Surgeon General described cigarette smoking as "the single most important preventable environmental factor contributing to illness, disability and death in the United States" (US DHEW 1979, p. vii). The 1982 Surgeon General's Report, citing an analysis by Doll and Peto (1981), estimated that for the year 1978, tobacco use caused 122,000 cancer deaths in men and women (US DHHS 1982). For 1982, the estimate for smoking-caused cancers was 129,000 (US DHHS 1982). The 1983 Surgeon General's Report estimated that 170,000 Americans died annually from CHD caused by cigarette smoking (US DHHS 1983). "During 1965–1977," the Report noted, "there were an estimated 2.8 million premature deaths from heart disease, primarily CHD, in American men and women attributable to the use of tobacco" (US DHHS 1983, p. 66).

The 1984 Report estimated that 80 to 90 percent of the 62,000 deaths from chronic obstructive lung disease (COLD), referred to later in this discussion as chronic obstructive pulmonary disease (COPD), in the United States in 1983 were attributable to cigarette smoking (US DHHS 1984). "Over 50,000 of the COLD deaths can therefore be considered preventable and premature since these individuals would not have died of COLD if they had not smoked" (US DHHS 1984, p. ii). In 1987, the Economic Report of the President stated, "Smoking presents the largest single source of health risk in America" (U.S. President 1987, p. 184).

This Chapter further delineates the mortality consequences of cigarette smoking in the United States. Deaths attributable to cigarette smoking are reported for two benchmark years—1965 and 1985. The Chapter focuses on the health consequences of smoking for current and former cigarette smokers. Deaths of nonsmokers caused by environmental tobacco smoke (National Research Council 1986; US DHHS1988a) and deaths from cigarette-related fires (Consumer Product Safety Commission 1987; Botkin 1988) are not discussed, nor are the morbidity consequences of cigarette smoking (US DHEW 1979; Rice et al. 1986).

A Twenty-Year Perspective: 1965–85

The two-decade interval, 1965–1985, was selected primarily for reasons of data availability. The year 1985 was the most recent one for which complete, nationwide, cause-specific mortality statistics were available from the National Center for Health Statistics (NCHS). Moreover, in both 1965 and 1985, questions on cigarette use were appended to the National Health Interview Survey (NHIS), a nationally representative, face-to-face interview survey that has been conducted annually by NCHS (Massey et al., 1987; NCHS 1986). In particular, 1985 was the most recent full year for which complete population-weighted data from the NHIS were available (see Chapter 5).

In addition, the years 1965 and 1985 represented the approximate midpoints of two large-scale prospective surveys of smoking and mortality among men and women in the United States, both sponsored by the American Cancer Society. In the first of these two prospective studies (Garfinkel 1980a,b, 1981; Hammond 1961, 1964a,b, 1966, 1968, 1969, 1972; Hammond and Garfinkel 1961, 1964, 1966, 1968, 1969, 1975; Hammond et al. 1976; Hammond and Seidman 1980; Lew and Garfinkel 1984, 1988), about 1 million persons were followed from 1959 through 1972. In the second study (Garfinkel 1985; Stellman and Garfinkel 1986; Stellman, Boffetta, Garfinkel 1988), about 1.2 million participants were followed from 1982 through 1988. The two studies will be referred to, respectively, as "Cancer Prevention Study I (CPS-I)" and "Cancer Prevention Study II (CPS-II)." In particular, this Chapter will present unpublished, preliminary results from the 4-year followup (1982–86) of CPS-II.

The theory, mathematics, limitations, and other methodological issues concerning the calculations of smoking-attributable mortality are described in the next section. The results of the analysis follow thereafter. Readers interested primarily in those results may proceed directly to the Section entitled "Populations at Risk: 1965 and 1985."

The Concept of Attributable Risk

In 1953, Levin estimated that 62 to 92 percent of all male lung cancers were "attributable to cigarette smoking" (Levin 1953). Levin's computations addressed the general problem: How many cases of a disease in a given population can be explained by the presence of a particular hazardous agent or a particular personal trait? Put differently, how many cases would have been avoided but for the presence of the agent or the trait (Doll and Peto 1981)?

In principle, the answer requires an experiment whereby disease rates are measured before and after the complete elimination of the hazardous agent or particular trait from the population of interest. Since this type of experiment is usually impractical, the most widely used approach is to estimate disease rates in representative sample populations of exposed and unexposed persons. The results are then extrapolated to the population of interest.

The phrase "cases *attributable* to agent A" is often used interchangeably with "cases *caused* by agent A." The latter term is meaningful so long as it is recognized that "caused" refers to an entire population rather than to any single, predetermined member of the population. Thus, the scientific validity of an estimate that 1,000 lives would be saved by the removal of some hazardous agent does not hinge upon naming the names of the people to be saved.

The population-based notion of causation is especially important for chronic diseases with multiple causes. Agent A, for example, may promote or enhance the disease-causing effect of agent B. A case-by-case analysis of afflicted individuals may never identify agent A as the primary cause in a single instance. Yet its elimination might substantially reduce disease incidence in the population under study.

Moreover, the concept of attributable risk generally requires a timeframe. In an assessment of the effects of removing a hazardous agent, a researcher could ask how many cases of a specific disease could be avoided in a specified time period, such as 1 year. When the disease has multiple causes, this quantity may differ from the number of cases of the disease that may eventually be avoided. By specifying a timeframe, the researcher inquires not whether such cases could be completely prevented, but whether their premature occurrence could be avoided.

For many diseases, death rates are more accessible and reliable than disease rates. Accordingly, computations of "attributable deaths" from a disease have been used in place of "attributable cases" of the disease. Because death from one cause or another is inevitable, such computations necessarily refer to a specific time period during which premature mortality may have been prevented.

Mathematics of Attributable Risk

Let d_1 and d_0, respectively, denote the incidence rates (in terms of new cases per unit time) of a particular disease among two sample cohorts—one exposed to a hazardous agent, the other unexposed. The two samples are assumed not to differ materially in any other respect, so that both would experience disease incidence d_0 in the absence of exposure. Accordingly, the difference $d_1–d_0$ measures the increase in disease incidence, or absolute risk, due to the agent. Moreover, the unitless ratio $r = d_1/d_0$, termed the relative risk, measures the degree to which the hazardous exposure multiplies the baseline incidence rate. It is often employed as a measure of the epidemiologic and biological significance of an observed association between an agent and a particular disease (Lilienfeld and Lilienfeld 1980; US DHEW 1979).

In the exposed cohort, the proportion of disease cases attributable to the hazardous agent is thus equal to $s=(d_1–d_0)d_1$ (which equals $(r–1)/r$). This quantity has been variously termed the assigned share or probability of causation or attributable proportion of risk among the exposed (Bond 1981; Oftedal, Magnus, Hvinden 1968; Black and Lilienfeld 1984; National Research Council 1984; Cox 1987).

For some hazardous agents, such as cigarette smoke, the disease incidence rates d_1 and d_0 and the relative risk r have been estimated directly from prospective longitudinal studies of exposed and unexposed cohorts. Alternatively, retrospective case–control studies do not provide estimates of d_1 and d_0 but yield a close approximation to the relative risk r when incidence of the disease is low (Cornfield 1951). Both types of studies provide estimates of the assigned share s.

The estimate of relative risk r, derived from epidemiologic studies, is then applied to the population of interest. Let p denote the proportion of exposed persons in the subject population, estimated independently from survey data. Then the quantity $f = pr/[p(r-1)+1]$ is the fraction of all cases of the disease (in a given time interval) that occurs among exposed persons in the subject population. This is sometimes called the "case fraction" (Miettinen 1974). Moreover, if fraction f of all cases occurs among exposed persons, and if fraction s of such exposed cases is attributable to the hazardous agent, then the fraction of all cases attributable to the agent is $a = fs$. From the definitions of f and s, the quantity a can be expressed as

$$a = \frac{p\,(r-1)}{p\,(r-1) + 1} \qquad (1)$$

This is Levin's measure of attributable risk, also termed etiologic fraction (Miettinen 1974), attributable fraction (CDC 1987b), and population-attributable risk (MacMahon and Pugh 1970). When a is expressed in percentage terms, it is often termed percent attributable risk or population-attributable risk percentage.

Equation (1) shows how the attributable risk a depends upon both the relative risk r and the proportion exposed p. Thus, an agent may be significant in the causation of disease among exposed persons so that its relative risk r greatly exceeds 1. Yet that agent may cause a small proportion of all cases of the disease because exposure rates p are low. Conversely, an agent that is widely prevalent (with large p) may contribute substantially to the total number of cases, even when its relative risk r is close to unity.

As a consequence of equation (1), the logistic transformation of a is

$$\log \frac{a}{(1-a)} = \log p + \log (r-1) \qquad (2)$$

where log denotes the natural logarithm. Equation (2) provides a convenient method of decomposing the uncertainty in the attributable risk a into two components—uncertainty in the proportion exposed p and uncertainty in the relative risk r.

Levin's measure of attributable risk can be generalized to cases where there are multiple levels of exposure, multiple causative agents, or confounding or stratifying variables, or when an agent can prevent a disease (Walter 1976; Miettinen 1974). In the case of multiple levels of exposure, it is convenient to let d_k denote the incidence rate and $r_k = d_k/d_0$ denote the relative risk for the k-th exposure level. Similarly, let p_k denote the proportion of the subject population exposed at the k-th level. Then $s_k = (r_k-1)/r_k$ is the assigned share among cases exposed at the k-th level. Likewise, the quantity $f_k = p_k r_k/[\Sigma_k p_k (r_k-1) + 1]$, where Σ_k denotes summation over exposure levels, is the fraction of all cases occurring among persons exposed at the k-th level. The generalized formula for attributable risk becomes $\Sigma_k f_k s_k$, which can be expressed as

$$a = \frac{\Sigma_k p_k \, (r_k-1)}{\Sigma_k p_k \, (r_k-1) + 1} \qquad (3)$$

Let D denote the total number of cases of disease in the population of interest in a given time interval. Then $A = aD$ is the estimated number of cases in the interval that are attributable to the agent. The quantity A is sometimes called "attributable cases." When relative risks or exposure rates vary by age, sex, or other stratifying variables, then separate estimates of A can be made for each combination of variables.

When there are multiple causative agents, attributable risks can be computed for each agent separately and for combined exposures. Thus, if agents X and Y both have a causal role in the development of a particular disease, then the relative risk for agent X may depend upon the presence or absence of exposure to agent Y. When X and Y act synergistically, some portion of the total risk attributable to X will reflect the combined contribution of X and Y. For example, indoor exposure to radon has recently been estimated to account for about 13,300 lung cancer deaths annually in the United States (Lubin and Boice 1988). Radon exposure and cigarette smoking interact synergistically in causing lung cancer (National Research Council 1988). Of the estimated 13,000 deaths attributable to radon exposure, about 11,000 would be due to the combined effect of smoking and radon, while about 2,000 would reflect radon exposure in nonsmokers (Lubin and Boice 1988).

Illustrative Calculation: Smoking and Lung Cancer in Women

Table 1 provides a detailed illustrative application of Levin's method to female deaths from lung cancer in the United States during 1985. The population of female smokers has been divided into ten exposure levels: five categories of current cigarette smokers based on the number consumed per day; and five categories of former cigarette smokers based on the length of time since quitting. For each exposure category, the upper panel shows the estimated prevalence p_k, derived from the 1985 NHIS. Also given are estimates of relative risk r_k derived from the 4-year followup (1982–86) of the second American Cancer Society prospective study (Garfinkel and Stellman 1988). At each exposure level, the upper panel also shows the assigned share s_k and the case fraction f_k.

The computations are summarized in the lower panel of Table 1. For both current and former smokers, as well as for all females at risk, the estimated prevalences p represent the corresponding sums $\Sigma_k\, p_k$ over the prevalence rates p_k in the individual subcategories. The case fractions f likewise represent sums of individual fractions f_k, while the attributable risks a are derived from the corresponding sums $\Sigma_k\, s_k f_k$. Attributable deaths A are derived from the products aD, where $D = 38{,}687$ lung cancer deaths among adult females in 1985.

Table 1 shows that almost two-thirds of all female lung cancer deaths occurred among women who currently smoke one pack or more daily or who have quit smoking within the last 5 years. Nine out of ten lung cancer deaths occurred in women with any history of regular cigarette use. Cigarette smoking accounted for an estimated 82 percent of lung cancer deaths in women, or 31,600 deaths in 1985. About 9,300 (or 29 percent) of the 31,600 female lung cancer deaths that were caused by smoking occurred among former smokers.

Both the prevalence rates and the relative risks in Table 1 are subject to sampling variability. By a formula analogous to equation (2), a standard error for the logistic transformation of a can be derived. Under the assumption that D has no sampling

TABLE 1.—Detailed computation of smoking-attributable lung cancer deaths among females, United States, 1985

Exposure category	Prevalence p (%)	Relative risk[a] r	Assigned share s (%)	Case fraction f (%)
Current smokers				
1–10 per day[b]	9.3	5.5	81.9	9.4
11–19 per day	3.3	11.3	91.1	6.7
20 per day	9.3	14.2	93.0	24.0
21–30 per day	3.2	20.4	95.1	11.8
≥31 per day	2.7	22.3	95.5	10.8
Former smokers				
0–2 years[c]	5.0	18.2	94.1	16.7
3–5 years	2.5	11.2	91.1	5.0
6–10 years	3.4	4.9	79.5	3.0
11–15 years	2.0	3.2	68.5	1.2
≥16 years	4.0	1.8	43.4	1.3

Exposure category	Prevalence p (%)	Case fractions f(%)	Attributable risk a (%)	Attributable deaths[d] A
Current smokers	27.8	62.7	57.7	22,300
Former smokers	16.9	27.2	24.1	9,300
Current and former smokers	44.7	89.9	81.8	31,600

[a]Ratio of age-adjusted death rates, where age adjustment was performed by direct standardization to the age distribution of woman-years of exposure among nonsmokers.
[b]Number of cigarettes smoked per day, as of the date of enrollment (September 1982).
[c]Number of years elapsed since last smoked regularly, as of the date of enrollment (September 1982).
[d]Attributable deaths A equal aD, where a is attributable risk and D equals 38,687 lung cancer deaths among adult females in 1985.
SOURCE: Garfinkel and Stellman (1988); NHIS 1985, unpublished tabulations; NCHS, Division of Vital Statistics, 1985, unpublished.

variability, statistical confidence bounds for A can also be calculated. For the calculation shown in Table 1, the estimated 95-percent confidence interval on a for all smokers was 72.1 to 88.6 percent. The corresponding confidence interval for D was 27,900 to 34,300 deaths. Only 2.6 percent of the variance of the logistic transformation of a was due to sampling variability of prevalence rates.

Uncertainties in Attributable Risk

Aggregation Bias Versus Statistical Precision

Sampling variation is not the sole source of uncertainty in estimates of attributable risk. The computations of Table 1 entail the assumption that the relative risks r_k depend only upon the specified indices of current and former smoke exposure.

Thus, for former cigarette smokers in Table 1, the degree of risk after cessation of smoking is shown as depending only upon the length of cessation. Yet the magnitude of the residual risk also depends upon the extent of prior cigarette smoke exposure (Hammond 1968; Lubin et al. 1984) and the reason for stopping (Kahn 1966). Also, some persons may have quit smoking after lung cancer had been diagnosed. As Table 1 shows, women who had stopped smoking for 16 or more years at the time of enrollment into CPS-II had a subsequent 4-year relative risk of lung cancer equal to 1.8. Within this group of long-term quitters, however, those women who had previously smoked 21 or more cigarettes daily had an estimated relative risk of 4.0 (Garfinkel and Stellman 1988).

Likewise, for current smokers in Table 1, the degree of lung cancer risk is shown as depending only upon the current number of cigarettes smoked per day. Yet the risk depends critically upon the lifetime dosage of cigarette smoking, especially the duration of cigarette use and the age of initiation of regular smoking (Brown and Kessler 1988; Doll and Peto 1978, 1981; Peto 1986; US DHHS 1982). While the relative risk r was 22.3 for all women currently smoking 31 or more cigarettes daily (Table 1), it was 18.9 for heavy smokers of 18 to 30 years' duration and 38.8 for heavy smokers of more than 40 years (Garfinkel and Stellman 1988).

A more detailed, multidimensional breakdown of exposure levels may minimize errors of classification, but such disaggregation also increases the sampling variability of the estimates. Conversely, increased aggregation of exposure levels will reduce sampling variability. Thus, if relative risk were assumed to depend only upon present smoking status (current versus former), then the estimated attributable risk for female lung cancer deaths in 1985 would be 80 percent, with a confidence range of 77 to 83 percent. The confidence range of attributable deaths A would be narrowed to 29,700 to 32,000.

Age-Standardization

The relative risks in Table 1 were estimated as a ratio of age-adjusted death rates, where the age adjustment was performed by direct standardization to the age distribution of nonsmokers' person-years at risk. In principle, if the relative risk is in fact age independent, then the estimate of relative risk in large samples should not be very sensitive to the choice of the standard population (Anderson et al. 1980). In practice, however, the estimates can depend strongly upon the standard population. For the illustrative calculation in Table 1, the use of the entire population of CPS-II woman-years at risk (rather than nonsmokers only) resulted in an attributable risk for lung cancer of 79 percent, with a confidence range of 75 to 82 percent (see Table 11).

Potential Biases in Applying the Results of Prospective Studies to the General Population

Subjects enrolled in the CPS-II prospective study constituted over 1.5 percent of all American adults age 45 and over (Stellman, Boffetta, Garfinkel 1988). Still, they differed from the U.S. population in a number of ways (Garfinkel 1985; Stellman and Garfinkel 1986). CPS-II entrants were more highly educated. The black and Hispanic populations were underrepresented, though less so than in CPS-I (Garfinkel 1985). As in CPS-I, institutionalized and seriously ill persons, as well as illiterate people who could not complete a questionnaire, were excluded (Lew and Garfinkel 1984). In both CPS-I and CPS-II, the overall mortality rates of the enrollees fell substantially below those of the general U.S. population (Hammond 1969; Lew and Garfinkel 1988).

These considerations do not by themselves invalidate the use of CPS-II to estimate smoking-attributable risks for the entire American population. The critical assumption in Table 1 above is whether the estimated relative risks r_k—not the absolute death rates d_k—are representative of the general population.

For CHD and for all-cause mortality, CPS-I subjects who were reportedly well at the time of enrollment showed higher estimated relative risks of cigarette smoking than those subjects who said they were sick or who gave a recent history of cancer, heart disease, or stroke (Hammond and Garfinkel 1969; Lew and Garfinkel 1988). A similar elevation of relative risk in well subjects has been found for lung cancer in CPS-II (Garfinkel and Stellman 1988). Since initially well persons had lower disease rates, the proportional effect of cigarette smoking appeared to be larger. While CPS-I and CPS-II excluded seriously ill and institutionalized persons, the magnitude of the resulting bias is unclear. In the 1980 U.S. Census, about 1.5 percent of the U.S. adult population was institutionalized. Among persons aged 65 years and over, the proportion was 5.3 percent (U.S. Bureau of the Census 1986).

Cigarette smoking has been found to act synergistically with certain workplace exposures (such as asbestos and ionizing radiation) in the development of lung cancer (US DHHS 1985; Saracci 1987; National Research Council 1988). Such interactions may also be present in the etiology of nonneoplastic lung disease. Alcohol and tobacco likewise interact synergistically in the etiology of oral and esophageal cancer (US DHEW 1979). Moreover, cigarette smoking has been found to interact synergistically with elevated serum cholesterol and elevated blood pressure in enhancing the risk of CHD (US DHHS 1983). Persons of lower socioeconomic status (SES) may be more likely to receive such workplace exposures, to consume alcohol heavily, or to have unfavorable CHD risk factors. However, if the effects of cigarette smoking are multiplicative, then exclusion of such persons from CPS-I and CPS-II would not bias the estimated relative risks of disease due to cigarette smoking. Conversely, if the effects of cigarette smoking are purely additive, rather than synergistic, then the exclusion of persons with elevated baseline disease rates would bias upward the estimated relative risks of disease due to smoking.

The estimated relative risks in Table 1 are specific to women and have been standardized for age. Standardization for other stratifying or confounding variables was not performed. In principle, failure to control for such variables could bias upward or downward the estimated relative risks due to cigarette use. As discussed in Chapter 2, numerous attempts to control statistically for confounding and stratifying variables have not materially altered the estimated relative risks for cigarette-related diseases.

In the illustrative computation of Table 1, no distinction among the races has been drawn. For both sexes, the prevalence of current cigarette use is higher for blacks than for whites. Conversely, smaller fractions of black men and women are former cigarette smokers (US DHHS 1988b). Black persons were underrepresented in CPS-II, constituting only 4 percent of entrants (Stellman and Garfinkel 1986). Hence, the relative risks reported in Table 1 may not be accurate for black women. Among the 38,687 adult female lung cancer deaths in 1985, a total of 3,392 (8.8 percent) occurred in black women. Hypothetically, if the attributable risks *a* among black women had been only half those of whites, then the smoking-attributable lung cancer deaths in Table 1 would be reduced from 31,600 to 30,300.

In prospective cohort studies, mortality rates tend to be reduced in the initial year or two of followup. This phenomenon of lower initial mortality results from a tendency to exclude persons who are sick at the outset of the study. In particular, the relative risks in Table 1 were derived from the 4-year followup (1982–86) of CPS-II subjects. Accordingly, it is possible that the planned 6-year followup of CPS-II (1982–88) will reveal somewhat lower relative risks than those reported for the first 4 years.

Conversely, measurements of exposure and other personal characteristics, typically obtained at the start of a prospective study, become less accurate as the duration of followup increases. The relative risks reported in Table 1, for example, have been classified according to the subjects' cigarette smoking practices upon enrollment in 1982. If many women who were current smokers in 1982 had in fact quit smoking by 1986, then the reported relative risks for "current" smokers are actually those of a mixture of current and former smokers.

In the analysis reported below, the 4-year followup of CPS-II is to be compared with the 6-year followup of CPS-I. Such a comparison needs to be interpreted in light of potential biases arising from short- and long-duration followup in prospective studies.

Uncertainties in Exposure

Potential errors in estimated exposure rates p_k are a further source of uncertainty in the computation of attributable risk *a*. In the illustrative calculation of Table 1, such exposure rates were derived from the 1985 NHIS, a large-scale, stratified, face-to-face household interview survey of the noninstitutionalized civilian population of the United States. Among the possible errors in NHIS estimates are: underreporting or misreporting of current cigarette use; inaccurate recall of past cigarette smoking; nonresponse biases due to exclusion of some persons not available for interview; and underrepresentation of certain population segments. These sources of uncertainty are discussed in Chapter 5. On the whole, NHIS-derived estimates of population smoking rates have been consistent with other face-to-face interview surveys (CDC 1987a).

Errors in the Classification of Causes of Death

The estimation of attributable deaths A requires information on total deaths D. For the computation in Table 1, the latter quantity was defined as deaths in 1985 whose underlying cause was primary lung cancer (International Classification of Diseases, Ninth Revision [ICD-9], Code 162). Deaths from the larger class of Respiratory Cancers (ICD-9 Codes 162–165) were not used because they include pleural mesotheliomas and secondary lung cancers. Still, the use of ICD-9 Code 162 alone may not eliminate all errors of death certification. In a review of over 1,300 thoracic cancer deaths in Minnesota between 1979 and 1981, Lilienfeld and Gunderson (1986) identified four cases of pleural malignant mesothelioma that had been classified as Code 162.9. Moreover, it is at least arguable that physicians in recent years have been reluctant to diagnose primary lung cancer in the absence of a history of cigarette smoking (McFarlane et al. 1986).

While errors in disease classification and death certification of lung cancer in 1985 may be relatively minor, the same cannot be said with assurance about other diseases caused by cigarette use. Thus, deaths certified as being caused by CHD (ICD-9 Codes 410–414) may not adequately reflect the lethal consequences of cigarette use on the cardiovascular system. Many deaths from Hypertensive Diseases (Codes 401–404, including Hypertensive Heart Disease, 402, and Hypertensive Disease, 404) may have been aggravated by cigarette use. Similarly, deaths certified as being caused by COPD (ICD-9 Codes 490–492 and 496) may incompletely reflect the numbers of deaths from nonneoplastic respiratory disease due to smoking. Many cases of Influenza and Pneumonia (ICD-9 Codes 480–487) may not have been lethal but for the coexistence of cigarette-induced lung damage.

The major prospective studies of cigarette smoking and mortality that were initiated in the 1950s relied upon the International Classification of Diseases, Seventh Revision (ICD-7) (Hammond 1966; Dorn 1959; Kahn 1966; Rogot 1974; Rogot and Murray 1980; Doll and Hill 1956, 1964, 1966; Doll et al. 1980; Doll and Peto 1976). Coding conventions have changed considerably since ICD-7 was adopted in 1955 (Klebba 1975, 1982; Klebba and Scott 1980). While ICD-7 Code 162 was reserved for lung cancer that was "specified as primary," a separate code 163 was allocated to lung cancers "not specified as primary or secondary." In practice, however, epidemiologists and vital statisticians recognized that the great fraction of lung cancer deaths certified under ICD-7 Code 163 were primary and that deaths certified under the two codes were in fact indistinguishable. Accordingly, it was standard procedure to report combined deaths for Codes 162 and 163—a practice adhered to in the analysis below. Still, the use of the combined category 162–163 in ICD-7 may have introduced greater diagnostic uncertainty than the current use of Code 162 in ICD-9.

Previous Estimates of Attributable Risk from Cigarette Smoking

Many authors have estimated the number or proportion of deaths attributable to cigarette use, either from a single cause, a group of causes, or all causes (Ravenholt 1964, 1984; Rice et al. 1986; McIntosh 1984; Whyte 1976; Hammond and Seidman

1980; Doll and Peto 1981; Garfinkel 1980a; U.S. Office of Technology Assessment (US OTA) 1985; Schultz 1986; Goldbaum et al. 1987; CDC 1987b). Doll and Peto (1981) estimated 83,000 smoking-attributable deaths from lung cancer in 1978. Rice and colleagues (1986, Table 5) estimated 270,000 smoking-attributable deaths among U.S. adults in 1980, including 86,000 from CHD, 75,000 from lung cancer, and 14,000 from "emphysema, chronic bronchitis." The Centers for Disease Control (1987b) estimated 315,000 smoking-attributable deaths for 1984, including 77,000 from CHD, 93,000 from lung cancer, and 51,000 from "chronic bronchitis, emphysema" combined with "chronic airways obstruction."

These studies differ with respect to specific causes of disease, the time period under consideration, the populations at risk, the sources of epidemiologic data, and the specific methodology for estimation of risk. Thus, some researchers have directly applied Levin's measure of attributable risk, as defined in equations (1) and (3) (Rice et al. 1986; McIntosh 1984; CDC 1987b; Goldbaum et al. 1987; Whyte 1976). In doing so, they assumed that estimates of relative risk r, derived from particular epidemiologic studies, could be extrapolated to the population under consideration. By contrast, Hammond and Seidman (1980) and Garfinkel (1980a) computed attributable risks directly for the CPS-I study population.

In an analysis of avoidable deaths from cancer, Doll and Peto (1981) employed a different model. Let N denote the size of the population at risk, while D denotes the total number of deaths from a specific cause. If d_0 denotes the cause-specific death rate among unexposed persons, then $D - d_0 N$ is an estimate of the number of deaths attributable to the exposure. To estimate attributable cancer risks for the United States in 1978, Doll and Peto (1981) then assumed that the age- and sex-specific cancer mortality rates for nonsmokers d_0 observed in CPS-I during 1959–72 could be applied to nonsmokers in the general population in 1978. In support of such an assumption, they note that for men, nonsmokers' cancer rates in other prospective studies (Kahn 1966; Doll and Peto 1976) closely matched those observed in CPS-I (Doll and Peto 1981). Moreover, CPS-I lung cancer rates of nonsmoking women were similar to those of U.S. women in 1950, before their lung cancer rates began to increase.

Doll and Peto's method was employed by OTA (1985) to estimate attributable deaths from CHD (US OTA 1985). For cancer, nonsmoker death rates in CPS-I may well approximate d_0 for the U.S. population. But the same conclusion does not appear to be warranted for CHD (Sterling and Weinkam 1987). In fact, the use of CPS-I nonsmoker death rates yielded an estimate of 142,000 smoking-attributable deaths from CHD in 1982. By contrast, application of the Levin method gave an estimate of 91,000 deaths (US OTA 1985).

Doll and Peto (1981) rejected the application of relative risks derived from CPS-I to the U.S. population in 1978. Their central concern was that such relative risks had increased in the two decades since the start of CPS-I in 1959. Among smokers aged 60 years or more in 1965, a much smaller fraction had smoked regularly during early life. For older women smokers, in particular, only one in eight had begun to smoke regularly as a teenager. This proportion increased markedly in subsequent decades (Chapter 5). In view of the importance of quantity and duration of smoking in determining lung cancer risk—and especially in view of the critical role of early-life smoking in the etiology of smoking-induced cancers (Peto 1986)—it was highly likely that the relative risks for smoking-induced cancers would have increased since the early 1960s. (See also Doll et al. 1980.)

Accordingly, there may be serious biases in the application of relative risks from 1960s prospective epidemiologic studies to 1980s populations. Such potential biases constitute the most serious criticism of prior studies of smoking-attributable deaths. Updated epidemiologic evidence for the 1980s is needed to address this criticism.

Populations At Risk: 1965 and 1985

Table 2 and Figures 1 through 5 describe the populations at risk in 1965 and 1985. While Table 2 reports the percentages of smokers, the figures show the absolute numbers of U.S. resident adults in each smoking category for each year. Children and young adults under age 18, who may also suffer adverse effects from cigarette use, are excluded from Table 2 and the figures.

In both 1965 and 1985, respondents to the NHIS were asked, "Have you smoked at least 100 cigarettes in your entire life?" Those who answered affirmatively were then asked how much they smoked currently or, if they were not current smokers, when they

TABLE 2.—Prevalence of cigarette smoking, persons aged 18 years or more, United States, 1965 and 1985

	1965[a] (%)	1985[b] (%)
Males		
Current smokers[c]	53.4	32.7
Former smokers	20.8	29.1
Never smoked regularly[d]	25.8	32.8
Females		
Current smokers[c]	34.1	27.5
Former smokers	8.1	17.1
Never smoked regularly[d]	57.8	55.4

NOTE: Prevalence estimates for 1965 and 1985 have been directly standardized to the age distributions of the U.S. resident populations in each year, respectively (U.S. Bureau of the Census 1974, 1986).

[a]Based upon 52,873 self-responses to the Cigarette Smoking Supplement to the 1965 National Health Interview Survey. Standard errors 0.3 to 0.4 percent for males, 0.1 to 0.2 percent for females. Inclusion of 33,422 additional proxy responses resulted in the following estimates: male current smokers, 51.9 percent; male former smokers, 19.0 percent; female current smokers, 33.6 percent; and female former smokers, 7.7 percent.

[b]Based upon 32,859 self-responses to the Cigarette Smoking Supplement to the 1985 National Health Interview Survey. Standard errors 0.4 percent for males, 0.3 percent for females.

[c]In 1965, current smokers included all respondents who reported a current number smoked per day, including "less than 1 per day." In 1985, current smokers included all respondents who answered affirmatively to the question "Do you smoke now?"

[d]In both 1965 and 1985, the category "never smoked regularly" included two groups of respondents: (1) those who answered negatively to the question "Have you ever smoked at least 100 cigarettes in your life?"; and (2) those who answered affirmatively but denied ever smoking cigarettes regularly. In 1965 and 1985, respectively, group 1 accounted for 99 percent and 97 percent of all respondents in the category "never smoked regularly."

last smoked regularly. While the NHIS for 1965 permitted proxy respondents, the estimates in both years have been derived from self-respondents only (see Note b of Table 2).

Table 2 shows the percentage distribution among adult men and women in three categories: current smokers, former smokers, and those who never smoked regularly. Between 1965 and 1985, the proportions of current smokers declined and the proportions of former smokers increased. The most marked change was the decline in the prevalence of current cigarette use among adult men.

In Figure 1, the responses have been further divided into four categories: current smokers of fewer than 25 cigarettes daily; current smokers of 25 or more cigarettes daily; former smokers who quit within the last 5 years; and former smokers who stopped for more than 5 years. The weighted proportions in each category, tabulated by age and sex, were then multiplied by the corresponding estimates of the U.S. resident population (U.S. Bureau of the Census 1974, 1986).

In 1965, there were an estimated 53.7 million adult current cigarette smokers (standard error, 0.2 million), which represented about 43 percent of all U.S. residents aged 18 years or more. By 1985, there were an estimated 53.5 million adult current smokers, composing 30 percent of U.S. adults. While the total number of current smokers stayed about the same, there was a shift in their distribution by sex. The number of adult male current smokers declined from 31.7 million (53.4 percent) in 1965 to 28.2 million (32.7 percent) in 1985, while adult female smokers increased from 22.0 million (34.1 percent) to 25.3 million (27.5 percent) (Figure 1).

In 1965, about 28 percent of adult male smokers who were nonproxy respondents to the NHIS consumed 25 or more cigarettes per day (Figure 1). By 1985, this proportion had risen to 32 percent. For women, the proportions of heavier current smokers rose from 14 percent of nonproxy respondents in 1965 to 21 percent of smokers in 1985. The true population prevalence of smoking 25 or more cigarettes per day in 1965 is somewhat uncertain because the elimination of proxy respondents may make the sample nonrepresentative. As shown in Chapter 5, however, there was no significant change in the proportion of heavy smokers between 1974 and 1985.

By contrast, the numbers of former smokers increased substantially between 1965 and 1985. Thus, in 1965, there were about 17.6 million adult former smokers (12.4 million men and 5.2 million women). By 1985, this number had risen to 40.9 million (25.2 million men and 15.7 million women). There was an increase in the proportion of former smokers who had stopped for more than 5 years (from 49 to 63 percent of male former smokers, and from 41 to 57 percent of female former smokers) (Figure 1).

Cigarette Smoking and Other Forms of Tobacco Use

Figure 2 shows the 1965 and 1985 adult populations broken down according to the type of tobacco used. In 1965, the NHIS included questions on cigar and pipe smoking as well as cigarette use. The 1985 questionnaire inquired only about cigarette smoking. However, questions about all forms of tobacco use, including smokeless tobacco, were included on a supplement to the 1985 Current Population Survey, performed by the U.S. Bureau of the Census (see Chapter 5).

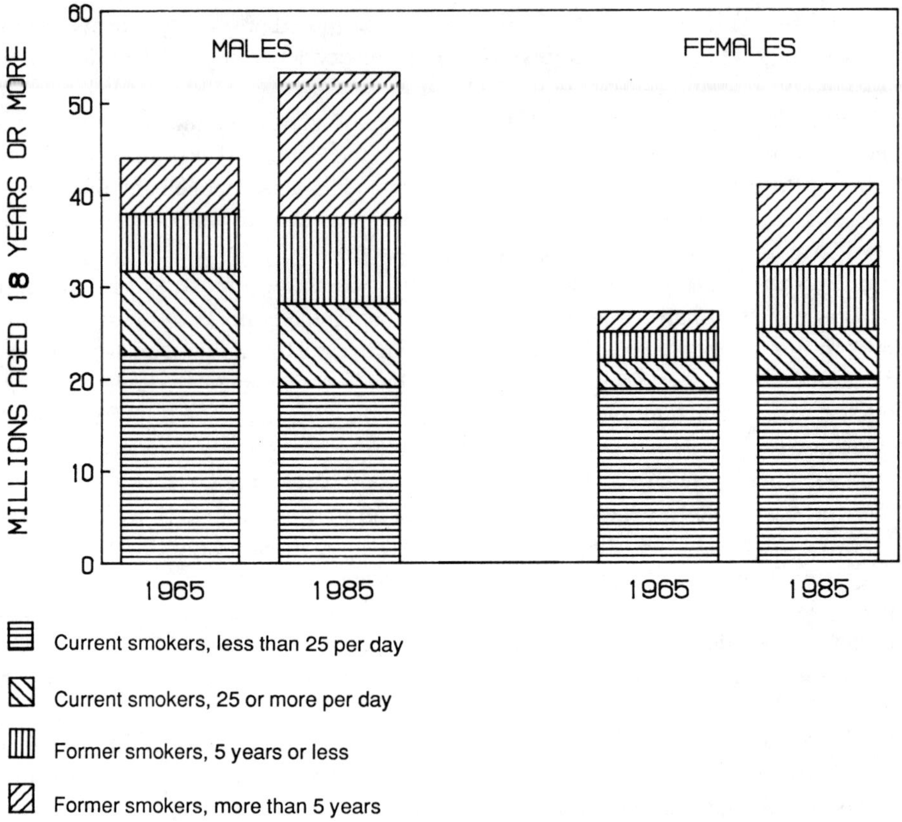

FIGURE 1.—Populations of current and former cigarette smokers, adult men and women, United States, 1965 and 1985

SOURCE: Estimated from unpublished tabulations, NHISs 1965 and 1985; and estimates of the resident populations of the United States by age and sex, 1965 and 1985 (US Bureau of the Census 1974, 1986).

Figure 2 shows a marked change over two decades in the forms of tobacco used by men. In 1965, 5.2 million men (9 percent) had a history of ever smoking pipes or cigars, but not cigarettes. In 1985, the number using noncigarette tobacco dropped to 2.7 million or 3 percent of the men. In 1965, 29 million men had a history of ever smoking cigarettes and other forms of tobacco, about two-thirds of all cigarette smokers. By 1985, the number had dropped to 5.6 million, only 1 in 10 of all cigarette smokers.

Older Cohorts of Cigarette Smokers

Figures 3 and 4 focus on persons aged 60 years and over, who suffer the highest incidence rates of smoking-related diseases. For 1965 and 1985, respectively, these groups of older persons were born before 1906 and before 1926. Among older men, as shown in Figure 3, the two-decade interval witnessed a 136-percent increase in the number of former cigarette smokers. Among older women, the number of current smokers

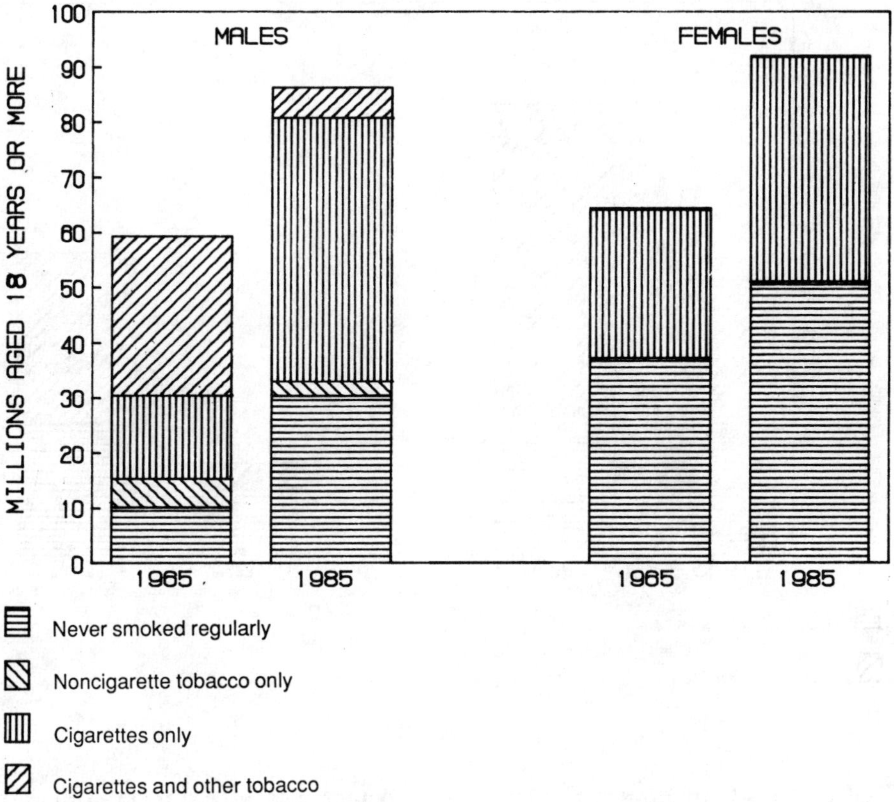

FIGURE 2.—Populations of adult men and women classified by history of tobacco use, United States, 1965 and 1985

SOURCE: Estimated from unpublished tabulations, NHISs 1965 and 1985; unpublished tabulations, CPS 1985; and estimates of the resident populations of the United States by age and sex, 1965 and 1985 (US Bureau of the Census 1974, 1986).

doubled, while the number of former smokers increased sixfold. Between 1965 and 1985, the population of older women with a history of regular cigarette use, past or present, increased over threefold.

The NHISs for 1965 and 1985 did not ask about the age of initiation of cigarette use. However, this information is available from other sources. For 1985, tabulations of the age of onset of regular cigarette use were made from the Current Population Survey. About 69 percent of older men with a history of cigarette use, past or present, began to smoke before age 20 (Figure 4). Among older women, the proportion was 39 percent.

For 1965, three sources of information provide the age of smoking initiation among cohorts born before 1906: the NHISs of 1978–80 (Harris 1983), the Current Population Survey of 1955 (Haenszel et al. 1956), and the initial 1959 questionnaire to CPS-I (Hammond 1966, Appendix tables). For older men with a history of cigarette use, about 60 percent started smoking before age 20 (range, 56 to 62 percent). For older women smokers, about 12 percent started in their teenage years (range, 9 to 15 percent).

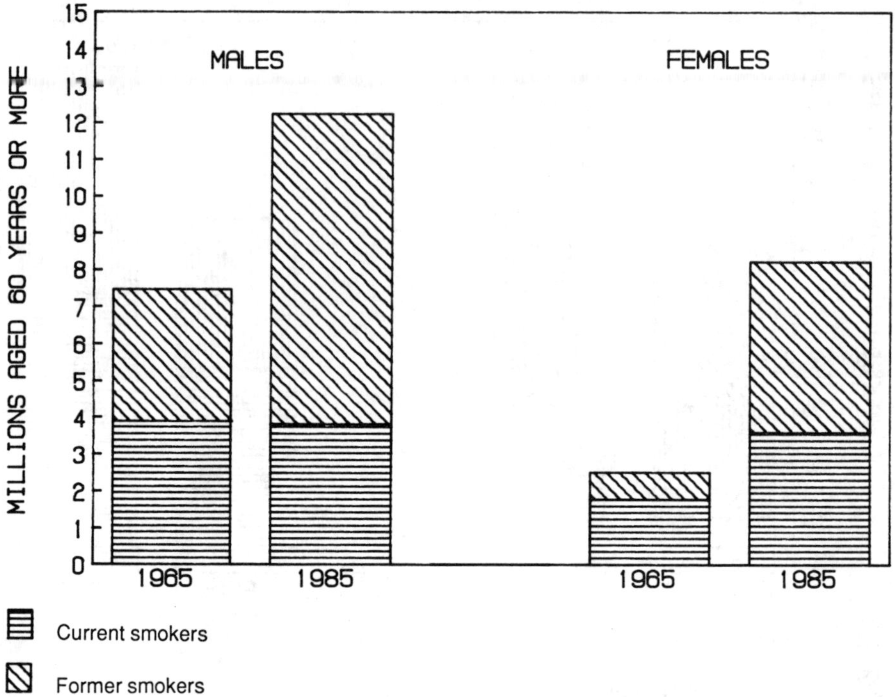

FIGURE 3.—Populations of current and former cigarette smokers, men and women aged 60 years or more, United States, 1965 and 1985

SOURCE: Estimated from unpublished tabulations, NHISs 1965 and 1985; and estimates of the resident populations of the United States by age and sex, 1965 and 1985 (US Bureau of the Census 1974, 1986).

Accordingly, the period between 1965 and 1985 saw a marked increase in the number of women smokers who reached the age of 60 years (Figures 3 and 4). Moreover, the number of such women who started smoking in their teens increased by about tenfold (Figure 4). Additional data on age of initiation are presented in Chapter 5.

Overlapping Populations at Risk

In 1965, a total of 71.3 million adults had a history of regular cigarette smoking, past or present. By 1985, this count had increased to 94.4 million. These two populations overlapped. Among the adult population at risk in 1985, about 54.8 million were born before 1948, and therefore they were also aged 18 years or more in 1965. About 95 percent of the latter group began to smoke during 1965 or earlier (Harris 1983; unpublished tabulations from the Current Population Survey 1985). This means that about 51.8 million adults, who had ever smoked in 1985, had also been at risk in 1965.

The overlap is depicted graphically in Figure 5, where the diagonal lines show the populations common to both years. Among 44.1 million adult men with a history of

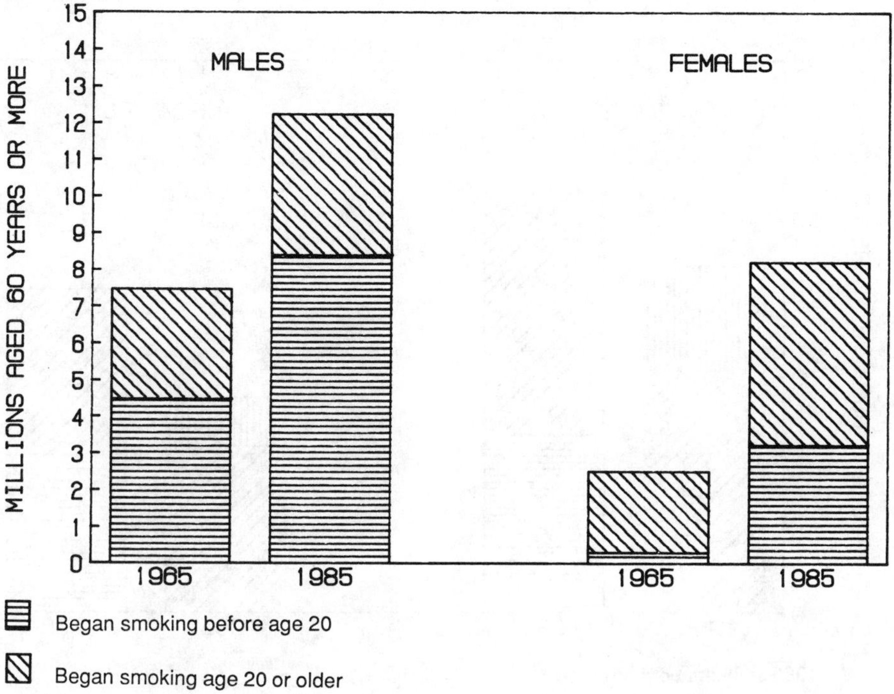

FIGURE 4.—Populations of men and women aged 60 years or more with a history of regular cigarette smoking, classified by age started to smoke regularly, United States, 1965 and 1985

SOURCE: Estimated from Harris (1983); Haenszel et al. (1956); Hammond (1966); unpublished tabulations, NHISs 1965 and 1985; unpublished tabulations, CPS 1985; and estimates of the resident populations of the United States by age and sex, 1965 and 1985 (US Bureau of the Census 1974, 1986).

cigarette smoking in 1965, about 30.8 million survived to 1985. The vertical lines show the remaining 13.3 million men who died before 1985 (standard error, 0.4 million). Likewise, among 27.2 million adult women with a smoking history in 1965 (diagonal lines and vertical lines combined), about 6.2 million died before 1985 (vertical lines). Not all of the decedents, however, died as a consequence of their cigarette use.

The horizontal lines in Figure 5 show the populations of adults at risk in 1985 who were not also at risk in 1965. The estimates are 22.6 million men and 20.0 million women. These counts do not include persons who may have taken up smoking after 1965 but died before 1985. Nor do they include smokers under age 18 in 1965 and 1985. Still, it appears that in the two-decade period following the 1964 Surgeon General's Report and the 1965 Federal Cigarette Labeling and Advertising Act, some 43 million Americans took up regular cigarette smoking, either temporarily or permanently. About two-thirds of them began to smoke by age 18.

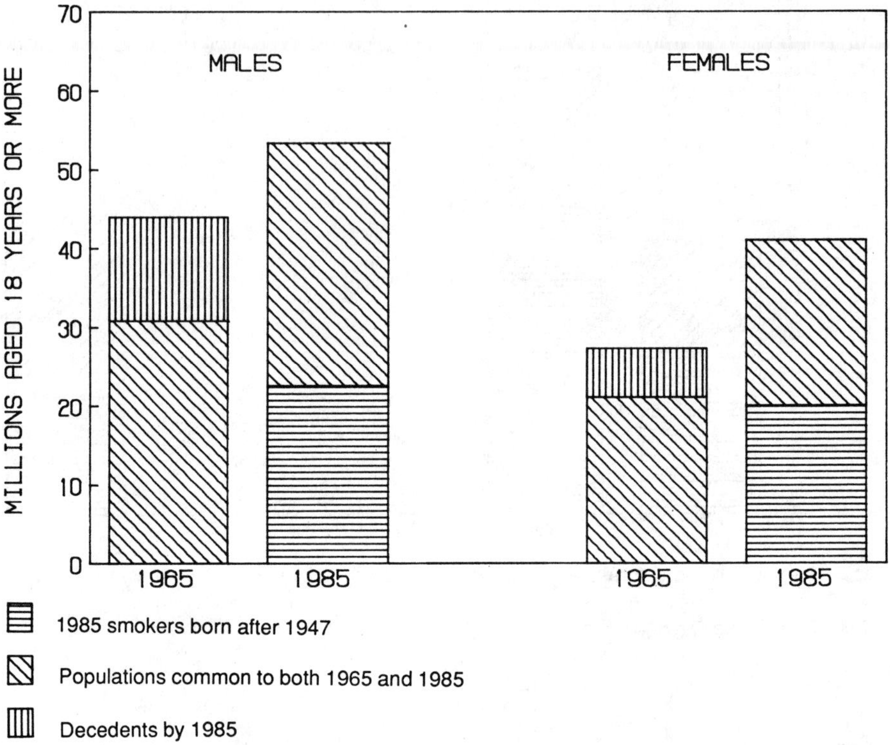

FIGURE 5.—Populations of adult men and women with a history of regular cigarette smoking, United States, 1965 and 1985

SOURCE: Estimated from Harris (1983); unpublished tabulations, NHISs 1965 and 1985; unpublished tabulations, CPS 1985; and estimates of the resident populations of the United States by age and sex, 1965 and 1985 (US Bureau of the Census 1974, 1986).

Changes in the Cigarette Product

The 1965 and 1985 population surveys did not elicit information on the type of cigarette smoked. However, there was a decline in the average tar and nicotine yield of cigarettes, at least as measured by the U.S. Federal Trade Commission (FTC) using smoking machines under standardized conditions (Chapters 2 and 5). Data on aggregate cigarette sales and other population surveys (US DHEW 1979; US DHHS 1980, 1981; Chapter 5) also show that the proportion of persons smoking filter-tipped cigarettes increased substantially. Among entrants into CPS-II in 1982, more than 90 percent were filter-tipped-cigarette smokers. In this group, there was an average of 18 years of filter-tipped-cigarette smoking prior to enrollment (Stellman and Garfinkel 1986). The majority of these persons had smoked nonfilter cigarettes earlier in life.

It remains problematic whether such changes in cigarette manufacture and patterns of cigarette smoking have substantially reduced risks to cigarette smokers. There is considerable evidence that the actual reduction in the dangerous chemicals in cigarette smoke is much smaller than implied by the FTC machine measurements (US DHHS 1988a). While there is evidence that the long-term use of filter cigarettes and low-tar cigarettes may somewhat reduce the risk of lung cancers, there are considerably fewer data on a protective effect for other smoking-induced diseases (Alderson et al. 1985; Castelli et al. 1981; Hawthorne and Fry 1978; Kaufman et al. 1983; Lee and Garfinkel 1981; Lubin et al. 1984; Hammond et al. 1976; Wynder and Stellman 1979; US DHHS 1981; Wilcox et al. 1988; Stellman 1986a,b).

During the 1965–85 period, numerous chemical treatments and additives have been applied to cigarettes during tobacco curing and storage, sheet reconstitution, puffing, casing, and cigarette assembly. The chemicals include humectants, pesticides, flavorings, plasticizers, ash adhesives, and other agents. Cigarette filters, plug wraps, and tipping papers have evolved. The mix of domestic tobaccos has also changed, and oriental varieties have been added increasingly to American cigarette blends. The details of these product changes remain proprietary (US DHHS 1981).

Other Changes in the Cigarette Smoking Population

The present comparison of populations at risk in 1965 and 1985 has been confined to sex, age, and history of tobacco use. Still, there may have been other changes in the characteristics of persons who smoke cigarettes.

Surveys such as the NHIS have consistently shown a socioeconomic gradient in current cigarette use, as measured by education, occupation, and other characteristics (US DHEW 1979; US DHHS 1980; Novotny et al. 1988; US DHHS 1988a; Brackbill, Frazier, Shilling 1988; Chapter 5). There is some evidence that socioeconomic differentials in smoking rates have widened. The proportionate decline in adult smoking rates between 1965 and 1985 was highest for people who had graduated from college and lowest for those who had not completed high school (Chapter 5). Between 1970 and 1980, white-collar men and women showed proportionately greater declines in smoking rates than their blue-collar counterparts (US DHHS 1985).

Among the factors that may influence the risks of cigarette smoking are: the coexistence of untreated hypertension; elevated serum cholesterol; consumption of oral contraceptives; alcohol use; diabetes mellitus; and workplace exposure to other toxic and carcinogenic agents such as asbestos and radon daughters. With respect to these factors, it needs to be determined whether the typical cigarette user of the 1980s differs from his or her counterpart of the 1960s.

Cigarette smokers have higher rates of alcohol use, are more sedentary, and are less likely to wear seat belts (Schoenborn and Benson 1988; Williamson et al. 1986). It is unknown whether these relationships have strengthened or weakened over the years. There is evidence in the American population of declines in dietary cholesterol, in dietary saturated fat as a percentage of total calories, and in serum cholesterol levels (Havlik and Feinbeib 1979). The prevalence of untreated and inadequately treated hypertension has also declined (Havlik and Feinleib 1979). However, detailed studies of the clustering of cigarette smoking with other risk factors for CHD are unavailable. It remains unclear whether the observed long-term declines in hypercholesterolemia and hypertension have been more or less pronounced in cigarette smokers than in nonsmokers. There is some evidence that cigarette smoking reduces therapeutic effectiveness of new pharmacologic and invasive treatments of CHD (Deanfield et al. 1984; Galan et al. 1988). Finally, in 1965, oral contraceptives were just coming into widespread use. By 1985, oral contraceptive use was prevalent among both smokers and nonsmokers (Goldbaum et al. 1987).

Those Smokers Most at Risk in 1985 Were Also Smokers in 1965

In sum, between 1965 and 1985, there have been major changes in the populations of smokers at risk for cigarette-related injury. In 1965, most men who smoked cigarettes had also used cigars and pipes. However, by 1985 the great majority smoked cigarettes exclusively. In 1965, about 40 percent of current smokers were women. By 1985, women numbered almost half of current smokers.

Moreover, the numbers of former smokers increased substantially in both sexes—especially in men. In 1965, about one-quarter of all living men (self-respondents to NHIS, age 18 or older) with a history of regular cigarette use were former smokers. By 1985, former smokers made up almost half of all living men age 18 or older who ever smoked. Finally, the two-decade interval witnessed a substantial increase in the number of women smokers reaching the age of 60 years, with a tenfold rise in the population of older women who had begun to smoke as teenagers.

These changes in the population at risk have also been observed in other, nonrandom samples of the U.S. smoking population, including a recent comparison of the 1959 entrants into CPS-I with the 1982 entrants into CPS-II (Stellman and Garfinkel 1986). The percentage of male smokers who smoked 20 or more cigarettes per day in CPS II (76 percent) was higher than in CPS-I (69 percent); the percentage of female smokers who smoked 20 or more cigarettes per day increased even more from CPS-I to CPS-II (43 percent to 61 percent).

Among the 94.4 million adults in 1985 with a history of cigarette use, about 51.8 million smoked cigarettes as adults before 1966. The youngest of these persons is now in his or her late thirties. This group represents the vast majority of persons who are now at risk for the fatal and nonfatal consequences of cigarette smoking.

Cancer Prevention Study I and Cancer Prevention Study II

CPS-I, formerly termed the American Cancer Society 25-State study, began in October 1959 and ended in October 1972. Over 1 million men and women, representing 3 percent of the population over the age of 45 years, were recruited in 1,121 counties (Hammond 1964a,b, 1966; Garfinkel 1985). Illiterate persons, institutionalized populations, itinerant workers, and illegal aliens were not recruited. More than 97 percent of enrollees were white. Enrollment was by family; an eligible family had to have one member over age 45. Once a family was eligible, every family member over the age of 35 was asked to participate. As a result of family-based recruitment, more than three-quarters of CPS-I subjects were married. As a consequence of the eligibility rules, the age distribution of entrants peaked at 45–49 years. More than one-third of participants had at least some college education.

CPS-II was instituted in September 1982. The study, conducted in all 50 States, had the same enrollment plan and organizational structure as CPS-I. Over 1.2 million persons were enrolled. As in CPS-I, subjects were predominantly white and more educated than the general population. While 2 percent of CPS-I participants were black, the proportion increased to 4 percent in CPS-II. Still, black persons were underrepresented. Like CPS-I participants, CPS-II enrollees were predominantly over 40 years of age. Unlike CPS-I, the mode of their age distribution was 50 to 59 years (Garfinkel 1985; Stellman and Garfinkel 1986).

CPS-II is planned to continue through 1988. Preliminary results of the first 4 years of followup (1982–86) are available. For these 4 years, ascertainment of the fact of death among enrollees is thought to be virtually complete. However, as of July 1988, the cause of death had not been ascertained for about 9 percent of male deaths and 13 percent of female deaths.

Comparison of the 6-year followup (1959–65) of CPS-I and the 4-year followup of CPS-II is reported below. For computation of relative risks, cause-specific death rates for CPS-I males and females have been standardized to the age distributions of man-years and woman-years of exposure during 1965–69. Relative risks in CPS-II were likewise computed as the ratios of age-adjusted death rates, where standardization was performed with respect to the age distributions of man- and woman-years of exposure during 1982–86.

For comparison of absolute death rates (as opposed to relative risks), the age-specific rates in both studies were standardized to the age distribution of U.S. resident white males and females in 1965. For CPS-II, absolute death rates have been corrected for underascertainment of causes of death. No such correction was made for CPS-I, where death certificate retrieval is virtually complete.

No attempt has been made to correct for possible noncomparability between ICD-7 (CPS-I) and ICD-9 (CPS-II). Studies of the transition between the Seventh and Eighth Revisions of the International Classification of Diseases have shown significant noncomparability (Klebba 1975, 1982). Similar results have been reported for the transition between the Eighth and Ninth Revisions (Klebba and Scott 1980). Comparison of the Seventh and Ninth Revisions, however, suggests that the combined changes have been self-cancelling (Personal communication, J. Klebba to J. Harris, June 1988).

Both CPS-I and CPS-II are more representative of middle-class white Americans than the U.S. population as a whole. Still, the two cohorts were derived from virtually identical sampling schemes, and analysis of the entrants has shown similar demographic characteristics (Stellman and Garfinkel 1986). These considerations enhance the validity of comparisons between the American Cancer Society studies.

Nonsmokers' Death Rates

Table 3 reports a comparison of the age-adjusted death rates for the three leading causes of death from cigarette smoking: CHD; chronic obstructive pulmonary disease

(COPD); and lung cancer. For COPD and lung cancer, in particular, there has been no discernible change in nonsmokers' death rates. The relatively small changes—less than 15 percent up or down—are all statistically insignificant. The absence of significant change in nonsmokers' lung cancer rates confirms and extends the findings of Doll and Peto (1981) and Garfinkel (1981). For COPD, the table presents the first information on trends in nonsmokers' death rates.

It needs to be emphasized, however, that the statistical test for a change in lung cancer or COPD rates is of relatively low power. For COPD, there are sufficient data to have detected an increase of 53 percent or more in males and an increase of 42 percent or more in females at the 0.05 level of significance. For lung cancer, increases of more than 37 and 24 percent for males and females, respectively, were detectable as statistically significant.

In contrast to lung cancer and COPD, Table 3 shows a very marked decline in CHD death rates in nonsmokers. Over an approximate 20-year period, nonsmokers' age-adjusted death rates dropped by 64 percent in men and 69 percent in women. The observed decline in nonsmokers' CHD death rates is in keeping with the CHD decline in the general population. However, the magnitude of the decline is larger in the American Cancer Society subjects. Among U.S. white males, the age-adjusted death rate from CHD (standardized to the 1965 population distribution) declined by 41 percent during 1965–85. For U.S. white females, the decline was 40 percent (NCHS 1967 and unpublished; U.S. Bureau of the Census 1974, 1986).

TABLE 3.—Age-adjusted annual death rates per 100,000 for CHD, COPD, and lung cancer among males and females, aged 35 years or more, who never smoked regularly, 6-year followup (1959–65) of CPS-I compared with 4-year followup (1982–86) of CPS-II

	Males		Females	
Disease	CPS-I	CPS-II[a b]	CPS-I	CPS-II[a b]
CHD	745	270	479	153
420[c]; 410–414[e]	(726–775)[d]	(256–284)	(467–491)	(146–159)
COPD	9.5	8.7	4.0	5.6
500–502, 527.1[c]; 490–492, 496[e]	(7.0–12.9)	(6.5–11.7)	(3.1–5.3)	(4.5–7.0)
Lung cancer	15.5	13.6	10.3	11.4
162–163[c]; 162[e]	(12.5–19.3)	(10.8–17.0)	(8.9–11.9)	(9.8–13.3)

[a]For both CPS-I and CPS-II, age adjustment of rates was performed by direct standardization to the age distributions of U.S. resident white males and females, respectively, in 1965 (U.S. Bureau of the Census 1974).

[b]For CPS-II, death rates were corrected for delayed ascertainment of causes of death. Among 4,959 known deaths during 1982–86 in male nonsmokers, death certificates had not been received for 439 by June 1988. Among 10,161 known deaths in female nonsmokers, 1,411 had not been received.

[c]CPS-I coding, International Classification of Diseases, Seventh Revision.

[d]Numbers in parentheses are 95-percent confidence intervals.

[e]CPS-II coding, International Classification of Diseases, Ninth Revision.

SOURCE: Unpublished tabulations, American Cancer Society.

Current Cigarette Smokers' Death Rates: Lung Cancer

Figures 6 and 7, respectively, show changes in the age-specific lung cancer death rates of men and women who described themselves as regular cigarette smokers on the original questionnaire for each prospective study. The death rates, depicted in each figure on a logarithmic scale, apply to all such current smokers. No adjustment has been made for differences in the number of cigarettes smoked or duration of cigarette use.

The age–incidence curves in both figures show a striking crossover effect. Among older male smokers, especially those aged 70 years or more, lung cancer death rates in CPS-II exceed those in CPS-I twofold to fourfold. By contrast, among younger male smokers, especially those less than 50 years old, CPS-II death rates are about 30 to 40 percent lower. The observed crossover phenomenon appears to be consistent with long-term changes in cigarette smoke exposure among successive cohorts. The increase in lung cancer among older male smokers reflects their increased frequency of cigarette use and increased cigarette smoking in early life. The decline in lung cancer among

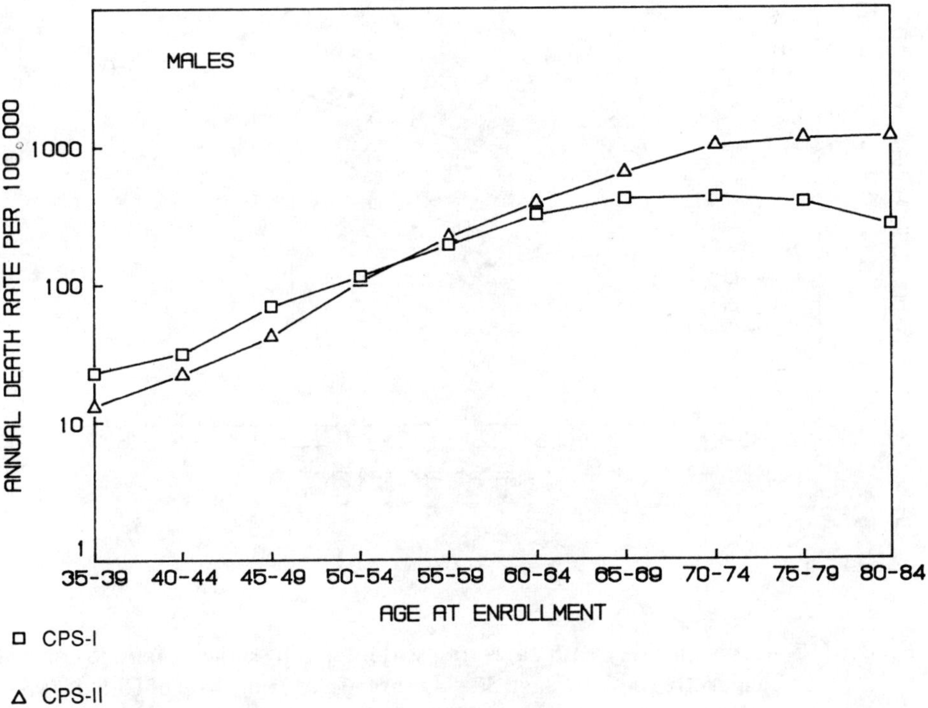

FIGURE 6.—Age-specific death rates (log scale) for lung cancer, male current cigarette smokers aged 35–84 years; 6-year followup of CPS-I (1959–65), compared with 4-year followup of CPS-II (1982–86)

SOURCE: Unpublished tabulations, American Cancer Society. Estimates for CPS-II are preliminary.

younger men may reflect their increased use of filter-tipped and low-tar cigarettes. Most currently smoking men aged 35 to 39 years in CPS-II, for example, were likely to have been lifelong filter-tipped cigarette smokers.

An even more striking crossover is shown for female current cigarette smokers in Figure 7. In particular, the age of crossover comes somewhat earlier. Among women smokers aged 45 years or more, lung cancer death rates have increased fourfold to sevenfold. (There were no deaths and a small number of person-years of exposure at ages 75 or more in CPS-I.) By contrast, lung cancer death rates in the very youngest cohorts, aged 35 to 44 years, have declined by 35 to 55 percent. As in the case of men, the crossover appears to reflect differential trends in cigarette smoking among successive cohorts of women.

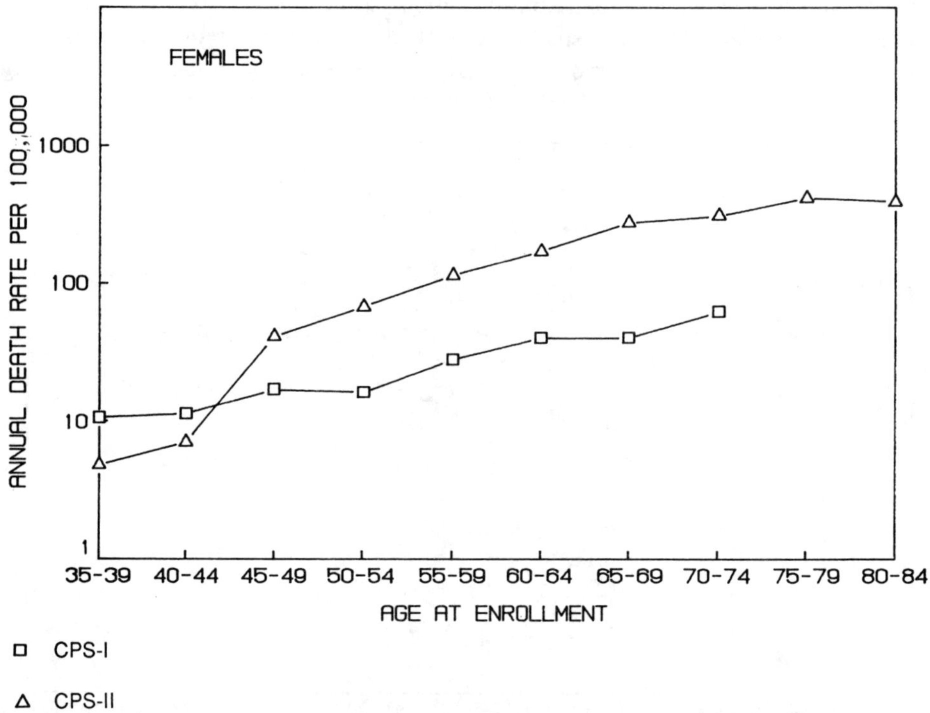

FIGURE 7.—Age-specific death rates (log scale) for lung cancer, female current cigarette smokers aged 35–84 years; 6-year followup of CPS-I (1959–65), compared with 4-year followup of CPS-II (1982–86)

SOURCE: Unpublished tabulations, American Cancer Society. Estimates for CPS-II are preliminary.

Current Cigarette Smokers' Death Rates: Coronary Heart Disease

Figure 8 shows the proportional decline from CPS-I to CPS-II in the age-adjusted CHD death rates of current smokers and nonsmokers. The relative declines are depicted separately for men and women, and for persons younger than 65, and 65 and older. CHD death rates have declined in both cigarette smokers and nonsmokers. For the predominantly white, middle-class populations under study in CPS-I and CPS-II, the overall decline among smokers and nonsmokers was greater than observed for the U.S. white population.

Still, the declines in CHD mortality rates among nonsmokers were notably greater than among current cigarette smokers. The disparity is seen at all ages, but appears somewhat greater among younger persons. In contrast to lung cancer (Figures 6 and 7), no crossover in age–incidence curves is observed. The increasing smoker–nonsmoker disparity at younger ages argues against a significant salutary effect of lifelong filter-tipped cigarette use. The possibility that changes in other coronary risk factors among cigarette smokers may explain their reduced decline in CHD rates needs further investigation.

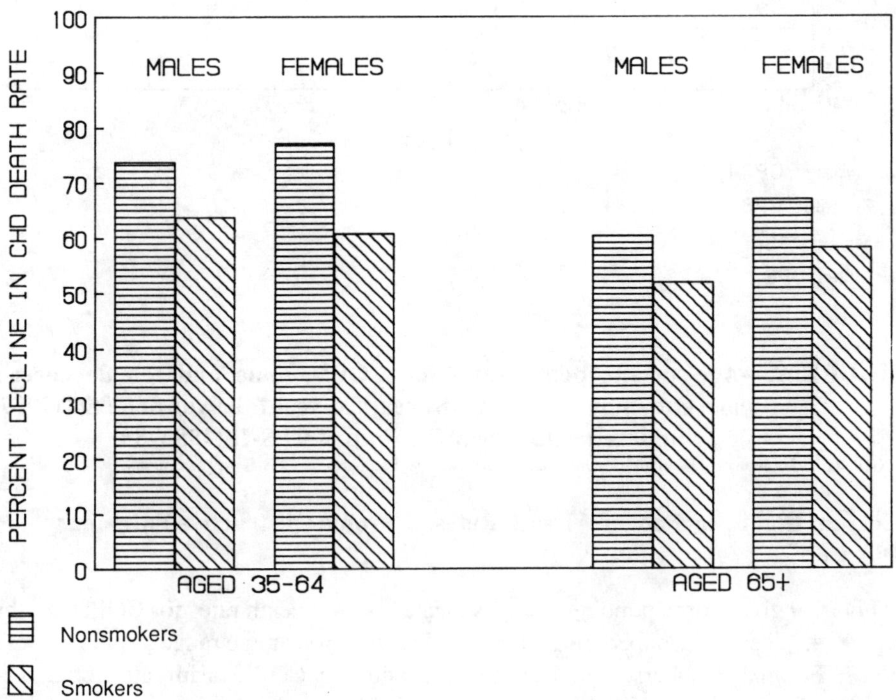

FIGURE 8.—Percentage decline in age-adjusted death rates for CHD; 6-year followup of CPS-I (1959–65), compared with 4-year followup of CPS-II (1982–86)

SOURCE: Unpublished tabulations, American Cancer Society. Estimates for CPS-II are preliminary.

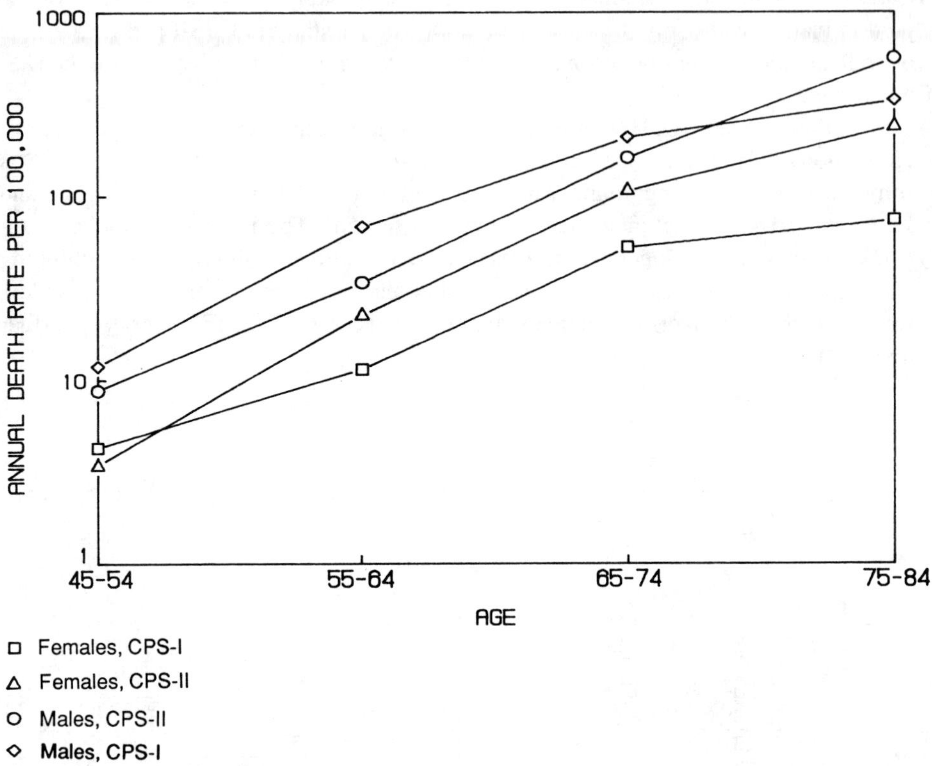

FIGURE 9.—Age-specific death rates for COPD, male and female current cigarette smokers aged 45–84 years; 6-year followup of CPS-I (1959–65), compared with 4-year followup of CPS-II (1982–86)

SOURCE: Unpublished tabulations, American Cancer Society. Estimates for CPS-II are preliminary.

Current Cigarette Smokers' Death Rates: Chronic Obstructive Pulmonary Disease

Figure 9 gives corresponding changes in age-specific death rates for COPD. In this figure, the ages are grouped into 10-year rather than 5-year age ranges as in Figures 6 and 7. For male smokers, there has been a reduction in COPD death rates for ages 45 to 74 years. For female smokers over 55 years old, there has been about a twofold to threefold increase in COPD rates.

Estimated Relative Risks from CPS-I and CPS-II

For men and women, respectively, Tables 4 and 5 depict estimated relative risks in the 6-year followup of CPS-I for all-cause mortality and for 14 specific causes of death (15 causes for women, including cervical cancer). For men in Table 4, the estimated relative risks for current and former cigarette smokers are given separately. For women in Table 5, the numbers of deaths and person-years of exposure among former smokers were too small to give reliable death rates for many causes. Accordingly, in conformity with earlier reports of CPS-I mortality, the death rates for current smokers are compared with those of women with any history of regular cigarette use, past or present.

For both men and women, the estimates in Tables 4 and 5 are in accord with earlier reports on CPS-I mortality (Garfinkel 1980b; Hammond 1964a,b, 1966, 1972; Hammond and Garfinkel 1969; Hammond and Seidman 1980). Among men, former smokers have lower mortality ratios. In both sexes, relative risks for CHD are higher at younger ages. Both sexes, but to a greater extent, men, show elevated risks of other cardiovascular diseases including stroke, hypertensive heart disease, and aortic aneurysm. In both sexes, smokers' death rates are higher for bronchitis and emphysema and for seven cancers including lung cancer. The relative risk of lung cancer among current smokers in CPS-I is about 11.3 for men and 2.7 for women.

The results for CPS-II, given in Tables 6 and 7, show substantial changes in the mortality risk of cigarette smoking over two decades. The all-cause relative risk for men has increased from 1.8 in CPS-I to 2.3 in CPS-II. For women, it has risen from 1.2 to 1.9. These increases in overall mortality are not an artifact of the method of age adjustment, because CPS-II contained proportionately fewer person-years of exposure at the youngest ages than CPS-I.

As reflected in Table 6 and Table 7, the relative risks for CHD death have increased for both men and women. The relative risks for men, in particular, are consistent with those reported from recent case–control studies (Kaufman et al. 1983; Rosenberg et al. 1985) and from the followup of the Multiple Risk Factor Intervention Trial (MRFIT) cohort, as described in Chapter 2. The markedly elevated relative risks for younger women in Table 7 are consistent with those reported in a recent case–control study (Slone et al. 1978) and in a prospective study of 120,000 female nurses (Willett et al. 1987). Such consistencies across epidemiologic studies—especially cohort and case–control studies reported during the 1980s—argue against any appreciable bias in the 4-year preliminary results of CPS-II given in Tables 6 and 7.

Tables 6 and 7 show consistently increased relative risks for cerebrovascular lesions among both men and women, particularly in the younger age groups. Among women under 65 years old, the estimated relative risk of death from stroke is 4.8, with a 95-percent confidence range of 3.5 to 6.5. The observed increases in risk for current smokers are reduced in former smokers.

The finding of an elevated risk of cerebrovascular disease among cigarette smokers is not new. Elevated death rates from stroke were reported in CPS-I (Hammond 1966; Hammond and Garfinkel 1969) and are reproduced in Tables 4 and 5. The 1983 Surgeon General's Report noted the association between stroke and cigarette use; no data on the effect of smoking cessation were available (US DHHS 1983). A recent prospective study of 8,000 men of Japanese origin (Abbott et al. 1986) showed an elevated risk of thromboembolic and hemorrhagic strokes among cigarette smokers. While there was no clear trend of increasing risk with higher daily smoking rates, subjects who quit smoking had reduced risks compared with continuing smokers. In the prospective study of 120,000 female nurses, Colditz et al. (1988) found a dose–response relationship be-

TABLE 4.—Estimated relative risks for current and former smokers of cigarettes, males aged 35 years or more, 6-year (1959–65) followup of American Cancer Society 25-State study (CPS-I)

Underlying cause of death	Current smokers[a]	Former smokers[a]
All causes	1.80 (1.75–1.85)[b]	1.38 (1.33–1.42)[b]
CHD, age ≥35 (420)[c]	1.83 (1.76–1.91)	1.42 (1.34–1.49)
CHD, age 35–64[d] (420)	2.25 (2.13–2.39)	1.56 (1.45–1.68)
CHD, age ≥65 (420)	1.39 (1.30–1.48)	1.27 (1.17–1.37)
Hypertensive Heart Disease (440–443)	1.63 (1.36–1.96)	1.19 (0.94–1.51)
Cerebrovascular Lesions, age ≥35 (330–334)	1.37 (1.25–1.49)	0.96 (0.85–1.08)
Cerebrovascular Lesions, age 35–64 (330–334)	1.79 (1.55–2.08)	1.02 (0.83–1.25)
Cerebrovascular Lesions, age ≥65 (330–334)	1.15 (1.02–1.30)	0.93 (0.80–1.08)
Aortic Aneurysm, Non-Syphilitic (451)	4.11 (3.13–5.40)	2.40 (1.73–3.34)
Ulcer, Duodenal, Gastric, and Jejunal (540–542)	3.06 (2.24–4.18)	1.49 (0.98–2.27)
Influenza and Pneumonia (480–481, 490–493)	1.82 (1.45–2.27)	1.62 (1.24–2.12)
Bronchitis and Emphysema (500–502, 527.1)	8.81 (6.40–12.13)	10.20 (7.34–14.17)
Cancer, Lip, Oral Cavity, and Pharynx (140–148)	6.33 (3.60–11.13)	2.73 (1.36–5.49)
Cancer, Esophagus (150)	3.62 (2.02–6.48)	1.28 (0.53–3.08)
Cancer, Pancreas (157)	2.34 (1.81–3.02)	1.30 (0.92–1.84)
Cancer, Larynx (161)	10.00 (3.51–28.51)	8.60 (2.87–25.74)
Cancer, Lung (162–163)	11.35 (9.10–14.15)	4.96 (3.86–6.38)
Cancer, Kidney (180)	1.84 (1.23–2.76)	1.79 (1.11–2.87)
Cancer, Bladder, Other Urinary Organs (181)	2.90 (2.01–4.18)	1.75 (1.07–2.87)

NOTE: Based upon 1,692,652 man-years of exposure among male subjects who never smoked regularly, or who smoked only cigarettes, present or past. Relative risks, estimated with respect to men who never smoked regularly, have been directly standardized to the age distribution of all man-years of exposure.

[a]Refers to cigarette smoking status at enrollment (October 1959–March 1960).

[b]Numbers in parentheses are 95-percent confidence intervals, computed on the assumption that the logarithm of relative risk was normally distributed.

[c]All disease codes refer to International Classification of Diseases, Seventh Revision.

[d]When an age range is given, it refers to the age at enrollment in 1959.

SOURCE: Unpublished tabulations, American Cancer Society.

TABLE 5.—Estimated relative risks for current cigarette smokers and for all subjects with a history of regular cigarette smoking, females aged 35 years or more, 6-year (1959–65) followup of American Cancer Society 25-State study (CPS-I)

Underlying cause of death	Current smokers[a]	Current and former smokers[a]
All causes	1.23 (1.18–1.28)[b]	1.24 (1.20–1.28)[b]
CHD, age ≥35 (420)[c]	1.40 (1.29–1.51)	1.38 (1.29–1.74)
CHD, age 35–64[d] (420)	1.81 (1.67–1.97)	1.74 (1.61–1.89)
CHD, age ≥65 (420)	1.24 (1.11–1.39)	1.25 (1.14–1.37)
Hypertensive Heart Disease (440–443)	1.31 (1.04–1.66)	1.27 (1.04–1.55)
Cerebrovascular Lesions, age ≥35 (330–334)	1.19 (1.06–1.35)	1.26 (1.13–1.80)
Cerebrovascular Lesions, age 35–64 (330–334)	1.92 (1.69–2.18)	1.80 (1.59–2.03)
Cerebrovascular Lesions, age ≥65 (330–334)	0.97 (0.81–1.16)	1.09 (0.95–1.26)
Aortic Aneurysm, Non-Syphilitic (451)	4.64 (3.00–7.20)	3.67 (2.46–5.48)
Ulcer, Duodenal, Gastric, and Jejunal (540–542)	1.37 (0.81–2.31)	1.52 (0.96–2.41)
Influenza and Pneumonia (480–481, 490–493)	0.91 (0.59–1.41)	0.96 (0.69–1.33)
Bronchitis and Emphysema (500–502, 527.1)	5.89 (3.97–8.76)	5.85 (4.02–8.53)
Cancer, Lip, Oral Cavity, and Pharynx (140–148)	1.96 (1.14–3.39)	1.89 (1.16–3.08)
Cancer, Esophagus (150)	1.94 (1.02–3.69)	2.15 (1.09–4.23)
Cancer, Pancreas (157)	1.39 (1.04–1.86)	1.38 (1.07–1.78)
Cancer, Larynx (161)	3.81 (0.78–18.52)	3.10 (0.65–14.99)
Cancer, Lung (162–163)	2.69 (2.14–3.37)	2.59 (2.04–3.30)
Cancer, Cervix Uteri (171)	1.10 (0.83–1.47)	1.32 (1.02–1.71)
Cancer, Kidney (180)	1.43 (0.89–2.31)	1.47 (0.97–2.23)
Cancer, Bladder, Other Urinary Organs (181)	2.87 (1.74–4.74)	2.31 (1.45–3.67)

NOTE: Based upon 3,325,989 woman-years of exposure among subjects who never smoked regularly, or who smoked only cigarettes, present or past. Relative risks, estimated with respect to women who never smoked regularly, have been directly standardized to the age distribution of all woman-years of exposure.

[a]Refers to cigarette smoking status at enrollment (October 1959–March 1960).

[b]Numbers in parentheses are 95-percent confidence intervals, computed on the assumption that the logarithm of relative risk was normally distributed.

[c]All disease codes refer to International Classification of Diseases, Seventh Revision.

[d]When an age range is given, it refers to the age at enrollment in 1959.

SOURCE: Unpublished tabulations, American Cancer Society.

TABLE 6.—Estimated relative risks for current and former smokers of cigarettes, males aged 35 years or more, 4-year (1982–86) followup of American Cancer Society 50-State study (CPS-II)

Underlying cause of death	Current smokers[a]	Former smokers[a]
All causes	2.34 (2.26–2.43)[b]	1.58 (1.53–1.64)[b]
CHD, age ≥35 (410–414)[c]	1.94 (1.80–2.08)	1.41 (1.33–1.50)
CHD, age 35–64[d] (410–414)	2.81 (2.49–3.18)	1.75 (1.55–1.99)
CHD, age ≥65 (410–414)	1.62 (1.48–1.77)	1.29 (1.20–1.38)
Other Heart Disease[e] (390–398, 401–405, 415–417, 420–429)	1.85 (1.63–2.10)	1.32 (1.18–1.48)
Cerebrovascular Lesions, age ≥35 (430–438)	2.24 (1.88–2.67)	1.29 (1.10–1.51)
Cerebrovascular Lesions, age 35–64 (430–438)	3.67 (2.51–5.36)	1.38 (0.91–2.07)
Cerebrovascular Lesions, age ≥65 (430–438)	1.94 (1.58–2.38)	1.27 (1.07–1.50)
Other Circulatory Disease[f] (440–448)	4.06 (3.08–5.35)	2.33 (1.81–3.01)
COPD (490–492,496)	9.65 (7.00–13.30)	8.75 (6.48–11.80)
Other Respiratory Disease[g] (010–012, 480–489,493)	1.99 (1.52–2.61)	1.56 (1.25–1.95)
Cancer, Lip, Oral Cavity, Pharynx (140–149)	27.48 (9.96–75.83)	8.80 (3.15–24.59)
Cancer, Esophagus (150)	7.60 (3.81–15.17)	5.83 (3.02–11.25)
Cancer, Pancreas (157)	2.14 (1.62–2.82)	1.12 (0.86–1.45)
Cancer, Larynx (161)	10.48 (3.61–30.43)	5.24 (1.83–14.99)
Cancer, Lung (162)	22.36 (17.77–28.13)	9.36 (7.43–11.77)
Cancer, Kidney (189)	2.95 (1.92–4.54)	1.95 (1.31–2.90)
Cancer, Bladder, Other Urinary Organs (188)	2.86 (1.85–4.44)	1.90 (1.28–2.82)

NOTE: Preliminary estimates, based upon 1,491,791 man-years of exposure among male subjects who never smoked regularly, or who smoked only cigarettes, present or past. Relative risks, estimated with respect to men who never smoked regularly, have been directly standardized to the age distribution of all man-years of exposure.

[a]Refers to cigarette smoking status at enrollment (September 1982).

[b]Numbers in parentheses are 95-percent confidence intervals, computed on the assumption that the logarithm of relative risk was normally distributed.

[c]All disease codes refer to International Classification of Diseases, Ninth Revision.

[d]When an age range is given, it refers to the age at enrollment in 1982.

[e]Includes Hypertensive Heart Disease (401–404).

[f]Includes Aortic Aneurysm, Non-Syphilitic, and General Arteriosclerosis (440–441).

[g]Includes Influenza and Pneumonia (480–487).

SOURCE: Unpublished tabulations, American Cancer Society.

TABLE 7.—Estimated relative risks for current and former cigarette smokers, females aged 35 years or more, 4-year (1982–86) followup of American Cancer Society 50-State study (CPS-II)

Underlying cause of death	Current smokers[a]	Former smokers[a]
All causes	1.90 (1.82–1.98)[b]	1.32 (1.27–1.37)[b]
CHD, age ≥35 (410–414)[c]	1.78 (1.62–1.97)	1.31 (1.19–1.44)
CHD, age 35–64[d] (410–414)	3.00 (2.50–3.59)	1.43 (1.15–1.77)
CHD, age ≥65 (410–414)	1.60 (1.42–1.80)	1.29 (1.16–1.43)
Other Heart Disease[e] (390–398, 401–405, 415–417, 420–429)	1.69 (1.44–1.99)	1.16 (1.00–1.34)
Cerebrosvascular Lesions, age ≥35 (430–438)	1.84 (1.56–2.16)	1.06 (0.88–1.27)
Cerebrovascular Lesions, age 35–64 (430–438)	4.80 (3.52–6.54)	1.41 (0.94–2.13)
Cerebrovascular Lesions, age ≥65 (430–438)	1.47 (1.19–1.81)	1.01 (0.83–1.24)
Other Circulatory Disease[f] (440–448)	3.00 (2.20–4.08)	1.34 (0.95–1.90)
COPD (490–492,496)	10.47 (7.78–14.09)	7.04 (5.33–9.30)
Other Respiratory Disease[g] (010–012,480–489,493)	2.18 (1.60–2.97)	1.38 (1.04–1.84)
Cancer, Lip, Oral Cavity, Pharynx (140–149)	5.59 (3.15–9.91)	2.88 (1.57–5.26)
Cancer, Esophagus (150)	10.25 (4.94–21.27)	3.16 (1.45–6.85)
Cancer, Pancreas (157)	2.33 (1.77–3.08)	1.78 (1.37–2.30)
Cancer, Larynx (161)	17.78 (3.45–91.74)	11.88 (2.46–57.34)
Cancer, Lung (162)	11.94 (9.99–14.26)	4.69 (3.86–5.70)
Cancer, Cervix Uteri (180)	2.14 (1.06–4.30)	1.94 (0.97–3.87)
Cancer, Kidney (189)	1.41 (0.86–2.30)	1.16 (0.72–1.87)
Cancer, Bladder, Other Urinary Organs (188)	2.58 (1.31–5.08)	1.85 (1.00–3.42)

NOTE: Preliminary estimates, based upon 2,418,909 woman-years of exposure among female subjects who never smoked regularly, or who smoked only cigarettes, present or past. Relative risks, estimated with respect to women who never smoked regularly, have been directly standardized to the age distribution of all woman-years of exposure.
[a]Refers to cigarette smoking status at enrollment (September 1982).
[b]Numbers in parentheses are 95-percent confidence intervals, computed on the assumption that the logarithm of relative risk was normally distributed.
[c]All disease codes refer to International Classification of Diseases, Ninth Revision.
[d]When an age range is given, it refers to the age at enrollment in 1982.
[e]Includes Hypertensive Heart Disease (401–404).
[f]Includes Aortic Aneurysm, Non-Syphilitic, and General Arteriosclerosis (440–441).
[g]Includes Influenza and Pneumonia (480–487).
SOURCE: Unpublished tabulations, American Cancer Society.

tween cigarette use and risk of stroke. They also noted a slight increase in risk among former cigarette smokers, especially for the first 2 years after cessation. The preliminary results from CPS-II, reported in Tables 6 and 7, further support a causal role for cigarette smoking in stroke.

The preliminary results of CPS-II also show significantly higher relative risks for cancers of the lip, oral cavity and pharynx, esophagus, and lung, as compared with CPS-I. The computed relative risk for lung cancer death has increased to 22 in men and 12 in women. While the relative risks for COPD death have not changed significantly among men, there is a trend toward increasing risk among women. The available data from CPS-II do not permit identification of specific mortality risks for hypertensive heart disease, aortic aneurysm, and influenza and pneumonia, as in CPS-I. However, among broader categories of cardiovascular and nonneoplastic respiratory disease, increased risks are likewise found in CPS-II.

Endocrine and Sex-Related Cancers in Women

A protective effect of smoking on cancer of the endometrium has been suggested in a recent case–control study (Lesko et al. 1985). For CPS-I, the relative risk for cancers of the uterine corpus (ICD-7 Codes 172-174) among current smokers was 0.94 (95-percent confidence interval, 0.57 to 1.53). Preliminary results for CPS-II suggest a reduced relative risk for endometrial cancer (ICD-9 Code 182).

Recent data on a possible protective effect of smoking for breast cancer have been contradictory (See Chapter 2; Rosenberg et al. 1984). For CPS-I, the relative risk for breast cancer (ICD-7 Code 170) among current smokers was 0.88 (95-percent confidence interval, 0.77 to 1.01), while the relative risk among former smokers was 1.20 (95-percent confidence interval, 1.15 to 1.35). Preliminary data from CPS-II have likewise been contradictory.

An increased risk of cervical cancer among cigarette smokers has been reported in case–control studies (LaVecchia et al. 1986; Nischan, Ebeling, Schindler 1988). For CPS-I, the relative risk for cervical cancer (ICD-7 Code 171) was 1.10 (95-percent confidence interval, 0.83 to 1.47). Data from CPS-II show a twofold increase in cervical cancer mortality among current smokers (relative risk 2.14, 95-percent confidence interval 1.06 to 4.30).

Summary

The relative risks for current smokers for selected comparable disease categories causally related to smoking in CPS-I and CPS-II are summarized and listed side by side in Table 8. These comparisons show substantial increases in the risk of death due to smoking for most of the disease categories listed between the years 1959 and 1965 and 1982 and 1986. Statistically significant increases in relative risks occurred in those disease categories for which 95-percent confidence limits around the estimated relative risks do not overlap between CPS-I and CPS-II. Compared with men during this period, women experienced greater increases in the relative risks of cerebrovascular lesions (ages 35 to 64 years), COPD, laryngeal cancer, and lung cancer.

TABLE 8.—Summary of estimated relative risks for current cigarette smokers, major disease categories causally related to cigarettes, males and females aged 35 years and older, CPS-I (1959–65) and CPS-II (1982–86)

Underlying cause of death[a]	Males		Females	
	CPS-I	CPS-II	CPS-I	CPS-II
CHD, age ≥35	1.83	1.94	1.40	1.78[b]
CHD, age 35–64	2.25	2.81[b]	1.81	3.00[b]
Cerebrovascular Lesions, age ≥35	1.37	2.24[b]	1.19	1.84[b]
Cerebrovascular Lesions, age 35–64	1.79	3.67[b]	1.92	4.80[b]
COPD	8.81	9.65	5.89	10.47
Cancer, Lip, Oral Cavity, and Pharynx	6.33	27.48	1.96	5.59
Cancer, Esophagus	3.62	7.60	1.94	10.25[b]
Cancer, Pancreas	2.34	2.14	1.39	2.33
Cancer, Larynx	10.00	10.48	3.81	17.78
Cancer, Lung	11.35	22.36[b]	2.69	11.94[b]

[a]See Tables 4–7 for International Classification of Disease codes.
[b]95-percent confidence intervals do not overlap between CPS-I and CPS-II.
SOURCE: Tables 4–7.

Smoking-Attributable Mortality in the United States, 1965 and 1985

Table 9 reports the attributable risks *a* from cigarette smoking during the year 1965. Ten causes of death are considered: CHD, COPD, cerebrovascular disease, and cancers of seven sites. The computations are based upon the age-adjusted relative risks reported in CPS-I and the prevalence rates reported in the 1965 NHIS. For men, the age-adjusted relative risks among present and past cigarette smokers with a history of pipe or cigar use were slightly lower than those for present and past smokers of cigarettes exclusively. While the latter are reported for comparison in Table 4, the former were used in the attributable risk computations. In 1965, as shown in Figure 2, about two-thirds of men with a history of regular cigarette smoking were also exposed to pipe or cigar smoke. (As noted in Note b of Table 10 below, the use of relative risks derived from the death rates of men who smoked cigarettes exclusively resulted in about a 5-percent increase in attributable deaths for 1965.) For women, the computation of attributable risks in 1965 did not distinguish between current and former smokers.

TABLE 9.—Estimated attributable risks for 10 selected causes of death from cigarette smoking, males and females, United States, 1965

Cause of death	Males[a] (%)	Females[b] (%)
CHD, age 35–64	42 (40–45)[c]	26 (23–30)
CHD, age ≥65	11 (9–14)	3.3 (2.1–5.1)
COPD	84 (79–88)	67 (57–76)
Cancer of lip, oral cavity, and pharynx	74 (59–85)	27 (12–51)
Cancer of larynx	84 (61–94)	47 (8–90)
Cancer of esophagus	57 (36–76)	14 (6–29)
Cancer of lung	86 (82–88)	40 (31–50)
Cancer of pancreas	41 (30–53)	14 (6–30)
Cancer of bladder	53 (39–66)	36 (20–56)
Cancer of kidney	36 (19–56)	17 (5–42)
Cerebrovascular disease, age 35–64	28 (21–36)	28 (22–33)
Cerebrovascular disease, age ≥65	2.0 (0.6–6.6)	1.3 (0.2–6.5)

[a]For males, computations based on prevalence rates in Table 2 and relative risks for male current and former cigarette smokers, with or without a history of pipe and cigar smoking, derived from CPS-I.
[b]For females, attributable risks computed from prevalence rates in Table 2 and relative risks for all female smokers, past and present, in Table 5.
[c]Numbers in parentheses are 95-percent confidence intervals.

In 1965, as Table 9 reveals, cigarette smoking was responsible for 42 percent of CHD deaths among younger men and 26 percent of deaths among younger women. For COPD deaths at all ages, the smoking-attributable risks were 84 percent for men and 67 percent for women. For lung cancer, the respective attributable risks were 86 percent and 40 percent for men and women. With the exception of deaths from stroke among younger persons, attributable risks were markedly higher for men.

Table 10 reports the corresponding smoking-attributable deaths, *A*, during the year 1965. Attributable deaths were computed by multiplying the attributable risk percentages in Table 9 by the corresponding cause-specific death rates among persons aged 20

TABLE 10.—Estimated deaths (in thousands) attributable to cigarette smoking, 10 selected causes, males and females, United States, 1965

Cause of death	Males	Females
CHD, age <65	51 (48–54)[a]	9.5 (8.2–10.8)
CHD, age ≥65	25 (20–30)	6.0 (3.9–9.4)
COPD	16 (15–17)	2.3 (2.0–2.7)
Cancer of lip, oral cavity, and pharynx	3.6 (2.9–4.2)	0.4 (0.2–0.8)
Cancer of larynx	1.9 (1.4–2.2)	0.1 (0.02–0.3)
Cancer of esophagus	2.4 (1.5–3.2)	0.1 (0.2–0.8)
Cancer of lung	35 (34–36)	3.1 (2.4–3.8)
Cancer of pancreas	3.8 (2.8–4.9)	0.9 (0.4–2.0)
Cancer of bladder	3.0 (2.2–3.7)	1.0 (0.5–1.5)
Cancer of kidney	1.2 (0.7–1.9)	0.3 (0.1–1.8)
Cerebrovascular disease, age <65	5.5 (4.2–7.2)	4.7 (3.8–5.6)
Cerebrovascular disease, age ≥65	1.5 (0.4–4.8)	1.0 (0.2–5.9)
Ten causes	150[b] (143–157)	30 (26–34)

NOTE: Computed from Table 9 and tabulations of deaths at ages 20 years or more by cause for 1965 (NCHS 1967). Sums may not equal totals because of rounding.

[a]Numbers in parentheses are 95-percent confidence intervals.

[b]When the attributable risk estimates given in Note a of Table 9 were used, the total attributable deaths for males were 158,000 (95-percent confidence interval, 151,000 to 166,000). Approximately two-thirds of the 8,000 additional deaths were from CHD.

years or more. For the 10 causes combined, cigarette smoking was responsible for 150,000 deaths among men and 30,000 deaths among women in 1965.

Among men, CHD deaths made up 51 percent of smoking-attributable mortality for the 10 causes combined. This proportion is consistent with the estimate of 45 percent reported by the 1964 Advisory Committee to the Surgeon General for excess mortality from all causes (US PHS 1964). Similarly, lung cancer accounted for 23 percent of the smoking-attributable mortality for the 10 causes combined—again consistent with the

1964 Report's estimate of 16 percent of deaths from all causes. Among women, CHD deaths made up 52 percent and lung cancer 10 percent of the smoking attributable mortality from the 10 causes combined.

Table 11 shows the estimated attributable risks *a* from cigarette smoking for the year 1985. For comparability with the 1965 calculations, the same 10 causes of death are considered. The computations are based upon the relative risks reported in CPS-II and the prevalence rates reported in the 1985 NHIS. For men, the computations employed the relative risks for past and present smokers of cigarettes exclusively, as shown in Table 6. As Figure 2 indicates, the proportion of male smokers who used other forms

TABLE 11.—Estimated attributable risks for 10 selected causes of death from cigarette smoking, males and females, United States, 1985

Cause of death	Males (%)	Females (%)
CHD, age <65	45 (40–50)[a]	41 (34–48)
CHD, age ≥65	21 (17–26)	12 (9–15)
COPD	84 (78–88)	79 (73–83)
Cancer of lip, oral cavity, and pharynx	92 (79–97)	61 (45–76)
Cancer of larynx	81 (57–93)	87 (56–97)
Cancer of esophagus	78 (62–89)	75 (57–87)
Cancer of lung	90 (88–92)	79 (75–82)
Cancer of pancreas	29 (18–43)	34 (25–44)
Cancer of bladder	47 (31–63)	37 (18–61)
Cancer of kidney	48 (32–64)	12 (3–43)
Cerebrovascular disease, age <65	51 (36–65)	55 (45–65)
Cerebrovascular disease, age ≥65	24 (16–35)	6 (2–14)

NOTE: Computed from Tables 2, 6, and 7. For adult men under 65, the proportions of current and former cigarette smokers in 1985 were, respectively, 34.7 and 25.8 percent. For men 65 or older, the prevalences of current and former cigarette smoking were, respectively, 19.4 and 51.1 percent. For adult women under 65, the corresponding proportions were 30.1 and 16.5 percent; for adult women 65 or older, 12.6 and 19.6 percent.

[a]Numbers in parentheses are 95-percent confidence intervals.

of tobacco was too small to affect significantly the results for 1985. For women, relative risks for current and former cigarette smokers were employed (Table 7).

Comparison of Tables 9 and 11 reveals significant increases in attributable risk from 1965–85. In 1985, smoking accounted for 21 percent of CHD deaths in older men, compared with 11 percent in 1965. The attributable risks for cancers of the lip, oral cavity and pharynx, esophagus, and lung increased significantly.

Changes in the attributable risk estimates for women are even more striking. Among younger women, smoking now accounts for an estimated 41 percent of CHD deaths and an estimated 55 percent of lethal strokes, compared with 26 and 28 percent, respectively, in 1965. Among women of all ages, 79 percent of lung cancers are attributable to cigarette use (see Table 11).

Overall, smoking accounted for 86.7 percent of all lung cancer deaths (95-percent confidence interval 84.9 to 88.4), 81.8 percent of all COPD deaths (95-percent confidence interval 78.3 to 85.3), and 21.5 percent of all CHD deaths (95-percent confidence interval 19.4 to 23.4). In addition, smoking accounted for 18.0 percent of all stroke deaths (95-percent confidence interval 14.2 to 22.9).

Table 12 reports estimated smoking-attributable deaths for the 10 causes during 1985. Total deaths have increased to 231,000 for men and 106,000 for women. As opposed to 1965, CHD in men now accounts for only one-third of the smoking-attributable mortality from the 10 causes combined. The proportion of these attributable deaths due to lung cancer has increased to one-third. Likewise, among women, smoking-attributable CHD fatalities now account for one-third of the 10-cause total; the relative importance of smoking-induced cancer fatalities has also increased.

The total 10-cause smoking-attributable mortality for 1985 was 337,000 deaths, compared with 183,000 in 1965. A portion of the observed 1965–85 increase, however, was the result of population growth. In addition, there were increases in the proportion of elderly persons who would be more at risk for smoking-induced death. For men and women, respectively, Figures 10 and 11 show the results of a correction for population increase and population aging. In each figure, three quantities are shown for each of four categories of smoking-attributable mortality: CHD deaths under age 65; CHD deaths age 65 years or more; COPD deaths; and lung cancer deaths. The first quantity is the estimated smoking-attributable deaths for 1965. The second bar shows smoking-attributable deaths for 1985. The third bar shows the estimated 1985 smoking-attributable deaths if the U.S. populations at each age had remained at 1965 levels. The latter quantities were computed as aD^*, where a is the attributable risk given in Table 11 and D^* is a population-corrected estimate of 1985 U.S. deaths. The latter quantity was computed by multiplying 1985 age-specific death rates by the populations at risk in 1965.

Figures 10 and 11 show that population growth and aging cannot explain the changes in smoking-attributable mortality between 1965 and 1985. In particular, the marked increases in smoking-attributable deaths from lung cancer and COPD in women are systematic consequences of the American woman's adoption of lifelong cigarette smoking, from teenage years onward.

For men, population-corrected deaths due to smoking in 1985 were 165,000, compared with 150,000 in 1965. For women, population-corrected deaths due to smoking

TABLE 12.—Estimated deaths (in thousands) attributable to cigarette smoking, 10 selected causes, males and females, United States, 1985

Cause of death	Males	Females
CHD, age <65	34 (30–38)[a]	11 (9–12)
CHD, age ≥65	44 (36–54)	26 (20–34)
COPD	37 (35–39)	20 (18–21)
Cancer of lip, oral cavity, and pharynx	5.1 (4.4–5.4)	1.6 (1.2–2.0)
Cancer of larynx	2.3 (1.6–2.7)	0.6 (0.4–0.7)
Cancer of esophagus	5.0 (4.0–5.7)	1.6 (1.3–1.9)
Cancer of lung	76 (74–77)	30 (29–32)
Cancer of pancreas	3.3 (2.1–5.0)	3.4 (2.8–5.1)
Cancer of bladder	3.1 (2.1–4.2)	1.1 (0.6–1.9)
Cancer of kidney	2.6 (1.8–3.5)	0.4 (0.1–1.5)
Cerebrovascular disease, age <65	5.5 (3.9–7.0)	5.2 (4.3–6.2)
Cerebrovascular disease, age ≥65	12 (8–17)	4.8 (1.9–11.4)
Ten causes	231 (220–242)	106 (98–115)

NOTE: Computed from Table 11 and unpublished tabulations of deaths at ages 20 years or more by cause from NCHS, 1985. Sum of individual causes may not equal totals because of rounding.
[a]Numbers in parentheses are 95-percent confidence intervals.

in 1985 were 67,000, compared with 30,000 in 1965. Even if the population had remained entirely stable during 1965 through 1985, the lethality of cigarette use in American women would have doubled.

Among men, the total of 231,000 smoking-induced deaths in 1985 represented 41 percent of total deaths from the 10 causes combined and 22 percent of all deaths among persons aged 20 years or more. Among women, the total of 106,000 smoking-induced deaths represented 25 percent of deaths from the 10 causes combined and 11 percent of deaths from all deaths among persons aged 20 years or more.

The computations in Tables 10 and 12 have omitted other causes of death that are likely to be attributable to cigarette use. If the relative risks given in Tables 6 and 7 for

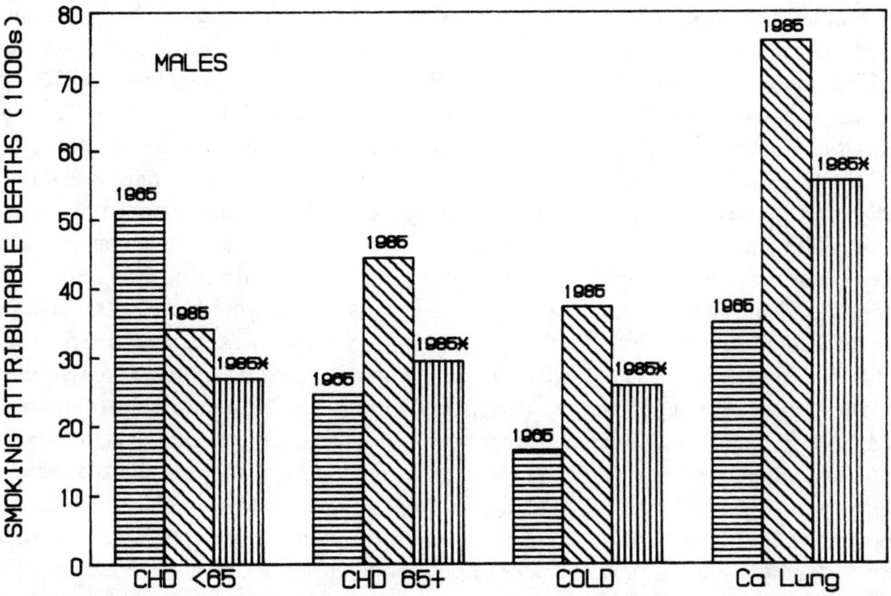

FIGURE 10.—Estimated cigarette-smoking-attributable deaths from CHD, COPD, and lung cancer, males aged 20 years or more, United States, 1965 and 1985

NOTE: For the bars marked 1985*, the estimated smoking-attributable deaths in 1985 have been corrected for population increases during 1965–85.

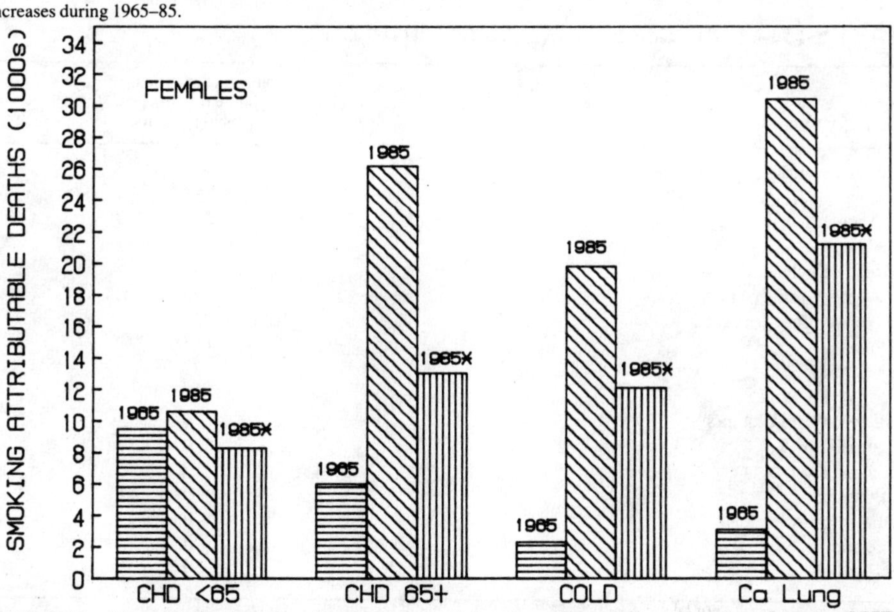

FIGURE 11.—Estimated cigarette-smoking-attributable deaths from CHD, COPD, and lung cancer, females aged 20 years or more, United States, 1965 and 1985

NOTE: For the bars marked 1985*, the estimated smoking-attributable deaths in 1985 have been corrected for population increases during 1965–85.

the broader categories of cardiovascular and nonneoplastic respiratory disease are applied to deaths from hypertensive heart disease, arteriosclerosis, aortic aneurysm, and influenza and pneumonia, then smoking-attributable deaths would increase to 256,000 among men and 126,000 among women. Inclusion of deaths among newborns and infants due to smoking during pregnancy would add an additional 2,500 to the total (CDC 1987b; McIntosh 1984; Kleinman et al. 1988); this does not include fetal loss due to smoking (Stein et al. 1981). Inclusion of lung cancer deaths among nonsmokers due to environmental tobacco smoke (NRC 1986) would add 3,800 and inclusion of deaths from cigarette-caused fires (Hall 1987) would add 1,700 to total attributable deaths. Inclusion of deaths due to cervical cancer caused by smoking would add 1,500. Including these additional causes of death, the smoking-attributable mortality in 1985 is then estimated to be approximately 390,000. Recent studies have also noted increased risks among smokers for hepatic cancer (Trichopoulos et al. 1987), penile cancer (Hellberg et al. 1987), leukemia (Kinlen and Rogot 1988), and anal cancer (Daling et al. 1987).

Among all persons at risk during 1985, an estimated 52 million were also cigarette smokers in 1965. The remaining 42 million were new cigarette smokers. In 1985, only about 4,400 deaths occurred among the latter group, which consists of persons in their teens, twenties, and thirties. Thus, 99 percent of deaths attributable to cigarette use in 1985 occurred among people who started smoking in 1965 or earlier. The vast majority of these people started smoking before the release of the 1964 Surgeon General's Report

TABLE 13.—Estimated risks of various activities

Activity or cause	Annual fatalities per 1 million exposed persons
Active smoking	7,000[a]
Alcohol	541
Accident	275
Disease	266
Motor vehicles	187
Alcohol-involved	95
Non-alcohol-involved	92
Work	113
Swimming	22
Passive smoking[b]	19
All other air pollutants[b]	6
Football	6
Electrocution	2
Lightning	0.5
DES in cattlefeed	0.3
Bee sting	0:2
Basketball	0.02

NOTE: Activities are not mutually exclusive; there are overlaps between categories. Differences in fatalities do not imply proportionate differences in years of life lost.

[a]Number of deaths per million smokers who began smoking before 1965.

[b]Cancer deaths only.

SOURCE: Active smoking, CPS-II; NHISs 1965, 1985; U.S. Bureau of the Census (1974, 1986). Other activities or causes, U.S. President (1987).

and before the 1965 Federal Cigarette Labeling and Advertising Act. For this group, the annual smoking-attributable fatality rate is about 7 deaths per 1,000 at risk, or about 7,000 deaths per 1 million persons. As shown in the Economic Report of the President (U.S. President 1987), this rate far exceeds the rates for other risks of death (Table 13).

Conclusions

1. Lung cancer death rates increased two- to fourfold among older male smokers over the two decades between the American Cancer Society's two Cancer Prevention Studies (CPS-I, 1959–65, and CPS-II, 1982–86). Lung cancer death rates for younger male smokers fell about 30 to 40 percent during this period.
2. Lung cancer death rates increased four- to sevenfold among female smokers aged 45 years or older in CPS-II compared with CPS-I, while lung cancer death rates among younger women declined 35 to 55 percent.
3. The two-decade interval witnessed a two- to threefold increase in death rates from chronic obstructive pulmonary disease (COPD) in female smokers aged 55 years or older.
4. There was no change in the age-adjusted death rates for lung cancer and COPD between CPS-I and CPS-II among men and women who never smoked regularly.
5. Overall death rates from coronary heart disease (CHD) declined substantially between CPS-I and CPS-II. The decline in CHD mortality among nonsmokers, however, was notably greater than among current cigarette smokers.
6. In CPS-II, the relative risks of death from cerebrovascular lesions were 3.7 and 4.8 for men and women smokers under age 65. Increased risks of stroke were also observed among older smokers and former smokers. Along with the recently reported results of other studies, these findings strongly support a causal role for cigarette smoking in thromboembolic and hemorrhagic stroke.
7. In 1985, smoking accounted for 87 percent of lung cancer deaths, 82 percent of COPD deaths, 21 percent of CHD deaths, and 18 percent of stroke deaths. Among men and women less than 65 years of age, smoking accounted for more than 40 percent of CHD deaths.
8. The large increase in smoking-attributable mortality among American women between 1965 and 1985 was a direct consequence of their adoption of lifelong cigarette smoking, especially from their teenage years onward.
9. In 1985, 99 percent of smoking-attributable deaths occurred among people who started smoking before the 1964 Surgeon General's Report. For this group, the annual smoking-attributable fatality rate is about 7,000 deaths per 1 million persons at risk.
10. For 10 causes of death, a total of 337,000 deaths were attributable to smoking in 1985. These represented 22 percent of all deaths among men and 11 percent among women. If other cardiovascular, neoplastic, and respiratory causes of death were included—as well as deaths among newborns and infants resulting from maternal smoking, deaths from cigarette-caused residential fires, and lung cancer deaths among nonsmokers due to environmental tobacco smoke—the total smoking-attributable mortality was about 390,000 in 1985.

References

ABBOTT, R.D., YIN, Y., REED, D.M., YANO, K. Risk of stroke in male cigarette smokers. *New England Journal of Medicine* 315(12):717–720, September 18, 1986.

ALDERSON, M.R., LEE, P.N., WANG, R. Risks of lung cancer, chronic bronchitis, ischaemic heart disease, and stroke in relation to type of cigarette smoked. *Journal of Epidemiology and Community Health* 39(4):286–293, December 1985.

AMERICAN CANCER SOCIETY. Unpublished tabulations.

ANDERSON, S., AUQUIER, A., HAUCK, W.W., OAKES, D., VANDAELE, W., WEISBERG, H.I. *Statistical Methods for Comparative Studies*. New York: John Wiley and Sons, 1980.

BLACK, B., LILIENFELD, D.E. Epidemiological proof in toxic tort litigation. *Fordham Law Review* 52:732–785, 1984.

BOND, V.P. The cancer risk attributable to radiation exposure: Some practical problems. *Health Physics* 40:108–111, January 1981.

BOTKIN, J.R. The fire-safe cigarette. *Journal of the American Medical Association* 260(2): 226–229, July 8, 1988.

BRACKBILL, R., FRAZIER, T., SHILLING, S. Smoking characteristics of US workers, 1978–1980. *American Journal of Industrial Medicine* 13:5–41, 1988.

BROWN, C.C., KESSLER, L.G. Projections of lung cancer mortality in the United States: 1985–2025. *Journal of the National Cancer Institute* 80(1):43–51, March 2, 1988.

CASTELLI, W.P., DAWBER, T.R., FEINLEIB, M., GARRISON, R.J., MCNAMARA, P.M., KANNEL, W.B. The filter cigarette and coronary heart disease: The Framingham Study. *Lancet* 2(8238):109–113, July 18, 1981.

CENTERS FOR DISEASE CONTROL. Cigarette smoking in the United States, 1986. *Morbidity and Mortality Weekly Report* 36(35):581–585, September 11, 1987a.

CENTERS FOR DISEASE CONTROL. Smoking-attributable mortality and years of potential life lost—United States, 1984. *Morbidity and Mortality Weekly Report* 36(42):693–697, October 30, 1987b.

COLDITZ, G.A., BONITA, R., STAMPFER, M.J., WILLETT, W.C., ROSNER, B., SPEIZER, F.E., HENNEKENS, C.H. Cigarette smoking and risk of stroke in middle-aged women. *New England Journal of Medicine* 318(15):937–941, April 14, 1988.

CONSUMER PRODUCT SAFETY COMMISSION. *Toward a Less Fire-Prone Cigarette: Final Report of the Technical Study Group on Cigarette and Little Cigar Fire Safety*. Consumer Product Safety Commission, October 1987.

CORNFIELD, J. A method of estimating comparative rates from clinical data. Applications to cancer of the lung, breast, and cervix. *Journal of the National Cancer Institute* 11:1269–1275, 1951.

COX, L.A. JR. Statistical issues in the estimation of assigned shares for carcinogenesis liability. *Risk Analysis* 7(1):71–80, 1987.

CURRENT POPULATION SURVEY. Unpublished tabulations, 1985.

DALING, J.R., WEISS, N.S., HISLOP, T.G., MADEN, C., COATES, R.J., SHERMAN, K.J., ASHLEY, R.L., BEAGRIE, M., RYAN, J.A., COREY, L. Sexual practices, sexually transmitted diseases, and the incidence of anal cancer. *New England Journal of Medicine* 317(16): 973–977, October 15, 1987.

DEANFIELD, J., WRIGHT, C., KRIKLER, S., RIBEIRO, P., FOX, K. Cigarette smoking and the treatment of angina with propranolol, atenolol, and nifedipine. *New England Journal of Medicine* 310(15):951–954, April 12, 1984.

DOLL, R., GRAY, R., HAFNER, B., PETO, R. Mortality in relation to smoking: 22 years' observations on female British doctors. *British Medical Journal* 280(6219):967–971, April 5, 1980.

DOLL, R., HILL, A.B. Lung cancer and other causes of death in relation to smoking. A second report on the mortality of British doctors. *British Medical Journal* 2:1071–1081, November 10, 1956.

DOLL, R., HILL, A.B. Mortality in relation to smoking: Ten years' observations of British doctors. *British Medical Journal* 1:1399–1410, May 30, 1964; 1460–1467, June 6, 1964.

DOLL, R., HILL, A.B. Mortality of British doctors in relation to smoking: Observations on coronary thrombosis. In: Haenszel, W. (ed.) *Epidemiological Approaches to the Study of Cancer and Other Chronic Diseases*, NCI Monograph 19. U.S. Department of Health, Education, and Welfare, Public Health Service, National Cancer Institute, January 1966, pp. 205–268.

DOLL, R., PETO, R. Mortality in relation to smoking: 20 years' observations on male British doctors. *British Medical Journal* 2:1525–1536, December 25, 1976.

DOLL, R., PETO, R. Cigarette smoking and bronchial carcinoma: Dose and time relationships among regular and lifelong non-smokers. *Journal of Epidemiology and Community Health* 32(4):302–313, December 1978.

DOLL, R., PETO, R. The causes of cancer: Quantitative estimates of avoidable risks of cancer in the United States today. *Journal of the National Cancer Institute* 66(6):1191–1308, June 1981.

DORN, H.F. Tobacco consumption and mortality from cancer and other diseases. *Public Health Reports* 74(7):581–593, July 1959.

GALAN, K.M., DELIGONUL, U., KERN, M.J., CHAITMAN, B.R., VANDORMAEL, M.G. Increased frequency of restenosis in patients continuing to smoke cigarettes after percutaneous transluminal coronary angioplasty. *American Journal of Cardiology* 61:260–263, 1988.

GARFINKEL, L. Cancer mortality in nonsmokers: Prospective study by the American Cancer Society. *Journal of the National Cancer Institute* 65(5):1169–1173, November 1980a.

GARFINKEL, L. Cardiovascular mortality and cigarette smoking. In: Ramstrom, L.M. (ed.) *The Smoking Epidemic. A Matter of Worldwide Concern. Proceedings of The Fourth World Conference on Smoking and Health.* Stockholm: Almqvist and Wiksell International, 1980b, pp. 41–44.

GARFINKEL, L. Time trends in lung cancer mortality among nonsmokers and a note on passive smoking. *Journal of the National Cancer Institute* 66(6):1061–1066, June 1981.

GARFINKEL, L. Selection, follow-up and analysis in the American Cancer Society prospective studies. In: Garfinkel, L., Ochs, O., Mushinski, M. (eds.) *Selection, Follow-up, and Analysis in Prospective Studies: A Workshop*, NCI Monograph 67. National Cancer Institute. NIH Publication No. 85-2713, 1985, pp. 49–52.

GARFINKEL, L., STELLMAN, S.D. Smoking and lung cancer in women. *Cancer Research* 48(23):6951–6955, December 1, 1988.

GOLDBAUM, G.M., KENDRICK, J.S., HOGELIN, G.C., GENTRY, E.M., BEHAVIORAL RISK FACTORS SURVEYS GROUP. The relative impact of smoking and oral contraceptive use on women in the United States. *Journal of the American Medical Association* 258(10):1339–1342, September 11, 1987.

HAENSZEL, W., SHIMKIN, M.B., MILLER, H.P., MILMORE, B.K., CONOVER, A.G. *Tobacco Smoking Patterns in the United States*, Public Health Monograph 45. U.S. Public Health Service, 1956.

HALL, J.R. JR. *Expected Changes in Fire Damages From Reducing Cigarette Ignition Propensity.* Quincy, Massachusetts: National Fire Protection Association, Fire Analysis Division, 1987.

HAMMOND, E.C. Smoking in relation to physical complaints. *Archives of Environmental Health* 3:146–164, August 1961.

HAMMOND, E.C. Some preliminary findings on physical complaints from a prospective study of 1,064,004 men and women. *American Journal of Public Health* 54(1):11–23, January 1964a.

HAMMOND, E.C. Smoking in relation to mortality and morbidity. Findings in the first thirty-four months of follow-up in a prospective study started in 1959. *Journal of the National Cancer Institute* 32(5):1161–1188, May 1964b.

HAMMOND, E.C. Smoking in relation to the death rates of one million men and women. In: Haenszel, W. (ed.) *Epidemiological Approaches to the Study of Cancer and Other Chronic Diseases*, NCI Monograph 19. U.S. Department of Health, Education, and Welfare, Public Health Service, National Cancer Institute, January 1966, pp. 127–204.

HAMMOND, E.C. Quantitative relationship between cigarette smoking and death rates. In: Wynder, E.L. (ed.) *Toward a Less Harmful Cigarette*, NCI Monograph 28. U.S. Public Health Service, National Cancer Institute, June 1968, pp. 3–8.

HAMMOND, E.C. Life expectancy of American men in relation to their smoking habits. *Journal of the National Cancer Institute* 43(4):951–962, October 1969.

HAMMOND, E.C. Smoking habits and air pollution in relation to lung cancer. In: Lee, D.H.K. (ed.) *Environmental Factors in Respiratory Disease*. New York: Academic Press, 1972.

HAMMOND, E.C., GARFINKEL, L. Smoking habits of men and women. *Journal of the National Cancer Institute* 27(2):419–442, August 1961.

HAMMOND, E.C., GARFINKEL, L. Changes in cigarette smoking. *Journal of the National Cancer Institute* 33(1):49–64, July 1964.

HAMMOND, E.C., GARFINKEL, L. The influence of health on smoking habits. In: Haenszel, W. (ed.) *Epidemiological Approaches to the Study of Cancer and Other Chronic Diseases*, NCI Monograph 19. U.S. Department of Health, Education, and Welfare, Public Health Service, National Cancer Institute, January 1966, pp. 269–285.

HAMMOND, E.C., GARFINKEL, L. Changes in cigarette smoking 1959–1965. *American Journal of Public Health* 58(1):30–45, January 1968.

HAMMOND, E.C., GARFINKEL, L. Coronary heart disease, stroke, and aortic aneurysm. Factors in etiology. *Archives of Environmental Health* 19:167–182, August 1969.

HAMMOND, E.C., GARFINKEL, L. Aspirin and coronary heart disease: Findings of a prospective study. *British Medical Journal* 2:269–271, May 3, 1975.

HAMMOND, E.C., GARFINKEL, L., SEIDMAN, H., LEW, E.A. "Tar" and nicotine content of cigarette smoke in relation to death rates. *Environmental Research* 12(3):263–274, December 1976.

HAMMOND, E.C., HORN, D. The relationship between human smoking habits and death rates. A follow-up study of 187,766 men. *Journal of the American Medical Association* 155:1316–1328, August 7, 1954.

HAMMOND, E.C., SEIDMAN, H. Smoking and cancer in the United States. *Preventive Medicine* 9(2):169–173, March 1980.

HARRIS, J.E. Cigarette smoking among successive birth cohorts of men and women in the United States during 1900–80. *Journal of the National Cancer Institute* 71(3):473–479, September 1983.

HAVLIK, R.J., FEINLEIB, M. (eds.) *Proceedings of the Conference on the Decline in Coronary Heart Disease Mortality*. U.S. Department of Health, Education, and Welfare, National Institutes of Health. DHEW Publication No. (NIH) 79-1610, 1979.

HAWTHORNE, V.M., FRY, J.S. Smoking and health: The association between smoking behaviour, total mortality, and cardiorespiratory disease in west central Scotland. *Journal of Epidemiology and Community Health* 32:260–266, 1978.

HELLBERG, D., VALENTIN, J., EKLUND, T., STAFFAN, N. Penile cancer: Is there an epidemiological role for smoking and sexual behaviour? *British Medical Journal* 295(6609): 1306–1308, November 21, 1987.

INTERNATIONAL CLASSIFICATION OF DISEASES. *International Classification of Diseases*, Seventh Revision (ICD-7).

INTERNATIONAL CLASSIFICATION OF DISEASES. *International Classification of Diseases*, Ninth Revision (ICD-9). U.S. Department of Health and Human Services, Public Health Service, Health Care Financing Administration. DHHS Publication No. (PHS) 80-1260, September 1980.

KAHN, H.A. The Dorn study of smoking and mortality among U.S. veterans: Report on eight and one-half years of observation. In: Haenszel, W. (ed.) *Epidemiological Approaches to the Study of Cancer and Other Chronic Diseases*, NCI Monograph 19. U.S. Department of Health, Education, and Welfare, Public Health Service, National Cancer Institute, January 1966, pp. 1–125.

KAUFMAN, D.W., HELMRICH, S.P., ROSENBERG, L., MIETTINEN, O.S., SHAPIRO, S. Nicotine and carbon monoxide content of cigarette smoke and the risk of myocardial infarction in young men. *New England Journal of Medicine* 308(8):409–413, February 24, 1983.

KINLEN, L.J., ROGOT, E. Leukaemia and smoking habits among United States veterans. *British Medical Journal* 297(6649):657–659, September 10, 1988.

KLEBBA, A.J. Comparability of mortality statistics for the seventh and eighth revisions of the International Classification of Diseases, United States. Vital and Health Statistics, Series 2, No. 66. U.S. Department of Health, Education, and Welfare. DHEW Publication No. (HRA) 76-1340, October 1975.

KLEBBA, A.J. Mortality from diseases associated with smoking: United States, 1960–77. *Vital and Health Statistics*, Series 20, No. 17. U.S. Department of Health and Human Services. DHHS Publication No. (PHS) 82-1854, January 1982.

KLEBBA, A.J., SCOTT, J.H. Estimates of selected comparability ratios based on dual coding of 1976 death certificates by the eighth and ninth revisions of the International Classification of Diseases. *Monthly Vital Statistics Report From the National Center for Health Statistics* 28(11):1–19, February 29, 1980.

KLEBBA, J. Personal communication to J. Harris, June 1988.

KLEINMAN, J.C., PIERRE, M.B. JR., MADANS, J.H., LAND, G.H., SCHRAMM, W.F. The effects of maternal smoking on fetal and infant mortality. *American Journal of Epidemiology* 127(2):274–282, 1988.

LAVECCHIA, C., FRANCESCHI, S., DECARLI, A., FASOLI, M., GENTILE, A., TOGNONI, G. Cigarette smoking and the risk of cervical neoplasia. *American Journal of Epidemiology* 123(1):22–29, January 1986.

LEE, P.N., GARFINKEL, L. Mortality and type of cigarette smoked. *Journal of Epidemiology and Community Health* 35(1):16–22, March 1981.

LESKO, S.M., ROSENBERG, L., KAUFMAN, D.W., HELMRICH, S.P., MILLER, D.R., STROM, B., SCHOTTENFELD, D., ROSENSHEIN, N.B., KNAPP, R.C., LEWIS, J., SHAPIRO, S. Cigarette smoking and the risk of endometrial cancer. *New England Journal of Medicine* 313(10):593–596, 1985.

LEVIN, M.L. The occurrence of lung cancer in man. *Acta-Unio Internationalis Contra Cancrum* 9:531–541, 1953.

LEW, E.A., GARFINKEL, L. Mortality at ages 65 and over in a middle-class population. *Transactions of the Society of Actuaries* 36:257–308, 1984.

LEW, E.A., GARFINKEL, L. Differences in mortality and longevity by sex, smoking habits and health status. *Transactions of the Society of Actuaries* 39:19–36, 1988.

LILIENFELD, D.E., GUNDERSON, P.D. The "missing cases" of pleural malignant mesothelioma in Minnesota, 1979–81: Preliminary report. *Public Health Reports* 101(4): 395–399, July–August 1986.

LILIENFELD, A.M., LILIENFELD, D.E. *Foundations of Epidemiology*, Second Edition. New York: Oxford University Press, 1980.

LUBIN, J.H., BLOT, W.J., BERRINO, F., FLAMANT, R., GILLIS, C.R., KUNZE, M., SCHMAHL, D., VISCO, D. Modifying risk of developing lung cancer by changing habits of cigarette smoking. *British Medical Journal* 288(6435):1953–1956, June 30, 1984.

LUBIN, J.H., BOICE, J.D. JR. Estimating radon-induced lung cancer in the U.S. Working paper, 1988.

MACMAHON, B., PUGH, T.F. *Epidemiology. Principles and Methods.* Boston: Little, Brown and Company, 1970.

MASSEY, M.M., BOYD, G., MATTSON, M., FEINLEIB, M.R. Inventory of surveys on smoking. *Public Health Reports* 102(4):430–438, July–August 1987.

MCFARLANE, M.J., FEINSTEIN, A.R., WELLS, C.K. Necropsy evidence of detection bias in the diagnosis of lung cancer. *Archives of Internal Medicine* 146(9):1695–1698, September 1986.

MCINTOSH, I.D. Smoking and pregnancy: Attributable risks and public health implications. *Canadian Journal of Public Health* 75(2):141–148, March–April 1984.

MIETTINEN, O.S. Proportion of disease caused or prevented by a given exposure, trait or intervention. *American Journal of Epidemiology* 99(5):325–332, 1974.

NATIONAL CENTER FOR HEALTH STATISTICS. *Vital Statistics of the United States 1965. Volume 2—Mortality, Part A.* U.S. Department of Health, Education, and Welfare, Public Health Service, National Center for Health Statistics, 1967.

NATIONAL CENTER FOR HEALTH STATISTICS. Unpublished tabulations, 1985.

NATIONAL CENTER FOR HEALTH STATISTICS. *Health, United States, 1986.* U.S. Department of Health and Human Services, Public Health Service, National Center for Health Statistics. DHHS Publication No. (PHS) 87-1232, December 1986.

NATIONAL HEALTH INTERVIEW SURVEY. Unpublished tabulations, 1965.

NATIONAL HEALTH INTERVIEW SURVEY. Unpublished tabulations, 1985.

NATIONAL RESEARCH COUNCIL. *Assigned Share for Radiation as a Cause of Cancer. Review of Radioepidemiologic Tables Assigning Probabilities of Causation.* Washington, D.C.: National Academy Press, 1984.

NATIONAL RESEARCH COUNCIL. *Environmental Tobacco Smoke. Measuring Exposures and Assessing Health Effects.* Washington, D.C.: National Academy Press, 1986.

NATIONAL RESEARCH COUNCIL. *Health Risks of Radon and Other Internally Deposited Alpha-Emitters. BEIR IV.* Washington, D.C.: National Academy Press, 1988.

NISCHAN, P., EBELING, K., SCHINDLER, C. Smoking and invasive cervical cancer risk. Results from a case–control study. *American Journal of Epidemiology* 128(1):74–77, July 1988.

NOVOTNY, T.E., WARNER, K.E., KENDRICK, J.S., REMINGTON, P.L. Smoking by blacks and whites: Socioeconomic and demographic differences. *American Journal of Public Health* 78(9):1187–1189, September 1988.

OFTEDAL, P., MAGNUS, K., HVINDEN, T. On the probability of radiation being the cause of leukaemia. (Letter.) *British Journal of Radiology* 41:711–712, 1968.

PEARL, R. Tobacco smoking and longevity. *Science* 87(2253):216–217, March 4, 1938.

PETO, R. Influence of dose and duration of smoking on lung cancer rates. In: Zaridze, D.G., Peto, R. (eds.) *Tobacco: A Major International Health Hazard.* Lyon, France: International Agency for Research on Cancer, 1986, pp. 23–33.

RAVENHOLT, R.T. Cigarette smoking: Magnitude of the hazard. (Letter.) *American Journal of Public Health* 54(11):1923–1926, November 1964.

RAVENHOLT, R.T. Addiction mortality in the United States, 1980: Tobacco, alcohol, and other substances. *Population and Development Review* 10(4):697–724, December 1984.

RICE, D.P., HODGSON, T.A., SINSHEIMER, P., BROWNER, W., KOPSTEIN, A.N. The economic costs of the health effects of smoking, 1984. *Milbank Quarterly* 64(4):489–547, 1986.

ROGOT, E. Smoking and mortality among U.S. veterans. *Journal of Chronic Diseases* 27:189–203, 1974.

ROGOT, E., MURRAY, J.L. Smoking and causes of death among U.S. veterans: 16 years of observation. *Public Health Reports* 95(3):213–222, May–June 1980.

ROSENBERG, L., KAUFMAN, D.W., HELMRICH, S.P., SHAPIRO, S. The risk of myocardial infarction after quitting smoking in men under 55 years of age. *New England Journal of Medicine* 313(24):1511–1514, December 12, 1985.

ROSENBERG, L., SCHWINGL, P.J., KAUFMAN, D.W., MILLER, D.R., HELMRICH, S.P., STOLLEY, P.D., SCHOTTENFELD, D., SHAPIRO, S. Breast cancer and cigarette smoking. *New England Journal of Medicine* 310:92–94, January 12, 1984.

SARACCI, R. The interactions of tobacco smoking and other agents in cancer etiology. *Epidemiologic Reviews* 9:175–193, 1987.

SCHOENBORN, C.A., BENSON, V. Relationships between smoking and other unhealthy habits: United States, 1985. *Advance Data From Vital and Health Statistics of the National Center for Health Statistics* 154:1–8, May 27, 1988.

SHULTZ, J.M. *SAMMEC. Smoking-Attributable Mortality, Morbidity, and Economic Costs.* Computer Software and Documentation. Minnesota Department of Health, Center for Nonsmoking and Health, 1986.

SLONE, D., SHAPIRO, S., ROSENBERG, L., KAUFMAN, D., HARTZ, S.C., ROSSI, A.C., STOLLEY, P.D., MIETTINEN, O.S. Relation of cigarette smoking to myocardial infarction in young women. *New England Journal of Medicine* 298(23):1273–1276, June 8, 1978.

STEIN, Z., KLINE, J., LEVIN, B., SUSSER, M., WARBURTON, D. Epidemiologic studies of environmental exposures in human reproduction. In: Berg, G.G., Maillie, H.D. (eds.) *Measurement of Risks.* New York: Plenum Press, 1981, pp. 163–183.

STELLMAN, S.D. Cigarette yield and cancer risk: Evidence from case–control and prospective studies. In: Zaridze, D.G., Peto, R. (eds.) *Tobacco: A Major International Health Hazard.* Lyon, France: International Agency for Research on Cancer, 1986a, pp. 197–209.

STELLMAN, S.D. Influence of cigarette yield on risk of coronary heart disease and chronic obstructive pulmonary disease. In: Zaridze, D.G., Peto, R. (eds.) *Tobacco: A Major International Health Hazard.* Lyon, France: International Agency for Research on Cancer, 1986b, pp. 237–249.

STELLMAN, S.D., BOFFETTA, P., GARFINKEL, L. Smoking habits of 800,000 American men and women in relation to their occupations. *American Journal of Industrial Medicine* 13:43–58, 1988.

STELLMAN, S.D., GARFINKEL, L. Smoking habits and tar levels in a new American Cancer Society prospective study of 1.2 million men and women. *Journal of the National Cancer Institute* 76(6):1057–1063, June 1986.

STERLING, T.D., WEINKAM, J.J. Errors in estimates of smoking-related deaths derived from nonsmoker mortality. *Risk Analysis* 7(4):463–475, 1987.

TRICHOPOULOS, D., DAY, N.E., KAKLAMANI, E., TZONOU, A., MUNOZ, N., ZAVITSANOS, X., KOUMANTAKI, Y., TRICHOPOULOU, A. Hepatitis B virus, tobacco smoking and ethanol consumption in the etiology of hepatocellular carcinoma. *International Journal of Cancer* 39(1):45–49, January 1987.

U.S. BUREAU OF THE CENSUS. *Estimates of the Population of the United States, by Age, Sex, and Race: April 1, 1960 to July 1, 1973. Current Population Reports*, Series P-25, No. 519. U.S. Bureau of the Census, April 1974.

U.S. BUREAU OF THE CENSUS. *Estimates of the Population of the United States, by Age, Sex, and Race: 1980 to 1985. Current Population Reports*, Series P-25, No. 985. U.S. Bureau of the Census, April 1986.

U.S. DEPARTMENT OF HEALTH AND HUMAN SERVICES. *The Health Consequences of Smoking for Women. A Report of the Surgeon General.* U.S. Department of Health and Human Services, Public Health Service, Office of the Assistant Secretary for Health, Office on Smoking and Health, 1980.

U.S. DEPARTMENT OF HEALTH AND HUMAN SERVICES. *The Health Consequences of Smoking. The Changing Cigarette: A Report of the Surgeon General.* U.S. Department of Health and Human Services, Public Health Service, Office of the Assistant Secretary for Health, Office on Smoking and Health. DHHS Publication No. (PHS) 81-50156, 1981.

U.S. DEPARTMENT OF HEALTH AND HUMAN SERVICES. *The Health Consequences of Smoking: Cancer. A Report of the Surgeon General.* U.S. Department of Health and Human Services, Public Health Service, Office on Smoking and Health. DHHS Publication No. (PHS) 82-50179, 1982.

U.S. DEPARTMENT OF HEALTH AND HUMAN SERVICES. *The Health Consequences of Smoking: Cardiovascular Disease. A Report of the Surgeon General.* U.S. Department of Health and Human Services, Public Health Service, Office on Smoking and Health. DHHS Publication No. (PHS) 84-50204, 1983.

U.S. DEPARTMENT OF HEALTH AND HUMAN SERVICES. *The Health Consequences of Smoking: Chronic Obstructive Lung Disease. A Report of the Surgeon General.* U.S. Department of Health and Human Services, Public Health Service, Office on Smoking and Health. DHHS Publication No. (PHS) 84-50205, 1984.

U.S. DEPARTMENT OF HEALTH AND HUMAN SERVICES. *The Health Consequences of Smoking: Cancer and Chronic Lung Disease in the Workplace. A Report of the Surgeon General.* U.S. Department of Health and Human Services, Public Health Service, Office on Smoking and Health. DHHS Publication No. (PHS) 85-50207, 1985.

U.S. DEPARTMENT OF HEALTH AND HUMAN SERVICES. *The Health Consequences of Involuntary Smoking. A Report of the Surgeon General.* U.S. Department of Health and Human Services, Public Health Service, Centers for Disease Control. DHHS Publication No. (CDC) 87-8398, 1986.

U.S. DEPARTMENT OF HEALTH AND HUMAN SERVICES. *The Health Consequences of Smoking: Nicotine Addiction. A Report of the Surgeon General, 1988.* U.S. Department of Health and Human Services, Public Health Service, Centers for Disease Control, Center for Health Promotion and Education, Office on Smoking and Health. DHHS Publication No. (CDC) 88-8406, 1988a.

U.S. DEPARTMENT OF HEALTH AND HUMAN SERVICES. *Health, United States, 1987.* U.S. Department of Health and Human Services, Public Health Service, Centers for Disease Control, National Center for Health Statistics. DHHS Publication No. (PHS) 88-1232, March 1988b.

U.S. DEPARTMENT OF HEALTH, EDUCATION, AND WELFARE. *Smoking and Health. A Report of the Surgeon General.* U.S. Department of Health, Education, and Welfare, Public Health Service, Office of the Assistant Secretary for Health, Office on Smoking and Health. DHEW Publication No. (PHS) 79-50066, 1979.

U.S. OFFICE OF TECHNOLOGY ASSESSMENT. *Smoking-Related Deaths and Financial Costs.* Health Program, Office of Technology Assessment, U.S. Congress, September 1985.

U.S. PRESIDENT. *Economic Report of the President. Transmitted to the Congress January 1987*. Washington, D.C., 1987.

U.S. PUBLIC HEALTH SERVICE. *Smoking and Health. Report of the Advisory Committee to the Surgeon General of the Public Health Service*. U.S. Department of Health, Education, and Welfare, Public Health Service, Center for Disease Control. PHS Publication No. 1103, 1964.

WALTER, S.D. The estimation and interpretation of attributable risk in health research. *Biometrics* 32:829–849, December 1976.

WHYTE, H.M. The relative importance of the major risk factors in atherosclerotic and other diseases. *Australian and New Zealand Journal of Medicine* 6(5):387–393, October 1976.

WILCOX, H.B., SCHOENBERG, J.B., MASON, T.J., BILL, J.S., STEMHAGEN, A. Smoking and lung cancer: Risk as function of cigarette tar content. *Preventive Medicine* 17(3):263–272, March 1988.

WILLETT, W.C., GREEN, A., STAMPFER, M.J., SPEIZER, F.E., COLDITZ, G.A., ROSNER, B., MONSON, R.R., STASON, W., HENNEKENS, C.H. Relative and absolute excess risks of coronary heart disease among women who smoke cigarettes. *New England Journal of Medicine* 317(21):1303–1309, November 19, 1987.

WILLIAMSON, D.F., FORMAN, M.R., BRADSTOCK, M.K., GENTRY, E., BINKIN, N.J. Behavioral Risk Factor Survey results for cigarette smoking and other health-risk behaviors among U.S. women, 1981–1983. (Abstract.) In: *Epidemic Intelligence Service 35th Annual Conference*. U.S. Department of Health and Human Services, Public Health Service, 1986.

WYNDER, E.L., STELLMAN, S.D. Impact of long-term filter cigarette usage on lung and larynx cancer risk: A case–control study. *Journal of the National Cancer Institute* 62(3):471–477, March 1979.

CHAPTER 4

TRENDS IN PUBLIC BELIEFS, ATTITUDES, AND OPINIONS ABOUT SMOKING

CONTENTS

Introduction

This Chapter analyzes trends in public beliefs, attitudes, and opinions about smoking. It is divided into three sections. The first describes trends in public beliefs regarding the health effects of smoking, the second describes trends in public attitudes about smokers and smoking, and the third describes trends in public opinion about smoking policies.

At the outset, it is important to define and clarify the important terms used in this Chapter. Terms such as knowledge, awareness, opinions, beliefs, and attitudes have commonsense meanings to the lay person, but more complex meanings to the social scientist. For example, Allport (1935) reviewed many definitions of attitude and constructed his own comprehensive definition: "An attitude is a mental or neural state of readiness, organized through experience, exerting a directive or dynamic influence upon the individual's response to all objects and situations with which it is related." Entire books have been devoted to the science of defining and measuring public attitudes, opinions, and beliefs (e.g., Oskamp 1977).

For sections two and three of this Chapter, which deal with attitudes and opinions, the commonplace understanding of these terms will suffice. For the first section, however, which covers beliefs about health effects, a more careful approach is warranted. This Section generally follows the construct described by Fishbein (1977), which embraces three levels of belief:

1. Level 1 (awareness): A person may believe that "the Surgeon General has determined that cigarette smoking is dangerous to health."
2. Level 2 (general acceptance): A person may believe that "cigarette smoking is dangerous to health."
3. Level 3 (personalized acceptance): A person may believe that "my cigarette smoking is dangerous to *my* health."

Most of the survey data presented in the first section address Level 2 beliefs. At times, the term public knowledge is used to refer to public beliefs (Level 2 beliefs at the population level). There are few data regarding Level 1 beliefs; consequently, use of the terms awareness and public awareness is generally avoided. Data pertinent to Level 3 beliefs are available from a few surveys in three forms: (1) questions asking whether smoking "is harmful to *your* health"; (2) questions asking whether respondents are "concerned" about the effects of smoking on *their* health; and (3) questions asking whether respondents believe that they are less likely, as likely, or more likely than other people to be adversely affected by smoking. These levels of beliefs are discussed in more depth later in this Chapter.

Data Sources

The information presented in this Chapter is derived from three principal sources:

1. Nationally representative surveys conducted by the U.S. Public Health Service from 1964–87, including the Adult Use of Tobacco Surveys (AUTSs) (1964, 1966, 1970, 1975, 1986) and the National Health Interview Surveys (NHISs) (1985, 1987). The NHIS questions were part of the Health Promotion and Dis-

ease Prevention Supplement in 1985 and the Cancer Control Supplement in 1987. The surveys for 1964–75 used, for the most part, the same methods and questionnaire wording. Different methods and questionnaires were used in subsequent surveys.

2. Nationally representative surveys conducted by private organizations, such as Gallup and Roper, and sponsored by various organizations.
3. National surveys of population *subgroups* or local surveys. These surveys were used, for the most part, only when nationally representative data were unavailable.

Data from these surveys are presented in several tables throughout this Chapter, each of which addresses beliefs or opinions about a particular smoking-related scientific fact or policy. When one of the primary data sources (e.g., the AUTS) is not included in a table, it is because the relevant question was not asked in the survey or survey year or because the data were not available.

Preliminary first-quarter estimates from the Cancer Control Supplement to the 1987 NHIS are provided in some tables (unpublished data, National Cancer Institute). These data are unweighted. When available, year-end weighted data are cited; in all cases, these figures are very similar to the first-quarter estimates.

The surveys used in this Chapter and in Chapter 5 are described in the Appendix to this Chapter. Table 1 provides basic information about the survey methodology. The amounts of information provided for the different surveys vary because certain

TABLE 1.—Methodology of surveys

Survey	Survey firm	Sample size	Age (years)	Response rate (%)	Mode[a]
AUTS 1964	National Analysts	5,794	≥21	76	P
AUTS 1966	National Analysts Opinion Research	5,768		72	P T[b]
AUTS 1970	Chilton	5,200	≥21		P(9%[c]) T(91%)
AUTS 1975	Chilton	12,000			T(96%) P(4%[c])
Roper 1978	Roper	2,511			P
NHIS 1985	Census Bureau	33,630	≥18	90	P
AUTS 1986	Westat	13,031	≥17	74	T
AMA 1986	Kane, Parsons	1,500			T
AMA 1987	Kane, Parsons	1,500			T
MTF[d] 1975–87	University of Michigan		18		Q

[a]P, personal interview; T, telephone interview; Q, self-administered questionnaire.
[b]Nonrespondents to personal interviews.
[c]Nontelephone households.
[d]Monitoring the Future Project, survey of high school seniors.

methodological details were available for some surveys but not for others. Additional information on the methodology of these surveys has been published elsewhere (Massey et al. 1987).

Issues in Comparing Surveys

When assessing trends from different surveys conducted at different times by different organizations, it is important to consider the following caveats. The response to each specific question depends upon multiple factors, including the mode of data collection (e.g., in person versus telephone), the sociodemographic representativeness of the sample, the exact wording of the question (e.g., bold, direct-sounding questions versus conservative-sounding statements), the type of response allowed or requested (e.g., open- versus closed-ended questions), the order of questions within the survey, and the content and nature of the rest of the survey (e.g., a survey specifically addressing smoking versus another of a general topic). Even minor changes in the survey methods or questionnaire wording may lead to markedly discrepant results for a specific question.

Additional precautions exist when interpreting surveys that assess public knowledge. When asked a knowledge question, respondents may attempt to answer it "correctly" in order to please the interviewer. The Health Promotion and Disease Prevention Supplement to the 1985 NHIS sheds light on this question. In this survey (NCHS 1986), respondents were asked whether smoking increases the risk of developing cataracts and gall bladder disease–two conditions not associated with smoking. The extent to which these types of questions (sometimes called "red herrings") are answered in the affirmative (and thus incorrectly) may reflect the respondents' general tendency to respond in the affirmative. More than 85 percent of respondents reported that smoking causes emphysema, chronic bronchitis, and laryngeal, esophageal, and lung cancer; however, 11 percent and 16 percent reported that smoking causes gallstones and cataracts, respectively. The responses indicating a connection between smoking and cataracts or gall bladder disease may represent misinformed beliefs or a bias from attempting to answer knowledge questions "correctly." There are other possible explanations, however. For instance, these responses (as well as other "correct" responses) may represent inferences that respondents have made, in some cases regarding questions they have never thought about. In these cases, some persons may be inclined to infer a connection between a known risk behavior and *any* disease outcome.

In the case of questions about public knowledge (e.g., "Do you think that smoking is or is not a cause of lung cancer?"), the "don't know" response should be included in the denominator when calculating the proportion of the population that believes a particular fact. This process was used for calculating unpublished data presented below.

When two surveys produce unexpected or discrepant results, a close inspection of the methods often explains the findings. Two examples involve surveys of public opinion about smoking policies. In one case, two separate national surveys conducted in 1986 regarding support for a ban on cigarette advertising provided apparently discrepant results (American Medical Association (AMA) 1986). A careful review of the questionnaire wording revealed marked differences in the remarks made just prior to each question. In a survey conducted for AMA, respondents were first informed about the AMA's support of a policy to ban advertising—67 percent subsequently responded that they were in favor of such a ban. In contrast, in a survey conducted for the American Cancer Society (ACS), the American Heart Association (AHA), and the American Lung Association (ALA), respondents were first informed that "some people feel that as long as cigarettes are legal, cigarette advertising should be permitted. Others feel that cigarette advertising should not be permitted." Thirty-three percent subsequently responded that cigarette companies should not be permitted to advertise in newspapers and magazines.

There are at least three reasons these questions might be expected to evoke different responses. First, the wording prior to each question may have biased the respondents—one to align with the sponsoring agency's policy and the other to consider the legal implications of such a ban. Second, the first survey asked whether cigarette advertising should be *banned* while the second asked whether cigarette advertising should be *permitted.* To the extent that some respondents may have a general inclination to answer in the affirmative, such wording differences could influence the results. Third, the word "ban" may have negative connotations for some respondents. Two national surveys (including one sponsored by AMA) conducted 1 year later, which provided no introductory comments, found that 49 percent of adults (Gallup 1987a) and 55 percent of adults (Harvey and Shubat 1987) were in favor of a ban on tobacco advertising (see Table 31).

A second example involves two surveys conducted in Michigan in 1986 regarding public opinion on smoking in public places (Perlstadt and Holmes 1987). A survey sponsored by the affiliates of ALA and AHA in Michigan revealed that 82 percent of adults favored restrictions on smoking in public places. In contrast, a survey conducted 2 months later and sponsored by the Michigan Tobacco and Candy Distributors and Vendors Association indicated that 82 percent of the public thought the legislature should refrain from further legislation restricting smoking. After assessing the survey methods and questionnaires, the Michigan Department of Public Health concluded that markedly different questionnaire wording and survey methods accounted for the discrepant results.

To assist in the interpretation of the data presented in this Report, data sources are described in Table 1 and in the Appendix to this Chapter, and the exact (or approximate) question wording and response choices are provided as a footnote to each table when available. Response choices, when obvious, are often omitted (e.g., simple yes–no questions). Although the same question wording may be used in different surveys, other factors may have important effects on the responses. The reader should therefore interpret with caution observed differences and trends presented in this Chapter because many of the potential factors that may affect responses are not known.

Trends in Public Beliefs About the Health Effects of Smoking

Overview

The health consequences of smoking are well documented and widely acknowledged in the scientific literature (see Chapter 2 in this Report). In 1964, the Surgeon General's Advisory Committee on Smoking and Health, after an extensive review of the literature, reported that cigarette smoking was causally associated with lung and laryngeal cancer in men, was the most important cause of chronic bronchitis, and was associated with esophageal cancer, bladder cancer, coronary artery disease, emphysema, peptic ulcer, and low-birthweight babies (US PHS 1964).

During the 25-year period since 1964, subsequent reports of the Surgeon General have updated and extended the findings of the Advisory Committee. The purpose of this Section is to determine the extent to which this information has been disseminated to and accepted by the U.S. public. Public knowledge of the health risks of smoking can be considered under three broad categories: whether smoking is harmful to health in general and whether smokers perceive *themselves* to be at risk from smoking, as well as the magnitude of risk from smoking and how this compares to other health risks. Because health concerns and risks among adolescents differ from those of adults, we have addressed surveys of their knowledge under a separate heading.

For each specific known health risk noted, the section below includes: (1) a description of the known medical or scientific facts; that is, a brief summary of the information known about the health risk (see Chapter 2 for a more detailed description of the information about health risks), (2) a report on the trends in the public's knowledge of this fact (if available), and (3) a brief description of the current status of knowledge with respect to smoking status. This Section concludes with a summary of the important gains in knowledge, the gaps that remain, the factors that may promote or interfere with change, and the relationship between these trends and the 1990 Health Objectives for the Nation.

In a few cases, published studies have analyzed public knowledge or beliefs by sociodemographic groupings (NCHS 1988; Folsom et al. 1988; Fox et al. 1987; Shopland and Brown 1987; Dolecek et al. 1986). Because these analyses were available only occasionally, and because some of these studies did not control for smoking status, sociodemographic correlation data are not presented below. Because smoking rates and socioeconomic status are inversely correlated (Chapter 5), differences in public knowledge or beliefs according to smoking status may reflect differences in socioeconomic status.

Is Cigarette Smoking Harmful to Smokers in General?

In 1964, 81 percent of adults strongly or mildly agreed that smoking is harmful to health (Table 2). An identical series of questions asked in the AUTSs from 1964–75 demonstrated an increase in this belief to 90 percent of adults. Public knowledge on this question increased during this period among current smokers (70 to 81 percent), as well as among never smokers (89 to 95 percent).

TABLE 2.—Trends in public knowledge about smoking and health

			Cigarette smoking is harmful to health (percentage who agree by smoking status)				
Survey	Year	Reference	Current smokers	Former smokers	Never smokers	All non-smokers	All adults
1. AUTS[a]	1964	US DHEW 1969	70	91	89	89	81
2. AUTS[a]	1966	US DHEW 1969	78	89	89	89	85
3. AUTS[a]	1970	US DHEW 1973	79	92	92	92	87
4. AUTS[a]	1975	US DHEW 1976a	81	95	95	95	90

[a]Percentages include those who "strongly agree" or "mildly agree."

NOTE: Actual questions:

1. Smoking cigarettes is harmful to health (strongly agree, mildly agree, no opinion, mildly disagree, strongly disagree).
2. Cigarette smoking is harmful to health (strongly agree, mildly agree, no opinion, mildly disagree, strongly disagree).

3–4. Smoking cigarettes is harmful to health (strongly agree, mildly agree, no opinion/don't know, mildly disagree, strongly disagree).

TABLE 3.—Trends in public beliefs regarding the relative hazards of different cigarette brands, 1970, 1975, 1986

	Percentage of current smokers		
	1970	1975	1986
Some kinds of cigarettes are probably more hazardous to health than others[a]			
Kind I smoke probably more hazardous than others[a]	(6)	(10)	(8)
Kind I smoke probably less hazardous than others[a]	(25)	(25)	(21)
Kind I smoke probably about the same as others[a]	(14)	(14)	(13)
Don't know	(2)	(2)	(2)
Subtotal	47	51	45
All cigarettes are probably about equally hazardous[a]	43	41	50
Cigarettes are probably not hazardous to health at all	4	5	2
Don't know or not stated if some are hazardous	6	4	3
Total	100	100	100

[a]The word "probably" was not used in the 1986 AUTS. The wording in the three surveys was otherwise similar.
SOURCE: AUTSs 1970, 1975, 1986 (US DHEW 1973, 1976a; US DHHS, in press).

Although smokers and nonsmokers acknowledge the health risks from smoking, certain types of smoking (such as light smoking or smoking low-tar cigarettes) or smoking for a limited period of time may be perceived as less hazardous. In general, there are few data to assess the degree to which these beliefs are held. According to the AUTSs in 1970, 1975, and 1986, 45 to 50 percent of current smokers believed that "some kinds of cigarettes are probably more hazardous than others," 40 to 50 percent believed that "all cigarettes are probably about equally hazardous," and 5 percent or less believed that "cigarettes are probably not hazardous to health at all" (Table 3). More specific data are reviewed below.

Heavy Versus Light Smoking

A large body of evidence has shown that light smoking, that is, 1 to 9 cigarettes per day, is associated with a significantly increased risk of overall morbidity and mortality from lung cancer, chronic obstructive pulmonary disease (COPD), heart disease, and other smoking-related diseases compared with never smoking (US DHEW 1979a; US DHHS 1982, 1983, 1984).

Between 1970 and 1978, national surveys conducted by the Roper Organization addressed beliefs regarding the health risks of heavy versus light smoking (FTC 1981). Respondents were asked how hazardous smoking is and were given three possible responses: any amount, only heavy smoking, and not hazardous. In 1970, 45 percent of respondents considered only heavy smoking to be hazardous (Table 4); by 1978, 31

TABLE 4.—Trends in public knowledge about the health hazards of smoking

Survey	Year	Reference	What amount of smoking is hazardous to health?[a,b] (percentage who responded for each amount)			
			Any amount	Only heavy smoking	Not hazardous	Don't know
1. Roper	1970	Roper 1978	47	45	5	3
2. Roper	1972	Roper 1978	48	42	6	4
3. Roper	1974	Roper 1978	54	39	4	3
4. Roper	1976	Roper 1978	54	38	4	4
5. Roper	1978	Roper 1978	61	31	5	4
6. AUTS	1986	US DHHS, in press	72	20		5 (current smokers)
			81	13		4 (former smokers)
			85	11		4 (never smokers)

[a]Respondents were allowed to choose only one answer. The "not hazardous" response was not available for the AUTS.

[b]Percentages of responses in Roper surveys refer to all respondents; in AUTS 1986, percentages represent current, former, and never smokers, respectively.

NOTE: Actual questions:

1–5. How hazardous is smoking? (any amount, only heavy smoking, not hazardous, don't know)

6. Do you think that only heavy smoking is hazardous or that *any* smoking is hazardous? (only heavy smoking, any smoking, don't know)

percent considered only heavy smoking to be hazardous. Corresponding increases occurred in those responding "any amount."

The 1986 AUTS posed a similar question but did not offer "not hazardous" as a possible response (Table 4). It showed that most respondents, given the two choices of "any amount" or "only heavy smoking," chose the former (85, 81, and 72 percent of never, former, and current smokers, respectively).

When asked, "How many cigarettes a day do you think a person would have to smoke before it would affect their (sic) health?" 49 percent of current smokers and 40 percent of never smokers cited 10 or more (Table 5), thus failing to recognize light smoking as a health risk. Twenty percent of current smokers cited 25 or more cigarettes as the minimum number necessary for adverse health effects (Table 5), which is identical to the proportion of current smokers who indicated, in response to the prior question, that only heavy smoking is hazardous to health (Table 4).

Tar Yield

Studies have shown that smoking filtered lower tar cigarettes reduces the risk of lung cancer compared with smoking unfiltered higher tar cigarettes. However, there is no conclusive evidence that the lower yield cigarettes are associated with reduced risk of overall mortality, cancers other than lung, COPD, or heart disease. Moreover, compensatory smoking behavior in response to lower nicotine intake might actually increase the intake of tobacco smoke toxins in some individuals (US DHHS 1981).

Very few surveys have assessed the perceived harmfulness of low-tar cigarettes versus high-tar cigarettes or never smoking. In the 1980 Roper Survey (FTC 1981), respondents were presented with the following false statement: "It has been proven that smoking low-tar, low-nicotine cigarettes does not significantly increase a person's risk of disease over that of a nonsmoker." Nine percent of smokers said they "know it's true," 27 percent said they "think it's true," and 32 percent said they did not know if it was true or not. The complicated wording of this question and use of the word "proven" make interpretation of these results difficult. Different results may have been obtained using a question such as, "Do you believe that smoking low-tar cigarettes is or is not harmful to health?"

The 1980 Roper survey also asked respondents their beliefs about the following statement: "Even if a woman smokes low tar, low nicotine cigarettes during pregnancy, she still significantly increases her risk of losing the baby before or during birth." Forty-three percent of all respondents and 37 percent of smokers said they "know it's true" or "think it's true" (unpublished data, FTC).

The 1987 NHIS asked respondents if they believed that "People who smoke low tar and nicotine cigarettes are less likely to get cancer than people who smoke high tar and nicotine cigarettes." A total of 30 percent agreed with the statement whereas 50 percent disagreed (year-end data).

Folsom and associates (1988) surveyed 1,252 blacks (aged 35 to 74 years) and 1,870 whites in the metropolitan Minneapolis/St. Paul area during 1985–86. Respondents were presented with the following statement: "If 'tar' and nicotine were removed from cigarettes, there would be no other chemicals in tobacco smoke that cause disease."

TABLE 5.—Public knowledge about the health hazards of smoking in relation to daily cigarette consumption, 1986

	How many cigarettes a day you think a person would have to smoke before it would affect their health?[a] (percentage indicating the following number of cigarettes per day)							
	1	2–4	5–9	10–14	15–24	25–39	≥40	Don't know
Current smokers	14	4	8	12	17	3	17	25
Former smokers	17	6	10	13	19	2	9	22
Never smokers	21	9	10	11	19	1	9	20

[a]The question was open ended. Responses were grouped in the categories 1–9, 10–24, and ≥25 cigarettes per day to conform to the common definitions of light, moderate, and heavy smoking.
SOURCE: AUTS 1986 (US DHHS, in press).

The percentages of those correctly identifying this statement as false were 59 percent of black men, 76 percent of white men, 42 percent of black women, and 60 percent of white women. Those who considered the statement to be true may believe low-tar and -nicotine cigarettes to be less hazardous.

Duration of Smoking

Overall mortality ratios for smokers compared with nonsmokers increase with the duration of smoking. Overall mortality rates among smokers are slightly above the rates of nonsmokers for the first 5 to 15 years of smoking but then increase more rapidly as the years of smoking increase (US DHEW 1979a). Mortality ratios for lung cancer, coronary heart disease (CHD), and COPD increase with decreasing age of initiation (US DHHS 1982, 1983, 1984). An increased risk of morbidity (e.g., as measured by days of hospitalization, bed disability, and work lost) among smokers may occur much earlier than increases in mortality ratios.

The 1964 AUTS asked respondents, "How many cigarettes a day for how many years might make a cigarette smoker more likely to get lung cancer?" Most of those who considered smoking to be a cause of lung cancer believed that smoking would increase the risk of lung cancer only after at least 10 years of smoking (regardless of the number of cigarettes smoked per day) (Table 6).

The 1986 AUTS asked respondents, "How long would a person have to smoke (number) of cigarettes each day before it would affect their (sic) health?" The number of cigarettes used in this question was the number identified by the respondent (in the previous question) as that which "a person would have to smoke before it would affect their (sic) health" (see Table 5). A majority of respondents in all smoking categories believed that smoking 10 or fewer years would affect a person's health. A higher percentage of never smokers (36 percent) than current smokers (23 percent) believed that smoking less than 1 year would affect a person's health. Correspondingly, a slightly higher percentage of current smokers (10 percent) than never smokers (5 percent) believed that health effects would occur only after at least 15 years of smoking (Table 7).

The wording in these two questions from the 1964 and 1986 AUTSs is substantially different, making any comparison difficult. In particular, the 1986 question may have favored responses indicating a shorter duration of smoking by referring to general effects on health (which could be interpreted as nothing more than a cough) whereas the 1964 question asked about the risk of lung cancer.

Does Cigarette Smoking Cause:

Lung Cancer?

Lung cancer, first correlated with smoking more than 50 years ago, is the single largest contributor to the total cancer death rate (US DHHS 1982). Lung cancer alone accounted for an estimated 139,000 (28 percent) of the estimated 494,000 total cancer deaths in the United States in 1988 (ACS 1988a). It is estimated that cigarette smoking

TABLE 6.—Public beliefs about the health effects of smoking in relation to duration of smoking, 1964

	How many cigarettes a day for how many years might make a cigarette smoker more likely to get lung cancer?[a] (percentage indicating the following number of years[b])					
	≤9	10–19	20–29	≥30	Don't know/ no answer	Smokers not more likely to get lung cancer
Current smokers	10	12	12	11	10	43
Former smokers	17	17	16	14	14	22
Never smokers	17	16	10	13	19	24

[a] Asked only of those who indicated in the previous survey question that smokers are more likely than nonsmokers to develop lung cancer. The denominators for these percentages include all respondents.

[b] Regardless of number of cigarettes per day.

SOURCE: AUTS 1964 (US DHEW 1969).

TABLE 7.—Public beliefs about the health effects of smoking in relation to duration of smoking, 1986

	How long would a person have to smoke (number) cigarettes[a] each day before it would affect their health? (percentage indicating the following years of smoking)							
	<1	1–2	3–5	6–10	11–15	>15	Never	Don't know
Current smokers	23	15	10	8	3	10	0.6	30
Former smokers	24	13	13	10	3	9	0.4	29
Never smokers	36	16	10	6	2	5	0.1	25

[a]The number of cigarettes used in this question was the number identified by the respondent (in the previous survey question) as that which "a person would have to smoke before it would affect their health." (See Table 6).

SOURCE: AUTS 1986 (US DHHS, in press).

causes approximately 90 percent of lung cancer deaths in men and 80 percent in women (see Chapter 3).

Surveys have addressed public knowledge about the relationship between smoking and lung cancer since 1954. In 1954, fewer than half of adults (41 percent) thought that smoking is one of the causes of lung cancer (Table 8). Since that time, public knowledge of the association between smoking and lung cancer has increased steadily. By 1964, a majority of adults (66 percent) believed that smoking causes lung cancer; surveys in 1985, 1986, and 1987 showed that this proportion had increased to between 87 and 95 percent.

Heart Disease?

The 1964 Report of the Surgeon General's Advisory Committee identified an association between smoking and CHD, although it did not consider the available data to be sufficient to establish a causal relationship (US PHS 1964). Since that time, evidence from numerous investigations has established cigarette smoking as the most important modifiable risk factor for CHD in the United States (US DHHS 1983). Cigarette smoking increases the risk of death from CHD approximately threefold in persons less than 65 years old and is responsible for 40 to 45 percent of CHD deaths in this age group (Chapter 3).

Public beliefs that smoking is associated with the risk of CHD have steadily increased since 1964, when fewer than half of adults (40 percent) thought that smokers were more likely than nonsmokers to develop heart disease (Table 9). Surveys in 1985, 1986, and 1987 showed that 77 to 90 percent of adults believed that smoking increases the risk of developing heart disease. Each of these recent surveys showed that current smokers were less likely to have this belief than former and never smokers.

In 1986, current smokers were less likely to acknowledge a relationship between smoking and heart disease (71 percent) than were former smokers (84 percent) and never smokers (80 percent).

Chronic Obstructive Pulmonary Disease?

The 1964 Report of the Surgeon General's Advisory Committee identified cigarette smoking as the most important cause of chronic bronchitis (US PHS 1964). Today, cigarette smoking has been identified as the major cause of chronic bronchitis and emphysema in the United States. Eighty to eighty-five percent of deaths from COPD are attributed to cigarette smoking (Chapter 3; also see US DHHS 1984).

Since 1964, the public belief that smoking is associated with an increased risk of COPD has increased. In 1964, half of adults (50 percent) thought that smokers were more likely to get chronic bronchitis and emphysema (Table 10). By 1986, most adults thought that cigarette smokers were more likely than nonsmokers to develop chronic bronchitis (81 percent) and emphysema (89 percent). The preliminary first-quarter 1987 NHIS estimates were similar.

In three surveys that asked identical questions regarding emphysema and chronic bronchitis (NHISs 1985 and 1987, AUTS 1986), there were consistent slightly higher proportions who believed that smoking is associated with emphysema compared with chronic bronchitis.

In 1986, smokers were less likely to acknowledge an association between smoking and chronic bronchitis (73 percent) than were former smokers (84 percent) and never

TABLE 8.—Trends in public knowledge about smoking and lung cancer

			Cigarette smoking causes lung cancer (percentage who agree by smoking status)				
Survey	Year	Reference	Current smokers	Former smokers	Never smokers	All nonsmokers	All adults
1. Gallup	1954	Gallup 1981					41
2. Gallup	1957	Gallup 1981					50
3. Gallup	1958	Gallup 1981					44
4. AUTS	1964	US DHEW 1969	53	75	75	75	66
5. AUTS	1966	US DHEW 1969	57	79	70	72	66
6. Gallup	1969	Gallup 1981					71
7. Gallup	1971	Gallup 1981					71
8. Gallup	1977	Gallup 1981					81
9. Gallup	1978	Gallup 1978	72			87	81
10. Gallup	1981	Gallup 1981	69			91	83

TABLE 8.—Continued

Survey	Year	Reference	Cigarette smoking causes lung cancer (percentage who agree by smoking status)				
			Current smokers	Former smokers	Never smokers	All nonsmokers	All adults
11. NHIS	1985	NCHS 1986[a]	92	96	96	96	95
12. AUTS	1986	US DHHS, in press	85	94	95	95	92
13. Gallup	1987	ALA 1987	75	90		94	87
14. NHIS[b]	1987		83	92	92		89

[a]And unpublished data.

[b]Preliminary first-quarter data (unpublished). Year-end percentage for all adults is 89 percent.

NOTE: Actual questions:

1–3. Do you think that cigarette smoking is or is not one of the causes of lung cancer? (yes, is a cause; no, is not a cause; no opinion)

4–5. Would you say that cigarette smoking is definitely, probably, probably not, or definitely not a major cause of lung cancer, or that you have no opinion either way?*

6–10. Do you think that cigarette smoking is or is not one of the causes of lung cancer? (yes, is a cause; no, is not a cause; no opinion)

11. Tell me if you think cigarette smoking definitely increases, probably increases, probably does not, or definitely does not increase a person's chances of getting the following problems . . . lung cancer.**

12. Do you think a person who smokes is any more likely to get lung cancer than a person who doesn't smoke? (much more likely, somewhat more likely, no, don't know)†

13. Do you think smoking is a cause of lung cancer? (yes, no, don't know)

14. People have differing beliefs about the relationship between smoking and health. Do you believe cigarette smoking is related to . . . lung cancer?

*Percentages include those who say smoking is "definitely" or "probably" a major cause of lung cancer.

**Percentages include those who believe smoking "definitely" or "probably" increases the risk.

†Percentages include those who believe smokers are "much more likely" or "somewhat more likely" to get lung cancer.

TABLE 9.—Trends in public knowledge about smoking and heart disease

Survey	Year	Reference	Smoking cigarettes causes heart disease (percentage who agree by smoking status)				
			Current smokers	Former smokers	Never smokers	All nonsmokers	All adults
1. AUTS	1964	US DHEW 1969	32	51	44	46	40
2. AUTS	1966	US DHEW 1969	33	53	43	47	42
3. AUTS	1966	US DHEW 1969	46	65	58	60	54
4. Gallup	1969	Gallup 1981					60
5. Gallup	1977	Gallup 1981					68
6. Gallup	1978	Gallup 1978	63			72	68
7. Gallup	1981	Gallup 1981	59			82	74
8. NHIS	1985	NCHS 1988	88	93	92	92	90
9. AUTS	1986	US DHHS, in press	71	84	80	81	78

TABLE 9.—Continued

Survey	Year	Reference	Smoking cigarettes causes heart disease (percentage who agree by smoking status)				
			Current smokers	Former smokers	Never smokers	All nonsmokers	All adults
10. NHIS[a]	1987		73	82	77		77

[a]Preliminary first-quarter data (unpublished). Year-end percentage for all adults is 76 percent.

NOTE: Actual questions:

1–2. Do you think the chances of getting coronary heart disease are the same for people who don't smoke cigarettes as they are for people who do smoke cigarettes? Who would be more likely to get it, people who don't smoke cigarettes or people who do smoke cigarettes?

3. Cigarette smokers are more likely to die from heart disease than people who don't smoke cigarettes. (strongly agree, mildly agree, no opinion, mildly disagree, strongly disagree)*

4–7. Do you think that cigarette smoking is or is not one of the causes of heart disease?

8. Do you think cigarette smoking definitely increases, probably increases, probably does not, or definitely does not increase a person's chances of getting heart disease?†

9. Do you think a person who smokes is any more likely to get heart disease than a person who doesn't smoke? (much more likely, somewhat more likely, no, don't know)**

10. People have differing beliefs about the relationship between smoking and health. Do you believe cigarette smoking is related to . . . heart disease?

*Percentages include those who "strongly agree" or "mildly agree."

†Percentages include those who believe that smoking "definitely" or "probably" increases the risk.

**Percentages include those who believe smokers are "much more likely" or "somewhat more likely" to get heart disease.

TABLE 10.—Trends in public knowledge about smoking and emphysema or chronic bronchitis

Survey	Year	Reference	Percentage who agree by smoking status				
			Current smokers	Former smokers	Never smokers	All nonsmokers	All adults
			Smoking is a cause of emphysema/chronic bronchitis				
1. AUTS	1964	US DHEW 1969	42	60	55	56	50
2. AUTS	1966	US DHEW 1969	46	60	52	54	51
			Smoking is a cause of emphysema				
3. NHIS	1985	NCHS 1986[b]	89	94	91	92	91
4. AUTS	1986	US DHHS, in press	85	92	90	91	89
5. Gallup	1987	ALA 1987	75	91		90	85
6. NHIS[a]	1987		79	87	84		84
			Smoking is a cause of chronic bronchitis				
7. AUTS	1966	US DHEW 1969	50	56	65	56	59
8. NHIS	1985	NCHS 1986[b]	82	89	88	88	86

TABLE 10.—Continued

Survey	Year	Reference	Percentage who agree by smoking status: Current smokers	Former smokers	Never smokers	All nonsmokers	All adults
9. AUTS	1986	US DHHS, in press	73	84	83	84	81
10. NHIS[a]	1987		71	81	79		77

[a]Preliminary first-quarter data (unpublished). Year-end percentages for all adults are 75 percent (chronic bronchitis) and 82 percent (emphysema).

[b]/And unpublished data.

NOTE: Actual questions:

1–2. Do you think the chances of getting emphysema and chronic bronchitis are the same for people who don't smoke cigarettes as they are for people who do smoke cigarettes? Who would be more likely to get it, people who don't smoke cigarettes or people who do smoke cigarettes?*

3. Tell me if you think cigarette smoking definitely increases, probably increases, probably does not, or definitely does not increase a person's chances of getting the following problems . . . emphysema.‡

4. Do you think a person who smokes is any more likely to get emphysema than a person who doesn't smoke? (much more likely, somewhat more likely, no, don't know)**

5. Do you think that smoking is a cause of emphysema? (yes, no, don't know)

6. Do you believe cigarette smoking is related to emphysema?

7. Cigarette smoking causes chronic bronchitis. (strongly agree, mildly agree, no opinion, mildly disagree, strongly disagree)†

8. Tell me if you think cigarette smoking definitely increases, probably increases, probably does not, or definitely does not increase a person's chances of getting the following problems . . . chronic bronchitis.‡

9. Do you think a person who smokes is any more likely to get chronic bronchitis than a person who doesn't smoke? (much more likely, somewhat more likely, no, don't know)**

10. People have differing beliefs about the relationship between smoking and health. Do you believe cigarette smoking is related to . . . chronic bronchitis?

*Percentages are those who believe that smokers are more likely to get emphysema and chronic bronchitis.

†Percentages include those who "strongly agree" or "mildly agree."

**Percentages include those who believe smokers are "much more likely" or "somewhat more likely" to get the disease.

‡Percentages include those who believe that smoking "definitely" or "probably" increases the risk.

smokers (83 percent). Similarly, smokers were less likely to acknowledge an association between smoking and emphysema (85 percent) than were former smokers (92 percent) and never smokers (90 percent). Similar patterns were seen in the earlier surveys.

Other Cancers?

Laryngeal and esophageal cancer: By 1964, smoking was identified as a cause of laryngeal cancer in men; an association between smoking and cancer of the esophagus was also noted, although the data were not considered sufficient to establish a causal relationship at that time (US PHS 1964). An estimated 75 to 90 percent of laryngeal and esophageal cancer deaths are attributed to smoking, and smokers have mortality rates from these diseases that are approximately 8 to 18 times higher than those of never smokers (Chapter 3).

Since 1977, public beliefs that smoking increases the risk of developing cancer of the larynx and esophagus have not changed substantially (Table 11). In 1977, 79 percent of adults reported that smoking is one of the causes of throat cancer. In 1985, 80 percent of adults thought that smoking increases a person's risk of developing esophageal cancer and 88 percent thought that smoking increases the risk of acquiring laryngeal cancer. Use of different wording to describe the cancer site (throat, laryngeal, esophageal, "mouth and throat") makes comparisons among these surveys difficult.

In 1986, current smokers were less likely to acknowledge a relationship between smoking and laryngeal cancer (82 percent) than were former smokers (91 percent) or never smokers (91 percent). Similar patterns were seen in the earlier surveys and in the preliminary 1987 NHIS data (Table 11).

Bladder cancer: The 1964 Report of the Surgeon General's Advisory Committee identified an association between smoking and cancer of the bladder, although the evidence was not considered sufficient to establish a causal relationship (US PHS 1964). Thirty-seven to forty-seven percent of bladder cancer deaths are now attributable to smoking (Chapter 3).

Few data are available on public knowledge about the association between smoking and cancer of the bladder. The 1979 Chilton Survey (Chilton 1980) showed that 25 percent of adult respondents (29 to 31 years of age) believed that "cancer of the bladder (has) been found to be associated with cigarette smoking." In the 1985 NHIS, 36 percent of adults thought that cigarette smoking definitely or probably increases a person's risk of developing bladder cancer. In the 1986 AUTS, 33 percent of adults thought that smokers are more likely than nonsmokers to develop bladder cancer. Current smokers were less likely to acknowledge this relationship (25 percent) than were former smokers (32 percent) and never smokers (38 percent).

What Are the Special Health Risks for Women?

The special health risks for women include effects of smoking on pregnancy outcome, increased risk of cardiovascular disease (CVD) among smokers who use oral contraceptives, and increased risk of cervical cancer in women who smoke (Chapters 2 and 3). Data exist on public beliefs regarding the first two of these three categories of risk.

TABLE 11.—Trends in public knowledge about smoking and cancer of the mouth/throat/larynx/esophagus

			Smoking causes cancer of the mouth/throat/larynx/esophagus (percentage who agree by smoking status)				
Survey	Year	Reference	Current smokers	Former smokers	Never smokers	All nonsmokers	All adults
1. Gallup	1977	Gallup 1981				79	
2. Gallup	1978	Gallup 1978	73			82	79
3. Gallup	1981	Gallup 1981	69		87	81	
4. NHIS	1985	NCHS 1986[b]	83	90	90	90	88
5. NHIS	1985	NCHS 1986[b]	75	83	82	82	80
6. AUTS	1986	US DHHS, in press	82	91	91	91	88
7. NHIS[a]	1987		73	85	83		80

[a]Preliminary first-quarter data (unpublished). Year-end percentage for all adults is 80 percent.

[b]And unpublished data.

NOTE: Actual questions:

1–3. Do you think that cigarette smoking is or is not one of the causes of cancer of the throat?

4–5. Tell me if you think cigarette smoking definitely increases, probably increases, probably does not, or definitely does not increase a person's chances of getting the following problems . . . cancer of the larynx or voice box (question 4) . . . cancer of the esophagus (question 5).*

6. Do you think a person who smokes is any more likely to get cancer of the larynx or voice box than a person who doesn't smoke?

7. People have differing beliefs about the relationship between smoking and health. Do you believe cigarette smoking is related to . . . cancer of the mouth and throat?

*Percentages include those who believe that smoking "definitely" or "probably" increases the risk.

Effects of Smoking on Pregnancy Outcome

In 1964, knowledge of the health consequences of smoking during pregnancy mostly concerned the increased risk of low-birthweight babies (US PHS 1964). Considerable evidence has accumulated since that time. In the 1980 Surgeon General's Report, smoking was identified as an important cause of premature births, miscarriages, and stillbirths, as well as low-birthweight babies (US DHHS 1980).

From the data available, it appears that the public has become more knowledgeable about the effects of smoking on premature births. In 1966, 34 percent of adults of *all* ages thought that women who smoke during pregnancy are more likely to have premature babies than women who do not smoke (Table 12). Fox and coworkers (1987) published data on beliefs about the risks of smoking during pregnancy among persons 18 to 44 years of age. By 1985, 70 percent of adults aged *18 to 44 years* thought that smoking during pregnancy definitely or probably increases the chances of premature birth.

Only recent data are available on public knowledge of the effects of smoking on spontaneous abortion (miscarriage), stillbirth, and low birthweight (Table 12). In 1985, 80 percent of adults (aged 18 to 44 years) thought that smoking during pregnancy definitely or probably increases the risk of having a low-birthweight baby; 74 percent of adults thought that smoking definitely or probably increases the risk of miscarriage; and 66 percent of adults thought that smoking during pregnancy definitely or probably increases the risk of stillbirth. The 1987 NHIS showed that 89 percent of respondents believed that smoking during pregnancy "may" harm the baby. The 1966, 1985, and 1987 surveys each showed that current smokers were less likely than nonsmokers to believe that smoking increases the risk of adverse pregnancy outcomes. The Federal Trade Commission (FTC) (1981) reviewed data from a 1979 Chilton survey and a 1980 Roper survey on public beliefs concerning the effects of smoking during pregnancy.

Risk of Cardiovascular Disease Among Smokers Who Use Oral Contraceptives

In 1964, the interactive effect of smoking and oral contraceptive use on the risk of CVD had not been established. The 1977/1978 Surgeon General's Report cited recent studies showing that oral contraceptive use potentiates the harmful effects of smoking on the cardiovascular system (US DHEW 1978). Since 1978, the package inserts for oral contraceptives have described this risk for users (see Chapter 7). It is now known that oral contraceptives or cigarettes, when used alone, increase the risk of heart attacks twofold; however, when used in combination, the increased risk is tenfold (US DHHS 1980). Smoking and oral contraceptive use also appear to interact synergistically to greatly increase the risk of subarachnoid hemorrhage (US DHHS 1983).

No trend data are available on the knowledge of health risks from the combined use of cigarettes and oral contraceptives. In 1985, 62 percent of adults aged 18 to 44 years believed that a woman who both takes oral contraceptives and smokes is more likely to have a stroke (Table 12). Nonsmokers were only slightly more likely than smokers to believe this (65 vs. 59 percent). Women were much more likely to believe this than were men (72 vs. 52 percent). In 1980, 64 percent of women believed that a woman who takes birth control pills further increases her risk of getting a heart attack if she also smokes.

TABLE 12.—Trends in public knowledge about the special health risks for women who smoke

Survey	Year	Percentage who agree by smoking status[a] Current smokers	Former smokers	Never smokers	All nonsmokers	All adults
Smoking during pregnancy increases the chances of premature birth						
1. AUTS	1966	25	43	34		
2. NHIS	1985 (all)	64	71	75		70
2. NHIS	1985 (men)					64
2. NHIS	1985 (women)					76
Smoking during pregnancy increases the chances of stillbirth						
3. NHIS	1985 (all)	57	67	72		66
3. NHIS	1985 (men)					63
3. NHIS	1985 (women)					68
Smoking during pregnancy increases the chances of miscarriage						
4. NHIS	1985 (all)	66	75	79		74
4. NHIS	1985 (men)					72
4. NHIS	1985 (women)					75
Smoking during pregnancy increases the chances of having a low-birthweight baby						
5. NHIS	1985 (all)	74	82	83		80
5. NHIS	1985 (men)					74
5. NHIS	1985 (women)					85
A woman taking birth control pills is more likely to have a stroke if she smokes						
6. NHIS	1985 (all)	59	67	64	65	62
6. NHIS	1985 (men)	48	57	54	55	52
6. NHIS	1985 (women)	70	80	72	74	72

TABLE 12.—Continued

Survey	Year	Percentage who agree by smoking status				
		Current smokers	Former smokers	Never smokers	All nonsmokers	All adults
A woman who takes birth control pills further increases her risk of getting a heart attack if she also smokes						
7. Roper	1980 (women)					64
Smoking by a pregnant woman may harm the baby						
8. NHIS[b]	1987	83	90	93		89

[a]Data for 1966 include all adults (US DHEW 1969). Data for 1985 are from Fox et al. (1987) and NCHS (1986) and include only those people 18 to 44 years of age. Roper data for 1980 are from the FTC (1981).

[b]Preliminary first-quarter data (unpublished). Year-end percentage for all adults is 89 percent.

NOTE: Actual questions:

1. Women who smoke during pregnancy are more likely to have premature babies than women who do not smoke (strongly agree, mildly agree, no opinion, mildly disagree, strongly disagree).*
2. Does cigarette smoking during pregnancy definitely increase, probably increase, probably not or definitely not increase the chances of premature birth?†
3. . . . of stillbirth?†
4. . . . of miscarriage?†
5. . . . of low birthweight of the newborn?†
6. If a woman takes birth control pills, is she more likely to have a stroke if she smokes than if she does not smoke?
7. A woman who takes birth control pills further increases her risk of getting a heart attack if she also smokes (know it's true, don't know if it's true, think it's true, think it's not true, know it's not true).‡
8. Smoking by a pregnant woman may harm the baby. (strongly agree, agree, disagree, strongly disagree)**

*Percentages include those who "strongly agree" or "mildly agree."

†Percentages include those who believe that smoking "definitely" or "probably" increases the risk.

‡Percentage includes those who "know it's true" or "think it's true."

**Percentages include those who "strongly agree" or "agree."

Involuntary (Passive) Smoking

In 1964, the health effects of environmental tobacco smoke (ETS) exposure were not established. Today, ETS has been identified as a cause of disease, including lung cancer, in healthy nonsmokers. In addition, compared with the children of nonsmoking parents, children of parents who smoke have an increased frequency of respiratory infections and slightly lower rates of increase in lung function as the lungs mature (US DHHS 1986a).

From the available data, it appears that the public is more likely to believe that there are health risks from ETS exposure. The percentage of adults who thought that smoking is hazardous to nonsmokers' health increased from 46 percent to 58 percent between 1974 and 1978 (Table 13). By 1986 (AUTS), 81 percent of adults thought that tobacco smoke is harmful for nonsmokers who live or work with smokers. Similarly, in 1987 (ACS 1988b), 81 percent thought that people's smoke is harmful to others nearby. The 1986 and 1987 surveys used wording corresponding to Level 2 (general acceptance) beliefs. The 1987 NHIS used wording corresponding to Level 3 (personalized acceptance) beliefs, but nevertheless obtained the same proportion (81 percent) (Table 13).

In the 1986 AUTS, former and never smokers were more likely to consider ETS to be *generally* harmful to health (82 and 87 percent, respectively), compared with current smokers (69 percent). Similar patterns were seen in the 1987 NHIS and 1988 Gallup survey. In the 1986 AUTS, when nonsmokers were asked whether they considered ETS to be harmful to *their* health, 69 percent responded that they thought so (62 percent of former smokers and 74 percent of never smokers).

Is Smoking an Addiction?

In 1964, the Surgeon General's Advisory Committee came to the following conclusion, based on the evidence available at that time: "The tobacco habit should be characterized as an habituation rather than an addiction." The Advisory Committee's Report, however, did note that tobacco use is "reinforced and perpetuated by the pharmacologic actions of nicotine on the central nervous system" (US PHS 1964). The 1979 Surgeon General's Report called smoking "the prototypical substance-abuse dependency" (US DHEW 1979a). The 1988 Surgeon General's Report reaffirmed that conclusion and provided a detailed review of the evidence (US DHHS 1988).

Only limited data are available to assess public knowledge of the addictive nature of tobacco use. In a 1978 survey conducted by the Roper Organization, 50 percent of adults (57 percent of smokers) considered smoking a habit, 29 percent (22 percent of smokers) thought it an addiction, and 17 percent (15 percent of smokers) believed it to be both (Roper 1978).

In a 1986 Gallup poll of 1,046 adults 18 years and older conducted in Canada by household interviews, 76.5 percent of respondents considered "cigarette smoking to be

TABLE 13.—Trends in public knowledge about the health risks of passive smoking

			Smoking is hazardous to nonsmokers' health (percentage who agree by smoking status)				
Survey	Year	Reference	Current smokers	Former smokers	Never smokers	All nonsmokers	All adults
1. Roper	1974	Roper 1978	30			57	46
2. Roper	1976	Roper 1978	38			61	52
3. Roper	1978	Roper 1978	40			69	58
4. AUTS[a]	1986	US DHHS, in press	69	82	87	85	81
5. NHIS[b]	1987		68	85	88		81
6. Gallup	1987	ACS 1988b	64	86	89		81

[a]Percentages presented here are slightly lower than those previously published (CDC 1988) because the latter did not include "don't know" responses in the denominator.

[b]Preliminary first-quarter data (unpublished). Year-end percentage for all adults is 81 percent.

NOTE: Actual questions:

1–3. Is smoking hazardous to nonsmokers' health? (probably is hazardous, probably doesn't have any real effect, don't know)

4. Think now for a moment about a nonsmoker who lives or works with smokers . . . . Do you think that exposure to tobacco smoke is harmful or not harmful to the nonsmoker's health?

5. The smoke from someone else's cigarette is harmful to you. (strongly agree, agree, disagree, strongly disagree)*

6. If people smoke, do you think that it *is* harmful or is *not* harmful to people who are near them? (yes, harmful; no, not harmful; can't say/no opinion)

*Percentages include those who "strongly agree" or "agree."

like a drug addiction." Of current smokers, 79.6 answered "yes" to the question, "Do you think you are addicted to cigarettes?" (Canadian Gallup 1986)

Interaction Between Smoking and Other Exposures

The 1985 Surgeons General's Report (US DHHS 1985) reviewed evidence regarding the interaction between smoking and a variety of occupational exposures in causing disease. With respect to the interaction between smoking and asbestos, the Report concluded that these two exposures act synergistically to increase the risk of lung cancer. The risk of lung cancer in cigarette-smoking asbestos workers is more than fiftyfold the risk in nonsmokers who have not been exposed to asbestos.

Few data are available on public knowledge of these interactions. The 1980 Roper survey (unpublished data, FTC) asked respondents about their belief concerning the following statement: "If you smoke and have worked with asbestos you are at least 50 times more likely to get lung cancer than if you have done neither." Seventy-four percent of respondents (and 69 percent of smokers) said that they "know it's true" or "think it's true."

Smokeless Tobacco

Smokeless tobacco (ST) use leads to increased risk of oral cancer and nicotine addiction (US DHHS 1986c).

No data are available to assess trends in public knowledge of the health risks of ST use. In the 1986 AUTS, 78 percent of adults thought that the use of chewing tobacco is harmful in any way to a person's health. Similarly, 73 percent thought that the use of snuff is harmful to a person's health. Current smokers were less likely to know about the health effects of using chewing tobacco and snuff (71 and 66 percent, respectively) compared with former smokers (79 and 75 percent, respectively) and never smokers (81 and 76 percent, respectively).

According to the 1987 NHIS (preliminary first-quarter estimates), 82 percent of adults thought that a relationship exists between chewing tobacco use and mouth and throat cancers. Seventy-seven percent thought that snuff use is related to these cancers (unpublished data, National Cancer Institute).

Personal Health Risks for Smokers

There have been few attempts to determine smokers' beliefs regarding their own personal risk. Several Gallup surveys conducted between 1977 and 1987 asked respondents, "Do you think cigarette smoking is or is not harmful to your health?" (Table 14). Data are available for current smokers for the years 1981 and 1985. The proportion of current smokers answering in the affirmative increased from 80 percent in 1981 to 90 percent in 1985. These data, at first glance, suggest that a high percentage of smokers

TABLE 14.—Trends in public beliefs about one's personal risk from smoking

			Cigarette smoking is harmful to YOUR health (percentage who agree by smoking status)				
Survey	Year	Reference	Current smokers	Former smokers	Never smokers	All nonsmokers	All adults
1. Gallup	1977	Gallup 1985					90
2. Gallup	1978	Gallup 1978	83			95	90
3. Gallup	1981	Gallup 1985	80			96	90
4. Gallup	1983	Gallup 1985					92
5. Gallup	1985	Gallup 1985	90	96		96	94
6. Gallup	1987	ALA 1987					94
7. NHIS[a]	1987		55				

[a]Preliminary first-quarter data (unpublished). Year-end percentage is 55 percent.

NOTE: Actual questions:

1–6. Do you think cigarette smoking is or is not harmful to your health?

7. Do you believe your smoking has affected your health in any way?

perceive a personalized risk from smoking. However, nonsmokers were asked to respond to the question, implying that the wording may not be understood by some respondents as referring to truly personalized health risks. Wording such as, "Do you think that *your* cigarette smoking is or is not harmful to your health?" might elicit different responses.

The 1987 NHIS (unpublished data, National Cancer Institute) showed that 55 percent of current smokers answered "yes" to the question, "Do you believe your smoking has affected your health in any way?" The principal reason this percentage is substantially lower than that obtained by the 1985 Gallup survey (90 percent) is probably that the former was likely to be understood as referring to overt symptoms or disease, while the latter was likely to be understood as referring to the risk of harm.

Another approach to measure perceptions of personalized risk has been to ask smokers whether they are "concerned" about the effects of smoking on *their* health. It appears that smokers are more likely today to be concerned that smoking is harmful to their own health. In 1964, 50 percent of current smokers were concerned about the possible effects of smoking on their own health (Table 15); this proportion increased to 75 percent by 1986. However, in 1986, only 18 percent of smokers were *very* concerned about the effects of smoking on their health; 56 percent of smokers were only fairly or slightly concerned; and 24 percent were not at all concerned.

From 1970–86, the percentage of smokers who were very concerned about the possible effects of smoking on their health decreased from 29 to 18 percent, while the percentage who were only slightly concerned increased from 19 to 34 percent. This redistribution within the population of smokers having any concern may have occurred because a much greater proportion of those who were very concerned may have quit smoking during this period; therefore, they would not have been included in subsequent surveys.

A third approach to assess personalized risk, or more correctly, the absence of personalized risk, is to ask smokers if they believe themselves to be at lower risk than other smokers. In 1986, 21 percent of adults thought that the cigarettes they smoked were less hazardous than other cigarettes (Table 3).

Other data pertaining to perceptions of personalized risk from ETS and from smoking among adolescents appear in the sections on Involuntary Smoking (above) and Adolescent Knowledge (below).

How Harmful Is Smoking?

The data presented above reveal that a vast majority of adults agree that smoking is hazardous to health and correctly recognize the conditions that are associated with smoking. However, these data do not address the depth of the public's understanding regarding the absolute risk of smoking, the relative risks of smoking, the population-attributable risk of smoking, and the risk of smoking in comparison with other risks. A more in-depth understanding of the risks of smoking may be much more important in promoting behavioral change than the more superficial beliefs measured by the data presented above. Unfortunately, only limited data are available to address the public's in-depth understanding of the risks of smoking.

TABLE 15.—Trends in smokers' concern about the effects of smoking on their own health

Survey	Year	Concern about the possible effects of cigarette smoking on your health (percentage who responded by level of concern)				
		Very concerned	Fairly concerned	Only slightly concerned	Not concerned	Any concern[a]
1. AUTS	1964	13	18	19	50	50
2. AUTS	1966	12	17	18	53	47
3. AUTS	1970	29	22	19	31	69
4. AUTS	1975	25	23	19	32	68
5. AUTS	1986	18	22	34	24	75

[a]Very, fairly, or only slightly concerned.

NOTE: Actual questions:

1–5. Are you in any way concerned about the possible effects of cigarette smoking on your health?

SOURCE: US DHEW (1969, 1973, 1976a); US DHHS, in press.

Absolute Risk

Absolute risks can be described by the proportion of those exposed to a given risk factor who will actually die or develop the particular condition, or by the reduction in life expectancy caused by exposure. As many as one-third of heavy smokers aged 35 years will die before age 85 of diseases caused by their smoking (Mattson, Pollack, Cullen 1987), and 30-year-old smokers will shorten their lives an average of 6 to 8 years if they smoke a pack a day (US DHEW 1979a).

From 1970–78, the proportion of adults who believed that smoking a pack of cigarettes a day made a great deal of difference in longevity increased slightly from 42 to 50 percent (FTC 1981). However, most adults underestimate the impact of smoking on longevity, according to a 1980 Roper survey. In this survey, 30 percent of the population and 41 percent of smokers did not know that a typical 30-year-old smoker shortened his life expectancy *at all* by smoking (FTC 1981). Among those who did know that smoking reduces one's life expectancy, many underestimated the degree to which this is true. On average, nonsmokers underestimated the loss in life expectancy by about 2 years and smokers underestimated it by more than 4 years.

Relative Risk

Relative risk describes the risk of dying or developing disease for a person exposed to a particular risk factor compared with someone not exposed. For example, male smokers are 22 times more likely and female smokers are 12 times more likely to develop lung cancer compared with nonsmokers of the same sex (Chapter 3).

In the 1980 Roper study, respondents were asked if smokers were specifically 10 times more likely to die from lung cancer (the estimated relative risk derived from the data available at that time); 23 percent of the general population and 39 percent of smokers did not believe this statement. Some of this lack of belief may be due to the use of a specific figure. However, using more general terms, 16 percent of adults and 25 percent of smokers did not think that smokers were "many times" more likely than nonsmokers to develop lung cancer (FTC 1981).

Attributable Risk and Smoking-Attributable Mortality

Attributable risk refers to that proportion of a disease that can be "attributed" to (or is caused by) a particular risk factor, such as smoking. For example, smoking accounts for about 80 to 90 percent of lung cancer deaths and 80 to 85 percent of deaths from COPD (Chapter 3).

Much of the information regarding the public's understanding of the magnitude of the risks of smoking comes from the Roper survey conducted in 1980. In this survey, 43 percent of adults and 49 percent of smokers did not know that smoking causes *most* of the cases of lung cancer and 22 percent of adults and 27 percent of smokers did not know that smoking even causes *many* cases of lung cancer (FTC 1981). In the 1987 NHIS (unpublished data, National Cancer Institute), 28 percent (preliminary first-quarter estimate) of smokers and 16 percent (year-end figure) of the general population disagreed with the statement, "Most deaths from lung cancer are caused by cigarette smoking."

Attributable risk figures can be used to calculate smoking-attributable mortality. The 1979 Surgeon General's Report (US DHEW 1979a, p. ii) attributed approximately 350,000 deaths each year to cigarette smoking. In 1985, an estimated 390,000 deaths in the United States were attributable to smoking (Chapter 3). In the 1979 Chilton survey, adults aged 29 to 31 years were asked: "In the United States, two million people die each year. About how many of these deaths are probably related to cigarette smoking?" The responses offered by the interviewer, along with the percentages chosen, were: 10,000 deaths, 22 percent; 50,000, 16 percent; 100,000, 16 percent; 300,000, 17 percent; don't know, 31 percent (Chilton 1980).

Comparative Risk

The risk of dying from smoking can be compared with the risk of dying from other behavioral risk factors, such as living under stress, eating high-cholesterol foods, or drinking heavily. The public's perception of these comparative risks was assessed by Roper surveys from 1970–78 (Table 16). In 1970, living under a lot of tension and stress and not getting regular exercise were considered by more adults to make a great deal of difference in longevity than was smoking a pack of cigarettes daily. In contrast, fewer adults considered regularly eating food high in cholesterol, consuming three or four drinks of liquor a day, or being 20 lb overweight to have an effect on longevity. In 1978, only stress was considered by more adults to make a great deal of difference on longevity.

In 1983, Louis Harris and Associates conducted a national telephone survey of 1,254 randomly selected adults for *Prevention* magazine (Harris 1983). Respondents were asked to rank 24 health and safety factors on a 1-to-10 (low-to-high) scale of importance. A sample of 103 health experts (medical school chairmen of preventive medicine, public health school deans, government officials, journal editors, and others) was also interviewed and was asked to make the same rankings. All of the public's mean rankings were in the top half of the scale; thus, none of the factors were seen as trivial in importance. "Not smoking" was ranked near the middle, below "keeping water quality acceptable," "having smoke detectors in the home," "taking steps to control stress," and "getting enough vitamins and minerals" (Figure 1). In contrast, the panel of experts ranked "not smoking" at the top of the list (Figure 2).

The 1986 AUTS asked five questions comparing the perceived risk of cigarette smoking with the perceived risk of drinking alcoholic beverages, smoking marijuana, being exposed to air pollution, driving without a seat belt, and being 20 lb overweight (Table 17). In each of the comparisons, never smokers were more likely to disagree than to agree that cigarette smoking is less harmful than the other risks. Only in the case of marijuana smoking are the percentages of those agreeing and disagreeing similar. On the other hand, current smokers were more likely to agree than to disagree that cigarette smoking is less dangerous than marijuana smoking and air pollution.

Dolecek and coworkers (1986) surveyed 973 adults in Chicago from a sample of family members of students who participated in AHA's Chicago Heart Health Cur-

TABLE 16.—Trends in public knowledge about the health risks of smoking compared to other risks, 1970–78

	It makes a great deal of difference in longevity if a person . . . (percentage who agree by year)				
Question	1970	1972	1974	1976	1978
lives under a lot of tension and stress	69	72	74	76	74
doesn't get regular exercise	49	38	38	33	34
smokes a pack of cigarettes a day	42	42	44	45	50
regularly eats a lot of food with high cholesterol	31	34	38	39	43
drinks 3 or 4 highballs a day	29	34	35	37	39
is 20 pounds overweight	23	26	25	24	24

SOURCE: Roper (1978).

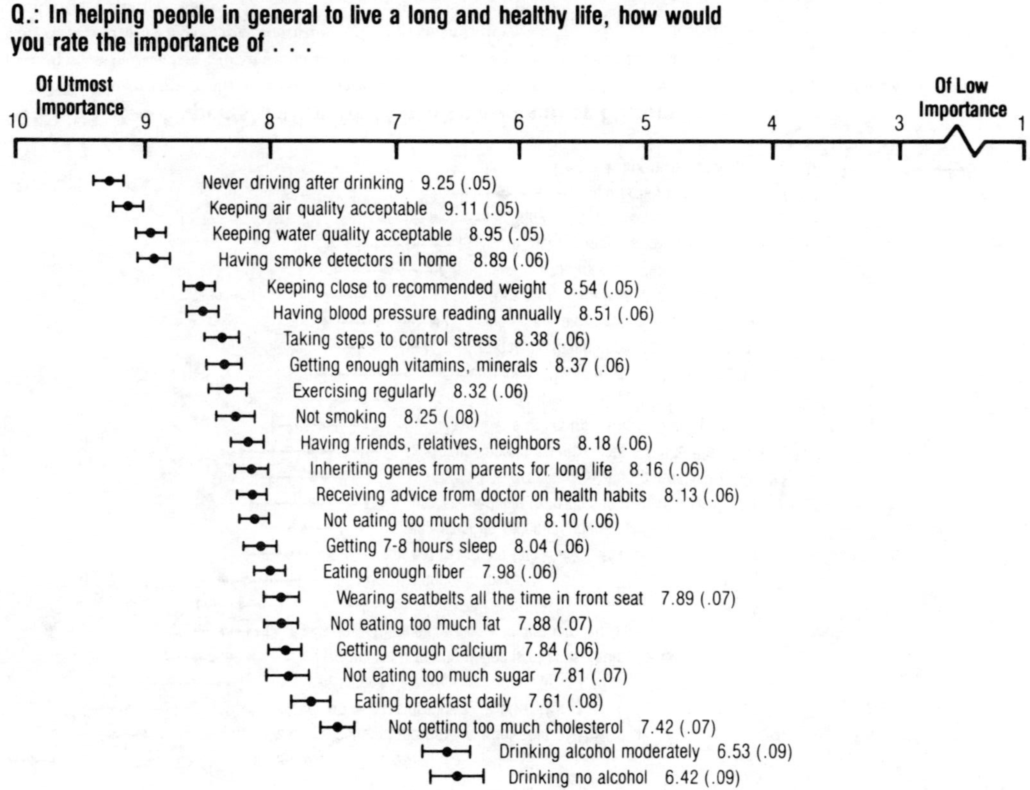

FIGURE 1.—Adult public's rating of 24 health and safety factors

NOTE: Shown above is the mean importance rating for each factor given by 1,254 adults using a 1 to 10 scale. Given in parentheses is the standard error of the mean. The 95-percent confidence interval around each mean is graphically displayed as a band or range consisting of ± two standard error values.

SOURCE: Harris (1983).

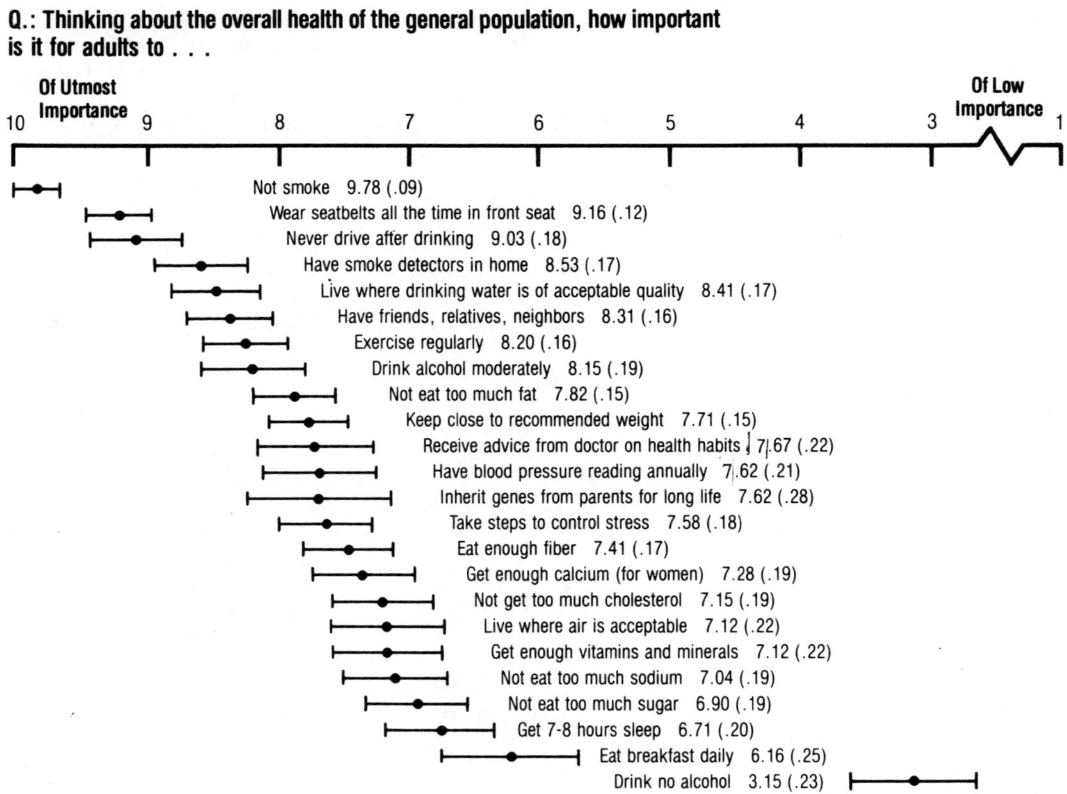

FIGURE 2.—Experts' rating of 24 health and safety factors

NOTE: Shown above is the mean importance rating for each factor given by 103 experts using a 1 to 10 scale. Given in parentheses is the standard error of the mean. An indicator of the variability of individual ratings around each mean is graphically displayed as a band or range consisting of ± two standard error values.

SOURCE: Harris (1983).

TABLE 17.—Public knowledge about the harmfulness of cigarette smoking compared with other risks, 1986

	Percentage who agree			Percentage who disagree		
	Current smokers	Former smokers	Never smokers	Current smokers	Former smokers	Never smokers
Moderate use of cigarettes is less harmful to health than moderate use of alcoholic beverages.	32	21	20	54	63	63
Smoking cigarettes is less harmful to health than smoking marijuana.	48	38	37	33	34	40
Air pollution is a greater health risk than cigarettes.	48	30	28	41	54	57
Smoking cigarettes is less dangerous than driving without a seat belt.	36	25	26	52	58	68
Smoking is less harmful than being 20 pounds overweight.	31	19	18	59	69	71

NOTE: Percentages of those who agree include those who "strongly agree" or "somewhat agree." Percentages of those who disagree include those who "strongly disagree" or "somewhat disagree."
SOURCE: AUTS 1986 (US DHHS, in press).

riculum Program during the 1980–81 school year. Respondents were asked to select the three major risk factors for CVD from a list of nine. The percentage responses for these risk factors were: high blood pressure, 25 percent; overweight, 22 percent; stress/tension/worry, 14 percent; *cigarette smoking*, 13 percent; heredity/family history, 7 percent; eating too much cholesterol (fat), 7 percent; not enough rest/working too hard, 6 percent; not enough exercise, 4 percent; and diabetes, 2 percent.

From 1982–86, Becker and Levine (1987) surveyed 90 adults with no known CHD who were siblings of patients hospitalized for recently documented CHD. Patients and siblings were all less than 60 years old. The siblings were randomized into an assessment group (interviewed within 2 weeks of the index patients' discharge and again 4 months later) and a control group (received only one interview at 4-month followup). Participants were asked in an open-ended question to name factors thought to cause or be associated with CHD. Smoking was identified by 81 percent of the control group (after stress, 91 percent) and was the risk factor most often cited by the assessment group (97 percent).

Folsom and others (1988) conducted two surveys in the metropolitan Minneapolis/St. Paul area during 1985–86. One survey sampled blacks aged 35 to 74 years, while the other sampled a primarily white population. Subjects were asked the open-ended question, "What do you think are the most important causes of cardiovascular diseases (heart attack or stroke)?" The percentage of blacks (total sample size=1,252) who identified smoking as one of the most important causes of CVD was 32 percent; stress/worry (54 percent) and improper diet (45 percent) ranked higher. Among whites (total sample size=1,870), smoking and improper diet were both ranked highest (54 percent).

In a survey conducted in 1987 by the Gallup Organization for ACS, 90 percent of adults reported that smoking cigarettes contributes to a higher risk of cancer. Lower percentages reported that a higher cancer risk is associated with suntan and sunburn (73 percent), alcohol (34 percent), high-fat diet (33 percent), and smoked and nitrite-cured meats (31 percent) (ACS 1988b).

For the studies reviewed above on comparative risk, data stratified by smoking status were available only from the 1986 AUTS.

Knowledge Among Adolescents About the Health Risks of Smoking

Because most regular cigarette smokers begin to smoke before age 21 (Chapter 5), it is important to consider teenagers' knowledge about the health effects of smoking. This knowledge can be addressed in the following categories: (1) general health effects of smoking, (2) personalized risk of smoking-related diseases, (3) risks of smoking compared with other health risks, (4) beliefs about addiction, and (5) health effects of ST use.

General Health Effects

Since 1975, beliefs among adolescents that cigarette smoking is harmful have increased. National data on knowledge of high school seniors about the health risks of smoking are available from the Monitoring the Future Project (sponsored by the Na-

TABLE 18.—Knowledge about the health risks of smoking among high school seniors, 1975–86, Monitoring the Future Project, National Institute on Drug Abuse

	How much do you think people risk harming themselves (physically or in other ways), if they smoke one or more packs of cigarettes per day? (percentage responding in each category)					
Survey year	Don't know	No risk	Slight risk	Moderate risk	Great risk	Any risk [a]
1975	2	3	9	35	51	95
1976	2	2	9	31	56	96
1977	2	2	9	29	58	96
1978	2	2	8	30	59	97
1979	1	2	7	27	63	97
1980	1	1	7	27	64	98
1981	1	1	6	28	63	98
1982	2	2	7	30	61	97
1983	1	2	7	29	61	97
1984	1	2	6	27	64	97
1985	2	2	6	24	67	97
1986	1	1	5	26	66	97

[a] Slight, moderate, or great risk of harm combined.

SOURCE: Bachman, Johnston, O'Malley (1980a,b, 1981, 1984, 1985, 1987); Johnston and Bachman (1980); Johnston, Bachman, O'Malley (1980a,b, 1982, 1984, 1986).

TABLE 19.—Perceived harmfulness of drugs among high school seniors, 1986; Monitoring the Future Project, National Institute on Drug Abuse

How much do you think people risk harming themselves (physically or in other ways), if they... (percentage of people responding)	Great risk
try one or two drinks of an alcoholic beverage (beer, wine, liquor)?	5
try marijuana (pot, grass) once or twice?	15
take one or two drinks nearly every day?	25
smoke marijuana occasionally?	25
try amphetamines (uppers, pep pills, bennies, speed) once or twice?	25
try barbiturates (downers, goofballs, reds, yellows, etc.) once or twice?	25
use smokeless tobacco regularly (chewing tobacco, plug, dipping tobacco, snuff)?	**26**
try cocaine once or twice?	34
have five or more drinks once or twice each weekend?	39
try LSD once or twice?	42
try heroin (smack, horse) once or twice?	46
take cocaine occasionally	54
smoke one or more packs of cigarettes per day?	**66**
take amphetamines regularly?	67
take barbiturates regularly?	67
take four or five drinks nearly every day?	67
take heroin occasionally?	68
smoke marijuana regularly?	71
take cocaine regularly?	82
take LSD regularly?	83
take heroin regularly?	87

NOTE: Possible responses included great risk, moderate risk, slight risk, no risk, don't know.
SOURCE: Bachman, Johnston, O'Malley (1987).

tional Institute on Drug Abuse) for every year since 1975. Although nearly all teenagers recognize some risk of harm from smoking, the proportion who think that smoking a pack or more a day causes great risk of harm increased from 51 percent in 1975 to 67 percent by 1985 (Table 18).

A 1975 survey (US DHEW 1975a) of teenagers who smoked revealed that many thought that the dangers of smoking were exaggerated for their age group (52 percent of girls; 54 percent of boys); that there was too much talk about things that were bad for them (43 percent of girls; 48 percent of boys); and that air pollution was just as important a cause of lung cancer as cigarettes (67 percent of girls; 51 percent of boys). In 1986, only 16 percent of high school seniors agreed with the statement, "The harmful effects of cigarettes have been exaggerated" (see Table 24; Bachman, Johnston, O'Malley 1987) (data stratified by smoking status were not published).

Personalized Risk

In a survey of 895 students in grades 2 through 12 in 134 public schools in Milwaukee, WI, during the 1979–80 academic year, Leventhal, Glynn, and Fleming (1987) assessed the degree to which the students personalized the health risk from smoking. When asked, "Do you think that smoking can injure or hurt the body?" 98 percent answered affirmatively and were able to accurately name one or more body parts that are adversely affected by smoking. A subsample of 622 subjects (smokers and nonsmokers) was asked whether they "would be less likely, about as likely, or more likely to get sick from smoking than other people." Those answering "less likely" accounted for 47 percent of the smokers but only 36 percent of the nonsmokers, 47 percent of those who intended to become adult smokers versus 36 percent of those who did not intend to become adult smokers, and 41 percent of those from smoking families versus 28 percent of those from nonsmoking families. These findings suggest that although children and adolescents recognize smoking as harmful, they may not personalize the risk. This failure to personalize the perception of risk may play a role in the initiation of smoking.

Some teenagers may minimize or deny their personal risk because of a belief that certain smoking patterns are safe. In the 1974 and 1979 Teenage Smoking Surveys conducted by the Department of Health, Education, and Welfare (US DHEW 1976b, 1979b), about one-quarter of teenagers agreed with the statement, "There's nothing wrong with smoking cigarettes if you don't smoke too many." About one-third agreed with the statement, "Cigarette smoking is harmful only if a person inhales."

Comparative Risk

In the 1979 Chilton Survey (Chilton 1980), teenagers were asked which of the following caused the most deaths during the past year: traffic accidents, fires, cigarette smoking, or drug overdose. Traffic accidents were cited by 44 percent of teenagers, followed by drug overdose (21 percent), cigarette smoking (19 percent), and fires (6 percent).

The High School Seniors Survey includes questions about the risks associated with using a variety of licit and illicit drugs at different levels of intake. In 1986, 66 percent of high school seniors thought that smoking one or more packs of cigarettes per day causes great risk of harming oneself. More students saw great risk in the regular use of marijuana, cocaine, LSD, and heroin (Table 19). In contrast, more teenagers saw great risk in regular smoking compared with trying amphetamines, barbiturates, cocaine, or LSD; in trying or using occasionally marijuana or cocaine; or in trying alcohol, having one to two drinks per day, or having five or more drinks one or two times per week.

The *Weekly Reader* magazine includes a survey twice a year in the periodical, which is distributed throughout the country to more than 10 million children in grades 2 through 9. Surveys are filled out in class by students under a teacher's supervision. The topics addressed are rotated so that the same survey is repeated every 4 years. The Spring 1986 survey covered safety and health (Weekly Reader 1986). Of an estimated 400,000 student responses for grades 2 through 6, 128,000 were randomly chosen for analysis. Although the respondents do not represent a randomly selected sample, results pertaining to tobacco are presented here because of the large sample size and the paucity of data available for young children.

The survey included the following question: "Many people say the following things are harmful for kids to do. How harmful do you think each is for kids your age? (very harmful, somewhat harmful, not harmful) . . . overeating, eating junk food, listening to very loud music, smoking, chewing tobacco, staying up late, failing to get enough exercise." Grade-specific results for students in grades 4 through 6 showed that smoking (90 to 95 percent) and chewing tobacco (80 to 90 percent) were much more likely to be perceived as "very harmful" compared with the other choices, all of which were considered to be "very harmful" by less than 40 percent of respondents (except for loud music, among fourth graders—70 percent). However, these results should be interpreted with caution because of the possibility of sampling bias and the leading nature of the question.

Addiction

Of particular concern are teenagers who are unaware of the addictive nature of cigarette smoking, and who, therefore, may be tempted to "experiment" with smoking. In the 1974 and 1979 DHEW Teenage Smoking Surveys (US DHEW 1976b, 1979b), about one-quarter of the teenagers agreed with the statement, "Teenagers who smoke regularly can quit for good any time they like." About 60 percent agreed that "It's okay for teenagers to experiment with cigarettes if they quit before it becomes a habit." In the 1979 survey, teenagers were asked, "What would you say is the possibility that 5 years from now you will be a cigarette smoker?" Fifty percent of the current regular smokers (48 percent of boys and 52 percent of girls) answered "definitely not" or "probably not." These findings suggest that a large proportion of new smokers are unaware of or underestimate the addictive nature of smoking.

In 1975, 56 percent of girls aged 13 to 17 years and 62 percent of young women aged 18 to 35 years thought that smoking was as addictive as illegal drugs (US DHEW 1975a).

In the study by Leventhal, Glynn, and Fleming (1987) of 895 students in grades 2 through 12 in Milwaukee, WI, subjects were asked how hard it is for heavy smokers and for light smokers to quit smoking, and how heavy and light smokers feel when they quit. Answers were used to construct a "knowledge of addiction" scale. The investigators found that young people who smoke or who have smoking family members have lower "knowledge of addiction" scores. The authors speculate that these individuals may be "defending against the thought that either they or a parent has an uncontrollable problem."

Information on teenage beliefs concerning the addictiveness of ST use is discussed below.

Smokeless Tobacco Use

In 1985, the Office of the Inspector General, Department of Health and Human Services, surveyed a nonrandom sample of 399 students in 11 junior high or middle schools and 20 high schools in 16 States regarding ST use (US DHHS 1986d). ST users were oversampled based on identification of users and nonusers by school officials. The sample was composed of 290 current ST users (73 percent) and 109 nonusers (27 percent). Eighty percent of junior high school users and 92 percent of high school users acknowledged that dipping snuff and chewing tobacco *can be* harmful to a person's health (Table 20). When asked about the extent of physical harm that may result from ST use, however, about half of users believed that there is no risk or only slight risk from regular use. One-third of junior high school users and only 5 percent of high school users thought that ST use may lead to mouth cancer. There was poor understanding of the effects of ST use on gum and dental conditions. One-quarter of junior high school users believed that regular ST use is not addictive, and more than one-third did not know that snuff contains nicotine. In summary, these findings suggest that users are substantially uninformed about the health effects and addictiveness of smokeless tobacco use. However, the degree to which these results can be generalized nationally is limited by the nonrepresentative nature of the sample.

Data from the Monitoring the Future Project showed that in 1986, a total of 59 percent of high school seniors believed that regular ST use poses a great (26 percent) or moderate (33 percent) risk of harm, compared with 36 percent who believed that ST use poses slight (28 percent) or no (8 percent) risk (Bachman, Johnston, O'Malley 1987).

Constituents of Tobacco Smoke

The estimated number of known compounds in tobacco smoke exceeds 4,000, including some that are pharmacologically active, toxic, mutagenic, carcinogenic, and antigenic (Chapter 2). One of these is carbon monoxide, whose presence in cigarette smoke is cited in one of the four health warnings rotated on cigarette packages and advertisements since 1985 (Chapter 7).

In a 1979 survey conducted by Chilton Research Services for the Federal Trade Commission (FTC 1981), respondents were asked, "Does cigarette smoke contain carbon monoxide?" Fifty-one percent of teenagers (aged 13–18) either did not know (21 percent) or said "no" (29 percent); 45 percent of adults (aged 29–31) either did not know (26 percent) or said "no" (19 percent).

In a 1980 Roper survey (FTC 1981), 53 percent of all respondents and 56 percent of smokers did not know or believe that "Cigarette smoke contains carbon monoxide, which is a dangerous gas."

In the 1986 AUTS, 62 percent of current smokers answered "yes" to the question, "As far as you know, does cigarette smoke contain carbon monoxide?" Thirteen percent said "no," and 25 percent did not know. Former and never smokers were not asked this question.

TABLE 20.—Beliefs about the health effects of smokeless tobacco (ST) use among 399 junior and senior high school students (percentage who agree) in 16 States, 1986

	Users		Nonusers
	Junior high school (N = 76)	High school (N = 214)	(N = 109)
ST use *can be* harmful	80	92	97
Risk from ST use			
None or slight	57	42	32
Moderate to great	43	58	68
Regular ST use may lead to mouth cancer	33	5	5
Gum and mouth problems among users are very rare	64	41	33
ST use increases risk of tooth stains, wear, and loss	24	11	16
Snuff does not contain nicotine	38	20	32
Regular ST use is not addictive	25	15	10
ST use is much more safe than cigarettes	81	81	59

NOTE: ST user defined as follows: has dipped or chewed more than 100 times, currently uses daily or at least 3 days per week, dipping at least three times on days of use. Nonuser defined as follows: has never dipped or chewed, or has only tried it a few times or more than a few times but fewer than 100 times.
SOURCE: US DHHS (1986d).

Health Benefits of Smoking Cessation

The overall mortality ratio of former smokers (compared with never smokers) declines with increasing years of abstinence. According to data reviewed in the 1979 Surgeon General's Report (US DHEW 1979a) from the U.S. Veterans Study and the British Doctors Study, overall mortality rates of former smokers are similar to those of never smokers 15 years after quitting (US DHEW 1979a). With respect to lung cancer mortality, the increased risk diminishes substantially by 5 to 9 years after quitting, but remains above the risk of never smokers for many more years except for those with fewer than 30 years of cigarette smoking (Chapter 2). A reduction in CHD mortality occurs within the first few years after cessation (US DHHS 1983). The risk of COPD mortality decreases eventually after smoking cessation but does not decline to equal that of never smokers, even after 20 years of cessation (US DHHS 1984).

In the 1986 AUTS, respondents were asked how long it takes before former smokers' chances of developing a disease return to normal. Slightly more than half believed that the risks return to normal within 5 years (Table 21). Results were similar when stratified by smoking status.

The 1987 NHIS included questions regarding the health benefits of quitting in terms of specific disease risks. These data were not available for inclusion in this Report.

Discussion

It has been 25 years since the release of the first Surgeon General's Report on smoking and health. During that time, a major public health effort has been made to educate the public regarding the health consequences of smoking (see Chapters 6–8).

Public knowledge of the health risks of smoking has improved as a result of this massive public health education campaign. The belief that smoking is harmful to health has increased since 1964. In 1964, a majority of adults acknowledged the general health risk of smoking and believed that smoking is a major cause of lung cancer, but a minority believed that smoking increases the risk of COPD, heart disease, and premature birth. By the mid-1980s, a substantial majority of adults (including nonsmokers and smokers) recognized the general health risks of smoking and believed that smoking increases the risk of lung cancer, COPD, and heart disease, and prematurity, low birthweight, miscarriage, and stillbirths.

Knowledge of the risks of exposure to ETS has also increased markedly since 1974; in fact, this high level of belief preceded the release of the 1986 Surgeon General's Report on the health consequences of involuntary smoking.

Current Gaps in Public Beliefs About the Health Effects of Smoking

Despite the growing level of public knowledge noted above, a substantial *number* of Americans are still uninformed about or do not believe the health risks of smoking. These gaps in knowledge or beliefs are more evident when one considers the proportion of adults who do not acknowledge certain health risks rather than the proportion who do. For example, among smokers—for whom this information is particularly

TABLE 21.—Public knowledge about the health benefits of smoking cessation in relation to years of abstinence, 1986

	If someone gives up smoking completely, how long do you think it will take before their chances of developing a disease return to normal? (percentage indicating the following number of years)							
	<1	1–2	3–5	6–10	11–15	15	Never	Don't know
Current smokers	17	23	16	8	1	1	7	27
Former smokers	14	23	20	8	1	1	7	26
Never smokers	16	23	16	6	1	1	12	25

SOURCE: AUTS 1986 (US DHHS, in press).

relevant—10 percent in 1985 did *not* believe that smoking is harmful to health. In 1986, 15 percent did *not* think that a person who smokes is more likely than a person who does not smoke to get lung cancer. Similar proportions of smokers did *not* believe that smokers are more likely to get heart disease (29 percent), chronic bronchitis (27 percent), emphysema (15 percent), and laryngeal cancer (18 percent). These percentages correspond to 8 million to 15 million adult smokers in the United States.

Another gap exists in the public's understanding of the special health risks of women who smoke. Compared with 1964, in 1985 smokers were more than twice as likely to recognize smoking as a cause of premature delivery. However, in 1985, 24 percent of all women (smokers and nonsmokers combined) 18 to 44 years of age did not recognize the risk of prematurity; 15 percent did not recognize the risk of low birthweight; 25 percent did not recognize the risk of miscarriage; and 32 percent did not recognize the risk of stillbirth (Table 12; Fox et al. 1987).

The fact that in 1985 10 percent of smokers did not indicate that smoking is harmful to health (Table 2), despite all efforts designed to impart such information (Chapters 6–8), suggests that this group of smokers may resist accepting any information on the health effects of smoking. This finding has important implications for smoking control efforts and for setting public health objectives. It implies that other techniques besides providing information (e.g., policy incentives—see Chapter 7) are necessary to persuade some smokers to quit. It also suggests that it is unrealistic to set a goal above 90 percent of smokers for public knowledge about any health effect of smoking.

Another gap in public knowledge involves teenagers. Youth may understand that smoking is generally harmful to health, but many may not appreciate the addictive nature of smoking or may deny a personal susceptibility (Leventhal, Glynn, Fleming 1987). In addition, data from one study (US DHHS 1986c) suggest that many ST users are not aware of the health effects and addictiveness of the product.

Fishbein (1977) described three different ways in which individuals may be informed of a given piece of information: (1) they may become aware that the information exists; (2) they may accept the information in general; or (3) they may accept the information at a personalized level. These three ways of being informed correspond to three levels of belief mentioned at the beginning of this Chapter: Level 1 (awareness), Level 2 (general acceptance), and Level 3 (personalized acceptance).

Persons may have knowledge or beliefs at one level, but not at another. For example, some smokers may be aware of the Surgeon General's Reports and accept the general fact that smoking is dangerous, but do not believe that they will be harmed by smoking. The data presented in this Report support this concept. Whereas in 1975 approximately 90 percent of smokers believed that smoking is harmful to health (Table 2), in 1986 only 75 percent were concerned about the effects of smoking on *their* health (Table 15). The recognition of a general risk but disbelief in a personal risk may result from several factors, including a belief that using low-tar cigarettes (see Table 3), smoking fewer cigarettes daily (see Table 5), or having certain genetic factors eliminates the personal risk.

In order to make a fully informed decision, a person should have complete and accurate Level 3 beliefs about the outcomes of each alternative action (Fishbein 1977). The personalization (perception of the personal relevance) of abstract information has been shown to be an important aspect of behavior change in general (Mahoney 1974) and of health-related behavior change in particular (Ben-Sira 1982; Schinke and Gilchrist 1984).

Factors Interfering With Changes in Knowledge

There is a vast body of literature pertaining to the acquisition of knowledge and the process of learning. Research in this area has identified many factors that enhance or interfere with this acquisition. The brief discussion below does not attempt to provide a comprehensive review of this literature, but rather attempts to identify a few of the more salient factors that may impede the development of accurate beliefs about the health risks of smoking. The importance of beliefs in determining smoking behavior is discussed in Part II of Chapter 5 (sections on Cognition and Decisionmaking).

Informing the public about the health risks of smoking is difficult to accomplish. Risk assessment is a complex discipline, not fully understood by its practitioners, much less the lay public (Slovic 1986). Risk judgments are influenced by the memorability of past events; as a result, any factor that makes a risk memorable—such as a recent disaster or heavy media coverage—seriously distorts the perception of risk. Risks from dramatic and sensational causes of death, such as injuries, homicides, and natural disasters, tend to be greatly overestimated. Risks from undramatic causes, such as bronchitis, emphysema, or cancer, which take one life at a time and which may be more common in nonfatal form, tend to be underestimated (Slovic 1986). News media coverage of health risks has been found to be biased in the same direction, thus contributing to the difficulties of obtaining proper perspective on risks (Slovic 1986).

The fact that perceptions of risk are often inaccurate may indicate the need for warnings and educational programs. Such programs, however, face the obstacle that information based on probability is likely to have less impact on recipients than information based on certainty. For example, the data presented herein indicate that the majority of smokers believe that smoking increases the *chance* of getting lung cancer. However, not all smokers develop lung cancer, and on occasion, a well-publicized case of lung cancer occurs in an individual who never smoked. These "exceptions" may provide smokers with a rationale to continue smoking despite their abstract belief of risk.

In addition to their difficulty with understanding risks, smokers may deny personal risk with respect to health effects of smoking and addiction. Some smokers incorrectly believe that while smoking may be hazardous to others, it is not hazardous to themselves because of the particular type of cigarette they smoke, the amount they smoke, or their family history of disease. Persons who are exposed to a health risk, such as smokers, may attempt to reduce the anxiety generated in the face of that risk by denying the existence or magnitude of the risk, thus making the risk seem so small that it can be safely ignored (Slovic 1986).

Teenagers pose a special challenge for sharing knowledge of the health risks of smoking. As mentioned above and as shown in Table 18, the majority of high school seniors do believe that smoking is generally harmful. However, the fact that the health risks are in the distant future for teenage smokers may make it difficult for them to fully appreciate those risks. In other words, this lag may reduce teenagers' likelihood to transform Level 2 beliefs to Level 3 beliefs. This is one reason smoking prevention efforts now tend to emphasize social influence approaches and to deemphasize communication of the long-term health risks of smoking (Chapter 6).

Although empirical evidence is sparse, tobacco industry activities in the form of advertising and promotion, public relations, and lobbying may interfere with public beliefs and personalized acceptance of the health risks of smoking. Because most individuals may not understand *how* smoking causes the diseases with which it is associated, many persons may be vulnerable to information that attempts to cast doubt on such relationships. These industry activities are reviewed in Chapters 6 and 7.

The 1990 Health Objectives for the Nation

In 1980, the U.S. Public Health Service established the 1990 Health Objectives for the Nation (US DHHS 1980). A midcourse review of progress toward meeting these objectives was published in 1986 (US DHHS 1986b). These objectives included five goals for public knowledge of the health consequences of smoking:

> Objective 1: By 1990, the share of the adult population aware that smoking is one of the major risk factors for heart disease should be increased to at least 85 percent.
>
> Objective 2: By 1990, at least 90 percent of the adult population should be aware that smoking is a major cause of lung cancer, as well as multiple other cancers including laryngeal, esophageal, bladder, and other types.
>
> Objective 3: By 1990, at least 85 percent of the adult population should be aware of the special risk of developing and worsening chronic obstructive lung disease, including bronchitis and emphysema, among smokers.
>
> Objective 4: By 1990, at least 85 percent of women should be aware of the special health risks for women who smoke, including the effect on outcomes of pregnancy and the excess risk of CVD with oral contraceptive use.
>
> Objective 5: By 1990, at least 65 percent of 12-year-olds should be able to identify smoking cigarettes with increased risks of serious disease of the heart and lungs.

For the purposes of these objectives, the term aware was not defined and no distinction was made between Level 1, Level 2, and Level 3 beliefs (see above).

Progress toward meeting the first two objectives cannot be assessed reliably because they refer to smoking as "one of the major risk factors" for heart disease and "a major cause" of lung cancer and other cancers. On the other hand, most surveys have assessed public beliefs about whether smoking increases the risk of or "is related to" heart disease or lung cancer (Tables 8 and 9). As mentioned above, such wording changes can markedly affect results of surveys assessing public beliefs.

The third objective appears to have been met in the case of emphysema and nearly met in the case of chronic bronchitis (Table 10). In 1985, the percentages of adults 18 to 44 years of age who acknowledged the various effects of maternal smoking on the fetus were generally 10 to 20 percentage points below the goals listed in the fourth objective, except that 85 percent of women believed that smoking during pregnancy increases the risk of having a low-birthweight baby (Table 12). The percentage who knew of the interactive effects of smoking and oral contraceptive use on CVD was also below the 1990 goal. No data exist to assess progress toward achieving the fifth objective.

Trends in Public Attitudes About Smoking and Smokers

This Section describes trends in public attitudes about smoking in general and about smokers.

Involuntary Smoking as an Annoyance

Since 1964, the population has become increasingly annoyed by exposure to ETS. In 1964, less than half of adults (46 percent) thought that it was annoying to be near a person smoking cigarettes (Table 22). Identical questions asked in surveys conducted in 1964, 1966, 1970, and 1975 reveal an increase in the proportion of adults who were annoyed by being near a person who is smoking (from 20 to 35 percent among smokers and from 64 to 77 percent among nonsmokers). By 1986, 42 percent of smokers and 80 percent of nonsmokers reported that they were annoyed by the smoke from another person's cigarette. The 1987 NHIS (preliminary first-quarter data) obtained results similar to those of the 1986 AUTS.

Nonsmokers' Rights

According to Gallup surveys, the proportion of adults who feel that smokers should refrain from smoking in the presence of nonsmokers increased slightly between 1983 and 1987. In 1983, 69 percent of adults thought that smokers should refrain from smoking in the presence of others (Table 23). By 1987, 77 percent of adults (64 percent of smokers and 86 percent of nonsmokers) thought that smokers should refrain from smoking in front of others.

In the 1987 Gallup survey, respondents were asked where smokers should refrain from smoking when nonsmokers are present. The proportions who believed that smokers should not smoke in the presence of nonsmokers were 62 percent with respect to public places, 34 percent with respect to work, and 19 percent with respect to the home (ALA 1987).

In a 1987 survey conducted for AMA, respondents were asked, "Which do you feel is a more important individual right, the right of smokers to smoke anywhere, or the right of nonsmokers to a smoke-free environment?" Three-quarters of respondents (76 percent) thought that nonsmokers had the right to a smoke-free environment (49 percent of smokers and 86 percent of nonsmokers), compared with 10 percent who thought that smokers had the right to smoke anywhere (25 percent of smokers and 5 percent of nonsmokers) (Harvey and Shubat 1987).

TABLE 22.—Trends in public attitudes about exposure to environmental tobacco smoke

			It is annoying to be near a person who is smoking cigarettes (percentage who agree by smoking status)				
Survey	Year	Reference	Current smokers	Former smokers	Never smokers	All nonsmokers	All adults
1. AUTS	1964	US DHEW 1969	20	49	69	64	46
2. AUTS	1966	US DHEW 1969	26	52	70		48
3. AUTS	1970	US DHEW 1973	34	63	78	73	59
4. AUTS	1975	US DHEW 1976	35	72	79	77	63
5. Roper	1978	Roper 1978	5			60	
6. AUTS	1986	US DHHS, in press	42	73	83	80	69
7. NHIS[a]	1987		34	73	85		67

[a]Preliminary first-quarter data (unpublished).

NOTE: Actual questions:

1–4. It is annoying to be near a person who is smoking cigarettes. (strongly agree, mildly agree, no opinion, mildly disagree, strongly disagree)*

6. Is the smoke from someone else's cigarette very annoying to you, somewhat annoying to you, or not annoying at all?†

7. In general, would you say the smoke from other people's cigarettes is very annoying to you, somewhat annoying to you, or not at all annoying?†

*Percentages include those who "strongly agree" or "mildly agree."

†Percentages include those who state that smoke from someone else's cigarette is "very annoying" or "somewhat annoying."

TABLE 23.—Trends in public attitudes about smoking in the presence of nonsmokers

			Smokers should refrain from smoking in the presence of nonsmokers (percentage who agree by smoking status)				
Survey	Year	Reference	Current smokers	Former smokers	Never smokers	All nonsmokers	All adults
1. Gallup	1983	ALA 1987	55	70		82	69
2. Gallup	1985	ALA 1987	62	78		85	75
3. Gallup	1987	ALA 1987	64	76		86	77
4. NHIS[a]	1987		65	81	89		80

[a]Preliminary first-quarter data (unpublished). Year-end percentage for all adults is 80 percent.

NOTE: Actual questions:

1–3. Should smokers refrain from smoking in the presence of nonsmokers? (strongly agree, agree, disagree, strongly disagree, no opinion)*

4. If people want to smoke, they should not do so in indoor public places where it might disturb others. (strongly agree, agree, disagree, strongly disagree)*

*Percentages include those who "strongly agree" or "agree."

Actions When Smokers Light Up

Surveys conducted by the Roper Organization in 1974, 1976, and 1978 (Roper 1978) assessed actions of smokers when they are indoors with other people and want a cigarette, and actions of nonsmokers in response. Although these questions technically pertain to smoking behavior, the subject of the next chapter, they are indicators of attitudes toward smoking.

Smokers were asked, "Do you light up a cigarette without really thinking about it, or do you look around and then decide whether it's okay, or do you ask if others would mind, or do you just not smoke?" In 1978, a total of 57 percent either looked around and then decided (27 percent), or asked others (26 percent), or did not smoke (4 percent). Slightly lower total percentages for these three actions were reported in 1976 (55 percent) and 1974 (53 percent). The 1987 NHIS indicated that 21 percent of smokers would light up in a public place, while 26 percent would look around first, 15 percent would ask others, and 31 percent would refrain from smoking.

A total of 58 percent of *nonsmokers* in 1978 said that when someone is smoking indoors, they either ask the smoker to stop smoking (6 percent), indicate disapproval without saying so (10 percent), or try to move away (42 percent). In both 1974 and 1976, the total percentage for these three actions was 53 percent; other possible responses were: "doesn't matter," "enjoy it," "it depends," "and "don't know." According to the 1987 NHIS, fewer than 5 percent of nonsmokers would ask a smoker in public not to smoke (preliminary first-quarter data).

Opinions of Teenagers

According to recent surveys from the Monitoring the Future Project, most high school seniors think that smokers their age are trying to appear mature and sophisticated, and about half of teenagers think that smoking makes them look insecure (Table 24). Only 5 to 10 percent of respondents thought that smokers look cool, calm, in control; rugged, tough, independent; or mature and sophisticated. Most teenagers prefer to date people who do not smoke. Most also consider smoking a dirty habit and think that becoming a smoker reflects poor judgment. In 1986, 45 percent of teenagers strongly disliked being near people who were smoking while 37 percent did not mind being around people who were smoking. There appears to have been little change in these attitudes from 1981–86.

In summary, smokers and nonsmokers, adults and teenagers alike, generally believe that smokers should refrain from smoking in the presence of others and that it is annoying to be near a person who is smoking. In addition, teenagers are more likely to associate smoking and smokers with negative attributes than positive ones.

TABLE 24.—Trends in attitudes about smoking and smokers among high school seniors, 1981–86, Monitoring the Future Project, National Institute on Drug Abuse

	In my opinion, when a guy my age is smoking a cigarette, it makes him look . . . (percentage who agree)	
	1981	1986
like he's TRYING to appear mature and sophisticated	61	63
insecure	42	44
conforming	25	21
rugged, tough, independent	9	10
cool, calm, in control	6	6
mature, sophisticated	5	5

	In my opinion, when a girl my age is smoking a cigarette, it makes her look . . . (percentage who agree)	
	1981	1986
like she's TRYING to appear mature and sophisticated	65	65
insecure	47	50
conforming	27	22
independent and liberated	11	10
mature, sophisticated	7	5
cool, calm, in control	6	5

TABLE 24.—Continued

	Do you agree or disagree . . . (percentage who agree)	
	1981	1986
I prefer to date people who don't smoke	66	71
Smoking is a dirty habit	66	69
I think that becoming a smoker reflects poor judgment	57	59
I strongly dislike being near people who are smoking		45
I personally don't mind being around people who are smoking	38	37
The harmful effects of cigarettes have been exaggerated	16	16
Smokers know how to enjoy life more than nonsmokers	3	2

NOTE: Possible responses included agree, mostly agree, disagree, mostly disagree, neither. Percentages include those who "agree" or "mostly agree."

SOURCE: Johnston, Bachman, O'Malley (1982); Bachman, Johnston, O'Malley (1987).

Trends in Public Opinion About Smoking Policies

Overview

Background

This Section describes trends in public opinion about smoking policies. Public opinion information is helpful to legislators, public health officials, and other policymakers who often wish to know the degree of public support for an issue under consideration. The results presented in this Section are taken primarily from public opinion polls sponsored by a variety of private health organizations (Appendix).

This Section uses the categorization of policies employed in Chapter 7, including the following categories: (1) smoking restrictions, (2) restrictions on the sale and distribution of cigarettes, (3) policies pertaining to information and education, and (4) economic policies. Each section reviews trends in public opinion toward the policy and briefly describes the current status of opinions toward the policy with respect to the smoking status of the respondents.

Limitations of the Surveys in Assessing Public Opinion About Smoking Policies

Assessing trends in public opinion regarding smoking policies is more difficult in some ways than assessing trends in public knowledge regarding the health effects of smoking. For instance, surveys that ask about public opinion often refer to the "current" situation. However, the "current" situation may change from year to year and from survey to survey. For example, in 1964, 52 percent of adults thought that smoking should be allowed in fewer places than it was at that time. By 1975, 70 percent of adults thought that smoking should be allowed in fewer places than it was at that time. However, the "current" situation changed from 1964–75, making the survey results difficult to compare. Because smoking was already allowed in fewer places by 1975, the results of the 1975 survey reveal even greater support for limitations on smoking than indicated by the difference in percentages.

Restrictions on Smoking

General

Between 1964 and 1975, adults increasingly favored restrictions on smoking. In 1964, about half (52 percent) thought that smoking should be allowed in fewer places than it was at that time, compared with 70 percent by 1975 (Table 25). Comparable questions have not been asked to assess more recent trends since 1975. However, in 1986, 50 percent of adults disagreed that there were already enough restrictions on where people can smoke.

TABLE 25.—Trends in public opinion about restrictions on smoking in public places

			Smoking should be allowed in fewer places than it is now (percentage who agree by smoking status)				
Survey	Year	Reference	Current smokers	Former smokers	Never smokers	All nonsmokers	All adults
1. AUTS	1964	US DHEW 1969	34	56	68	65	52
2. AUTS	1966	US DHEW 1969	35	58	67	65	52
3. AUTS	1970	US DHEW 1973	42	61	68	66	57
4. AUTS	1975	US DHEW 1976a	51	77	82	80	70
			There are already enough restrictions on where people can smoke (percentage who DISAGREE by smoking status)				
Survey	Year	Reference	Current smokers	Former smokers	Never smokers	All nonsmokers	All adults
5. AUTS	1986	US DHHS, in press	23	53	63	59	50

NOTE: Actual questions:

1–4. The smoking of cigarettes should be allowed in fewer places than it is now. (strongly agree, mildly agree, no opinion, mildly disagree, strongly disagree)*

5. There are already enough restrictions on where people can smoke. (strongly agree, somewhat agree, neutral, somewhat disagree, strongly disagree)†

*Percentages include those who "strongly agree" or "mildly agree."

†Percentages include those who "strongly disagree" or "somewhat disagree."

Public Places

Table 26 presents data from five surveys conducted since 1978 that asked about opinions regarding restrictions on smoking in public places. Differences in the wording of the questions make comparisons among the surveys difficult. Two surveys solicited opinions about three mutually exclusive options (total ban on smoking, separate sections for smokers and nonsmokers, and no restrictions at all), two surveys asked for an opinion only about a total ban, and the fifth asked for an opinion only about "no smoking" sections.

The 1978 Gallup survey and the 1987 Harris survey both presented three options. The proportion of respondents favoring *either* a total smoking ban or separate sections was 84 percent in both. However, the percentage favoring a total ban increased from 16 to 23 percent. The 1987 and 1988 Gallup surveys showed that the percentages favoring a total ban were 55 and 60 percent, respectively (69 and 75 percent of nonsmokers, respectively); the option of separate sections was not presented in these surveys (Table 26).

Workplace

Questions used to assess opinions regarding smoking restrictions in the workplace have varied from year to year. It is not possible, therefore, to identify a clear trend, but the public has consistently shown support for policies that limit smoking in the workplace.

In 1966, 92 percent of adults thought that an employer had a right to tell employees when or where they can smoke while on the job (US DHEW 1969). In 1975, 78 percent of adults thought that management had the right to *prohibit* smoking in a place of business (US DHEW 1976a). By 1985, 87 percent of adults thought that companies should have a policy on smoking (80 percent of current smokers, 92 percent of nonsmokers). Most adults (79 percent) preferred assigning certain areas for smoking and nonsmoking as opposed to totally banning smoking at work (8 percent) (Gallup 1985).

Airplanes

Since 1978, it appears that more adults favor restricting smoking on airline flights. In a 1978 Gallup survey, 43 percent of adults thought a smoking ban should be imposed on commercial airline flights (Table 27). A 1987 AMA survey reported that 67 percent of adults thought that cigarette smoking should not be allowed on commercial airline flights. A 1987 survey conducted by the American Association for Respiratory Care (AARC) of 33,242 airline passengers in 39 States and 89 airports in the United States yielded similar results (AARC 1987) (Table 27).

According to the 1986 AUTS, 61 percent of respondents (82 percent of never smokers, 69 percent of former smokers, and 14 percent of current smokers) ask to be seated in the no-smoking sections of airplanes, restaurants, and other public places when given a choice (CDC 1988).

TABLE 26.—Trends in public opinion about restrictions on smoking in public places

			Smoking in public places[a]		
Survey	Year	Reference	% favoring total ban	% favoring separate sections	Total % favoring ban or sections
1. Gallup	1978	Gallup 1978	16 (22/8)	68 (67/70)	84 (89/78)
2. Lieberman	1986	Lieberman 1986		94 (95/93)	
3. Harris	1987	Harris 1988	23	61	84
4. Gallup	1987	Gallup 1987a	55 (69/25)		
5. Gallup	1988	Gallup 1988b	60 (75/26)		

[a]Percentages in parentheses refer to nonsmokers and current smokers, respectively.

NOTE: Actual questions:

1. In your opinion, which of the policies on this card should be followed with regard to smoking in such places as trains, buses, airplanes, restaurants, and offices? (There should be no restrictions at all on smoking in public places such as these; Special sections for smokers should be set aside in public places such as these; Smoking should not be allowed at all in public places such as these.)

2. Should public places have "no smoking" sections? (yes, no, no opinion)

3. Do you think that laws should prohibit smoking in public places, or should they require separate smoking and nonsmoking sections, or should smoking in public places not be regulated by law?

4-5. Would you favor or oppose a complete ban on smoking in all public places?

TABLE 27.—Trends in public opinion about restrictions on smoking in airplanes

			Smoking should not be allowed on commercial airline flights (percentage who agree by smoking status)				
Survey	Year	Reference	Current smokers	Former smokers	Never smokers	All nonsmokers	All adults
1. Gallup	1978	Gallup 1978	55			23	43
2. AMA	1987	Harvey and Shubat 1987	40			78	67
3. AARC[a]	1987	AARC 1987	30			74	64

[a]Survey of 33,242 airline passengers conducted in 39 States and 89 airports in the United States.

NOTE: Actual questions:

1. Do you think that cigarette smoking on commercial airplanes should or should not be banned completely?*
2. Do you feel that cigarette smoking should or should not be allowed on commercial airline flights?**

*Percentages are those who believe that cigarette smoking should be banned on flights.

**Percentages are those who believe that cigarette smoking should not be allowed on flights.

Restaurants

In four surveys, conducted between 1976 and 1987, approximately 20 percent of respondents favored a total ban on smoking in restaurants (Table 28). In contrast, most adults are in favor of *limiting* smoking in restaurants. A 1976 Roper poll indicated that 57 percent believed smoking should be restricted to certain areas in restaurants, while 22 percent favored a total ban on smoking. In a 1987 Gallup survey conducted for ALA, 74 percent of adults thought that certain areas should be set aside for smoking and 17 percent thought that smoking should be banned completely (ALA 1987; Gallup 1987a).

As mentioned above, 61 percent of respondents to the 1986 AUTS choose no-smoking sections of restaurants and other public places when given a choice (CDC 1988). In a survey conducted by the Gallup Organization for the National Restaurant Association in 1987, adults were asked about various opinions regarding smoking in restaurants: 61 percent overall said that they prefer to sit in a no-smoking section (83 percent of never smokers, 65 percent of former smokers, and 20 percent of current smokers) (Gallup 1987d).

Other Places

A Gallup survey conducted for the ALA in 1983 showed that 54 percent of adults favored setting aside certain areas for smoking in hotels and motels and 12 percent favored a total smoking ban. In a similar survey in 1987, these percentages were 67 percent and 10 percent, respectively, and were slightly higher for nonsmokers than for current smokers (Gallup 1988a).

Restrictions on the Sale and Distribution of Cigarettes

Complete Ban on Sales

The questions used to assess opinion regarding the outright ban of cigarette sales have varied considerably in wording. In 1964, respondents were asked if they agreed that "The selling of cigarettes should *not* be stopped completely." In 1970, respondents were asked if they agreed that "The selling of cigarettes *should* be stopped completely." Despite these differences, the responses consistently indicated little sympathy for this most stringent policy: approximately 30 percent of adults supported a ban in 1964, compared with 20 percent in 1981 (Table 29).

Limiting Sales to Minors

Most adults favor limiting cigarette sales to minors. In 1964, only 9 percent of adults thought that sales of cigarettes to people under a certain age should *not* be against the law. In 1970, 88 percent thought that such sales *should be* against the law (Table 30).

TABLE 28.—Trends in public opinion about restrictions on smoking in restaurants

			Smoking should be banned (or limited) in restaurants[a] (percentage who agree by smoking status)				
Survey	Year	Reference	Current smokers	Former smokers	Never smokers	All nonsmokers	All adults
1. Roper	1976	Roper 1978					22 (57)
2. Roper	1978	Roper 1978					23 (73)
3. Gallup	1983	ALA 1987	12 (74)	19 (71)		26 (65)	19 (69)
4. Gallup	1987	ALA 1987	7 (79)	19 (74)		23 (71)	17 (74)

[a]Percentages represent those who favor a total smoking ban. Percentages *in parentheses* represent those who favor setting aside certain areas for smoking.

NOTE: Actual questions:

1–2. Should smoking be permitted only in separate sections or should it be permitted anywhere . . . in eating places?

3–4. What is your opinion regarding smoking in these public places . . . restaurants? (set aside certain areas, totally ban smoking, or no restrictions)

TABLE 29.—Trends in public opinion about banning the sale of cigarettes

			Percentage who agree by smoking status				
Survey	Year	Reference	Current smokers	Former smokers	Never smokers	All nonsmokers	All adults
			The selling of cigarettes SHOULD BE stopped completely				
1. AUTS	1970	US DHEW 1973	27	36	48	44	38
2. Roper	1970	Roper 1978					15
3. Roper	1972	Roper 1978					13
4. Roper	1974	Roper 1978					12
5. Roper	1976	Roper 1978					12
6. Roper	1978	Roper 1978					16
7. Gallup	1977	Gallup 1981					19
8. Gallup	1978	Gallup 1978	11			23	19
9. Gallup	1981	Gallup 1981	10			26	20
			The selling of cigarettes should NOT be stopped completely				
10. AUTS	1964	US DHEW 1969	83	74	57	61	70
11. Gallup	1978	Gallup 1978					75

NOTE: Actual questions:
1. The selling of cigarettes should be stopped completely. (strongly agree, mildly agree, no opinion, mildly disagree, strongly disagree)*
2–6. A law should be passed against the sale of all cigarettes (agree, disagree, don't know)
7–9. Do you think the sale of cigarettes should or should not be banned completely?
10. The selling of cigarettes should *not* be stopped completely.
11. Cigarette sales should *not* be banned completely.
*Percentages include those who "strongly agree" or "mildly agree."

TABLE 30.—Trends in public opinion about restrictions on the sale or distribution of cigarettes

			Percentage who agree by smoking status				
Survey	Year	Reference	Current smokers	Former smokers	Never smokers	All nonsmokers	All adults
		Sales of cigarettes to people under a certain age should NOT be against the law					
1. AUTS	1964	US DHEW 1969	12	7	7	7	9
		Sales of cigarettes to people under a certain age SHOULD BE against the law					
2. AUTS	1970	US DHEW 1973	87	87	90	89	88
		Cigarette companies should not be permitted to distribute free cigarettes on public streets					
3. Lieberman	1986	Lieberman 1986	48			67	61

NOTE: Actual questions:

1. Sales of cigarettes to people under a certain age should *not* be against the law. (strongly agree, mildly agree, no opinion, mildly disagree, strongly disagree)*
2. Sales of cigarettes to people under a certain age should be against the law. (strongly agree, mildly agree, no opinion, mildly disagree, strongly disagree)*
3. Should cigarette companies be permitted to distribute free cigarettes on public streets?†

*Percentages include those who "strongly agree" or "mildly agree."

†Percentages are those who believe cigarette companies should not be permitted to distribute free samples.

Banning Free Samples

In a 1986 survey conducted by Lieberman Research, Inc. (1986) (New York City) for ACS, AHA, and ALA, 61 percent of adults said that the distribution of free cigarette samples should not be permitted (67 percent of nonsmokers, 48 percent of smokers) (Table 30).

Policies Pertaining to Information and Education

Restricting or Prohibiting Tobacco Advertising

Since 1964, several surveys have investigated public opinion regarding a cigarette advertising ban, with marked differences in the wording of questions. Taken together, they do not seem to indicate any trend in public opinion (Table 31). However, separate examinations of surveys using identical questions over time indicate increasing support for an advertising ban. A series of identical questions from the AUTSs from 1964 and 1975 showed an increase in support for a complete ban between 1964 and 1970. In 1964, 36 percent of adults thought that cigarette advertising should be stopped completely. This increased to 61 percent in 1970 and 56 percent in 1975 (Table 31). Support for an advertising ban may have increased by 1970 because Congress had already banned cigarette advertising on television and radio in 1969 (effective on January 2, 1971) (see Chapter 7). Another series of identical questions used in Gallup surveys after the broadcast advertising ban showed an increase in the proportion of the public favoring a cigarette advertising ban, from 36 percent in 1977 to 43 percent in 1981 to 49 percent in 1987 to 55 percent in 1988.

Since 1975, surveys have provided conflicting results regarding public support for a complete ban, most likely as a result of differences in the wording of questions. In the two Gallup surveys conducted in 1977 and 1981, support *for a complete ban on cigarette advertising* increased from 36 to 43 percent (Gallup 1987a). In a 1985 Gallup survey, adults were asked which statement best described the respondent's opinion regarding cigarette advertising: "There should be a total ban on cigarette advertising." "There should be a curb on some types or forms of cigarette advertising." "There should be no ban whatsoever on cigarette advertising in newspapers, magazines, or billboards." The public was divided in their responses: about a third favored each option (32, 36, and 31 percent, respectively) (Gallup 1985).

As mentioned at the beginning of this Chapter, two surveys conducted in 1986 reported different results. One, conducted by AMA, reported that almost two-thirds of adults favored such a ban whereas another, sponsored by ACS, AHA, and ALA, reported that only one-third of Americans supported such a ban for newspapers and magazines (see the earlier discussion of these discrepant results). Four more recent surveys, conducted in 1987 and 1988, revealed that about half of adults favor a complete ban on advertising (Table 31).

TABLE 31.—Trends in public opinion about restricting or banning cigarette advertising

Survey	Year	Reference	Cigarette advertising should NOT be permitted (percentage who agree by smoking status)				
			Current smokers	Former smokers	Never smokers	All nonsmokers	All adults
1. AUTS	1964	US DHEW 1969	23	37	46	44	36
2. AUTS	1970	US DHEW 1973	50	64	68	67	61
3. AUTS	1975	US DHEW 1976a	43	59	64	63	56
4. Gallup	1977	Gallup 1987a	28			41	36
5. Gallup	1978	Gallup 1978	28			41	36
6. Gallup	1981	Gallup 1987a	27			53	43
7. Lieberman	1986	Lieberman 1986	21 (23)			38 (38)	33 (33)
8. AMA	1986	Harvey and Shubat 1986	48			71	64
9. AMA	1987	Harvey and Shubat 1987	42			61	55[a]
10. Gallup	1987	Gallup 1987a	30			57	49[a]
11. Gallup	1987	ACS 1988	37	53	59	57	51[a]
12. Gallup	1988	Gallup 1988b	34			64	55[a]

[a]The percentages who believe that cigarette advertising *should* be permitted were 36 percent (Harvey and Shubat 1987), 47 percent (Gallup 1987a), 33 percent (ACS 1988), and 40 percent (Gallup 1988b). Remaining respondents indicated no opinion.

NOTE: Actual questions:

1–3. Cigarette advertising should be stopped completely. (strongly agree, mildly agree, no opinion, mildly disagree, strongly disagree)*

4–6,10,12. Do you think there should or should not be a complete ban on cigarette advertising?

7. Some people feel that, as long as cigarettes are legal, cigarette advertising should be permitted. Others feel that cigarette advertising should not be permitted. Should cigarette companies be permitted to advertise . . . in magazines? . . . in newspapers?†

8. The American Medical Association called for a ban on tobacco advertising. Do you favor or oppose such an advertising ban?

9. Do you favor or oppose a ban on advertising of all tobacco products?

11. Some people feel that cigarette advertising *should* be permitted; others feel that cigarette advertising *should not* be permitted. Do you feel that cigarette advertising *should be* or should *not* be permitted?

*Percentages include those who "strongly agree" or "mildly agree."

†Percentages in parentheses are for newspapers (otherwise for magazines).

Warning Labels for Cigarettes

Recent data are not available on public opinion about warning labels. However, from 1964–70, support for these appeared to increase. In 1964, 28 percent of adults thought that cigarette advertising or commercials should *not* be required to carry a warning statement to the effect that smoking may be harmful to health; in 1970, 88 percent thought that cigarette advertising or commercials *should* be required to carry such a warning statement (Table 32).

Several surveys have assessed opinions regarding the need to strengthen the then existing health warning on packages and/or advertisements (e.g., Roper 1978). Some of these surveys tested specifically worded warnings that had been produced as an alternative to the existing warning. Because these data over time are difficult to compare and were most relevant at the time of the survey, they are not presented here.

Survey data from Lieberman Research, Inc. (1986) pertaining to recall of warning statements are presented in Chapter 7.

Economic Policies

Taxation

Questions regarding taxation of cigarettes are referenced to the taxation level at the time of the interview. This level varies with time, so it is difficult to delineate trends in opinion regarding taxation. Nevertheless, national surveys indicate an increase in public acceptance of increased cigarette taxation (Table 33).

In 1964, 30 percent of adults thought that taxes on cigarettes should be much higher than they were at the time of the interview. Similar questions asked in 1977 and 1981 revealed an increase in this proportion to 39 and 46 percent, respectively (Gallup 1981) (Table 33). In 1987, 79 percent of adults (75 percent of smokers and 80 percent of nonsmokers) favored an increase in the tax on tobacco products if the money from the increase went to medicare (Harvey and Shubat 1987). These recent data are of particular interest in light of the prevailing sentiment opposing increases in taxes in general.

Hiring

A minority of adults feel that employers should be allowed to refuse to hire cigarette smokers. In the 1978 Roper survey, 22 percent of adults thought that an employer has the right to refuse to hire someone who smokes cigarettes. In a 1986 survey (Lieberman Research 1986), 21 percent of adults (27 percent of nonsmokers, 7 percent of current smokers) believed that employers should be allowed to turn down job applicants who smoke.

TABLE 32.—Trends in public opinion concerning cigarette warning labels

Survey	Year	Reference	Percentage who agree by smoking status: Current smokers	Former smokers	Never smokers	All nonsmokers	All adults
		Cigarette advertising should NOT be required to carry a warning statement					
1. AUTS	1964	US DHEW 1969	38	27	19	21	28
		Cigarette packages should NOT be required to carry a warning statement					
2. AUTS	1964	US DHEW 1969	42	27	21	22	30
		Cigarette advertising SHOULD BE required to carry a warning statement					
3. AUTS	1970	US DHEW 1973	83	90	91	91	88

NOTE: Actual questions:

1. Cigarette advertising or commercials should *not* be required to carry a warning statement to the effect that smoking may be harmful to health. (strongly agree, mildly agree, no opinion, mildly disagree, strongly disagree)*

2. Cigarette manufacturers should *not* be required to put on the outside package a warning label like "Cigarette smoking is dangerous to health." (strongly agree, mildly agree, no opinion, mildly disagree, strongly disagree)*

3. Cigarette advertising or commercials should be required to carry a warning statement to the effect that smoking may be harmful to health.*

*Percentages include those who "strongly agree" or "mildly agree."

TABLE 33.—Trends in public opinion about increasing cigarette taxes

			Taxes on cigarettes should be increased (percentage who agree by smoking status)				
Survey	Year	Reference	Current smokers	Former smokers	Never smokers	All nonsmokers	All adults
1. AUTS	1964	US DHEW 1969	14	33	44	42	30
2. Roper	1970	Roper 1978	20			46	36
3. Roper	1972	Roper 1978	13			44	32
4. Roper	1974	Roper 1978	14			42	31
5. Roper	1976	Roper 1978	12			46	33
6. Gallup	1977	Gallup 1981					39
7. Roper	1978	Roper 1978	16			50	38
8. Gallup	1978	Gallup 1978	45			57	45
9. Gallup	1981	Gallup 1981	23			59	46
10. AMA	1987	Harvey and Shubat 1987	75			80	79

NOTE: Actual questions:

1. Taxes on cigarettes should be much higher than they are now. (strongly agree, mildly agree, no opinion, mildly disagree, strongly disagree)*

2–5, 7. The tax on cigarettes should be sharply increased to reduce their sale. (agree, disagree, don't know)

6, 9. Do you think federal and state taxes on cigarettes should or should not be increased?

8. Do you think the present 8 cents/pack federal tax on cigarettes should or should not be increased?

10. Would you favor or oppose an increase in the tax on tobacco products if the money from the increase went to Medicare?

*Percentages include those who "strongly agree" or "mildly agree."

Conclusions

1. In the 1950s, 40 to 50 percent of adults believed that cigarette smoking is a cause of lung cancer. By 1986, this proportion had increased to 92 percent (including 85 percent of current smokers).
2. Between 1964 and 1986, the proportion of adults who believed that cigarette smoking increases the risk of heart disease rose from 40 to 78 percent. A similar increase occurred among smokers, from 32 to 71 percent.
3. The proportion of adults who believed that cigarette smoking increases the risk of emphysema and chronic bronchitis rose from 50 percent in 1964 to 81 percent (chronic bronchitis) and 89 percent (emphysema) in 1986. These proportions increased among current smokers from 42 percent in 1964 to 73 percent (chronic bronchitis) and 85 percent (emphysema) in 1986.
4. Despite these impressive gains in public knowledge, substantial numbers of smokers are still unaware of or do not accept important health risks of smoking. For example, the proportions of smokers in 1986 who did not believe that smoking increases the risk of developing lung cancer, heart disease, chronic bronchitis, and emphysema were 15 percent, 29 percent, 27 percent, and 15 percent, respectively. These percentages correspond to between 8 and 15 million adult smokers in the United States.
5. In 1985, substantial percentages of women of childbearing age did not believe that smoking during pregnancy increases the risk of stillbirth (32 percent), miscarriage (25 percent), premature birth (24 percent), and having a low-birthweight baby (15 percent). Of women in this age group, 28 percent did not believe that women taking birth control pills have a higher risk of stroke if they smoke.
6. Some smokers today do not recognize their own personal risk from smoking or they minimize it. In 1986, only 18 percent of smokers were "very concerned" about the effects of smoking on their health, and 24 percent were not at all concerned.
7. In 1986, about half of current smokers and 40 percent of never smokers incorrectly believed that a person would have to smoke 10 or more cigarettes per day before it would affect his or her health.
8. A national survey conducted in 1983 by Louis Harris and Associates found that the public underestimates the health risks of smoking compared with many other health risks.
9. Many smokers underestimate the population impact of smoking. In 1987, 28 percent of smokers (and 16 percent of the general population) disagreed with the statement, "Most deaths from lung cancer are caused by cigarette smoking."
10. The proportion of high school seniors who believe that smoking a pack or more of cigarettes per day causes great risk of harm increased from 51 percent in 1975 to 66 percent in 1986.
11. In 1986, about three-quarters of adults believed that using chewing tobacco or snuff is harmful to health.
12. The social acceptability of smoking in public is declining, as measured by the proportion of adults who find it annoying to be near a person smoking cigarettes. This proportion increased from 46 percent in 1964 to 69 percent in 1986.

13. A majority of the public favors policies restricting smoking in public places and worksites, prohibiting the sale of cigarettes to minors, and increasing the cigarette tax to fund the medicare program. Recent surveys indicate that about half the public supports a ban on cigarette advertising.

Appendix

Description of Primary Data Sources for Chapters 4 and 5

Adult Use of Tobacco Survey, 1964

This was the first AUTS sponsored by the U.S. Public Health Service. The survey was conducted by National Analysts, Inc., under contract with the National Clearinghouse for Smoking and Health in the fall of 1964. The data for this survey were collected using area probability sampling techniques and stratifying by the type of population and geographic area. Approximately 5,794 adults 21 years and older were interviewed in person. The response rate was 76 percent. Detailed methods have been published elsewhere (US DHEW 1969).

Adult Use of Tobacco Survey, 1966

This was the second AUTS sponsored by the U.S. Public Health Service. The survey was conducted by two research firms: National Analysts, Inc., and Opinion Research Corporation, under contract with the National Clearinghouse for Smoking and Health in the spring of 1966. The data were collected using area probability sampling techniques and stratifying by the type of population and geographic area. The 1964 AUTS questionnaire was used with minor changes. Approximately 5,768 adults were interviewed. Interviews were primarily in person, although telephone interviews were used for nonrespondents. The response rate was 72 percent. Detailed methods have been published elsewhere (US DHEW 1969).

Adult Use of Tobacco Survey, 1970

This was the third AUTS sponsored by the U.S. Public Health Service. The survey was conducted by Chilton Research Services under contract with the National Clearinghouse for Smoking and Health in the spring of 1970. The data were collected from a probability sample of households in the contiguous United States. Approximately 5,200 individuals were surveyed; 91 percent were interviewed by telephone and 9 percent, from nontelephone households, were interviewed face to face. Of the total number of respondents, 44 percent were male and 56 percent were female; all were at least 21 years old. The methods have been described elsewhere in detail (US DHEW 1973).

Adult Use of Tobacco Survey, 1975

This was the fourth AUTS sponsored by the U.S. Public Health Service. The survey was conducted by Chilton Research Services under contract with the National Clearinghouse for Smoking and Health in 1975. The data were collected from a probability sample of telephone numbers in the contiguous United States, with a separate survey of nontelephone households. Approximately 12,000 individuals were surveyed. The methods have been described elsewhere in detail (US DHEW 1976a).

Adult Use of Tobacco Survey, 1986

In 1986, 13,031 members of the civilian, noninstitutionalized population of the United States 17 years of age and older were surveyed by telephone on their smoking history, attitudes, and beliefs (CDC 1986).

A 2-stage sampling procedure was used within a computer-assisted telephone interview format. The first stage involved selecting a random sample of telephone exchanges within the United States. The sampling procedure was balanced for the number of telephones within the exchange. Clusters of between 10 and 15 households within each exchange were contacted using random-digit dialing. Households were enumerated and smoking status of members ascertained. Up to 27 callbacks were made to obtain a total of 36,405 households, with a response rate of 85.5 percent.

A further stratified random sampling procedure was used to provide an approximate equal proportion of respondents in each smoking category (current, former, never). The stratification variable was the number of smokers in the household. Up to 10 callbacks were made to interview the selected respondent, with a response rate of 86.9 percent. The overall response rate from the two stages of sampling was 74.3 percent (85.5 percent times 86.9 percent).

Quality control procedures in the survey involved 26 hours of survey-specific training and practice for interviewers and a silent monitoring of 10 percent of all interviews by supervisory staff. Data obtained were weighted to reflect the U.S. population in 2 stages. A base weight was calculated, which was the product of the weighting for cluster (completed screeners within cluster), household (telephone numbers within household), and person (to account for selection based on smoking status). Poststratification weighting was then undertaken for region, education, race, sex, and age.

American Medical Association, 1986, 1987

The data were gathered in telephone interviews with approximately 1,500 adults, conducted during May–June 1986 and January–February 1987. The surveys were conducted by Kane, Parsons and Associates of New York City. The samples were generated by Survey Sampling, Inc. (Westport, Connecticut) using a multistage probability method to provide a random sample of all residential telephones in the United States. Sampling error was an estimated plus or minus 2.5 percentage points at the 95-percent confidence level (Harvey and Shubat 1986, 1987).

Behavioral Risk Factor Surveillance System

Between 1981 and 1983, the U.S. Centers for Disease Control (CDC) collaborated with 29 State health departments (including the District of Columbia) to conduct one-time random-digit-dialed telephone surveys of adults 18 years of age and older. Standard methods and questionnaires were used to assess the prevalence of personal health practices and behaviors related to the leading causes of death, including cigarette smoking. Beginning in 1984, the surveys evolved into an ongoing surveillance system when States began collecting data throughout the year. For each State, approximately 1,200 (range 600–3,000) interviews are completed each year. The raw data are weighted to the age, race, and sex distribution for each State from the 1980 Census. This weighting accounts for the underrepresentation of men, blacks, and younger persons (18–24 years of age). A detailed review of the survey design and methods of analyzing the data has been published (Remington et al. 1985).

Chilton Survey, 1979

This survey was conducted by Chilton Research Services (Radnor, PA) for the FTC from December 21, 1978 through February 4, 1979. A random-digit-dialing procedure was used to collect interviews from 1,211 teenagers aged 13 to 18 years and from 407 adults aged 29 to 31 years in a national probability sample of telephone households. The 1,618 completed interviews represented 81 percent of the number of usable household telephone numbers (Chilton 1980).

Current Population Surveys

The U.S. Bureau of the Census regularly collects information as part of its Current Population Survey (CPS). Households are selected for survey via a sampling procedure designed to accurately reflect the U.S. population, and information is collected in person during a home visit. In 1955, 1966, 1967, 1968, and 1985, the CPS included a supplement that asked questions on current smoking practices. For 1985, 114,342 individuals, 16 years and older, were surveyed on smoking and smokeless tobacco use. Approximately 55 percent of the sample consisted of self-respondents while the remaining 45 percent were proxy respondents. The 1985 CPS sample was initially selected from the 1980 census files with coverage in all 50 States and the District of Columbia. This sampling methodology allows for State-specific analysis of smoking practices.

The estimation procedure used in this survey involves the inflation of the weighted sample results to independent estimates of the total civilian, noninstitutional population of the United States by age, race, sex, and Hispanic/non-Hispanic categories. These independent estimates are based on statistics on births, deaths, immigration, and emigration, as well as statistics on the strength of the Armed Forces. Based on the use of a special weighting algorithm developed by the Bureau of the Census, the CPS household sample estimates are considered to be representatitve of the United States. However, one potential problem with the CPS is the effect of proxy reports on sample estimates of smoking status. This may result in an underreporting bias.

Gallup Surveys

Gallup surveys are conducted using personal (face-to-face) or telephone interviews.

Personal surveys. The design of the sample for personal surveys is that of a replicated area probability sample down to the block level in the case of urban areas and to segments of townships in the case of rural areas.

After the Nation has been stratified geographically and by size of community according to information derived from the most recent census, more than 350 different sampling locations are selected on a mathematically random basis from within cities, towns, and counties that have in turn been selected on a mathematically random basis.

The interviewers are given no leeway in selecting the areas in which they are to conduct their interviews. Each interviewer is given a map on which a specific starting point is marked, and is instructed to contact households according to a predetermined travel pattern. At each occupied dwelling unit, the interviewer selects respondents by following a systematic procedure. This procedure is repeated until the assigned number of interviews has been completed.

Telephone surveys. The national Gallup telephone samples are based on the area probability sample used for personal surveys. In each of the sampling locations selected (as described above for personal surveys), a set of telephone exchanges that falls within the geographic boundaries of the sampling location is first identified. Listed telephone numbers in these exchanges are selected randomly and used as "seed numbers" for randomly generating telephone numbers. The result of this procedure is a sample of listed and unlisted telephone numbers assigned to households within telephone exchanges serving the sampling locations. The final sample of numbers thus reflects the stratification and selection of sampling locations.

After the survey data have been collected and processed, each respondent is assigned a weight so that the demographic characteristics of the total weighted sample of respondents match the latest estimates of the demographic characteristics of the appropriate adult population available from the U.S. Census Bureau. Telephone surveys are weighted to match the characteristics of the adult population living in households with access to a telephone. The weighting of personal interview data includes a factor to improve the representation of the kinds of people who are less likely to be found at home. The procedures described above are designed to produce samples approximating the adult civilian population (18 and older) living in private households (excluding those in prisons, hospitals, hotels, and religious and educational institutions, and those living on reservations or military bases)—and in the case of telephone surveys, households with access to a telephone (Gallup 1987a).

Lieberman Research Inc., 1986

The study was based on telephone interviews in a nationwide sample of 1,025 persons 18 years of age and older in the contiguous United States (Alaska and Hawaii were not included). A random-digit-dialed sample was used. Interviews were conducted from June 26 through July 10, 1986. The study was jointly sponsored by the American Cancer Society, the American Heart Association, and the American Lung Association; neither interviewers nor respondents were aware of the sponsors.

National Adolescent Student Health Survey, 1987

The National Adolescent Student Health Survey was initiated in 1985 by three national health organizations: the American School Health Association, the Association for the Advancement of Health Education, and the Society for Public Health Education. Funding for the survey was provided by the following agencies of the Public Health Service: the Office of Disease Prevention and Health Promotion (Office of the Assistant Secretary for Health), the Center for Chronic Disease Prevention and Health Promotion (CDC), and National Institute on Drug Abuse (Alcohol, Drug Abuse, and Mental Health Administration).

A two-stage cluster sampling procedure was used to survey 5,859 8th graders and 5,560 10th graders from 112 public and private schools. Twenty-four percent of the original sample of schools did not agree to participate and each was replaced by another randomly selected school from the same geographic area. Parents were informed of the content and purpose of the survey and were provided the opportunity to exclude their children from the survey. Students were informed that participation was voluntary and that all information provided would be strictly confidential. Parental requests for exclusion, student absenteeism, and voluntary nonparticipation reduced the survey response rate to 87.5 percent (88.9 percent for 8th grade and 86.0 percent for 10th grade).

During October to December 1987, trained survey administrators collected data from three randomly selected classes of 8th or 10th grade students at each participating school. Each student responded to one of three survey forms. The 30-day prevalence of cigarette smoking and smokeless tobacco use appeared on all survey forms. The item nonresponse on these questions was 0.2 percent of those who were surveyed.

National Health Interview Surveys

The National Health Interview Survey (NHIS), which is conducted regularly by the National Center for Health Statistics, uses a sampling frame developed by the U.S. Bureau of the Census and is based on a multistaged random probability sampling design. Information is collected in face-to-face household interviews using one adult per household and using proxy reporting for other members of the household. Since 1974, information on smoking has been obtained only by self-report. This has entailed telephone followup to selected household members who were not personally interviewed. Basic smoking information has been collected for several years, including 1965, 1966, 1970, 1974, 1976–80, inclusive, 1983, 1985, and 1987 (data prior to 1974 are based on both self-reports and proxy reporting; all of the more recent surveys were based on self-reports). Sample sizes for smoking data have ranged from 10,000 to 50,000 persons. There has been an overall consistency in the smoking questions asked in the different surveys. Beginning in 1985, an adequate sample of blacks was ensured by the survey design (using the technique of oversampling). The NHIS generally has a response rate of 96 percent (NCHS 1987). However, the extra step in converting proxy response to self-report leads to a decrease in the response rate to approximately 90 percent.

The data presented in this Chapter were taken from the Health Promotion and Disease Prevention Supplement to the 1985 NHIS and the Cancer Control Supplement to the 1987 NHIS.

National Health and Nutrition Examination Survey and Hispanic Health and Nutrition Examination Survey

Since 1960, the National Center for Health Statistics has conducted periodic health surveys that have included physical examinations and laboratory tests. Initially called the National Health Examination Survey (NHES), the name of this survey was changed to the National Health and Nutrition Examination Survey (NHANES) in 1970 when a nutrition component was added. The NHES was conducted in 1960, 1963, and 1966, and the NHANES in 1971, 1976, and 1988.

Although the NHANES as a population survey included all of the Nation's major subpopulations including Hispanics, the sample sizes were insufficient to produce reliable estimates of health status, particularly if the three major Hispanic subgroups—Mexican-Americans, Cuban-Americans, and Puerto Ricans—were considered separately. Therefore, the Hispanic Health and Nutrition Examination Survey (HHANES) was developed by the National Center for Health Statistics. The HHANES was designed to provide sufficient samples of each Hispanic subgroup. The survey not only produces reliable estimates of health status for each subgroup but also permits cross-cultural comparisons within the broader Hispanic cultural context.

The HHANES was a probability-based survey of three distinct subgroups of a major U.S. minority group rather than of a national sample. The sampling methodology used complex, multistaged, stratified, clustered samples of the defined population. When weighted, the sample data represent the targeted population. For HHANES, the targeted population consisted of three groups of civilian, noninstitutionalized persons, aged 6 months to 74 years from three areas of the country that had a sufficient number or proportion of Hispanics to render it economically feasible to screen households and to operate an examination center: (1) Mexican-Americans residing in selected areas of Texas, California, Colorado, New Mexico, and Arizona; (2) Cuban-Americans residing in Dade County, Florida; and (3) Puerto Ricans residing in the New York City area. Data were collected from 1982 through 1984 via in-person household interviews and via examination at a local examination center. Information was collected regarding a number of health issues, including the use of tobacco.

NIDA High School Seniors Surveys on Drug Use

Each year since 1975, the Monitoring the Future project has conducted surveys of representative national samples of high school seniors in the United States (Johnston, O'Malley, Bachman 1987). Monitoring the Future is conducted by the University of Michigan Institute for Social Research and receives its core funding from the National Institute on Drug Abuse.

Each year, a multistage sampling procedure is used to identify approximately 135 public and private schools (the number of private schools has varied from 14 to 22) that represent an accurate cross-section of high school seniors throughout the coterminous United States. The first stage involves the use of 74 primary sampling units developed by the University of Michigan Survey Research Center for use in its nationwide interview surveys.

The second sampling stage involves choice of a single high school from most geographic areas (more than one is chosen in major metropolitan areas). The probability of selection of any school is proportional to the size of the senior class. When a sampled school is unwilling to participate, a replacement school is selected from the same geographic area. Response rate of schools has been from 66 to 80 percent throughout the survey period.

Up to 400 seniors are surveyed from each school. In schools with more than 400 seniors, a random sampling system convenient for the school (provided it results in an unbiased sample) is used to choose the 400 students to be interviewed. Most schools use the classroom as the basis for this selection. The total number of students interviewed each year has been between 15,700 and 19,000. The student response rate has varied from 77 percent to 84 percent throughout the survey period.

The questionnaire administration in each school is carried out by local Survey Research Center representatives and their assistants following standardized procedures detailed in a project manual. Questionnaires are generally delivered in classrooms during normal class periods, although in some instances larger groups are used. Because of the range of topics, five different questionnaire forms are used in the survey. These are distributed to participants in an ordered sequence to produce identical subsamples. All five forms contain core data on demographics and some drug use (about one-third of the form); all other questions are asked of subsamples of the total respondents. Basic questions on cigarette usage have been included in the core for all years.

Followup surveys by mail are conducted annually using representative subsamples from each of the previously participating classes, that is, the classes of 1976 through 1987. Thus, long-term panel data are collected on individuals, and analyses aimed at separating secular, age, and cohort effects are possible. (See O'Malley, Bachman, Johnston 1988.)

NIDA National Household Surveys on Drug Abuse

NIDA conducted household surveys on drug use in 1979, 1982, and 1985. Data were obtained from a stratified random sample of 8,000 U.S. households; approximately 2,000 in-person interviews were conducted with respondents in the 12- to 17-year-old age group. Questions included whether any cigarettes were smoked within 30 days as well as within the previous year.

Roper Survey, 1978

This survey was conducted for the Tobacco Institute via face-to-face interviewing with 2,511 subjects. Other methodological details are unavailable.

Roper Survey, 1980

The 1980 Roper Survey used face-to-face interviews to test a nationally representative sample of 2,000 adults for knowledge about the health hazards of smoking. The study was commissioned by the FTC and was conducted in November 1980. The total sample was split into two halves, and one set of questions was varied between the two. Thus, the sample size for several of the questions on the health effects of smoking was approximately half the total sample size.

US DHEW Teenage Smoking Surveys

In 1968, 1970, 1972, 1974, and 1979, random samples of teenagers aged 12 to 18 years were surveyed by telephone in December–January (US DHEW 1972, 1976b, 1979b). The first stage of the 3-stage sampling plan involved grouping and selecting telephone exchanges and was designed to eliminate geographic bias. Within the selected exchanges, equal numbers of random-digit-dialed telephone numbers were generated and contacted. Household enumeration was undertaken with an adult respondent and if more than one person aged between 12 and 18 years lived in the house, random selection was used to choose the study participant.

In 1968, the sample size was 4,931, 89 percent of whom were interviewed by telephone. The other 11 percent lived in nontelephone households and were interviewed in their homes. As exclusion of the nontelephone households did not substantially affect prevalence estimates, later surveys did not include household interviewing of nontelephone households. The sample size in 1970 was 2,640; in 1972, it was 2,790; in 1974, it was 2,553; and in 1979, it was 2,639. In 1979, a followup survey was also undertaken of 1,194 (46.8 percent) of the 1974 respondents. Approximately 12,000 households were contacted in 1979, from which 2,639 people aged 12 to 18 years were interviewed. In no survey was there any attempt to validate the smoking status indicated.

References

ALLPORT, G.W. Attitudes. In: Murchison, C. (ed.) *A Handbook of Social Psychology*. Worcester, Massachusetts: Clark University Press, 1935.

AMERICAN ASSOCIATION FOR RESPIRATORY CARE. Majority of airline passengers want smoking ban; National health group calls for action. Press release. Dallas: American Association for Respiratory Care, September 1, 1987.

AMERICAN CANCER SOCIETY. Release of the Lieberman Survey. Press release. New York: American Cancer Society. November 10, 1986.

AMERICAN CANCER SOCIETY. *Cancer Facts and Figures—1988*. New York: American Cancer Society, 1988a.

AMERICAN CANCER SOCIETY. *The 1987 Survey of Public Awareness and Use of Cancer Tests*. Sponsored by the American Cancer Society, conducted by the Gallup Organization, analyzed by Lieberman Research, 1988b.

AMERICAN LUNG ASSOCIATION. Americans want smoke-free air at work. Press release. New York: American Lung Association, December 5, 1985.

AMERICAN LUNG ASSOCIATION. Smokers know risks but don't say "no" to cigarettes. Press release. New York: American Lung Association, December 4, 1987.

AMERICAN MEDICAL ASSOCIATION. Americans favor tobacco advertising ban, says AMA survey. Press release. Chicago: American Medical Association, October 29, 1986.

BACHMAN, J.G., JOHNSTON, L.D., O'MALLEY, P.M. *Monitoring the Future. Questionnaire Responses From the Nation's High School Seniors, 1976*. Ann Arbor, Michigan: University of Michigan, 1980a.

BACHMAN, J.G., JOHNSTON, L.D., O'MALLEY, P.M. *Monitoring the Future. Questionnaire Responses From the Nation's High School Seniors, 1978*. Ann Arbor, Michigan: University of Michigan, 1980b.

BACHMAN, J.G., JOHNSTON, L.D., O'MALLEY, P.M. *Monitoring the Future. Questionnaire Responses From the Nation's High School Seniors, 1980*. Ann Arbor, Michigan: University of Michigan, 1981.

BACHMAN, J.G., JOHNSTON, L.D., O'MALLEY, P.M. *Monitoring the Future. Questionnaire Responses From the Nation's High School Seniors, 1982*. Ann Arbor, Michigan: University of Michigan, 1984.

BACHMAN, J.G., JOHNSTON, L.D., O'MALLEY, P.M. *Monitoring the Future. Questionnaire Responses From the Nation's High School Seniors, 1984*. Ann Arbor, Michigan: University of Michigan, 1985.

BACHMAN, J.G., JOHNSTON, L.D., O'MALLEY, P.M. *Monitoring the Future. Questionnaire Responses From the Nation's High School Seniors, 1986*. Ann Arbor, Michigan: University of Michigan, 1987.

BECKER, D.M., LEVINE, D.M. Risk perception, knowledge, and lifestyles in siblings of people with premature coronary disease. *American Journal of Preventive Medicine* 3(1):45–50, 1987.

BEN-SIRA, Z. Health promoting function of mass media and reference groups: Motivating or reinforcing of behavior change. *Social Science and Medicine* 16(7):825–834, 1982.

CANADIAN GALLUP POLL, October 1986.

CENTERS FOR DISEASE CONTROL. Survey to assess the prevalence, attitudes, knowledge, and beliefs about smoking behavior among the adult population. Survey questionnaires. Prepared by Westat for the Office on Smoking and Health, Rockville, Maryland, August 1986.

CENTERS FOR DISEASE CONTROL. Passive smoking: Beliefs, attitudes, and exposures—United States, 1986. *Morbidity and Mortality Weekly Report* 37(15):239–241, April 22, 1988.

CHILTON RESEARCH SERVICES. *A Survey of Adolescent and Adult Attitudes, Values, Behavior, Intentions and Knowledge Related to Cigarette Smoking. Final Report*. Submitted to the Federal Trade Commission, June 25, 1980.

DOLECEK, T.A., SCHOENBERGER, J.A., OMAN, J.K., KREMER, B.K., SUNSERI, A.J., ALBERTI, J.M. Cardiovascular risk factor knowledge and belief in prevention among adults in Chicago. *American Journal of Preventive Medicine* 2(5):262–267, 1986.

FEDERAL TRADE COMMISSION. *Federal Trade Commission Staff Report on the Cigarette Smoking Advertising Investigation*. Federal Trade Commission, May 1981.

FISHBEIN, M. *Consumer Beliefs and Behavior With Respect to Cigarette Smoking: A Critical Analysis of the Public Literature. A Report Prepared for the Staff of the Federal Trade Commission*. Federal Trade Commission, May 1977.

FOLSOM, A.R., SPRAFKA, M., LUEPKER, R.V., JACOBS, D.R. JR. Beliefs among black and white adults about causes and prevention of cardiovascular disease: The Minnesota Heart Study. *American Journal of Preventive Medicine* 4(3):121–127, 1988.

FOX, S.H., BROWN, C., KOONTZ, A.M., KESSEL, S.S. Perceptions of risks of smoking and heavy drinking during pregnancy: 1985 NHIS findings. *Public Health Reports* 102(1):73–79, January–February 1987.

GALLUP. *Smoking in America. Public Attitudes and Behavior. Gallup Report No. 155*. Princeton, New Jersey: Gallup Organization, June 1978.

GALLUP. *Gallup Smoking Audit. The Gallup Report. Report No. 190*. Princeton, New Jersey: Gallup Organization, July 1981.

GALLUP. Survey of attitudes toward smoking. Conducted for the American Lung Association. Princeton, New Jersey: Gallup Organization, July 1985.

GALLUP. *Majority Backs Ban on Smoking in Public Places. Gallup Report No. 258*. Princeton, New Jersey: Gallup Organization, March 1987a.

GALLUP. Majority backs ban on smoking in public places. Press release. Princeton, New Jersey: Gallup Organization, April 3, 1987b.

GALLUP. Survey of attitudes toward smoking. Conducted for the American Lung Association. Princeton, New Jersey: Gallup Organization, 1987c.

GALLUP. Attitudes toward smoking in restaurants and fast food establishments. Conducted for the National Restaurant Association. Princeton, New Jersey: Gallup Organization, February 1987d.

GALLUP. On-the-go Americans prefer smoke-free air. *American Journal of Public Health* 78(5):563, May 1988a.

GALLUP. Majorities now support ban on public smoking, cigarette ads. Press release. Princeton, New Jersey: Gallup Organization, September 4, 1988b.

HARRIS, L. *Prevention in America: Steps People Take—Or Fail to Take—for Better Health*. Louis Harris and Associates, 1983.

HARRIS, L. *The Prevention Index, 1988*. Louis Harris and Associates, May 13, 1988.

HARVEY, L., SHUBAT, S. Public opinion on health care issues, 1986. In: *AMA Surveys of Physician and Public Opinion, 1986*. Chicago: American Medical Association, October 1986.

HARVEY, L., SHUBAT, S. Public opinion on health care issues. In: *AMA Surveys of Physician and Public Opinion on Health Care Issues, 1987*. Chicago: American Medical Association, April 1987.

JOHNSTON, L.D., BACHMAN, J.G. *Monitoring the Future. Questionnaire Responses From the Nation's High School Seniors, 1975*. Ann Arbor, Michigan: University of Michigan, 1980.

JOHNSTON, L.D., BACHMAN, J.G., O'MALLEY, P.M. *Monitoring the Future. Questionnaire Responses From the Nation's High School Seniors, 1977*. Ann Arbor, Michigan: University of Michigan, 1980a.

JOHNSTON, L.D., BACHMAN, J.G., O'MALLEY, P.M. *Monitoring the Future. Questionnaire Responses From the Nation's High School Seniors, 1979*. Ann Arbor, Michigan: University of Michigan, 1980b.

JOHNSTON, L.D., BACHMAN, J.G., O'MALLEY, P.M. *Monitoring the Future. Questionnaire Responses From the Nation's High School Seniors, 1981.* Ann Arbor, Michigan: University of Michigan, 1982.

JOHNSTON, L.D., BACHMAN, J.G., O'MALLEY, P.M. *Monitoring the Future. Questionnaire Responses From the Nation's High School Seniors, 1983.* Ann Arbor, Michigan: University of Michigan, 1984.

JOHNSTON, L.D., BACHMAN, J.G., O'MALLEY, P.M. *Monitoring the Future. Questionnaire Responses From the Nation's High School Seniors, 1985.* Ann Arbor, Michigan: University of Michigan, 1986.

JOHNSTON, L.D., O'MALLEY, P.M., BACHMAN, J.G. *National Trends in Drug Use and Related Factors Among High School Students and Young Adults, 1975–1986.* U.S. Department of Health and Human Services, Public Health Service, Alcohol, Drug Abuse, and Mental Health Administration, National Institute on Drug Abuse. DHHS Publication No. (ADM) 87-1535, 1987.

LEVENTHAL, H., GLYNN, K., FLEMING, R. Is the smoking decision an 'informed choice'? Effect of smoking risk factors on smoking beliefs. *Journal of the American Medical Association* 257(24):3373–3376, June 26, 1987.

LIEBERMAN RESEARCH. *A Study of Public Attitudes Toward Cigarette Advertising and Promotion Programs—Conducted for American Cancer Society, American Heart Association, American Lung Association.* Lieberman Research, October 1986.

MAHONEY, M.J. *Cognition and Behavior Modification.* Cambridge, Massachusetts: Ballinger Publishing, 1974.

MASSEY, M.M., BOYD, E., MATTSON, M., FEINLEIB, M.R. Inventory of surveys on smoking. *Public Health Reports* 102(4):430–438, July–August 1987.

MATTSON, M.E., POLLACK, E.S., CULLEN, J.W. What are the odds that smoking will kill you? *American Journal of Public Health* 77(4):425–431, April 1987.

NATIONAL CENTER FOR HEALTH STATISTICS, THORNBERRY, O.T., WILSON, R.W., GOLDEN, P.M. Health promotion data for the 1990 objectives, estimates from the National Health Interview Survey of Health Promotion and Disease Prevention, United States, 1985. *Advance Data From Vital and Health Statistics*, No. 126. U.S. Department of Health and Human Services, Public Health Service. DHHS Publication No. (PHS) 86-1250, September 19, 1986.

NATIONAL CENTER FOR HEALTH STATISTICS, THORNBERRY, O. An experimental comparison of telephone and personal health interview surveys. *Vital and Health Statistics*, Series 2, No. 106. U.S. Department of Health and Human Services, Public Health Service. DHHS Publication No. (PHS) 87-1380, August 1987.

NATIONAL CENTER FOR HEALTH STATISTICS, SCHOENBORN, C.A. Health promotion and disease prevention: United States, 1985. *Vital and Health Statistics*, Series 10, No. 163. Public Health Service. DHHS Publication No. (PHS) 88-1591, February 1988.

O'MALLEY, P.M., BACHMAN, J.G., JOHNSTON, L.D. Period, age, and cohort effects on substance use among young Americans: A decade of change, 1976–86. *American Journal of Public Health* 78(10):1315–1321, October 1988.

OSKAMP, S. *Attitudes and Opinions.* Englewood Cliffs, New Jersey: Prentice-Hall, 1977.

PERLSTADT, H., HOLMES, R.E. The role of public opinion polling in health legislation. *American Journal of Public Health* 77(5):612–614, May 1987.

REMINGTON, P.L., FORMAN, M.R., GENTRY, E.M., MARKS, J.S., HOGELIN, G.C., TROWBRIDGE, F.L. Current smoking trends in the United States. The 1981–1983 Behavioral Risk Factor Surveys. *Journal of the American Medical Association* 253(20):2975–2978, May 24–31, 1985.

ROPER. *A Study of Public Attitudes Toward Cigarette Smoking and the Tobacco Industry in 1978*, Volume 1. Roper Organization, May 1978.

SCHINKE, S.P., GILCHRIST, L.D. Preventing cigarette smoking with youth. *Journal of Primary Prevention* 5(1):48–56, Fall 1984.

SHOPLAND, D.R., BROWN, C. Toward the 1990 objectives for smoking: Measuring the progress with 1985 NHIS data. *Public Health Reports* 102(1):68–73, January–February 1987.

SLOVIC, P. Informing and educating the public about risk. *Risk Analysis* 6(4), 1986.

STEWART, P.J., DUNKLEY, G.C. Smoking and health care patterns among pregnant women. *Canadian Medical Association Journal* 133(10):989–994, November 15, 1985.

U.S. DEPARTMENT OF HEALTH AND HUMAN SERVICES. *The Health Consequences of Smoking for Women. A Report of the Surgeon General.* U.S. Department of Health and Human Services, Public Health Service, Office of the Assistant Secretary for Health, Office on Smoking and Health, 1980.

U.S. DEPARTMENT OF HEALTH AND HUMAN SERVICES. *The Health Consequences of Smoking. The Changing Cigarette: A Report of the Surgeon General.* U.S. Department of Health and Human Services, Public Health Service, Office of the Assistant Secretary for Health, Office on Smoking and Health. DHHS Publication No. (PHS) 81-50156, 1981.

U.S. DEPARTMENT OF HEALTH AND HUMAN SERVICES. *The Health Consequences of Smoking: Cancer. A Report of the Surgeon General.* U.S. Department of Health and Human Services, Public Health Service, Office on Smoking and Health. DHHS Publication No. (PHS) 82-50179, 1982.

U.S. DEPARTMENT OF HEALTH AND HUMAN SERVICES. *The Health Consequences of Smoking: Cardiovascular Disease. A Report of the Surgeon General.* U.S. Department of Health and Human Services, Public Health Service, Office on Smoking and Health. DHHS Publication No. (PHS) 84-50204, 1983.

U.S. DEPARTMENT OF HEALTH AND HUMAN SERVICES. *The Health Consequences of Smoking: Chronic Obstructive Lung Disease. A Report of the Surgeon General.* U.S. Department of Health and Human Services, Public Health Service, Office on Smoking and Health. DHHS Publication No. (PHS) 84-50205, 1984.

U.S. DEPARTMENT OF HEALTH AND HUMAN SERVICES. *The Health Consequences of Smoking: Cancer and Chronic Lung Disease in the Workplace. A Report of the Surgeon General.* U.S. Department of Health and Human Services, Public Health Service, Office on Smoking and Health. DHHS Publication No. (PHS) 85-50207, 1985.

U.S. DEPARTMENT OF HEALTH AND HUMAN SERVICES. *The Health Consequences of Involuntary Smoking. A Report of the Surgeon General.* U.S. Department of Health and Human Services, Public Health Service, Centers for Disease Control. DHHS Publication No. (CDC) 87-8398, 1986a.

U.S. DEPARTMENT OF HEALTH AND HUMAN SERVICES. *The 1990 Health Objectives for the Nation: A Midcourse Review.* U.S. Department of Health and Human Services, Public Health Service, Office of Disease Prevention and Health Promotion, November 1986b.

U.S. DEPARTMENT OF HEALTH AND HUMAN SERVICES. *The Health Consequences of Using Smokeless Tobacco. A Report of the Advisory Committee to the Surgeon General, 1986.* U.S. Department of Health and Human Services, Public Health Service. NIH Publication No. 86-2874, April 1986c.

U.S. DEPARTMENT OF HEALTH AND HUMAN SERVICES. *Youth Use of Smokeless Tobacco: More Than a Pinch of Trouble.* U.S. Department of Health and Human Services, Office of Inspector General, Office of Analysis and Inspections, January 1986d.

U.S. DEPARTMENT OF HEALTH AND HUMAN SERVICES. *The Health Consequences of Smoking: Nicotine Addiction. A Report of the Surgeon General, 1988.* U.S. Department of Health and Human Services, Public Health Service, Centers for Disease Control, Center for Health Promotion and Education, Office on Smoking and Health. DHHS Publication No. (CDC) 88-8406, 1988.

U.S. DEPARTMENT OF HEALTH AND HUMAN SERVICES. *Adult Use of Tobacco, 1986.* U.S. Department of Health and Human Services, Public Health Service, Centers for Disease Control, Office on Smoking and Health, in press.

U.S. DEPARTMENT OF HEALTH, EDUCATION, AND WELFARE. *Use of Tobacco. Practices, Attitudes, Knowledge, and Beliefs. United States—Fall 1964 and Spring 1966.* U.S. Department of Health, Education, and Welfare, Public Health Service, Health Services and Mental Health Administration, National Clearinghouse for Smoking and Health, July 1969.

U.S. DEPARTMENT OF HEALTH, EDUCATION, AND WELFARE. *Teenage Smoking. National Patterns of Cigarette Smoking, Ages 12 Through 18, in 1968 and 1970.* U.S. Department of Health, Education, and Welfare, Health Services and Mental Health Administration, National Clearinghouse for Smoking and Health. DHEW Publication No. (HSM) 72-7508, 1972.

U.S. DEPARTMENT OF HEALTH, EDUCATION, AND WELFARE. *Adult Use of Tobacco, 1970.* U.S. Department of Health, Education, and Welfare, Public Health Service, Center for Disease Control, National Clearinghouse for Smoking and Health, June 1973.

U.S. DEPARTMENT OF HEALTH, EDUCATION, AND WELFARE. *Cigarette Smoking Among Teen-agers and Young Women.* U.S. Department of Health, Education, and Welfare, Public Health Service, National Institutes of Health. DHEW Publication No. (NIH) 77-1203, 1975a.

U.S. DEPARTMENT OF HEALTH, EDUCATION, AND WELFARE. *The Health Consequences of Smoking. 1975.* U.S. Department of Health, Education, and Welfare, Public Health Service, Center for Disease Control. HEW Publication No. (CDC) 77-8704, 1975b.

U.S. DEPARTMENT OF HEALTH, EDUCATION, AND WELFARE. *Adult Use of Tobacco—1975.* U.S. Department of Health, Education, and Welfare, Public Health Service, Center for Disease Control, 1976a.

U.S. DEPARTMENT OF HEALTH, EDUCATION, AND WELFARE. *Teenage Smoking: National Patterns of Cigarette Smoking, Ages 12 Through 18, in 1972 and 1974.* U.S. Department of Health, Education, and Welfare, Public Health Service, National Institutes of Health. DHEW Publication No. (NIH) 76-931, 1976b.

U.S. DEPARTMENT OF HEALTH, EDUCATION, AND WELFARE. *The Health Consequences of Smoking, 1977–1978.* U.S. Department of Health, Education, and Welfare, Public Health Service, Office of the Assistant Secretary for Health, Office on Smoking and Health. DHEW Publication No. (PHS) 79-50065, 1978.

U.S. DEPARTMENT OF HEALTH, EDUCATION, AND WELFARE. *Smoking and Health. A Report of the Surgeon General.* U.S. Department of Health, Education, and Welfare, Public Health Service, Office of the Assistant Secretary for Health, Office on Smoking and Health. DHEW Publication No. (PHS) 79-50066, 1979a.

U.S. DEPARTMENT OF HEALTH, EDUCATION, AND WELFARE. *Teenage Smoking. Immediate and Long-Term Patterns.* U.S. Department of Health, Education, and Welfare, National Institute of Education, November 1979b.

U.S. PUBLIC HEALTH SERVICE. *Smoking and Health. Report of the Advisory Committee to the Surgeon General of the Public Health Service.* U.S. Department of Health, Education, and Welfare, Public Health Service, Center for Disease Control. PHS Publication No. 1103, 1964.

U.S. PUBLIC HEALTH SERVICE. *The Health Consequences of Smoking. 1969 Supplement to the 1967 Public Health Service Review.* U.S. Department of Health, Education, and Welfare, Public Health Service. PHS Publication No. 1696-2 (Supplement), 1969.

WEEKLY READER. *Weekly Reader National Survey on Safety and Health.* Middletown, Connecticut: Field Publications, 1986.

CHAPTER 5

CHANGES IN SMOKING BEHAVIOR AND KNOWLEDGE ABOUT DETERMINANTS

CONTENTS

INTRODUCTION

This Chapter reviews two major aspects of smoking behavior since release of the first Surgeon General's Report on smoking and health in 1964: (1) changes in smoking behavior in the United States (Part I) and (2) changes in our knowledge about the determinants of smoking during this period (Part II).

During the past 25 years, the prevalence of cigarette smoking has declined in virtually every major sociodemographic group, including men and women, adults and adolescents, blacks and whites, and persons with and without college education. This decline has been particularly evident among men, in whom the prevalence of smoking declined from 50 percent in 1965 to 32 percent in 1987. The first part of this Chapter analyzes trends in smoking prevalence, cessation, and initiation, and examines smoking patterns among different sociodemographic groups and other special populations. These analyses are based, for the most part, on cross-sectional population-based data collected periodically since 1964.

At the same time, our knowledge about determinants of smoking has increased substantially. Physiological, behavioral, and social factors that may influence the initiation and maintenance of smoking have been extensively researched. Many important predictors of initiation, quitting, and relapse have been identified. The development of this body of knowledge is reviewed in the second part of this Chapter. Information reviewed in that part of the Chapter is primarily derived from research studies and intervention trials that employ smaller sample sizes than the population-based surveys used in Part I. These studies, however, usually collect more detailed information and often obtain longitudinal followup data.

PART I. CHANGES IN SMOKING BEHAVIOR

Trends in Cigarette Smoking

Introduction

Accurate information on trends in smoking prevalence in the major sociodemographic groups in the United States is of interest to public health officials, policymakers, researchers, clinicians, and news media. These data are important for estimating the magnitude of the problem of smoking and for targeting public health interventions to those at highest risk of smoking.

Accurate data on trends in smoking (including initiation and quitting) are necessary to be able to project future smoking patterns. Accurate projections must be available, in turn, to set appropriate but realistic goals for key future years (e.g., 1990, 2000). This Section analyzes trends in smoking prevalence, quitting, and initiation during the past quarter century. Data on smoking prevalence in the 1940s and 1950s from Gallup surveys and the Current Population Survey have been cited elsewhere (CDC 1987a; US DHHS 1988, Appendix A).

Changes in measures of smoking behavior (e.g., prevalence, quitting, initiation), like any quantitative variables, can be calculated as absolute or relative changes. For changes in percentages, the absolute change would be in percentage points; the relative (percent) change would be calculated by subtracting the "new" percentage from the base percentage, dividing the difference by the base percentage, and multiplying the quotient by 100. Each measure of change has advantages and disadvantages. Throughout Part I of this Chapter, changes in smoking prevalence, quitting, and initiation are described primarily in terms of absolute changes.

Nature and Quality of Data

A number of sources of information provide insight into smoking behavior in the United States. These sources fall into two main categories: those based on excise taxation of cigarettes and those based on population surveys of self-reported smoking.

Excise Tax and Sales Data

The Economic Research Service of the U.S. Department of Agriculture (USDA) has estimated total and adult per capita consumption of cigarettes for a number of years. These estimates are based on data from the Bureau of Alcohol, Tobacco and Firearms (Department of Treasury), the Bureau of Commerce (Department of Commerce), the Tobacco Institute, and other private and industry sources.

The Tobacco Institute reports the number of packs of cigarettes on which State taxes are paid; the Bureau of Alcohol, Tobacco and Firearms reports the number of cigarettes on which Federal taxes are paid; and the Bureau of Commerce reports the number of cigarettes imported into the United States. Both Federal and State taxes are excise taxes collected at the wholesale level (on removals) and are not standard sales taxes.

The estimated level of consumption is based on both Federal and State taxes on removals, as well as on imports, and is adjusted for estimated inventory changes. Adult per capita consumption is customarily calculated in the United States by dividing total consumption by the total estimated population 18 years of age and older. (The World Health Organization (1988) has published per capita cigarette consumption figures for countries throughout the world based on the population 15 years of age and older.)

Self-Reported Survey Data

A number of different data sources are available to assess national trends in smoking during the past 25 years. These surveys differ on the basis of sample size, method of data collection (telephone interview versus face-to-face household interview versus questionnaire administered in school), population (adults versus adolescents), sampling frame (national versus State based), and the extent of information collected on tobacco use. Details of the methodology for the various surveys are provided in the Appendix to Chapter 4 and in Table 1 of that chapter. The amount of information provided varies from survey to survey depending on the availability of information.

Validity of Self-Reported Survey Data

The validity of self-reports of smoking status from surveys may affect the usefulness of these data in reporting historical trends. Respondents' sensitivity to the social stigma associated with smoking has been cited as a reason persons might underreport their smoking status (Warner 1978; Kozlowski 1986). Whereas biochemical assessment is generally more reliable than self-report in assessing level of nicotine intake (US DHHS 1988), self-reported data appear valid for estimating prevalence of smoking in the population. For example, studies of patients in several settings (Petitti, Friedman, Kahn 1981; Pojer et al. 1984), as well as two large community studies (Fortmann et al. 1984; Pierce, Dwyer et al.1987b),have shown that measurement of smoking by self-report or by biochemical markers gives approximately the same estimates of prevalence. A more recent study of 1,317 Hispanics, however, showed that self-reported cigarette use underestimated biochemically validated use (Coultas et al. 1988).

It is possible that the accuracy of self-reported data will vary depending on whether the data collection method is face to face or by telephone interview. Although biochemical-validation data do not exist to allow the quantification of such a difference, comparisons of smoking prevalence estimates derived from surveys using telephone versus in-person interviews have shown that the former are generally 1 to 3 percentage points below the latter (CDC 1987a; see below and NCHS 1987). In addition, concerns have been expressed about the validity of data reported by one person on behalf of another ("proxy response") (NCHS 1985, p. 54). For adults, these concerns relate more to measures of the number of cigarettes smoked per day than to the classification of whether a person is a current smoker (US DHEW 1969, p. 794; Rogot and Reid 1975; National Research Council 1986, pp. 110–112). For adolescents, proxy reporting may also affect prevalence estimates (Millar 1985).

Correlation Between Self-Reported Survey Data and Sales Data

Warner (1978) compared self-reported data on cigarette consumption with USDA consumption data for the years 1964–75. He found that self-reported cigarette consumption increasingly underestimated the USDA estimates, possibly because of the increasing social stigma associated with smoking. Changing social acceptability of smoking would not be expected to affect the USDA estimates. To the extent that a "social acceptability" bias in self-reported data may have increased in recent years, the dramatic decrease in smoking prevalence observed during the past 25 years could be in part artifactual.

Hatziandreu et al. (in press) analyzed more recent data to determine whether the trend reported by Warner (1978) has continued. Self-reported consumption data for adults and teenagers were obtained from the National Health Interview Survey (NHIS) (National Center for Health Statistics (NCHS)) and the National Household Survey on Drug Abuse (National Institute on Drug Abuse (NIDA)). Self-reported cigarette consumption was estimated based on the smoking prevalence, the average self-reported number of cigarettes smoked per day, and the U.S. population size each year. A "consumption ratio" was calculated by dividing self-reported consumption by USDA estimates obtained from cigarette tax data. This ratio has been relatively stable recently, varying from 0.73 in 1974 to 0.69 in 1976 with a mean of 0.72 (Table 1). A least-squares regression analysis was used to identify any trend. The slope of the regression line was not significantly different from zero (p=0.85), countering the hypothesis that self-reported data are increasingly underestimating actual cigarette consumption. These results suggest that national surveys provide a reliable estimate of U.S. smoking trends. The reasons for the consistent difference between cigarette consumption based on excise tax data versus self-reported data are unclear; one possible explanation would be a systematic bias from "rounding down" of self-reported daily consumption to the nearest multiple of a half-pack (see Table 14 and related discussion and Kozlowski 1986).

TABLE 1.—Estimates of cigarette consumption in the United States, based on cigarette excise taxes and self-reports, 1974–85

Year	Excise taxes (billions)	Self-reported (billions)	Fraction
1974	599.0	434.9	0.73
1976	613.5	424.4	0.69
1978	616.0	438.4	0.71
1979	621.5	441.2	0.71
1980	631.5	459.1	0.73
1983	600.0	467.8	0.78
1985	594.0	414.4	0.70

NOTE: Estimated by the U.S. Department of Agriculture. Self-reported consumption includes estimated consumption for adults (NHIS, NCHS) and estimated consumption for adolescents (National Household Survey on Drug Abuse, NIDA).
SOURCE: Hatziandreu et al., in press.

The difference in the findings reported by Hatziandreu et al. (in press) and Warner (1978) may relate to differences in methodology. For example, Warner used data from the 1964, 1966, 1970, and 1975 Adult Use of Tobacco Surveys (AUTSs). He found that the major decrease in the consumption ratio occurred between 1966 and 1970. This may have occurred because the 1964 and 1966 AUTSs were in-person surveys, whereas the 1970 and 1975 AUTSs were telephone surveys. As mentioned above, telephone surveys generally provide slightly lower estimates of smoking prevalence than in-person surveys. On the other hand, Hatziandreu et al. (in press) used only in-person interview data (NHIS) for adults and the NIDA Household Interview Survey on Drug Use for adolescents. The consumption ratios obtained by Warner for 1964 and 1966 (0.73 and 0.72, respectively) using in-person survey data were similar to the mean ratio (0.72) reported by Hatziandreu et al. for the period 1974–85. In addition, the 1974 in-person estimate was 0.73 (Hatziandreu et al., in press), whereas the 1975 telephone estimate was 0.64 (Warner 1978). This difference provides further evidence that the decrease in the consumption ratio reported by Warner was an artifact of the change in the AUTS methodology.

Trends in Cigarette Sales

Total cigarette consumption in the United States (as estimated by sales data) increased steadily from 1900 until 1981, when an estimated total of 640 billion cigarettes were smoked (Table 2). Since 1981, there has been a steady decline in consumption despite increasing population size. The number of cigarettes smoked in 1987 is estimated at 574 billion.

These figures refer to manufactured cigarettes and do not include roll-your-own cigarettes. Roll-your-own cigarettes have accounted for a declining proportion of total cigarettes consumed through the 20th century. By 1950, the estimated per capita consumption of roll-your-own cigarettes was 126, or 3.4 percent of total cigarettes consumed; in 1987, these figures were 23 and 0.7 percent, respectively (USDA, unpublished data).

Cigarette consumption data are divided by the population of adults 18 years of age and older to give an estimate of adult per capita consumption. This estimate represents the average number of cigarettes sold per adult in the population, not per smoker. It should be noted that trends in adult per capita consumption are somewhat biased because there has been a trend over time for more people to start smoking regularly under age 18 (see section below on Trends in the Initiation of Smoking).

Per capita consumption of manufactured cigarettes increased dramatically from its level of 54 cigarettes in 1900 to 4,171 cigarettes in 1960 (Table 2). From 1960–73, this figure remained relatively stable (compared with the previous rates of change) at about 4,000 cigarettes per year. Since 1973, there has been a yearly decline in per capita consumption. From 1973–87, this figure fell more than 23 percent to 3,196 cigarettes per year. Although there has been a decline in every one of these 15 years, the rate of decline has varied. From 1974–79, the magnitude of the yearly change increased rapidly until it reached a 2-percent decrease per year. In the 10 years since 1979, this decrease has fluctuated with a mean of 2.4 percent per year (standard deviation (S.D.) = 1.9). The large drop from 1982–83 (7.2 percent) was more than two standard deviations above the mean and is thought to be related, to a significant degree, to the March 1983 increase in the Federal cigarette excise tax from 8 cents per pack to 16 cents per pack (see Chapter 7).

Trends in cigarette sales are also presented in Chapter 8 (Figure 3).

Trends in Smoking Prevalence Among Adults

Cigarette Smoking by Sex, Race (Whites and Blacks), and Educational Attainment (National Health Interview Surveys: 1965–87)

Table 3 presents smoking prevalence from NHIS data for the years 1965, 1966, 1970, 1974, 1976–80 inclusive, 1983, and 1985, and preliminary data for 1987. These data are presented for the total adult population (aged 20 years and older) and by sex, race (whites and blacks), and educational attainment. They differ slightly from estimates published by NCHS (NCHS 1988c) because the data presented here are adjusted to the

TABLE 2.—Total manufactured U.S. cigarette consumption and per capita consumption, adults aged 18 years and older, 1900–87

Year	Total consumption (billions)	Per capita consumption	Percentage change in per capita consumption from previous year
1900	2.5	54	
1910	8.6	151	+10.8[a]
1920	44.6	665	+16.0[a]
1930	119.3	1,185	+5.9[a]
1940	181.9	1,976	+5.2[a]
1950	369.8	3,552	+6.0[a]
1960	484.4	4,171	+1.6[a]
1961	502.5	4,266	+2.3
1962	508.4	4,266	0
1963	523.9	4,345	+1.9
1964	511.3	4,194	–3.5
1965	528.8	4,258	+1.5
1966	541.3	4,287	+0.7
1967	549.3	4,280	–0.2
1968	545.6	4,186	–2.2
1969	528.0	3,993	–4.6
1970	536.5	3,985	–0.2
1971	555.2	4,037	+1.3
1972	566.8	4,043	+0.1
1973	589.7	4,148	+3.0
1974	599.0	4,141	–0.2
1975	607.2	4,123	–0.4
1976	613.5	4,092	–0.8
1977	617.0	4,051	–1.0
1978	616.0	3,967	–2.1
1979	621.5	3,861	–2.7
1980	631.5	3,844	–0.4
1981	640.0	3,836	–0.2
1982	634.0	3,739	–2.6
1983	600.0	3,488	–7.2
1984	600.4	3,446	–1.2
1985	594.0	3,370	–2.3
1986	583.8	3,274	–2.9
1987 (estimate)	574.0	3,196	–2.4

[a]Annualized rate of change during preceding decade.
SOURCE: USDA (1987).

TABLE 3.—Trends in smoking prevalence (%), NHISs, United States, 1965–87, adults aged 20 years and older

		Sex		Race		Educational level			
Year	Overall population	Males	Females	Whites	Blacks	Less than high school graduate	High school graduate	Some college	College graduate
1965[a]	40.4	50.2	31.9	40.0	43.0				
1966	40.7	50.8	32.0	40.4	42.9	36.5	41.1	42.5	33.7
1970	37.0	44.3	30.8	36.5	41.4	34.8	38.3	36.7	28.1
1974	36.9	43.4	31.4	36.1	44.0	36.5	37.6	36.9	28.3
1976	36.1	42.1	31.3	35.6	41.2	35.8	37.8	36.4	27.4
1977	35.6	40.9	31.4	34.9	41.8	35.8	38.4	35.2	25.6
1978	34.0	39.0	29.6	33.6	38.2	35.3	36.5	32.7	23.8
1979	33.5	38.4	29.2	33.2	36.8	34.9	35.4	33.3	23.4
1980	33.3	38.5	29.0	32.9	37.2	35.5	35.7	31.2	24.6
1983	31.8	35.5	28.7	31.4	36.6	34.7	35.6	30.0	19.9
1985	30.4	33.2	28.0	29.9	36.0	35.7	34.2	28.1	18.4
1987[b]	29.1	31.7	26.8	28.8	34.0	35.7	33.1	26.1	16.3
Trend information (1965–85)									
Change[c]/year	–0.50	–0.84	–0.21	–0.50	–0.39	–0.06	–0.32	–0.70	–0.76
Standard error	0.03	0.04	0.03	0.03	0.08	0.03	0.05	0.07	0.08
R^2	0.97	0.98	0.81	0.97	0.74	NA[d]	0.87	0.94	0.93

[a]For 1965, data stratified by education were not available.
[b]Provisional data only.
[c]In percentage points.
[d]The slope of the regression line was not significantly different from zero, making the R^2 computation inappropriate.
SOURCE: NHISs 1965–87; unpublished data, Office on Smoking and Health.

1985 age distribution, whereas the previously published figures were adjusted to the 1970 age distribution.

For each group, observed smoking prevalence for each survey year is reported. Additionally, to assess time trends from 1965–85, weighted least-squares regression analyses have been applied to these data. The 1987 data were not included in the regression analyses because these data are preliminary estimates. These estimates can be used to provide a measure of predictive validity of the model; in general, the preliminary 1987 estimates are similar to projections from the model (Pierce, Fiore et al. 1989a).

The R^2 statistic was used for each trend analysis and is a measure of how well the linear model fits the observed data values. R^2 values may range from 0 (no linear trend) to 1.0 (a perfect fit between the observed values and a linear model).

The data on overall smoking prevalence, as well as for each sex and racial group presented in Table 3, demonstrate linear trends with R^2 values ranging from 0.74 to 0.98; thus, the models fit the data very well. Trends for three of the four educational categories are also fitted well by a linear model. For one category, less than high school graduation, no R^2 value is reported because the rate of change is very close to zero (making the R^2 statistic inappropriate as an index of the amount of variation explained by the model). The change (in percentage points) per year is the slope of the line of best fit calculated by the model. The standard error of the slope allows confidence limits to be placed around the estimate of change per year. Ninety-five-percent confidence limits around the estimate of a slope are approximately equal to the slope plus or minus two times the standard error.

Overall smoking prevalence declined from 40.4 percent in 1965 to 29.1 percent in 1987. The trend from 1965–85 is fitted almost exactly by a linear model (R^2=0.97). Smoking prevalence in the United States adult population is decreasing at a rate of 0.50 percentage points per year with a standard error of 0.03. Thus, the 95-percent confidence interval for the change per year is 0.44 to 0.56. There is no evidence of any sudden deviations from the identified trend such as that seen in the per capita consumption data in 1983 (Table 2).

The prevalence of smoking among men has decreased steadily from 50.2 percent in 1965 to 31.7 percent in 1987. The rate of decline between 1965 and 1985 was 0.84 percentage points per year (95-percent confidence limits, 0.76, 0.92). Female smoking prevalence remained stable at 31 to 32 percent from 1965–77. Subsequently, prevalence began to decline slowly and reached 26.8 percent in 1987. The overall rate of decline from 1965–85 was 0.21 percentage points per year (95-percent confidence limits, 0.15, 0.27). Fiore and coworkers (1989) have examined more recent trends in smoking by gender in greater detail. This analysis showed a rate of decline in prevalence among women of 0.33 percentage points per year between 1974 and 1985 (95-percent confidence limits, 0.21, 0.45) (R^2=0.88).

Although there has been a difference in smoking prevalence between blacks and whites, it may be explained by socioeconomic status (Novotny, Warner et al. 1988), and the rate of change in smoking prevalence in recent years has been similar between the races (Fiore et al. 1989). Smoking among whites decreased from 40.0 percent in 1965 to 28.8 percent in 1987. The rate of decline from 1965–85 was 0.50 percentage points per year (95-percent confidence limits, 0.44, 0.56; R^2=0.97).

For blacks the R^2 value for the simple linear model is 0.74, suggesting that the data should be reviewed more carefully. In 1965, 43.0 percent of blacks smoked. This number had changed little by 1977 when 41.8 percent smoked. From 1977–87, there was a considerable drop in smoking prevalence to 34.0 percent. Thus, the data suggest that there may be two trends among blacks. Fiore et al. (1989) fitted a linear model to the data for 1974–85 and reported a rate of change among blacks of –0.67 percentage points per year with 95-percent confidence limits of 0.37 and 0.97 (R^2=0.80). This rate of change was not significantly higher than that among whites for the same period (–0.57 percentage points per year). However, smoking prevalence among black men was decreasing at a faster rate than among white men (1.15 percentage points per year compared with 0.87, p=0.03). There were no significant differences noted in the rates of decrease among women of either race (blacks, 0.26 percentage points per year; whites, 0.32).

Trends in smoking among the various educational groups have differed markedly since 1966 (Pierce, Fiore et al. 1989b). College graduates have decreased their smoking level from 33.7 percent in 1966 to 16.3 percent in 1987. The rate of decline from 1966–85 was 0.76 percentage points per year (95-percent confidence limits, 0.60 to 0.92). Smoking prevalence in respondents who reported having attended some college decreased from 42.5 percent in 1966 to 26.1 percent in 1987 at a slightly lower rate of change (–0.70 percentage points per year) than that of college graduates. High school graduates who did not attend college reduced their smoking from 41.1 percent in 1966 to 33.1 percent in 1987 at a rate (–0.32 percentage points per year) less than half that for respondents who had attended college. Smoking prevalence in those respondents without a high school diploma did not change appreciably from 1966 (36.5 percent) to 1987 (35.7 percent); the rate of decline between 1966 and 1985 was only 0.06 percentage points per year. Thus, there is a twelvefold difference in rate of decline in smoking prevalence between the most and least educated groups in our society. The increasing gap in smoking prevalence by educational attainment is particularly evident when comparing the difference in smoking prevalence between the most and least educated groups in 1966 with the difference in 1987. In 1966, the prevalence rates were similar (33.7 and 36.5 percent, respectively); in 1987, prevalence in the most educated group (16.3 percent) was less than half that in the least educated group (35.7 percent).

Adult Use of Tobacco Surveys: 1964–86

In 1964, 1966, 1970, 1975, and 1986, the Office on Smoking and Health (formerly the National Clearinghouse for Smoking and Health) conducted detailed surveys of a representative sample of the U.S. adult population. The purpose of these surveys has been to study the population's knowledge, attitudes, and practices regarding the use of tobacco. The first two surveys primarily used in-person household interviews while the last three used telephone interviews. Prevalence of cigarette smoking in the United States as measured by the AUTSs has declined from 40.3 percent in 1964 to 26.5 percent in 1986 (Table 4). This decrease represents an overall decline in smoking of more than 34 percent during this 22-year period.

TABLE 4.—Trends in smoking prevalence (%), AUTS versus NHIS

Survey year	AUTS[a]	Estimated NHIS[b]	Difference (NHIS–AUTS)
1964	40.3	40.4	0.1
1966	42.2	39.4	–2.8
1970	36.2	37.4	1.2
1975	33.8	34.9	1.1
1986	26.5	29.4	2.9

[a]For all survey years, includes respondents aged 21 years and older except 1986, which includes respondents aged 17 years and older. All data weighted.
[b]Includes respondents aged 20 years and older. Values for each year are determined by extrapolating expected prevalence values based on regression analysis from Table 3.
SOURCE: Office on Smoking and Health (US DHEW 1969, 1973a, 1976; CDC 1987a).

Unlike the NHIS, for which data are collected during an in-person household interview, AUTSs collected data via telephone interviews in 1970, 1975, and 1986. The three AUTSs conducted since 1970 all produced prevalence estimates below those estimated (by regression analysis) from the NHISs (Table 4). The largest difference between the two surveys was 2.9 percentage points in 1986. The 95-percent confidence limits around the NHIS projection for 1986 are 27.8 to 31.7 compared with limits of 25.8 to 27.3 from the 1986 AUTS; thus, the difference in estimates between the two surveys is statistically significant. A difference in sampling modalities is among the most likely explanations for this discrepancy in prevalence estimates. A similar finding has been noted in State-specific prevalence estimates (see below). Telephone surveys have a small sampling bias by excluding households lacking telephones and may have a greater nonresponse bias because of generally lower response rates compared with household surveys (CDC 1987a).

Cigarette Smoking Among Different Occupational Groups

NHIS data have been published on smoking prevalence by occupation for the years 1970, 1978–80 combined, and 1985 (Table 5). There is a consistent pattern of higher smoking rates among blue-collar and service workers than among white-collar workers for all these survey years. For example, in 1985, the prevalence of smoking among blue-collar and white-collar workers was 40 and 28 percent, respectively. This difference was greater among males (14 percentage points) than among females (6 percentage points). Detailed data on smoking prevalence, percentage of former smokers, quitting attempts, and age of initiation within specific occupational categories for 1978–80 were published in the 1985 Surgeon General's Report (US DHHS 1985). Weinkam and Sterling (1987) also provided a detailed analysis of smoking by occupation using the 1970 and 1979–80 NHIS data.

Novotny, Warner, and colleagues (1988) performed multivariate logistic regression analyses on data from the 1985 NHIS (ages 25 to 64 years) to examine the independent

TABLE 5.—Prevalence of smoking (%) by occupation, 1970, 1978–80, and 1985

	1970[a]		1978–80[a]		1985[b]		
Occupation	Males	Females	Males	Females	Males	Females	Total
Currently employed	47.9	36.5	39.9	33.3	33.8	30.0	32.1
White collar	40.8	36.1	33.0	31.9	26.4	28.0	27.5
Blue collar	55.0	37.7	47.1	38.1	40.1	33.9	39.7
Service	53.3	39.4	47.5	37.4	40.3	35.4	37.2
Unemployed	55.9	42.3	53.1	39.6	44.3	28.0	36.1

[a]Aged 20 to 64 years.
[b]Aged 20 years and older.
SOURCE: NHISs 1970, 1978–80 (combined), and 1985, NCHS (US DHHS 1985, 1988).

effects of socioeconomic status (SES) and selected demographic factors on the odds of ever smoking (versus never smoking) and current smoking (versus former smoking). The SES/demographic factors included in the models were: sex, employment status, occupation, education, marital status, and poverty status. The investigators found that when they simultaneously controlled for the effects of these factors, unemployed persons were more likely than employed persons to be ever smokers or current smokers. However, blue-collar and service workers were not found to have significantly increased odds of ever or current smoking compared with white-collar workers. Employed persons were more likely to have quit smoking than unemployed persons.

Special Populations: Hispanics

Information on smoking among Hispanics was collected as part of the Hispanic Health and Nutrition Examination Survey (HHANES) between 1982 and 1984. This was a geographically based sample of Hispanics from three areas of the United States designed to represent three large Hispanic groups (Puerto Ricans in the New York City area; Cuban-Americans in Dade County, Florida; and Mexican-Americans in the Southwest). Sample sizes were 9,000 Mexican-Americans, 4,000 Puerto Ricans, and 1,500 Cuban-Americans.

According to the HHANES, the age-adjusted smoking rates for males aged 20 to 74 years were 43 percent for Mexican-Americans, 42 percent for Cuban-Americans, and 40 percent for Puerto Ricans. Among females, the smoking prevalence was 24 percent for Mexican-Americans and Cuban Americans and 30 percent for Puerto Rican Americans (Haynes 1987). A birth-cohort analysis of these data showed that smoking rates have decreased among successive cohorts of men, but increased among successive cohorts of women (Escobedo and Remington 1989).

These rates are higher than those obtained from the NHISs for the years 1979 and 1980 (Marcus and Crane 1985; Rogers and Crank 1988) and 1985 (Marcus and Crane 1987). However, the number of Hispanics in these NHIS samples was small, making prevalence estimates less reliable. Haynes (1987) suggests that NHIS data may underestimate smoking prevalence among Hispanics because questions about smoking were not asked in Spanish. The first estimates of smoking behavior among Hispanics that are both national and statistically reliable will be available from the 1987 NHIS, which oversampled for this population group.

Special Populations: American Indians and Alaskan Natives

There are no reliable national estimates of smoking prevalence among American Indians. Several surveys have assessed smoking rates among specific Indian tribes or on certain Indian reservations (CDC 1987b). Smoking prevalence is highest among Northern Plains Indians (42 to 70 percent) and Alaskan Natives (56 percent), where rates greatly exceed the rate in the general U.S. population. Much lower rates have been reported for Indians from the Southwest (13 to 28 percent). High rates of smokeless tobacco use have also been reported among some American Indian groups, especially in Indian youth. According to a survey of approximately 5,000 children 5 to 18 years of age in rural Alaska conducted by the Indian Health Service, 28 percent of girls and 34 percent of boys reported using smokeless tobacco products (CDC 1987c). Similar findings were obtained in other surveys of Native Americans (Schinke et al. 1987; CDC 1988; Hall and Dexter 1988).

Special Populations: Asian Americans

There are no reliable national estimates of smoking prevalence among Asian Americans. A few local surveys provide estimates of smoking prevalence among Asian Americans in specific geographic regions.

The State of Hawaii has a population composed of 29 percent Caucasian, 26 percent Japanese, 15 percent Hawaiian, and 15 percent Filipino. The State conducted a Behavioral Risk Factor Survey (see below) of 1,002 people by telephone in 1984. Smoking prevalence estimates were 28 percent for Caucasians, 27 percent for both Hawaiians and Filipinos, and 23 percent for Japanese (Hawaii State Department of Health 1984). A similar survey of 1,557 residents of the State was completed in 1986. Prevalence estimates from this second survey were 29.3 percent for Caucasians, 28.8 percent for Hawaiians, 25.1 percent for Filipinos, and 20.6 percent for Japanese (Chung 1986).

Special Populations: Pregnant Women

National data on smoking during pregnancy are scarce, especially prior to 1980. Since 1980, several national surveys have directed smoking questions to previously pregnant women, but survey methodologies vary widely and it is not possible to study secular changes in behavior.

Probably the best source of national data on smoking among pregnant women has been the National Natality Surveys (NNSs), which were conducted among national samples of married mothers of live infants born in 1967 and 1980. Data from these surveys were used by Kleinman and Kopstein (1987) to document changes in smoking behavior during pregnancy over that period of time. Among teenagers, smoking rates remained fairly constant over time at about 38 percent among whites and 27 percent among blacks. Among women over age 20, there were decreases in smoking prevalence that varied markedly by race and by educational attainment of the mother. Smoking prevalence among white women over age 20 declined from 40 percent in 1967 to 25 percent in 1980; among black women over age 20, it declined from 33 percent to 23 percent. Among white women over age 20, there was an increase in the proportion quitting smoking during pregnancy (11 percent to 16 percent), while among blacks the proportion quitting actually decreased (17 percent to 11 percent). Among white women with less than 12 years of education, the prevalence of smoking during pregnancy declined from 48 percent to 43 percent, while for women with 16 or more years of education, it declined from 34 percent to 11 percent. Among white smokers with less than 12 years of education, there was relatively little change in the proportion quitting during pregnancy (11 percent to 9 percent), but among smokers with 16 years or more of education, the proportion more than doubled (12 percent to 27 percent). Insufficient numbers of black women were sampled to study trends by education among blacks.

A study similar to the NNS, the National Maternal and Infant Health Survey, was begun in 1988. Data from that study will provide the best estimates of smoking during pregnancy for the late 1980s. At this time, however, no comparable national data exist to study women after 1980. Studies that have asked about smoking behavior during pregnancy have not asked about behavior during specific years, so it is not possible to calculate estimates of the prevalence of smoking in any particular time period. However, it is possible to use these data sources to examine general patterns of smoking during pregnancy. In general, women in the lowest age and socioeconomic categories have the highest likelihood of smoking during pregnancy.

The earliest data available to examine these patterns are from the Collaborative Perinatal Study (Niswander and Gordon 1972), which included women who obtained prenatal care at selected university centers in the early 1960s. White women were more likely to smoke than black women (53 percent versus 43 percent), and among smokers, whites smoked more cigarettes per day than blacks. By comparison, the national prevalence of smoking among women 25 to 44 years of age was 44 percent in 1965 (NCHS 1988c).

The National Survey of Family Growth (NSFG) collected data in 1982 on the smoking behavior of women, 15 to 44 years of age, during their most recent pregnancy, regardless of when the pregnancy occurred (NCHS 1988a). Of these women, 32 percent smoked during the pregnancy. Women who were aged 15 to 19 years when pregnant, who had less than 12 years of education, who were at 149 percent or less of poverty level, or who were unmarried had the highest smoking rates.

In the 1985 NHIS, questions related to smoking were asked of women aged 18 to 44 years who had given birth within the past 5 years (NCHS 1988b). Of these women, 32 percent reported having smoked during the 12 months preceding the birth; 21 percent of smokers reported quitting smoking and 36 percent reported reducing the number of cigarettes smoked after learning they were pregnant. Women under 25 years of age, with low income, of black race, unmarried, or unemployed were more likely to smoke than others. These same groups of women were less likely to quit smoking or to reduce the number of cigarettes smoked.

The 1990 Health Objectives for the Nation (US DHHS 1980a) state that "The proportion of women who smoke during pregnancy should be no greater than one-half the proportion of women overall who smoke." At the time of the midcourse review of the objectives (US DHHS1986c), no data were available to evaluate progress directly. According to the 1985 NHIS, approximately 31 percent of women aged 18 to 44 years smoked cigarettes in 1985 (31.7 percent of 18- to 29-year-olds and 31.2 percent of 30- to 44-year-olds) (NCHS 1988c). In the same survey, as mentioned above, 32 percent of women who had given birth in the preceding 5 years reported smoking in the 12 months preceding the birth, 21 percent of whom reportedly quit after learning they were pregnant. This indirect evidence seems to indicate that the smoking prevalence among pregnant women was much more than half the prevalence among nonpregnant women in the early 1980s. Unless major changes in smoking behavior have occurred in the latter half of the decade, the 1990 objective will not be met. Analysis of data from the Behavioral Risk Factor Surveillance System supports this conclusion (Williamson et al. 1989).

Special Populations: Military Personnel

In 1980, 1982, 1985, and 1988, the Department of Defense (DOD) performed worldwide surveys of alcohol and nonmedical drug use among military personnel.

These surveys assessed cigarette smoking among personnel by asking, "During the past 30 days, how many packs of cigarettes did you usually smoke during a typical day?" (The 1980 survey question used the phrase "in one day.") There were five possible responses: 3 or more packs; 2 or more, but less than 3 packs; 1 or more, but less than 2 packs; less than 1 pack, but smoked some; did not smoke in the past 30 days. Sample sizes ranged from 15,000 to 21,000. The number of military installations participating in the surveys ranged from 58 to 81. The surveyed population was proportionally representative of all DOD active duty members for sex, race/ethnicity, marital status, education, and age (Herbold 1987; US DOD 1987, 1988).

Overall smoking prevalence among military personnel declined steadily from 53 percent in 1982 to 46 percent in 1985 to 42 percent in 1988 (Table 6). These prevalence figures, although declining, are considerably higher than among all males or young males in the general population (Tables 3 and 18). This disparity may reflect socioeconomic differences between military personnel and the general population, although one study suggests that smoking initiation may often occur among recruits after entering the military (see below). The 1988 estimates for the individual military branches were: Air Force, 37 percent; Marine Corps, 42 percent; Army, 44 percent; and Navy, 45 percent (US DOD 1988).

TABLE 6.—Prevalence of cigarette smoking among U.S. military personnel, 1980, 1982, 1985, and 1988

	Percentage of current smokers[a]			
Rank[b]	1980 (N=15,016)	1982 (N=21,412)	1985 (N=17,328)	1988[c] (N=18,673)
E1–3	55	56	47	47
E4–6	55	55	52	45
E7–9	56	61	56	48
W1–4			40	34
O1–O3				19
O1–O2	24	25	17	
O3	23	24	18	
O4–O10			21	20
O4–O6	27	28		
Total	52	53	46	42

[a]Persons who had smoked cigarettes during the past 30 days.
[b]In ascending rank, from enlisted personnel (E1–9) to warrant officers (W1–4) to commissioned officers (O1–O10).
[c]Preliminary data (not adjusted for nonrespondents).
SOURCE: Herbold (1987); US DOD (1986, 1987, 1988).

Smoking prevalence rates among enlisted personnel (ranks E1–9) are at least twice the rates among commissioned officers in each survey year (Table 6). In 1988, for instance, smoking prevalence estimates ranged from 47 percent for the lowest ranks of enlisted personnel (E1–3) to 20 percent for the higher ranks of commissioned officers (O4–O10). The proportion of smokers smoking a pack or more a day was 55 percent; there was no consistent association between this proportion and military rank (US DOD 1988).

Cronan and Conway (1987) collected smoking information from 687 recruits entering the Navy and from 1,357 Navy servicemen stationed aboard ships in the San Diego area. The prevalence of smoking was 27.6 percent among recruits and 49.8 percent among shipboard men. The investigators concluded that the Navy is not attracting a higher than expected percentage of smokers from the U.S. population, but that many men start to smoke after they enter the Navy.

Reasons for higher smoking rates among military personnel include the inexpensive price of cigarettes in military facilities, peer pressure heightened by conditions of group living, stress, boredom, and lack of other forms of recreation (Cronan and Conway 1987; Blake 1985). In addition, there has been a historical connection between cigarettes and the military: cigarettes have been a part of the K-rations and C-rations provided to soldiers and sailors, and cigarette advertisements on radio and in the print media during World War II commonly featured military themes (Blake 1985). Cigarette advertising continues to appear in military-oriented publications (Davis 1987). In September 1988, Philip Morris Tobacco Company began to publish a monthly newsletter, "Military Smoker," which features articles opposing restrictions on smoking and on cigarette sales in military facilities; readers are urged to call a toll-free "Military Smoker" hotline telephone number (Philip Morris 1988).

Recent DOD initiatives to reduce smoking among military personnel are described in Chapter 6.

State-Specific Smoking Prevalence

Behavioral Risk Factor Surveillance System: 1982–87

The Behavioral Risk Factor Surveillance System (BRFS) has provided State-specific smoking prevalence estimates for adults 18 years of age and older for about half of the States since 1982 (Table 7). Data are collected through random-digit-dialed telephone interviews. Since 1984, the number of States participating in this surveillance system has increased steadily. For reporting States, median prevalence declined from 37 percent in 1982 to 24 percent in 1987. This decline exceeded the decline in national prevalence in the NHIS (Table 3), probably because of the nonrepresentative mix of States included in the BRFS in different years. In 1987, prevalence ranged from 15 percent in Utah to 32 percent in Kentucky.

Current Population Survey: 1985

In 1985, the Current Population Survey (CPS), a population-based, in-person household survey of more than 114,000 adult Americans, conducted by the U.S. Bureau of the Census, collected information about smoking and smokeless tobacco use. About 45 percent of interviews were conducted with proxy respondents. The survey estimated adult smoking prevalence (20 years of age and older) at 29.5 percent. Table 8 presents estimates of prevalence of cigarette smoking according to region of the country, census division, and State. Among the nine census divisions, prevalence was lowest in the Pacific (26.3 percent) and Mountain (27.2 percent) divisions and was highest in the East South Central (31.8 percent) and South Atlantic (31.3 percent) divisions.

Overall gender-specific prevalence was reported as 32.9 percent for males and 26.5 percent for females. Prevalence of smoking among males exceeded that among females in all States except Oregon and Wyoming (where the prevalence rates among men and women were either very similar or the same). Overall education-specific prevalence was 35.4 percent for persons with 12 years or less education (high school diploma or less) and 22.2 percent for persons with 13 or more years of education (some college or more education). Persons with 13 or more years of education reported lower smoking prevalence rates than those with 12 years or less education in all 50 States by a range of 20.2 percentage points in Tennessee to 5.7 percentage points in Hawaii.

TABLE 7.—State-specific smoking prevalence (%), Behavioral Risk Factor Surveillance System, adults aged 18 years and older, 1982–87

State	1982	1984	1985	1986	1987
Alabama	31			25	27
Alaska	36	34			
Arizona	32	28	26	24	26
Arkansas	27				
California	28	26	26	25	21
Colorado	34				
Connecticut			27		
Delaware	31				
District of Columbia	33	38	26	27	24
Florida	32		27	28	28
Georgia	29	37	29	27	25
Hawaii				25	23
Idaho		25	24	23	21
Illinois		34	26	28	26
Indiana	33	28	32	27	29
Iowa	30				
Kansas	22				
Kentucky	37		29	35	32
Maine					28
Maryland					25
Massachusetts				27	25
Michigan	31				
Minnesota		27	28	25	24
Missouri				26	29
Montana	26	29	25	23	22
Nebraska	23				
New Hampshire	29				
New Jersey	32				
New Mexico	29			26	21
New York			31	27	23
North Carolina	38	31	27	27	26
North Dakota		28	26	26	24
Ohio	30	29	29	28	27

TABLE 7.—Continued

State	1982	1984	1985	1986	1987
Pennsylvania	34				
Rhode Island		31	29	39	
South Carolina		26	29	27	25
South Dakota					25
Tennessee	32	32	28	28	28
Texas	30				
Utah		16	16	18	15
Virginia	34				
Washington					24
West Virginia	32	33	27	29	29
Wisconsin		27	25	26	26
Minimum	22	16	16	18	15
Maximum	38	38	32	35	32
Median	37	29	27	26	24
Number of States[a]	27	19	22	26	29

[a]Includes the District of Columbia.

NOTE: No data were available for the following States: LA, MS, NV, OK, OR, VT, and WY.

SOURCE: CDC (1986a,b, 1987f, unpublished data).

BRFS and CPS Comparison

In 1985, both the BRFS and the CPS collected State-specific information on adult smoking prevalence. Among the 22 States (including the District of Columbia) where comparisons can be made, the CPS (an in-person household survey) estimated higher smoking prevalence in 13 States and lower prevalence in 8 States than the BRFS (a telephone survey). The median difference in smoking prevalence between the CPS and the BRFS was +1.8 percentage points. This pattern is similar to that observed in comparisons between the in-person NHIS and the telephone AUTS (see above).

TABLE 8.—Smoking prevalence rates according to region of the country, census division, and State, adults aged 20 years and older, by gender and education, United States, CPS, 1985

	Overall	Males	Females	Education ≤12 years	Education >12 years
United States	29.5	32.9	26.5	35.4	22.2
Northeast Region	28.9	31.3	26.8	34.5	22.1
New England Division	29.5	30.6	28.6	36.3	22.5
Maine	30.3	31.8	29.1	37.0	17.3
New Hampshire	30.7	35.2	26.7	37.4	21.0
Vermont	30.7	31.8	29.7	37.7	21.4
Massachusetts	28.2	28.4	28.1	35.0	22.9
Rhode Island	34.4	35.8	33.3	39.9	26.3
Connecticut	29.6	30.9	28.5	36.3	23.1
Mid-Atlantic Division	28.7	31.6	26.2	34.0	22.0
New York	28.7	31.4	26.3	34.1	22.3
New Jersey	27.9	31.0	25.2	33.6	21.7
Pennsylvania	29.3	32.3	26.6	34.0	21.7
North Central Region	30.2	32.4	28.1	36.2	22.2
East North Central Division	31.0	33.0	29.3	37.5	22.5
Ohio	32.2	34.4	30.3	38.6	22.0
Indiana	32.8	35.7	30.1	38.4	23.8
Illinois	28.7	31.5	26.3	35.0	22.7
Michigan	34.0	34.4	33.7	40.9	24.7
Wisconsin	26.3	27.6	25.2	32.6	17.9
West North Central Division	28.1	31.1	25.4	33.1	21.7
Minnesota	28.7	30.0	27.4	34.6	21.6
Iowa	28.1	33.0	23.7	31.8	22.2
Missouri	27.7	31.1	24.6	32.0	21.4
North Dakota	26.4	28.3	24.7	31.3	21.8
South Dakota	28.6	30.7	26.8	34.5	21.0
Nebraska	24.9	26.6	23.6	29.2	19.4
Kansas	30.2	34.6	26.6	37.1	23.1
South Region	31.2	36.4	26.8	36.5	23.3
South Atlantic Division	31.3	36.3	27.1	36.6	24.0
Delaware	31.8	34.9	29.1	39.1	19.0
Maryland	29.7	31.5	28.1	36.3	20.1

TABLE 8.—Continued

	Overall	Males	Females	Education ≤12 years	Education >12 years
District of Columbia	31.4	34.2	29.3	38.5	24.2
Virginia	32.7	37.8	28.5	38.5	26.3
West Virginia	34.0	38.6	30.0	38.1	22.9
North Carolina	31.6	39.7	24.6	37.0	24.0
South Carolina	27.1	34.2	21.5	31.7	18.4
Georgia	31.8	38.5	26.5	36.4	25.1
Florida	31.7	35.5	28.4	36.8	25.4
East South Central Division	31.8	37.6	26.9	37.3	21.8
Kentucky	35.3	37.8	33.4	40.2	22.5
Tennessee	30.8	36.6	26.0	38.6	18.4
Alabama	30.6	38.5	23.5	35.3	23.6
Mississippi	31.1	38.8	24.8	34.9	25.3
West South Central Division	30.6	35.5	26.3	35.9	22.8
Arkansas	31.3	37.2	26.5	34.8	25.0
Louisiana	29.1	35.4	23.8	34.1	21.1
Oklahoma	33.0	35.7	30.4	41.5	22.7
Texas	30.6	35.5	26.3	35.9	22.8
West Region	26.5	29.3	23.9	32.8	20.9
Mountain Division	27.2	30.1	24.6	34.7	20.2
Montana	25.9	26.1	25.9	32.2	19.3
Idaho	24.1	26.6	21.7	29.6	17.8
Wyoming	31.7	31.9	31.9	40.9	21.0
Colorado	28.6	30.6	26.9	37.9	21.9
New Mexico	28.5	32.6	24.3	32.8	24.4
Arizona	29.5	34.3	25.3	37.4	21.5
Utah	14.1	18.2	10.2	22.5	8.0
Nevada	35.7	37.6	33.9	39.0	31.4
Pacific Division	26.3	29.0	22.7	32.0	21.1
Washington	28.6	29.9	27.4	36.1	21.8
Oregon	27.1	26.8	27.5	34.7	21.2
California	25.6	28.9	22.5	28.3	20.8
Alaska	34.3	40.9	28.0	41.1	27.2
Hawaii	27.6	30.7	24.7	30.6	24.9

NOTE: Percentages are age adjusted to the total U.S. population.
SOURCE: Office on Smoking and Health, unpublished data.

Summary

A number of national and State-based surveys provide information on cigarette smoking. These surveys have varying methodologies and response rates. The data of highest quality (large sample size, high response rate) are from the NHIS, and this source also has the best series of data for analyzing trends in smoking prevalence since 1965. Trend analysis demonstrates that smoking prevalence among adults overall is declining by 0.50 percentage points per year and this rate of decline has been consistent since 1965. If this rate of change continues for the next few years, overall prevalence will be 27 to 28 percent in 1990, which is higher than the 1990 Health Objective for the Nation (less than 25 percent) (US DHHS 1980a; see Chapter 1). Although there are differences between whites and blacks in smoking prevalence, the rate of change within each race has been similar in recent years. The decline has been much higher in men than in women and much higher in the more educated than in the less educated.

The consistency of the trends in these smoking prevalence data contrasts with the lack of year-to-year consistency in the consumption (excise tax) data presented in an earlier section. Given that both data sets report cigarette usage in the population, reasons for this difference need to be addressed. Each data set has its advantages. Excise tax data have the advantage of being an objective measure of manufactured-cigarette sales and are not subject to questions of validity that must be addressed with self-reported smoking from survey data. On the other hand, survey data provide information on smoking behavior in specific subpopulations within society.

Cigarette sales data, and trend analyses of these data, reflect both the number of people who smoke and the number of cigarettes each smoker consumes (plus a wastage and stock error term). On the other hand, trend analyses of self-reported smoking prevalence reflect only the number of people who smoke. Antismoking interventions may affect an individual's smoking status or daily cigarette consumption. For example, worksite smoking restrictions may induce some smokers to quit, whereas others who continue to smoke may smoke fewer cigarettes per day because of fewer opportunities to smoke. Similarly, increases in cigarette price (e.g., mediated by increased excise taxation) may induce price-sensitive smokers to quit or to reduce daily consumption.

While consumption data are often used as a more sensitive index of the relative impact of differing antismoking strategies, the primary goal of these strategies is a change in smoking prevalence. Smokers who reduce their daily cigarette consumption will reduce their health risks, but to a lesser extent compared with quitting entirely (see Chapters 2 and 3).

Trends in Quitting

Introduction

As the 1988 Surgeon General's Report documented (US DHHS 1988), cigarettes and other forms of tobacco are addicting. This addiction, including both pharmacologic and behavioral components, helps to explain the difficulty that most smokers experience in quitting and then maintaining abstinence. Smokers can be on a quitting cycle in which they are abstinent for a while, followed by a relapse to smoking for a period of time, after which they may quit again, and so on. Given this pattern, no single statistic can fully describe trends in quitting activity. Three interrelated statistics are:

1. *Percentage of former smokers.* The percentage of the population who are former smokers has been used as one indicator of quitting activity. For example, the total number of living persons who have quit smoking is often cited and is calculated by multiplying the proportion of the population who are former smokers by the size of the population. This figure, as calculated from the 1986 AUTS, is 43.2 million adults 17 years of age and older. However, the prevalence of former smokers is of limited value in assessing quitting activity because it does not take into account the number of people in the population who have ever smoked, because it does not include former smokers who have died, and because of marked differences in the initiation of smoking between males and females in different birth cohorts (Harris 1983; Warner and Murt 1982).
2. *Quit ratio.* This statistic is defined as the proportion of people who have ever smoked who are former smokers at a specific point in time; that is, the number of former smokers divided by the number of ever smokers (Pierce et al.1987a). Thus, this statistic is to quitting activity what smoking prevalence is to smoking activity. Both statistics consider the size of the population undertaking a behavior as a proportion of those who could undertake that behavior.

   However, the quit ratio does not provide all the information needed when describing quitting activity. It does not distinguish between a person who has been a former smoker for 3 days and a person who has been off cigarettes for 10 years. It does not distinguish between a current smoker who has just relapsed after 6 years of abstinence and a current smoker who has never tried to quit. In addition, the quit ratio does not reflect the magnitude of smoking prevalence; for example, a group in which 10 percent are current smokers and 10 percent are former smokers has the same quit ratio as a group in which 30 percent are current smokers and 30 percent are former smokers.
3. *The smoking continuum.* This is a 10-category index of the total population derived from the smoking status variable (current, former, or never smoker) and timing and duration of quit attempts. This index is particularly relevant for describing which segments of the population are trying to quit.

Trends in the quit ratio using NHIS data and an analysis of the smoking continuum using data from the 1986 AUTS are presented below.

Trends in the Proportion of Smokers Quitting (Quit Ratio) (NHIS)

Quit ratios for the total U.S. adult population and stratified by sex, race, and education, as derived from the 1965–87 NHISs, are presented in Table 9. Linear regression analyses of the weighted data from those surveys conducted between 1965 and 1985 are also provided to assess time trends. The 1987 data are not used in the regression analyses because they are preliminary. The linear models for the observed data in the subpopulations defined by sex, race, and education had R^2 values all between 0.78 and 0.95.

In 1965, 29.6 percent of ever smokers had quit. By 1987, this proportion had increased to 44.8 percent. The rate of increase in the quit ratio between 1965 and 1985 is 0.68 percentage points per year. Almost half (48.7 percent) of male smokers had quit by 1987 compared with 40.1 percent of female smokers. The rate of increase in the quit ratio is the same among men and women.

Regarding racial differences, 46.4 percent of whites who had been smokers had quit by 1987 compared with 31.5 percent of blacks. For whites, the rate of change in the quit ratio from 1965–85 was 0.72 percentage points per year, and the linear model fits the data exceedingly well. For blacks, the rate of change during this period was 0.43 percentage points per year. As with smoking prevalence, the quit ratio for blacks did not change between 1965 and 1974 but did change between 1974 and 1985. Fiore and colleagues (1989) have reported trends from 1974–85; during this period the rate of increase in the quit ratio among blacks (0.75 percentage points per year) was similar to that among whites (0.77). However, this similarity masks a difference between the sexes. The change in the quit ratio among blacks from 1974–85 was mainly seen in males, where the rate increased at 1.04 percentage points per year (compared with 0.67 in white males). Among black females, the quit ratio increased at 0.46 percentage points per year from 1974–85 (compared with 0.95 in white females). Thus, in recent years, black males have been quitting smoking at a significantly higher rate of change than white males ($p=0.01$). The difference in the rate of change between black and white females is in the opposite direction but is not statistically significant ($p=0.31$) because of the reduced linearity of the trends and smaller sample sizes of ever smokers among females than among males.

In 1966, about 40 percent of college graduates who had ever been smokers had quit. This proportion was 20 to 40 percent higher than the other educational groups. By 1987, the quit ratio among college graduates had risen to 61 percent, and the rate of change from 1966–85 (+0.85 percentage points per year) was greater than in any other educational category. Quitting has been increasing in all the other educational categories, with the slowest rate of change (0.41 percentage points per year) among persons without a high school diploma.

Smoking Continuum (AUTS)

The process of quitting smoking has been categorized by Prochaska and DiClemente (1983) according to smokers' intention to quit and the status of their most recent quit attempt. They labeled five stages of the quitting process as follows: precontemplation,

TABLE 9.—Trends in smoking quit ratio (%), NHISs, United States, 1965–87, adults aged 20 years and older

		Sex		Race		Educational level			
Year	Overall population	Males	Females	Whites	Blacks	Less than high school graduate	High school graduate	Some college	College graduate
1965[a]	29.6	31.4	24.6	30.5	22.8				
1966	29.5	31.4	24.2	30.4	22.6	33.3	28.0	28.7	39.7
1970	35.3	37.9	29.2	36.7	23.2	38.1	33.6	34.9	48.2
1974	36.3	39.3	30.8	38.0	21.8	38.0	35.2	36.6	47.9
1976	37.1	39.9	32.1	38.4	26.3	39.5	35.0	37.2	46.1
1977	36.8	40.3	31.3	38.2	24.8	38.3	34.0	36.8	48.6
1978	38.5	41.3	33.8	39.9	27.5	38.7	36.3	41.0	49.7
1979	39.0	41.5	34.0	40.3	28.0	40.8	36.7	37.5	50.6
1980	39.0	41.5	34.0	40.4	27.7	39.4	36.5	40.6	48.7
1983	41.8	44.1	37.6	43.3	29.3	42.1	38.7	41.2	54.9
1985	45.0	49.0	40.0	46.7	31.8	41.3	40.5	46.0	61.1
1987[b]	44.8	48.7	40.1	46.4	31.5	39.7	40.9	46.9	61.4
Trend information (1965–85)									
Change[c]/ year	+0.68	+0.73	+0.73	+0.72	+0.43	+0.41	+0.57	+0.73	+0.85
Standard error (±)	0.05	0.06	0.05	0.06	0.07	0.06	0.07	0.10	0.16
R^2	0.95	0.94	0.96	0.94	0.82	0.85	0.89	0.88	0.78

NOTE: Quit ratio = (Former Smokers/Current + Former Smokers)

[a]For 1965, data stratified by education were not available.

[b]Provisional data only.

[c]In percentage points.

SOURCE: NHISs 1965–87; unpublished data, Office on Smoking and Health.

contemplation, action, maintenance, and relapse. This categorization has proven useful in longitudinal research studies (see Part II of this Chapter and also Chapter 6); however, for cross-sectional population studies, this process of quitting can be analyzed according to current smoking status and the timing and duration of previous quit attempts. Thus, everyone can be classified on a smoking continuum.

This continuum is presented in Table 10. It is based on questions from the AUTS (see Appendix to this Chapter). Ten different categories are presented as percentages of the total population and as percentages of ever smokers. Categories of current smokers can also be described as percentages of all current smokers. These percentages are not provided below because of the possibility of misinterpretation. In particular, the percentage of those attempting to quit during the past year should not be calculated using current smokers as the denominator because this percentage excludes those who *successfully* quit during the past year. Instead, a more appropriate denominator (used below) would be those who were smokers at any time during the past year (including former smokers who quit during the past 12 months).

TABLE 10.—Smoking continuum, adults aged 17 years and older, United States, 1986

		Percentage of population	Percentage of ever smokers
Category 1	Never smokers	47.3	
Category 2	Former smokers who had quit 5 or more years ago	14.7	27.9
Category 3	Former smokers who had been abstinent for 1 to 5 years	5.7	10.8
Category 4	Former smokers who had been abstinent for 3 to 12 months	2.0	3.8
Category 5	Former smokers who had quit within the last 3 months	3.2	6.1
Category 6	Current smokers who had quit for 7 or more days in the past year	3.9	7.4
Category 7	Current smokers who had quit for 1–6 days in the past year	2.0	3.8
Category 8	Current smokers who had quit previously but not in the last year	11.6	22.0
Category 9	Current smokers who had never tried to quit but who had thought about it or would quit if there was an easy way to do so	5.4	10.2
Category 10	Current smokers who had never tried to quit, had not thought about it, and would not try to quit even if there was an easy way to do so	4.5	8.5

SOURCE: AUTS 1986 (US DHHS, in press, a).

The first category on this continuum includes those who have never smoked cigarettes. In 1986, 47.3 percent of the U.S. population 17 years of age and older was in this category. Former smokers who had quit smoking 5 or more years previously made up 14.7 percent of the population and 27.9 percent of ever smokers. Those in this category can be considered to be confirmed ex-smokers who are unlikely to relapse. Former smokers who had been abstinent for 1 to 5 years represented 10.8 percent of ever smokers. Former smokers who had been abstinent for less than a year represented 9.9 percent of ever smokers (categories 4 and 5 combined). Current smokers who had quit smoking for 7 or more days during the past year made up 7.4 percent of ever smokers. Another 3.8 percent of ever smokers had quit during the past year but were not able to stay off cigarettes for a week or more. Combining categories 4 through 7, 21.1 percent of ever smokers stopped smoking for at least 1 day during the year prior to the 1986 survey. This is 34 percent of all those who smoked that year.

Of ever smokers, 22.0 percent were current smokers who had previously made a serious quit attempt but not during the past year. Approximately 19 percent of ever smokers were current smokers who had never tried to quit; 45 percent of these have never thought about quitting and say that they would not quit even if there was an easy way to do so. Of those who had smoked during the past year, 70 percent had made at least one quit attempt (categories 4 through 8 divided by categories 4 through 10).

For the sake of convenience, category 10 is referred to below as the "hard-core smokers" category. However, it should be noted that others might also use this term to describe smokers who have failed to quit despite repeated attempts.

Tables 11 and 12 give the distribution for this smoking continuum by gender, education, race, and age. There are large differences between the subgroups in the proportion of ever smokers who are long-term abstainers (category 2). Males are more likely to be in this category than females, whites more than blacks, older people more than younger people, and the most highly educated more than the less well educated. The percentages of ever smokers in the categories reflecting recent quitting activity (4 through 7) and no recent quitting activity (8 through 10) were slightly higher for women than for men, probably resulting from the higher percentage of men in the combined categories 2 and 3 (abstinence for a year or more).

Educational differences in the smoking continuum are generally consistent with educational differences in smoking prevalence and quit ratio mentioned above. The proportion of ever smokers who have *not* tried to quit during the past year (categories 8 through 10) is 43.5 percent for the least educated group compared with 29.1 percent for the most educated group. The proportion in the hard-core smokers category is 9.8 percent for the least educated group compared with only 5.7 percent for the most educated group. However, the proportion of those who *have* made a quit attempt during the past year (categories 4 through 7) is also higher for the least educated group than for the most educated group (21.8 percent and 17.2 percent, respectively); this latter difference may reflect a lower success rate for quitting attempts among the least educated group. The differences between the least and most educated in these categories (4 through 7) become progressively smaller and then disappear as one moves from failed quit attempts during the past year (categories 6 and 7) to successful quit attempts

TABLE 11.—Smoking continuum by sex and education, percentage of ever smokers, United States, 1986

	Sex		Education			
	Males (%)	Females (%)	≤11 years (%)	12 years (%)	13–15 years (%)	≥16 years (%)
Smoking continuum						
Smokers who never tried to quit (10)[a]	8.3 (8.3)[b]	9.1 (9.1)	9.8 (9.8)	9.5 (9.5)	7.7 (7.7)	5.7 (5.7)
Smokers who never tried to quit (9)	9.1 (17.4)	9.6 (18.7)	9.8 (19.6)	9.5 (19.0)	10.9 (18.6)	5.7 (11.4)
Smokers not quitting in the last year (8)	21.5 (38.9)	23.9 (41.7)	23.9 (43.5)	22.5 (41.5)	22.5 (41.1)	17.7 (29.1)
Smokers quitting 1–6 days in the last year (7)	3.4 (42.3)	4.6 (46.3)	4.4 (47.9)	4.9 (46.4)	2.6 (43.7)	1.5 (30.6)
Smokers quitting 7 or more days in the last year (6)	6.5 (48.8)	8.6 (54.9)	7.4 (55.3)	7.9 (54.3)	8.6 (52.3)	5.0 (35.6)
Ex-smokers 0–3 months (5)	6.8 (55.6)	5.2 (60.1)	6.6 (61.9)	5.4 (59.7)	6.0 (58.3)	7.0 (42.6)
Ex-smokers 3–12 months (4)	3.6 (59.2)	4.3 (64.4)	3.4 (65.3)	4.1 (63.8)	4.7 (63.0)	3.7 (46.3)
Ex-smokers 1–5 years (3)	10.9 (70.1)	10.7 (75.1)	7.8 (73.1)	10.7 (74.5)	12.8 (75.8)	14.0 (60.3)
Ex-smokers ≥5 years (2)	30.1 (100)	25.1 (100)	27.2 (100)	25.3 (100)	24.4 (100)	39.2 (100)

[a]Category on the smoking continuum (see Table 10 for definitions).

[b]Numbers in parentheses are cumulative percentages.

SOURCE: AUTS 1986 (US DHHS, in press, a).

TABLE 12.—Smoking continuum by race and age, percentage of ever smokers, United States, 1986

	Race		Age			
	Whites (%)	Blacks (%)	18–24 years (%)	25–44 years (%)	45–64 years (%)	≥65 years (%)
Smoking continuum						
Smokers who never tried to quit (10)[a]	8.7 (8.7)[b]	8.6 (8.6)	9.1 (9.1)	6.9 (6.9)	8.3 (8.3)	7.4 (7.4)
Smokers who never tried to quit (9)	8.9 (17.6)	12.3 (20.9)	18.4 (27.5)	10.6 (17.5)	7.5 (15.8)	3.6 (11.0)
Smokers not quitting in the last year (8)	22.2 (39.8)	22.2 (43.1)	16.3 (43.8)	26.4 (43.9)	21.6 (37.4)	14.5 (25.5)
Smokers quitting 1–6 days in the last year (7)	3.6 (43.4)	6.9 (50.0)	7.2 (51.0)	4.4 (48.3)	3.2 (40.6)	2.1 (27.6)
Smokers quitting 7 or more days in the last year (6)	7.0 (50.4)	10.7 (60.7)	19.3 (70.3)	8.6 (56.9)	4.7 (45.3)	2.0 (29.6)
Ex-smokers 0–3 months (5)	5.9 (56.3)	7.5 (68.2)	7.2 (77.5)	5.8 (62.7)	6.2 (51.5)	8.2 (37.8)
Ex-smokers 3–12 months (4)	4.0 (60.3)	3.3 (71.5)	9.0 (86.5)	4.3 (67.0)	3.2 (54.7)	2.5 (40.3)
Ex-smokers 1–5 years (3)	10.8 (71.1)	9.4 (80.9)	10.3 (96.8)	11.4 (78.9)	9.9 (64.6)	10.1 (50.4)
Ex-smokers ≥5 years (2)	28.8 (100)	19.0 (100)	3.0 (100)	20.6 (100)	35.6 (100)	49.7 (100)

[a]Category on the smoking continuum (see Table 10 for definitions).
[b]Numbers in parentheses are cumulative percentages.
SOURCE: AUTS 1986 (US DHHS, in press, a).

during the past year (categories 4 and 5). For prolonged abstinence (1 or more years) (categories 2 and 3), the proportions then become greater for the more educated.

Among ever smokers, about two-fifths of both blacks and whites have not tried to quit during the past year, with 9 percent in the hard-core smokers category. Twenty-one percent of white ever smokers have made a quit attempt during the past year compared with 28 percent of blacks.

A person's likelihood of being in different categories of the smoking continuum differs considerably with age. About 44 percent of ever smokers between the ages of 25 and 44 years are smokers who have not made an attempt to quit during the past year, compared with 26 percent of those 65 years of age and older. However, there are roughly equal proportions of each age group in the hard-core smokers category. The proportion of ever smokers who made a quit attempt in the last year was highest (42.7 percent) in the youngest age group (18 to 24 years old) and is progressively smaller for each older age group (23.1 percent, 17.3 percent, and 14.8 percent, respectively, in those aged 25 to 44 years, 45 to 64 years, and 65 years and older).

Summary

As with trends in smoking status, trends in quitting activity have exhibited a consistent pattern since 1965. Almost half of the population who have ever been smokers have quit. Although the proportion of males who have quit is higher than that of females and the proportion of whites who have quit is higher than that of blacks, the rate of increase in the quit ratio is similar between these categories. The only diverging trend over time is the quitting activity for the less educated compared with the more educated.

One-third of those who smoked during the year prior to the 1986 AUTS quit smoking for at least 1 day during that year. Health education and motivational campaigns targeted at these individuals could help maintain them in "contemplation" and "action" stages (Prochaska and DiClemente 1983) and move them toward repeated quit attempts (see Part II).

Trends in the Proportion of Smokers Who Are Heavy Smokers

Although all the NHISs have included information on the number of cigarettes smoked per day, respondent rules on this question changed in 1974. Prior to that date, smoking information was obtained from either the sampled individual or a proxy adult living in the same household. For each survey since the 1974 NHIS, smoking information has been accepted only from the sampled individual. Proxy respondents have been shown to be less accurate in reporting daily cigarette consumption than self-respondents (US DHEW 1969, p. 794; Rogot and Reid 1975; National Research Council 1986, pp. 110–112). Proxy responses can be eliminated from analyses of the pre-1974 data to examine long-term trends in daily cigarette consumption. However, excluding proxy responses may make the sample nonrepresentative (see Chapter 3). Accordingly, in considering trends in the proportion of the smoking population who smoke 25 or more cigarettes per day, only NHIS data from 1974–85 are used here.

The proportion of smokers who smoked 25 or more cigarettes per day in each survey is presented in Table 13 and is shown in Figure 1. This proportion ranged from 25.5 to 29.8 percent and did not change significantly from 1974 through 1985 (p=0.4). In addition, this proportion did not change among sex- and race-specific subgroups of the smoking population (Figure 2) or in different age groups (NCHS 1988c). Heavy smoking has been consistently more common among whites compared with blacks, and among men compared with women; the differential by race has been greater than the differential by sex (Figure 2).

TABLE 13.—Self-reported cigarettes smoked per day (percentage of current smokers), United States, aged 20 years and older, 1974–85

	Number of cigarettes smoked per day		
Year	1–14	15–24	≥25
1974	30.8	43.2	26.0
1976	30.1	44.4	25.5
1977	30.3	43.2	26.5
1978	28.1	42.8	29.1
1979	28.2	43.0	28.8
1980	27.6	42.6	29.8
1983	28.5	44.9	26.6
1985	31.0	41.9	27.1

SOURCE: NHISs 1974–85; unpublished data, Office on Smoking and Health.

It is theoretically possible that the proportion of the "heaviest" smokers is increasing even though the proportion of "heavy" smokers (25 or more cigarettes per day) has not changed. However, no major increase occurred from 1974–85 in the proportion of smokers smoking 40 or more cigarettes per day (Table 14). The overall proportion smoking 40 or more cigarettes per day was 12.6 percent in 1974 and 13.2 percent in 1985. Table 14 also demonstrates respondents' inclination to report their daily cigarette consumption in round numbers related to the size of a cigarette pack (e.g., 10 or 20 cigarettes per day) (see Kozlowski 1986).

Because the sales-weighted average nicotine yield declined from 1974–83 (see Figure 14 in Chapter 2), one might expect to have observed an increase in average daily cigarette consumption. Compensatory changes in smoking behavior to maintain relatively constant nicotine intake have been shown to occur when smokers switch from high-yield to lower yield cigarettes (US DHHS 1988). Although daily cigarette consumption did not increase from 1974–85, other compensatory changes may have occurred (e.g., increased frequency of puffing or depth of inhalation) as the smoking population moved toward lower yield brands.

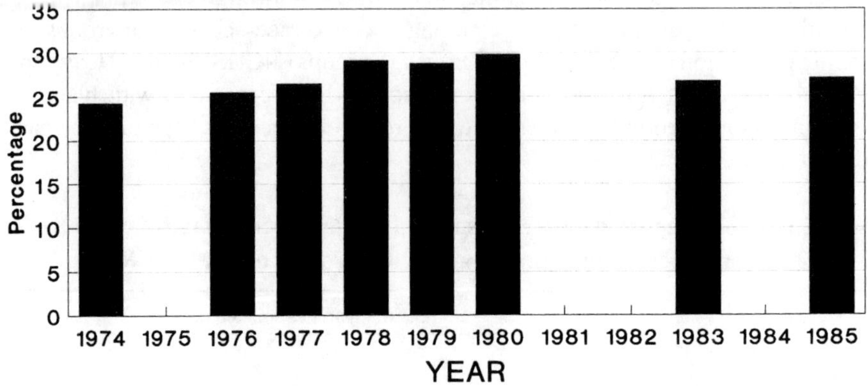

FIGURE 1.—Percentage of current smokers smoking ≥25 cigarettes per day, adults aged 20 years and older, United States, 1974–85

SOURCE: NHISs 1974–85; unpublished data, Office on Smoking and Health.

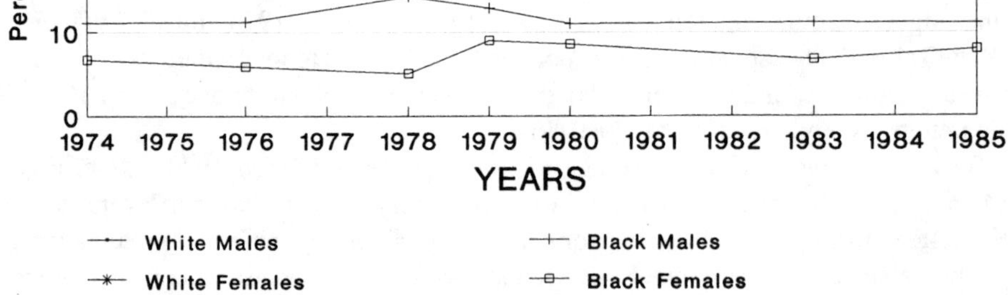

FIGURE 2.—Percentage of current smokers smoking ≥25 cigarettes per day, by race and gender, adults aged 20 years and older, United States, 1974–85

SOURCE: NHISs 1974–85; unpublished data, Office on Smoking and Health.

TABLE 14.—Self-reported cigarettes smoked per day (percentage of current smokers) by sex and race, United States, aged 20 years and older, 1974 and 1985

			Sex				Race			
	Overall		Males		Females		Blacks		Whites	
Cigarettes per day	1974	1985	1974	1985	1974	1985	1974	1985	1974	1985
1–9	15.0	15.0	12.0	12.5	18.3	17.7	30.0	28.1	12.7	12.8
10	12.6	12.6	9.9	10.2	15.6	15.1	21.9	21.3	11.4	11.2
11–19	10.9	11.3	10.0	10.9	12.0	11.7	14.8	14.1	10.3	10.9
20	35.1	32.9	35.5	32.4	34.5	33.5	23.9	26.1	36.7	33.9
21–39	13.8	15.0	16.8	17.2	10.7	12.6	5.1	5.8	15.1	16.6
40	10.1	9.5	12.3	11.9	7.5	7.0	3.7	3.0	11.0	10.6
≥41	2.5	3.7	3.5	4.9	1.4	2.4	0.6	1.6	2.8	4.0

SOURCE: NHISs 1974, 1985 (unpublished data, Office on Smoking and Health).

Trends in the Initiation of Smoking

Information on smoking patterns during adolescence is important because smoking initiation usually occurs during this age. Presented below are data concerning three measures of smoking behavior during adolescence: (1) age of smoking initiation; (2) trends in smoking prevalence among persons 20 to 24 years of age, used as an indicator of smoking initiation; and (3) smoking prevalence among adolescents.

Data on age of initiation provide information on the ages during which initiation usually occurs, but provide no information on the extent of tobacco use within the adolescent population. The prevalence of smoking among those 20 to 24 years of age serves as an indicator of smoking initiation among adolescents during the several years preceding a particular survey. This measure offers the advantages that smoking initiation is relatively complete by the time one enters this age group, and a survey sample representative of the total age-specific population can be obtained readily. However, these data offer no information on the ages during which smoking initiation actually occurred and do not necessarily reflect the most current initiation patterns among adolescents. Data on smoking prevalence among adolescents provide direct and current information on smoking behavior in the population of concern. However, interpretation of adolescent survey data is complicated by the use of different definitions of regular and experimental smoking in different surveys and by the failure of some surveys (e.g., school surveys of high school seniors) to include groups known to smoke at higher rates (e.g., high school dropouts).

Age of Initiation

Age of smoking initiation is a critical variable in targeting prevention efforts. Information on self-reported age of initiation is available from surveys of adolescents and adults. Adolescent surveys offer the advantage of providing current information on age of initiation without concerns of recall bias. However, these surveys cannot provide complete information on age of initiation because the samples exclude those who may start smoking at older ages. Adult surveys provide complete information on age of initiation, but recall bias may occur because adults are asked about an event (smoking initiation) that typically occurred decades earlier. A major value of an adult survey is that, by using birth cohorts, one can assess whether smoking initiation has changed over time.

In the 1986 High School Seniors Survey sponsored by NIDA (see below), seniors who had ever smoked were asked the grade in which they had smoked their first cigarette. About one-quarter of seniors smoked their first cigarette by grade 6, one-half by grade 8, three-fourths by grade 9, and 94 percent by grade 11 (Table 15). Males and whites were more likely to smoke their first cigarette at earlier grades than females and blacks, respectively. The pattern of smoking initiation was similar for those with and without plans for higher education.

In addition, the 1987 National Adolescent Student Health Survey (NASHS) (see below) collected information on the grade in which 8th and 10th grade students had smoked their first cigarette. Data are presented in Table 16 for 10th graders only. Ap-

TABLE 15.—Grade by which ever smokers smoked their first cigarette (%), reported by high school seniors, United States, 1986

Grade	Total	Males	Females	Whites	Blacks	Higher education plans	
						Yes	No
6	25.8	31.1	20.7	26.8	23.3	25.3	25.7
8	57.3	59.5	55.3	59.0	50.2	56.5	58.0
9	72.5	72.7	72.5	74.0	65.8	70.8	75.3
10	84.2	83.8	84.7	85.0	78.4	83.0	86.7
11	94.3	93.8	95.0	95.3	89.9	93.5	95.9
12	100.0	100.0	100.0	100.0	100.0	100.0	100.0
Sample size	3,079	1,423	1,526	2,308	302	1,791	972

SOURCE: Institute for Social Research, University of Michigan (Bachman, Johnston, O'Malley 1987).

proximately one-quarter of smokers reported that they had started smoking by grade 6 and approximately one-half of smokers had started by grade 7 or 8. Males were somewhat more likely than females to start smoking prior to grade 7, but females caught up by grade 9 due to their higher initiation rates in grades 7 to 9.

TABLE 16.—Recall of grade at smoking initiation by 10th-grade students, United States, 1987

	Males		Females	
	%	Cumulative %	%	Cumulative %
By grade 4	11.0	11.0	8.5	8.5
Grades 5 or 6	17.9	28.9	14.0	22.5
Grades 7 or 8	24.1	53.0	26.1	48.6
Grade 9	6.9	59.9	10.9	59.5
Grade 10	2.1	62.0	4.6	64.1
Not smoking by grade 10	38.1	100.0	35.9	100.0

SOURCE: National Adolescent Student Health Survey 1987 (US DHHS, in press, b).

Information on age of initiation is available for adults from NHISs conducted in 1978, 1979, 1980, and 1987. The 1987 data were not available for inclusion in the data presented below. The 1978–80 data are derived from responses to the question, "About how old were you when you first started smoking cigarettes fairly regularly?" These data have been used in previously published analyses of age of smoking initiation(US DHHS 1985; Harris 1983; McGinnis, Shopland, Brown 1987) and are again used below. The populations from the three NHISs were combined and grouped by 5-year birth cohorts. In the total sample, the average age of initiation among ever smokers (aged 20 to 64 years) was 17.2 for men and 19.1 for women (US DHHS 1985). The proportion of ever smokers (20 years of age and older) within each birth cohort who had started smoking before different ages is presented separately for males and females in Table 17 and Figures 3 and 4.

Among smokers born since 1935, more than four-fifths started smoking before age 21 and almost half started before age 18. The data reveal few differences across birth cohorts in age of initiation before age 16. However, for more recent birth cohorts, there has been a tendency for a higher percentage of ever smokers to have initiated smoking before age 18 or 21. The proportion starting before age 18 has increased from 38 percent of ever smokers born from 1910–14 to approximately half of ever smokers born between 1950 and 1954. The proportion starting before age 21 has increased between these two birth cohorts from 66 to 87 percent (Table 17). Stratifying by sex shows that this tendency for more recent birth cohorts to initiate smoking at a younger age has occurred among both sexes but has been more striking among females (Figures 3 and 4).

The data from the earliest birth cohorts may be biased somewhat by differential mortality among smokers with different ages of initiation. Mortality rates for smoking-related diseases are higher for smokers with younger ages of initiation (US DHHS 1982, 1983, 1984). Thus, the age of initiation data may be biased upward among, for example, the 1910–19 birth cohort, whose members were 61 to 70 years old in the last survey year included in these data (1980). However, the trend noted above toward declining age of initiation, especially among females, is still apparent when considering only those born since 1930. As pointed out above, the decline in age of initiation among males is only seen in the proportion of ever smokers starting before age 21.

In summary, these data indicate that uptake of smoking is now a phenomenon that occurs almost entirely during the teenage years and that the initiation of smoking is occurring at younger ages among more recent birth cohorts, especially among females. Data from the 1986 AUTS on age of initiation of smokeless tobacco use are presented in the Section on Smokeless Tobacco later in this Chapter.

Prevalence in 20- to 24-Year Age Group

The most complete ascertainment of smoking initiation would involve the collection of longitudinal data on children from the ages of about 9 to 21 years. Such complete population-based information for the United States is not available. However, trends in smoking prevalence in the 20- to 24-year age group (Table 18), as determined by the NHIS, provide an indirect measure of trends in smoking initiation. Using this measure has the advantage that smoking initiation is relatively complete by age 20. However, there is a lag of several years between actual initiation during adolescence and prevalence in this group. The R^2 values for the regression lines derived from these data are above 0.70 for sex-, race-, and education-specific groups, except for females overall, among whom initiation rates varied considerably.

From 1965–87, smoking initiation, as measured by prevalence among those aged 20 to 24 years, decreased from 47.8 percent to 29.5 percent, at a rate of decline from 1965–85 of 0.69 percentage points per year. There are marked gender differences in this measure of initiation. Smoking prevalence among young males has fallen from 56.3 percent in 1965 to 31.1 percent in 1987 at a rate of change (1965–85) of –1.19 percentage points per year. In contrast, smoking prevalence among young females has fallen

TABLE 17.—Proportion of ever smokers (%) who started smoking before various ages, by gender, birth cohorts from NHISs

Age at smoking initiation		Year of birth								
		1910–14	1915–19	1920–24	1925–29	1930–34	1935–39	1940–44	1945–49	1950–54
<14	Overall	8.9	11.0	9.2	8.1	8.8	8.3	8.5	8.5	8.6
	Male	13.0	16.3	12.5	11.7	12.8	11.1	11.1	10.1	10.3
	Female	2.6	3.4	4.2	2.7	3.7	4.7	5.1	6.1	6.6
<16	Overall	20.0	21.6	19.5	19.1	22.2	21.3	23.0	23.7	23.8
	Male	28.4	30.3	25.7	25.5	30.1	25.9	27.7	28.2	26.8
	Female	7.2	9.5	9.7	9.8	11.9	15.6	17.1	17.9	20.2
<18	Overall	38.3	42.1	40.0	42.9	45.0	46.0	48.5	47.2	52.0
	Male	49.9	53.1	48.7	54.0	56.9	53.8	55.6	52.2	56.6
	Female	20.6	26.7	26.2	26.8	29.8	35.6	40.1	40.9	46.7
<21	Overall	66.2	70.8	70.7	76.5	75.6	81.7	83.1	83.8	87.3
	Male	76.5	78.8	79.9	85.4	83.1	85.9	86.1	87.3	90.3
	Female	50.3	59.5	56.0	63.5	66.3	75.9	79.5	79.1	83.8
<25	Overall	78.0	83.2	86.9	88.8	90.0	92.7	93.8	95.5	97.7
	Male	88.7	90.4	93.8	95.2	95.0	95.0	96.3	97.8	98.5
	Female	61.9	72.6	75.8	79.5	83.7	89.5	90.9	92.7	96.7

SOURCE: NHISs 1978, 1979, 1980 combined (unpublished data, Office on Smoking and Health).

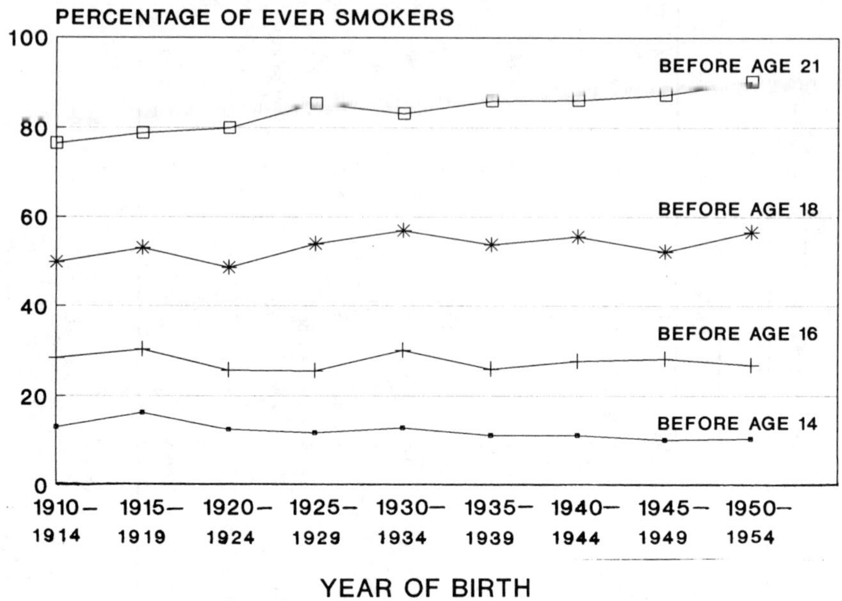

FIGURE 3.—Age by which males started smoking, by birth cohort

SOURCE: NHISs 1978–80, combined (unpublished data, Office on Smoking and Health).

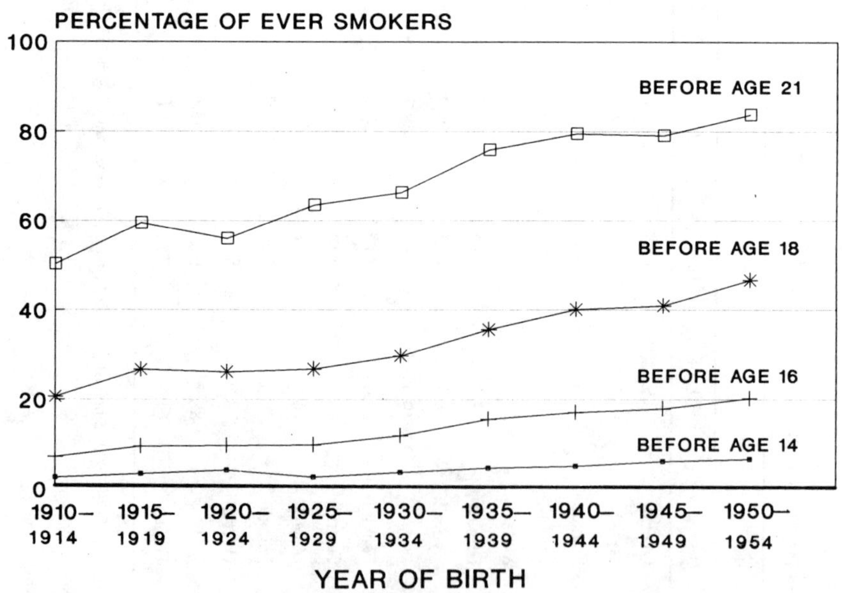

FIGURE 4.—Age by which females started smoking, by birth cohort

SOURCE: NHISs 1978–80, combined (unpublished data, Office on Smoking and Health).

TABLE 18.—Trends in smoking initiation, NHISs, United States, 1965–87

	Smoking prevalence (%), ages 20–24								
						Education level			
		Sex		Race		High school graduate or less		Some college or more	
Year	Overall population	Males	Females	Whites	Blacks	Males	Females	Males	Females
1965	47.8	56.3	40.5	47.5	50.8	63.6	42.6	42.7	34.5
1966	47.7	57.7	39.5	48.2	45.5	65.1	41.3	43.5	34.7
1970	41.5	48.5	35.8	41.2	45.2	60.0	40.2	33.2	26.8
1974	39.5	44.3	35.4	38.6	47.1	52.7	40.1	34.7	26.4
1976	39.6	45.9	34.2	39.5	42.3	54.1	41.0	34.4	23.0
1977	38.8	40.4	37.4	38.5	41.5	52.2	43.0	24.0	27.5
1978	35.4	38.5	32.5	35.7	34.8	46.8	39.3	25.9	21.1
1979	35.8	37.7	34.0	35.6	36.7	47.1	41.9	23.8	22.1
1980	36.1	40.0	32.5	35.9	37.9	50.1	40.3	20.1	19.4
1983	36.9	36.9	37.0	36.8	38.7	49.1	45.5	16.2	22.9
1985	31.8	31.0	32.5	32.5	28.2	43.0	43.6	15.5	17.2
1987[a]	29.5	31.1	28.1	30.5	25.6	43.8	37.6	16.3	15.1
Trend information (1965–85)									
Change[b]/year	–0.69	–1.19	–0.28	–0.68	–0.79	–1.00	0.10	–1.51	–0.72
Standard error	0.09	0.10	0.12	0.09	0.17	0.13	0.10	0.13	0.15
R^2	0.86	0.94	0.40	0.85	0.71	0.87	NA[c]	0.95	0.75

[a]Provisional data only.

[b]In percentage points.

[c]The slope of the regression line was not significantly different from zero, making the R^2 computation inappropriate.

SOURCE: NHISs 1965–87; unpublished data, Office on Smoking and Health.

only from 40.5 percent in 1965 to 28.1 percent in 1987 at a rate of change (1965–85) one-quarter that of young males (–0.28 percentage points per year). The slower rate of decline among women is due, in large part, to the increase in initiation rates in less educated young women (Pierce, Fiore et al. 1989b).

Smoking initiation patterns among whites and blacks have been similar during the past 20 years. From 1965–87, smoking prevalence among whites aged 20 to 24 years has decreased from 47.5 percent to 30.5 percent, while for blacks the decline has been from 50.8 percent to 25.6 percent. The rates of change between 1965 and 1985 among whites and blacks were similar (–0.68 and –0.79 percentage points per year, respectively). The prevalence of smoking had been higher among young blacks than among young whites for most survey years between 1965 and 1983, but whites had a higher prevalence in 1985 and 1987.

Marked differences in smoking initiation rates based on educational level have occurred. From 1965–87, the smoking initiation rate as measured by prevalence, ages 20 to 24, fell among males with 12 or fewer years of schooling (high school graduate or less) from 63.6 percent to 43.8 percent (–1.00 percentage point per year from 1965–85). In contrast, for males with 13 or more years of schooling (some college or more), prevalence has fallen from 42.7 percent to 16.3 percent, at a rate of decline (1965–85) of 1.51 percentage points per year. A similar difference in initiation rates by education was seen among women, although the rate of decline between 1965 and 1985 was less among women than among men of equivalent education. In the overall sample (men and women combined), the rate of decrease in initiation among persons with 13 or more years of education (1.10 percentage points per year) was three times that among persons with 12 or fewer years of education (0.35).

Trends in Adolescent Smoking

Several surveys have provided national estimates of smoking prevalence among adolescents. Because these surveys differ in terms of the definitions of smoking, ages of respondents, sample size, method of data collection (household versus school versus telephone interview), years in which the surveys were conducted, and overall results, the findings of the major surveys are presented below.

NIDA High School Seniors Surveys on Drug Use, 1976–87

Data from the NIDA-sponsored High School Seniors Surveys have been collected annually since 1975 and are presented in Table 19. These surveys have been carried out by the University of Michigan Institute for Social Research (Johnston, O'Malley, Bachman 1987). This data set is most useful for examining trends in smoking. Individual prevalence figures probably underestimate actual adolescent smoking prevalence because the survey does not include high school dropouts, who are known to have much higher smoking rates (Pirie et al. 1988; Yates et al. 1988).

Reported daily smoking of cigarettes has decreased among high school seniors from a peak prevalence of 29 percent in 1976 to 19 percent in 1987. However, the trend has not been linear. The majority of the change occurred between 1978 and 1980, after

TABLE 19.—Smoking status (%) of high school seniors, United States, 1975–87

Year	Daily smokers	Less than daily smokers	Previous smokers, not in last month	Never smokers
1975	27	10	37	26
1976	29	10	36	25
1977	29	10	38	24
1978	28	9	38	25
1979	26	9	40	26
1980	21	9	41	29
1981	20	9	42	29
1982	21	9	40	30
1983	20	9	41	29
1984	18	11	41	30
1985	19	11	39	31
1986	18	11	38	32
1987	19	11	38	33

SOURCE: Institute for Social Research, University of Michigan (Bachman, Johnston, O'Malley 1980a,b, 1981, 1984, 1985, 1987; Johnston and Bachman 1980; Johnston, Bachman, O'Malley 1980a,b, 1982, 1984, 1986, and unpublished data, 1987).

which prevalence has remained relatively stable. The proportion of high school seniors who have smoked within the last month, although not on a daily basis, has not changed substantially during this period. There is also rather little change in the proportion of this population who has previously smoked but not in the last 30 days. The proportion of high school seniors who have never smoked increased from 26 percent to 33 percent between 1975 and 1987.

Trends in smoking status by sex, race, and educational plans are presented in Table 20. The prevalence of daily smoking decreased in all major subcategories of high school seniors between 1976 and 1987. Daily smoking among males decreased from a peak prevalence of 28 percent in 1976 to 16 percent in 1987; most of this drop occurred between 1977 and 1980. Daily smoking among females decreased from a peak prevalence of 30 percent in 1977 to 20 percent in 1987, with the largest decrease occurring from 1979–81. Since 1981, the prevalence of daily smoking among high school students has remained fairly constant for both males and females. In each year since 1977, the prevalence of daily smoking has been higher in females than in males (median difference=4 percentage points).

The prevalence of daily smoking fell substantially among blacks, from 26 percent in 1976 to 8 percent in 1987. During the same period, prevalence declined among whites from 29 percent to 20 percent. The reasons for the dramatic decline among blacks are unclear. It does not appear to be due to increasing sampling bias over time—survey methods and sample sizes by race have been consistent. A substantial decrease in smoking initiation among blacks also occurred, as measured in the NHIS by prevalence in persons 20 to 24 years of age, between 1983 (38.7 percent) and 1985 (28.2 percent) (Table 18). This figure declined further to a preliminary estimate of 25.6 percent in 1987.

Students with plans to pursue higher education were much less likely to be daily smokers in 1976 than those without such plans (21 percent versus 37 percent). The ab-

TABLE 20.—Smoking status (%) of high school seniors by sex, race, and educational plans, United States, 1975–87

	Daily smokers						Less than daily smokers					
	Sex		Race		Plans for higher education		Sex		Race		Plans for higher education	
Year	M	F	W	B	Yes	No	M	F	W	B	Yes	No
1975	27	26					10	10				
1976	28	28	29	26	21	37	10	10	10	13	10	10
1977	28	30	28	25	20	38	10	10	9	11	10	9
1978	26	29	27	22	18	36	9	10	9	9	9	9
1979	22	28	26	19	17	35	9	9	9	9	9	9
1980	18	24	22	16	14	31	8	10	9	10	9	10
1981	18	22	20	13	13	30	8	10	9	9	9	9
1982	18	24	23	12	13	30	9	9	9	9	9	9
1983	19	23	22	12	14	30	9	10	9	9	10	9
1984	16	21	20	8	11	29	10	11	11	9	11	11
1985	17	21	20	11	13	31	10	11	11	8	10	11
1986	17	20	21	8	12	29	11	11	12	7	11	10
1987	16	20	20	8	14	30	11	11	12	6	11	11

TABLE 20.—Continued

	Previous smokers, not in last month						Never smokers					
	Sex		Race		Plans for higher education		Sex		Race		Plans for higher education	
Year	M	F	W	B	Yes	No	M	F	W	B	Yes	No
1975	38	36					24	28				
1976	38	36	37	36	39	35	24	25	25	24	31	19
1977	39	35	37	49	41	35	24	25	25	26	30	19
1978	40	38	38	40	42	35	26	24	25	29	31	20
1979	42	38	39	41	42	37	27	25	26	30	32	20
1980	43	39	40	45	44	37	30	28	29	30	34	23
1981	43	41	41	45	45	38	31	27	29	33	33	24
1982	41	39	40	43	43	37	32	28	29	36	35	24
1983	41	40	40	45	43	38	31	28	29	34	34	24
1984	41	39	40	42	42	38	33	29	29	40	35	24
1985	39	39	38	42	41	36	33	30	30	39	36	24
1986	38	38	38	41	39	37	34	31	30	44	37	25
1987	38	38	38	41	39	35	35	31	30	45	37	25

SOURCE: Institute for Social Research, University of Michigan (See Table 19 for citations).

solute difference (in percentage points) between the two groups remained constant between 1976 and 1987. In 1987, the prevalence of daily smokers among those with plans for higher education was less than half the prevalence among those without such plans (14 percent versus 30 percent).

The percentage of blacks who smoke on less than a daily basis exceeded the percentage of whites in 1976 (13 and 10 percent, respectively) but was lower than the percentage of whites in 1987 (6 and 12 percent, respectively). The percentage who have previously smoked but not in the past month has consistently been slightly higher among blacks than among whites and among those with plans for higher education than among those without college plans. Besides these findings, there have been few differences between subgroups and few changes between 1976 and 1987 in the proportion of high school seniors who are in these categories.

As mentioned above, the decrease in the proportion of high school seniors who smoke on a daily basis is reflected by a complementary increase in the proportion of high school seniors who have never smoked. This increase has been more marked among males compared with females and among blacks compared with whites.

1987 National Adolescent Student Health Survey

The 1987 NASHS collected data on prevalence of smoking within the last 30 days (US DHHS, in press,b). Respondents to this survey composed a random sample of the Nation's students in 8th and 10th grades. Sixty-three percent of the 8th graders were 13 years old and 27 percent were 14 years old. Sixty-two percent of the 10th graders were 15 years old and 28 percent were 16 years old. For each grade, 68 percent were white, 17 percent were black, and 9 percent were Hispanic.

Prevalence data are presented in Table 21. Eighty-four percent of the eighth graders reported that they had not even puffed on a cigarette in the last 30 days, with little difference between the sexes. Forty-nine percent of all eighth graders reported never having smoked a cigarette, with no difference between the sexes. Among 10th graders, the proportion not having puffed on a cigarette in the last 30 days was slightly lower: 76 percent among males and 71 percent among females. Thirty-eight percent of males and 36 percent of females in this grade reported that they had never had a cigarette.

TABLE 21.—30-day prevalence of smoking (%), United States, 1987, 8th and 10th grades

	8th grade		10th grade	
	Males	Females	Males	Females
Not even a puff	84.9	83.0	75.9	71.3
1–4 cigarettes	7.1	8.2	7.8	10.4
5–19 cigarettes	2.7	3.4	4.8	5.1
1–5 packs	2.4	3.5	5.6	7.4
More than 5 packs	2.9	1.9	6.0	5.8

SOURCE: National Adolescent Student Health Survey 1987 (US DHHS, in press, b).

Approximately equal proportions (7 to 8 percent) of males and females in the eighth grade reported smoking a pack or more in the last month. Among 10th graders, this proportion was more than twice as high, with 17 percent of males and 19 percent of females reporting that they smoked a pack or more in the last month.

US DHEW Teenage Smoking Surveys, 1968–79

Detailed questions on smoking were asked in five national telephone surveys of adolescents (ages 12 to 18 years) conducted by Chilton Research Services for the U.S. Department of Health, Education, and Welfare from 1968 through 1979 (US DHEW 1979b). Adolescents were classified by smoking status as follows: *never smokers*, had not taken even a few puffs of a cigarette; *experimental smokers*, had had a few puffs but had not smoked as many as 100 cigarettes; *ex-smokers*, had smoked at least 100 cigarettes but no longer smoked; *current occasional smokers*, smoked less than one cigarette per week; and *current regular smokers*, smoked at least one cigarette per week. In published results for these surveys, data for never smokers and experimental smokers were generally aggregated.

Summary data from each of the surveys are presented in Table 22 (males) and Table 23 (females). The proportion of both males and females of each age group who are classified as either never smokers or experimental smokers is substantially higher than the proportion of never smokers reported by other surveys. For example, the 1979 Teenage Smoking Survey showed that 75 percent of males and 82 percent of females aged 15 to 16 years had never smoked or had only experimented with cigarettes; in contrast, the 1987 NASHS (above) showed that only 38 percent of males and 36 percent of females in the 10th grade (15 to 16 years old) had never had a cigarette. Similarly, the 1979 Teenage Smoking Survey showed that 68 percent of males and 64 percent of females aged 17 to 18 years were either never smokers or experimental smokers; in contrast, the 1979 High School Seniors Survey showed that 27 percent of males and 25 percent of females were never smokers.

There are at least two possible explanations for the consistently and surprisingly high proportion of teenagers in the categories of never smokers and experimental smokers. First, 100 cigarettes may be too high a cutoff to use for classifying teenagers as never smokers or experimenters. Second, telephone interviewing may lead to more underreporting of cigarette smoking behavior than other survey modalities. Underreporting may be more important for some smoking categories than others—for instance, occasional smokers might be particularly sensitive about their smoking behavior and might be more likely to underreport the total number of cigarettes they have ever smoked.

Current smoking rates can also be compared between the Teenage Smoking Surveys and the High School Seniors Surveys. In the 1979 telephone survey, teenagers were classified on their reported smoking on a weekly basis. Of males aged 17 to 18 years, 19.3 percent were classified as current regular smokers (one or more cigarettes per week) and another 0.3 percent were classified as current occasional smokers (less than one cigarette per week). For females aged 17 to 18 years, these figures were 26.2 percent and 0.8 percent, respectively. In the High School Seniors Survey, students are

TABLE 22.—Cigarette smoking among teenage males, United States, 1968–79

		Age							
		12–14 years		15–16 years		17–18 years		Total	
Smoking status	Year	N	%	N	%	N	%	N	%
Never smoked or	1968	876	93.1	465	75.2	344	54.7	1,685	77.0
experimented only	1970	512	90.5	268	70.5	178	48.1	958	72.8
	1972	533	91.1	273	68.3	211	54.4	1,017	74.1
	1974	496	90.7	253	69.5	202	55.3	951	74.5
	1979	527	92.8	284	75.3	254	68.1	1,065	80.8
Former smoker	1968	25	2.7	34	5.5	71	11.3	130	5.9
	1970	21	3.7	35	9.2	52	14.1	108	8.2
	1972	20	3.4	50	12.5	56	14.4	126	9.2
	1974	28	5.1	45	12.4	44	12.1	117	9.2
	1979	23	4.0	38	10.1	46	12.3	107	8.1
Current occasional	1968	13	1.4	14	2.3	24	3.8	51	2.3
smoker	1970	1	0.2	3	0.8	2	0.5	6	0.5
	1972	5	0.9	6	1.5	4	1.0	15	1.1
	1974	0	0.0	0	0.0	6	1.6	6	0.5
	1979	0	0.0	4	1.1	1	0.3	5	0.4

TABLE 22.—Continued

		Age							
		12–14 years		15–16 years		17–18 years		Total	
Smoking status	Year	N	%	N	%	N	%	N	%
Current regular smoker	1968	27	2.9	105	17.0	190	30.2	322	14.7
	1970	32	5.7	74	19.5	138	37.3	244	18.5
	1972	27	4.6	71	17.8	117	30.2	215	15.7
	1974	23	4.2	66	18.1	113	31.0	202	15.8
	1979	18	3.2	51	13.5	72	19.3	141	10.7
Total	1968	941	100	618	100	629	100	2,188	100
	1970	566	100	380	100	370	100	1,316	100
	1972	585	100	400	100	388	100	1,373	100
	1974	547	100	364	100	365	100	1,276	100
	1979	568	100	377	100	373	100	1,318	100

SOURCE: US DHEW Teenage Smoking Surveys, 1968, 1970, 1972, 1974, 1979 (US DHEW 1979b).

TABLE 23.—Cigarette smoking among teenage females, United States, 1968–79

		Age							
		12–14 years		15–16 years		17–18 years		Total	
Smoking status	Year	N	%	N	%	N	%	N	%
Never smoked or	1968	919	97.9	552	84.4	462	73.0	1,933	86.8
experimented only	1970	536	95.0	312	81.5	264	70.0	1,112	84.0
	1972	569	95.3	312	77.0	277	66.7	1,158	81.7
	1974	495	90.2	250	69.3	228	62.1	973	76.2
	1979	514	92.3	319	81.8	239	63.9	1,072	81.2
Former smoker	1968	7	0.7	25	3.8	38	6.0	70	3.1
	1970	8	1.4	15	3.9	22	5.8	45	3.4
	1972	11	1.8	26	6.4	30	7.2	67	4.7
	1974	26	4.7	33	9.1	42	11.4	101	7.9
	1979	19	3.4	23	5.9	34	9.1	76	5.8
Current occasional	1968	7	0.7	14	2.1	15	2.4	36	1.6
smoker	1970	3	0.5	1	0.3	5	1.3	9	0.7
	1972	0	0.0	1	0.2	3	0.7	4	0.3
	1974	1	0.2	5	1.4	2	0.5	8	0.6
	1979	0	0.0	2	0.5	3	0.8	5	0.4

TABLE 23.—Continued

		Age							
		12–14 years		15–16 years		17–18 years		Total	
Smoking status	Year	N	%	N	%	N	%	N	%
Current regular	1968	6	0.6	63	9.6	118	18.6	187	8.4
smoker	1970	17	3.0	55	14.4	86	22.8	158	11.9
	1972	17	2.8	66	16.3	105	25.3	188	13.3
	1974	27	4.9	73	20.2	95	25.9	195	15.3
	1979	24	4.3	46	11.8	98	26.2	168	12.7
Total	1968	939	100	654	100	633	100	2,226	100
	1970	564	100	383	100	377	100	1,324	100
	1972	597	100	405	100	415	100	1,417	100
	1974	549	100	361	100	367	100	1,277	100
	1979	557	100	390	100	374	100	1,321	100

SOURCE: US DHEW Teenage Smoking Surveys, 1968, 1970, 1972, 1974, 1979 (US DHEW 1979b).

classified based on their reported smoking during the past 30 days. In the 1979 High School Seniors Survey (Table 22), 22 percent of males were classified as daily smokers and another 9 percent reported having smoked in the last month but not on a daily basis. In the same year, 29 percent of females were daily smokers and 9 percent smoked on less than a daily basis.

Comparing these two data sets shows that the telephone survey obtained lower estimates for *weekly* smoking than the school survey obtained for *daily* smoking (19 vs. 22 percent for males, 26 vs. 28 percent for females). The remaining current smokers (defined as less than one cigarette per week in the telephone survey and less than one per day in the school survey) were also estimated at lower rates in the telephone survey (0.3 vs. 9 percent for males, 0.8 vs. 9 percent for females). This suggests that the telephone survey underestimated both the number of daily smokers and the number of less-than-daily smokers. Most of the discrepancy appears to be due to a failure to identify the latter. It is unclear whether this difference is related to the system of classifying smokers or the telephone survey methodology.

NIDA National Household Surveys on Drug Abuse, 1979–85

NIDA conducted household surveys on drug abuse in 1979, 1982, and 1985. For each of these surveys, data were obtained from a stratified random sample of 8,000 U.S. households; approximately 2,000 in-person interviews were conducted with respondents in the 12- to 17-year-old age group. Questions included whether any cigarettes were smoked within 30 days as well as within the previous year. These surveys indicated that approximately 26 percent of the teenage population surveyed smoked at least one cigarette at some time during 1985 (Table 24). In 1985, 15.6 percent of this population had smoked within the previous month. Comparisons between data from the 1979 household survey and data from the more recent surveys are not appropriate, because in 1979 prevalence of use within the past year or past month was reported only for those who had smoked 100 cigarettes in their lifetime; this lifetime cutoff was not used in the later surveys.

TABLE 24.—Prevalence (%) of cigarette use among youth 12 to 17 years of age, 1979, 1982, and 1985, United States

Survey year	Any use in last year	Used in last 30 days
1979[a]	13.3	12.1
1982	24.8	14.7
1985	26.0	15.6

[a]The 1979 estimates are not necessarily comparable to later estimates because the 1979 survey asked questions only of those who had smoked 100 cigarettes in their lifetime.

SOURCE: NIDA National Household Surveys on Drug Abuse 1979, 1982, 1985 (US DHHS 1988).

Summary

Several national surveys provide information on adolescent smoking. These surveys vary substantially in sample size, methodology, definitions of smoking, ages of respondents, and other factors that may appreciably affect prevalence estimates.

The best trend data are available from the annual high school seniors survey. This survey shows that prevalence of daily cigarette consumption declined from 29 percent of seniors in 1976 to 21 percent in 1980, after which prevalence leveled off at 18 to 21 percent. Smoking prevalence among females has consistently exceeded that among males since 1977. The leveling off of smoking prevalence among high school seniors raises concern that the steadily declining initiation rates as determined by prevalence among adults aged 20 to 24 (NHIS) may soon level off as well.

Smoking prevalence has been consistently lower for high school seniors with plans to pursue higher education than for those without such plans. In 1987, smoking rates were 14 and 30 percent in these two groups, respectively.

Differences in prevalence of smoking and smokeless tobacco use (see below) between young males and young females suggest that the prevalence of any tobacco use is similar in these two groups. Whereas the prevalence of smoking is higher among female high school seniors than among males, the prevalence of smokeless tobacco use is higher among young males than among young females.

Changes in the Types of Cigarettes Smoked

Data on the market share of filter and nonfilter cigarettes, cigarettes of different machine-determined "tar" and nicotine yields, menthol and nonmenthol cigarettes, and cigarettes of different length have been published by the Federal Trade Commission (FTC) from information supplied to the agency by the major cigarette companies.

Filtered Cigarettes

Filters are the design characteristic of commercial cigarettes that most affects their machine-measured yield of harmful constituents (US DHHS 1981). Filters selectively remove nitrosamines and semivolatile phenols from smoke. Thus, filters affect not only the absolute amounts of these constituents delivered in smoke but also their relative concentrations in cigarette "tar."

Since the early 1950s, the proportion of cigarettes in the United States sold as filtered cigarettes has increased steadily. In 1950, less than 1 percent of cigarettes sold in the United States were filtered. That proportion rose to 19 percent in 1955, 51 percent in 1960, and 94 percent in 1986 (Table 25).

Low-Tar, Low-Nicotine Cigarettes

Trends in the sales-weighted average yield of tar and nicotine for cigarettes sold in the United States are shown in Figure 14 of Chapter 2. The sales-weighted average is based on the tar and nicotine yield of specific brands (as measured by the FTC machine-

TABLE 25.—Domestic market share of filter cigarettes as a proportion of total cigarettes sold, United States, 1950–86

Year	Market share (%)	Year	Market share (%)
1950	0.6	1969	77
1951	0.7	1970	80
1952	1	1971	82
1953	3	1972	84
1954	9	1973	85
1955	19	1974	86
1956	28	1975	87
1957	38	1976	88
1958	45	1977	90
1959	49	1978	90
1960	51	1979	91
1961	52	1980	92
1962	55	1981	92
1963	58	1982	93
1964	61	1983	93
1965	64	1984	93
1966	68	1985	94
1967	72	1986	94
1968	74		

SOURCE: FTC (1988).

testing method) multiplied by the quantity of sales for those brands. The sales-weighted average yield of tar fell from 35 mg in 1957 to 13 mg in 1987. For nicotine, the sales-weighted average fell from 1.3 mg in 1968 to 1.0 mg in 1985. However, the sales-weighted average yield of tar and nicotine leveled off between 1981 and 1987. As pointed out in Chapter 2, modifications in the makeup of commercial cigarettes have profoundly influenced these yields; for example, the steepest declines occurred in the late 1950s after introduction of filter tips.

Trends in the percentage of domestic sales of cigarettes yielding lower tar levels are shown in Table 26. The domestic market share of cigarettes yielding 15 mg or less tar increased from 2.0 percent in 1967 to 56.0 percent in 1981. Since 1981, this proportion has fallen slightly and has stabilized at 51 to 53 percent. About two-thirds of these cigarettes have tar yields between 9 and 15 mg.

It should be noted that the parameters used in the FTC machine-testing method (developed in the 1960s) do not necessarily reflect current smoking patterns. For example, the FTC method uses one puff per minute (Pillsbury et al. 1969), whereas human

TABLE 26.—Domestic market share of cigarettes with reduced tar, percentage of total cigarettes sold, United States, 1967–86

	Tar Yield				
Year	≤15 mg	≤12 mg	≤9 mg	≤6 mg	≤3 mg
1967	2.0				
1968	2.5				
1969	3.0				
1970	3.6				
1971	3.8				
1972	6.6				
1973	8.9				
1974	8.9				
1975	13.5				
1976	15.9				
1977	22.7				
1978	27.5				
1979	40.9		10.6	5.8	2.7
1980	44.8		16.8	7.3	3.3
1981	56.0		24.6	9.6	3.7
1982	52.2	43.8	27.8	8.9	2.9
1983	53.1	44.9	27.9	9.4	3.1
1984	51.0	43.4	26.3	9.4	2.9
1985	51.9	43.1	25.3	8.4	2.3
1986	52.6	44.5	22.3	9.9	2.6

SOURCE: FTC (1988); Kozlowski (1989).

studies of smoking patterns show an average interpuff interval of 34 seconds (that is, about two puffs per minute) (US DHHS 1988, Chapter 4, Table 2).

According to the 1986 AUTS, 41 percent of smokers smoke cigarettes yielding 15 mg or less tar (Table 27). The proportion of smokers smoking cigarettes yielding more than 15 mg tar is higher among males, blacks, and persons with less education compared with females, whites, and more educated persons, respectively. This proportion decreases with age; the higher proportion among those 17 to 19 years of age probably reflects the popularity of the higher tar Marlboro brand among adolescents (Hunter et al. 1986; Goldstein et al. 1987; Glantz 1985).

Increased consumer demand for lower yield cigarettes during the past two decades is probably attributed to consumer beliefs that lower yield brands are less hazardous. This impression may have resulted in part from cigarette advertising implying that low-yield brands are less hazardous or are safe (Davis 1987). According to the 1986 AUTS, 45 percent of current smokers believe that some kinds of cigarettes are probably more hazardous than others (see Chapter 4).

TABLE 27.—Percentage of current smokers, aged 17 years and older, who use cigarettes of varying tar yields and who use menthol cigarettes, by sex, race, and education, 1986

	Percentage of current smokers				
	Tar yield (mg/cigarette)				Menthol cigarette smokers
	≤10	>10–15	>15	Total	
Total	29.6	11.6	58.8	100	29.2
Sex					
Males	26.8	8.0	65.2	100	29.9
Females	32.7	15.6	51.7	100	34.0
Age					
17–19	31.7	2.7	65.6	100	29.3
20–24	30.4	4.9	64.8	100	24.1
25–44	31.5	8.8	59.7	100	34.4
45–64	26.3	17.8	55.9	100	23.7
≥65	26.3	22.6	51.1	100	21.1
Race					
White	31.8	12.3	55.9	100	23.1
Black	14.5	7.6	78.0	100	75.5
Other	26.2	5.3	68.5	100	24.9
Education					
≤11 years	23.5	11.6	64.8	100	27.6
12 years	29.4	11.9	58.7	100	29.7
13–15 years	36.8	9.7	53.5	100	32.0
≥16 years	36.4	13.2	50.4	100	27.1

SOURCE: Self-reported data on cigarette brand use, AUTS 1986 (US DHHS, in press, a). Sample sizes for each stratum are shown in Table 34.

The 1981 Surgeon General's Report (US DHHS 1981) concluded that although smoking lower yield cigarettes appears to reduce the risk of lung cancer, the benefits are minimal compared with giving up cigarettes entirely. Moreover, there is no definitive evidence that smoking lower yield cigarettes is associated with reduced risks of other cancers, cardiovascular disease, and fetal damage. Switching to low-yield brands may even increase the health risk for smokers who compensate for reduced nicotine intake by increasing the number of cigarettes smoked per day, the frequency of puffing, and the depth and duration of inhalation (US DHHS 1988).

The leveling off of sales-weighted tar and nicotine yields may be related to one or a combination of the following factors (US DHHS 1988): (1) a persistent brand loyalty of some smokers to moderate- or high-yield brands because of brand image; (2) a diminishing perception that low-yield brands are less hazardous (see Chapter 4); and (3) a tendency of some smokers to smoke cigarettes of such low tar and nicotine yields that further reductions in those yields may be unacceptable; that is, the "lower boundary" of comfortable cigarette use has been reached (Kozlowski 1987, 1989).

Menthol Cigarettes

From 1963–76, the domestic market share of menthol cigarettes increased gradually from 16 percent to 28 percent. Since 1976, this proportion has remained at 28 percent (FTC 1988). According to the 1986 AUTS, 29 percent of current smokers smoke menthol cigarettes. Seventy-six percent of black smokers smoke menthol cigarettes compared with 23 percent of whites (Table 27). Similar findings were reported by Cummings and colleagues (1987).

Menthol in cigarettes provides a sensation of cooling, which may promote deeper, prolonged inhalation of cigarette smoke. This may help to explain why blacks (who are much more likely to smoke menthol cigarettes) have higher mortality rates from certain smoking-related diseases (e.g., lung cancer, heart disease, and cerebrovascular disease) than whites despite smoking fewer cigarettes per day (Novotny, Warner et al. 1988). Increased lung cancer mortality rates among blacks may also relate to increased occupational or environmental exposures among blacks that promote the carcinogenic effects of smoking, or to the fact that blacks are more likely to smoke higher tar brands (Table 27), which are associated with higher lung cancer mortality rates (US DHHS 1981). There does not appear to be a positive correlation between the presence of menthol and higher tar yields in cigarette brands: in the FTC's 1985 list of 207 brands (FTC 1985), 67 percent (51/76) of menthol brands had tar yields of less than 13 mg, compared with 56 percent (73/131) of nonmenthol brands.

Cigarette Length

From 1967–86, the domestic market share of cigarettes 68 to 88 mm in length decreased from 91 percent to 60 percent. During the same time, the domestic market share of cigarettes 94 to 101 mm in length increased from 9 to 37 percent (Table 28).

Because of the dose–response relationship between smoking and risk of disease (see Chapter 2), this increase in the average length of cigarettes has potentially important public health implications. However, smokers tend to compensate for changes in cigarette length by changing the number of cigarettes smoked per day, puffing frequency, and other measures of smoking behavior so as to minimize the change in overall nicotine intake (US DHHS 1988).

TABLE 28.—Domestic market share of cigarettes (%), by cigarette length, percentage of total cigarettes sold, United States, 1967–86

Year	68–72 mm	79–88 mm	94–101 mm	110–121 mm
1967	14	77	9	
1968	12	74	13	
1969	11	74	16	
1970	9	73	18	
1971	8	72	20	
1972	8	71	21	
1973	7	71	22	
1974	6	71	23[a]	
1975	6	69	24	1
1976	5	69	24	2
1977	5	67	26	2
1978	5	65	27	2
1979	4	65	30	2
1980	3	63	32	2
1981	3	62	33	2
1982	3	61	34	2
1983	3	60	34	2
1984	3	59	36	2
1985	3	58	37	2
1986	2	58	37	3

NOTE: Because of rounding, the total of the individual percentages may not equal 100 percent in some instances.
[a]The 110- to 121-mm length was combined with the 94- to 101-mm length.
SOURCE: FTC (1988).

Summary and Comment

During the past 40 years, filtered cigarettes have virtually replaced nonfiltered cigarettes in the United States. The domestic market shares of lower (15 mg or less) tar cigarettes and menthol cigarettes have increased during the past two decades but have leveled off in recent years. The domestic market share of longer (94–101 mm) cigarettes has increased substantially since the mid-1960s and still appears to be rising slowly.

Continued health concerns among smokers are likely to encourage the cigarette industry to continue to design new cigarettes that are perceived as less hazardous. Besides filtered, low-yield cigarettes, other "high-tech" cigarettes have been marketed that may appear to smokers to be less hazardous. These include one brand with a recessed filter and another with a "flavor-control filter" that apparently allows the smoker to regulate the tar yield of individual cigarettes (Davis 1987). The R.J. Reynolds Tobacco Company announced in September 1987 plans to market a new product that heats rather than burns tobacco. R.J. Reynolds asserts that the product is a cigarette, and it has commonly been referred to in the press as a "smokeless cigarette." In a press release, the company's chief executive officer stated that "a majority of the compounds produced by burning tobacco are eliminated or greatly reduced, including most compounds that are often associated with the smoking and health controversy" (R.J. Reynolds 1987). The American Medical Association (1988) and the Coalition on Smoking OR Health (1988) have filed petitions with the U.S. Food and Drug Administration (FDA) seeking FDA regulation of this new product as a drug or medical device based on implicit health claims, among other reasons. As of November 1988, these petitions were under review by the FDA. In October 1988, R.J. Reynolds began test marketing the product, named Premier, in three cities (Phoenix and Tucson, AZ, and St. Louis, MO). (See Chapter 7.)

Other Types of Tobacco Use

Smokeless Tobacco Use

Smokeless tobacco (ST) use, including snuff and chewing tobacco, became a subject of concern in the United States during the 1980s (US DHHS 1986). Cross-sectional national surveys and various regional surveys have identified several demographic categories at high risk for the use of these products, including young white males, persons living in the Southern and North Central United States, American Indians, and Alaskan Natives (Rouse, in press; Boyd et al. 1987; CDC 1987c, 1988; Schinke et al. 1986). Trend data on ST use are available primarily through the AUTSs, which included persons aged 21 years or older in 1964, 1966, 1970, and 1975 (US DHEW 1969, 1973a, 1976), and persons aged 17 years and older in 1986 (Novotny, Pierce et al., in press). In addition, the 1970 and 1987 NHISs included data on ST use among persons aged 17 years and older and aged 18 years and older, respectively. The Behavioral Risk Factor Surveillance System of the Centers for Disease Control collected State-specific data on ST use among persons aged 18 years and older beginning in 1986 (CDC 1987d). The 1985 CPS of the U.S. Bureau of the Census included questions about ST use among persons aged 17 years and older (Marcus et al., in press). This survey also produced State-specific estimates for prevalence of use of these products. Definitions of ST use and questions asked about ST use in these surveys are listed in the Appendix to this Chapter.

Figure 5 compares age-specific data for men from the 1970 NHIS and the 1986 AUTS. Between 1970 and 1986, snuff use increased fifteenfold and chewing tobacco use more than fourfold among males aged 17 to 19 years. Smaller increases were observed among the middle-aged groups, and a decrease in the use of both products was noted for older men (age 50 and above). The NHIS used household interviews, and the AUTS used telephone interviews as their primary mode of data collection; however, this difference in methodology is unlikely to account for the substantial increase in ST use among teenage males.

Data on ST use among persons aged 21 years or older are presented below from the 1964–86 AUTSs. These surveys were based on in-person interviews in 1964 and 1966 and telephone interviews in 1970, 1975, and 1986. State-specific data from the 1985

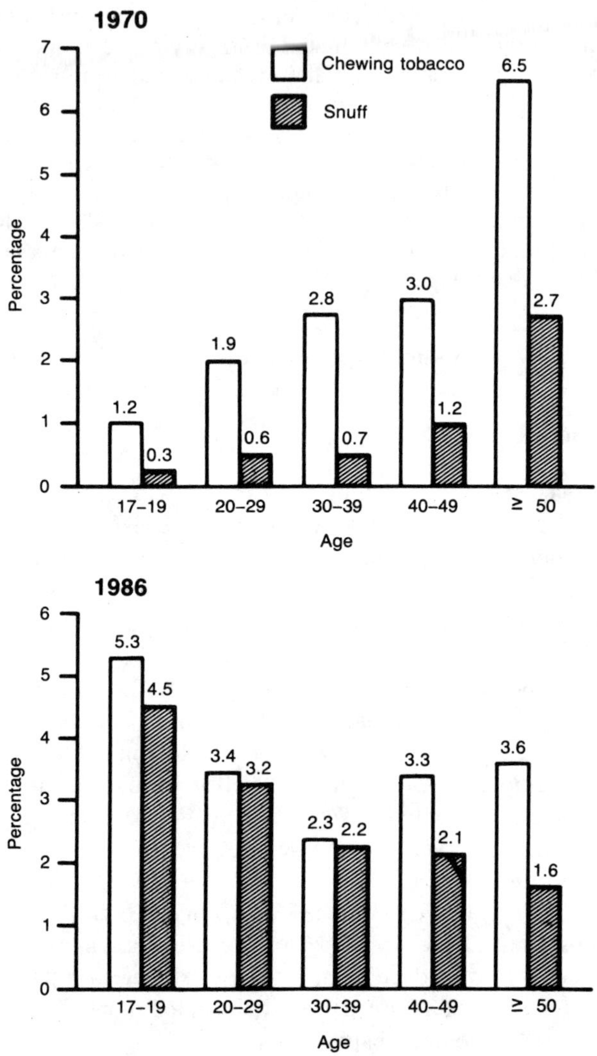

FIGURE 5.—Prevalence of chewing tobacco and snuff use among men, 1970 (NHIS) and 1986 (AUTS)

SOURCE: US DHHS (1986a); Novotny, Pierce et al., in press.

CPS are reported. Finally, data from a more detailed analysis of ST use from the 1986 AUTS for men aged 17 years and older (Novotny, Pierceet al., in press) are described.

The prevalence of current ST use from 1964–86 among persons aged 21 years and older, stratified by product and sex, is shown in Figure 6. For both products, there has been a steady overall decline in use by both men and women. It is possible that this decline is due in part to the change in the AUTS interview technique from in-person

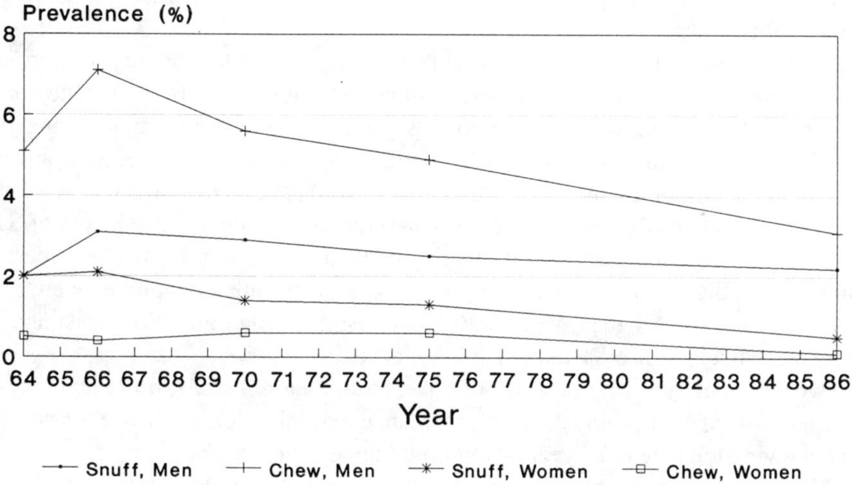

FIGURE 6.—Smokeless tobacco use among adults 21 years of age and older, United States, 1964–86

SOURCE: AUTSs (Novotny, Pierce et al., in press).

interview (1964 and 1966) to telephone interview (1970, 1975, 1986); telephone surveys generally provide slightly lower smoking prevalence estimates than in-person surveys (see above). The prevalence of ST use among women has consistently been very low. However, the use of snuff by older black women in the South is much more common than among women in the general population (Rouse, in press).

In 1986, the weighted prevalence of snuff use was 2.2 percent for men and 0.5 percent for women, and of chewing tobacco use, 3.1 percent for men and 0.1 percent for women among adults aged 21 years and older. For 1986, overall prevalence of ever and current use of ST among males, aged 17 years and older, is shown in Table 29. More than 10 percent of male respondents had ever used ST products; chewing tobac-

TABLE 29.—Prevalence (%) of ever use and current use of smokeless tobacco, males aged 17 years and older, United States, 1986

Product used	Ever use	Current use
Any smokeless tobacco	12.6	5.2
Snuff[a]	5.8	2.4
Chewing tobacco[b]	9.9	3.3
Both	3.1	0.5

[a]Includes those who also use chewing tobacco.

[b]Includes those who also use snuff.

SOURCE: AUTS 1986 (Novotny, Pierce et al., in press).

co appears to be used slightly more commonly than snuff. Few men (0.5 percent) use both products.

The prevalence of ever use and current use of any ST product by males, stratified by selected sociodemographic variables, is shown in Table 30. The prevalence of both current and ever use was highest among younger men, whites, men living in the Southeast, less educated men, men below the poverty level, unemployed men, and lower income men. Among males 17 to 19 years of age, 8.2 percent were current ST users. In a multivariate model using the sociodemographic variables as predictors of ST use (Table 31), white men were more than twice as likely to use ST as black men; men employed in blue-collar or service/laborer jobs or who were unemployed were 3 times more likely to use ST than white-collar workers; and men in the Southeast and West were more likely to use ST than men in other regions.

Two-thirds of men who ever used ST began use before age 21; more than one-third began before age 16 (Table 32). The median age of initiation of ST use for both snuff and chewing tobacco is 19 years (Novotny, Pierce et al., in press).

The State- and region-specific prevalence of current snuff and chewing tobacco use among men aged 16 years and older is shown in Table 33. These data are from the 1985 CPS. As mentioned earlier, 45 percent of interviews in the CPS were with proxy respondents. Proxy responses are known to affect the accuracy of information on smoking behavior, especially daily cigarette consumption (see above). The effect of proxy responses on data relating to ST use is unknown.

Overall prevalence for males in the 1985 CPS was 1.9 percent for snuff and 3.9 percent for chewing tobacco. Use of ST was lowest in the Northeast and highest in the South, with intermediate values reported for the North Central and Western regions. Among women, the overall prevalence of snuff use was only 0.5 percent, with all regions having prevalence rates of 0.5 percent or less except the South (1.4 percent). Prevalence of chewing tobacco use among women was 0.2 percent overall.

In summary, ST use is increasing among adolescent males and is decreasing slightly overall among men aged 21 years and older in the United States. It continues to be a rare behavior among women. According to national surveys, sociodemographic correlates of use include blue-collar and service/laborer employment, unemployment, and residence in the South. Local surveys have also shown high usage rates among American Indian youth (CDC 1987c, 1988; Schinke et al. 1987; Hall and Dexter 1988). Because ST use is more common among young males than among young females, while the prevalence of smoking among high school seniors is higher among females than among males (see above), the prevalence of any tobacco use may be similar among young males and young females.

Cigar and Pipe Smoking

Table 34 presents data from the 1986 AUTS for cigar and pipe smoking. Cigar and/or pipe smoking mainly occurs among men, in whom prevalence of use is 8.7 percent. The highest proportion of users are between the ages of 45 and 64 years. Usage is slightly higher in the most and least educated groups than in the intermediate education categories.

TABLE 30.—Prevalence (%) of smokeless tobacco use by sociodemographic categories, males aged 17 years and older, United States, 1986

Category	Ever use	Current use
Age group		
17–19	12.3	8.2
20–29	11.4	5.9
30–39	7.3	4.1
40–49	9.7	5.0
≥50	11.5	4.8
Race		
White	11.1	5.6
Black	6.6	3.0
Other	7.7	2.9
Geographic area		
Southeast	14.5	7.5
West	9.6	4.5
Midwest	9.5	4.3
Northeast	5.5	3.0
Completed years of school		
≤11	14.6	7.3
12	11.1	5.6
13–15	9.1	3.8
≥16	4.8	2.9
Poverty level		
Below	16.1	8.5
Above	9.9	4.9
Employment		
Unemployed	13.0	8.3
Service/laborer	12.3	6.4
Blue collar	7.0	3.6
White collar	2.3	1.0
Household income (dollars per year)		
<10,000	16.1	8.6
10,000–29,999	4.7	2.2
≥30,000	3.0	1.6

SOURCE: AUTS 1986 (Novotny, Pierce et al., in press).

TABLE 31.—Significant sociodemographic correlates of current use of any smokeless tobacco, males aged 17 years and older, United States, 1986

Parameter	Odds ratio	95% confidence limits
Region		
Southeast	3.0	1.8, 4.8
West	1.9	1.1, 3.3
Midwest	1.4	0.8, 2.5
Northeast	Referent	
Race		
White	2.4	1.3, 4.3
Black	Referent	
Employment		
Unemployed	3.8	1.9, 7.6
Service/laborer	2.9	1.8, 4.6
Blue collar	3.0	2.1, 4.3
White collar	Referent	

SOURCE: AUTS 1986 (Novotny, Pierce et al., in press).

TABLE 32.—Reported age of initiation and median age of initiation of smokeless tobacco use among ever users, males aged 17 years and older, United States, 1986

	Age group at initiation (percentage reporting)				
Product	<16	16–18	19–20	≥21	Median
Any smokeless tobacco	37.1	7.8	21.4	33.8	19
Snuff[a]	35.5	8.6	23.0	32.8	19
Chewing tobacco[b]	36.6	6.7	20.3	36.3	19

[a]Includes those who also use chewing tobacco.
[b]Includes those who also use snuff.
SOURCE: AUTS 1986 (Novotny, Pierce et al., in press).

TABLE 33.—Prevalence (%) of current use of snuff and chewing tobacco by region, division, and State, males aged 16 years and older, United States, 1985

	Snuff use	Chewing tobacco use	Any smokeless tobacco use
United States	1.9	3.9	5.5
Northeast Region	1.0	1.4	2.3
New England Division	0.4	0.8	1.2
Maine	0.9	1.5	2.3
New Hampshire	1.2	1.5	2.7
Vermont	0.9	4.7	5.5
Massachusetts	0.2	0.4	0.5
Rhode Island	0.5	0.6	0.9
Connecticut	0.3	0.5	0.8
Mid-Atlantic Division	1.2	1.6	2.7
New York	0.5	1.2	1.6
New Jersey	0.1	0.6	0.7
Pennsylvania	3.0	2.9	5.6
North Central Region	2.1	3.4	5.3
East North Central Division	1.8	2.9	4.4
Ohio	2.2	3.2	5.0
Indiana	2.6	3.2	5.6
Illinois	1.1	2.5	3.3
Michigan	0.8	2.7	3.4
Wisconsin	2.9	2.9	5.8
West North Central Division	2.9	4.7	7.5
Minnesota	3.5	2.8	6.1
Iowa	1.8	4.6	6.4
Missouri	3.1	3.6	6.7
North Dakota	6.1	5.1	10.7
South Dakota	1.9	6.1	7.9
Nebraska	1.4	6.8	8.0
Kansas	3.3	8.6	11.7
South Region	2.7	6.0	8.3
South Atlantic Division	1.8	5.2	6.7
Delaware	0.6	2.4	3.0
Maryland	0.4	2.1	2.4
District of Columbia	0.0	0.4	0.4
Virginia	2.3	6.2	7.8
West Virginia	11.5	13.5	23.1
North Carolina	1.8	8.6	9.8

TABLE 33.—Continued

	Snuff use	Chewing tobacco use	Any smokeless tobacco use
South Carolina	0.7	5.3	6.1
Georgia	1.4	7.3	8.7
Florida	1.1	1.9	2.9
East South Central Division	2.7	9.4	11.6
Kentucky	3.2	11.2	13.6
Tennessee	1.7	9.3	10.3
Alabama	1.7	6.6	8.3
Mississippi	5.7	11.4	16.5
West South Central Division	4.0	5.5	9.1
Arkansas	6.0	9.5	14.7
Louisiana	2.5	5.8	8.0
Oklahoma	4.8	6.7	11.0
Texas	4.0	4.6	8.2
West Region	1.4	3.3	4.5
Mountain Division	2.3	5.4	7.5
Montana	5.5	8.3	13.7
Idaho	2.3	6.7	8.7
Wyoming	3.4	13.0	15.8
Colorado	1.2	6.4	7.5
New Mexico	5.3	5.2	10.2
Arizona	2.0	3.8	5.4
Utah	0.9	3.0	3.7
Nevada	1.5	2.8	4.3
Pacific Division	1.0	2.6	3.4
Washington	1.8	6.1-	7.1
Oregon	2.7	5.4	7.6
California	0.7	1.7	2.3
Alaska	2.5	6.3	8.8
Hawaii	0.2	0.4	0.7

SOURCE: CPS 1985 (Marcus et al., in press.)

From 1964–86, there was an 80-percent decline in prevalence of both cigar and pipe smoking among men (Figure 7). The prevalence of cigar smoking declined from 29.7 to 6.2 percent; the prevalence of pipe smoking declined from 18.7 to 3.8 percent. Reasons cited to explain the drop in cigar sales include the effects of the antismoking campaign (several airlines have completely banned cigar and pipe smoking on all flights for many years, but only one airline has done so for cigarette smoking), declining image of cigar smoking, failure to attract new smokers, insufficient free-sample distribution, mediocre advertising and promotional activities, and declining quality of the product (Lazarus 1979).

TABLE 34.—Cigar/pipe smoking status (%) by major sociodemographic variables, United States, 1986

	Cigar/pipe smoking status				
	Current user	Former user	Never user	Total	Sample size
Total	4.3	22.2	73.5	100	13,031
Sex					
Male	8.7	41.8	49.6	100	6,377
Female	0.3	4.5	95.2	100	6,654
Age					
17–19	1.5	13.6	85.0	100	560
20–24	2.0	16.6	81.4	100	1,086
25–44	4.4	22.2	73.3	100	5,802
45–64	5.9	26.5	67.6	100	3,616
≥65	3.9	22.6	73.5	100	1,967
Race					
White	4.4	23.4	72.2	100	11,563
Black	3.7	13.9	82.4	100	1,096
Other	3.5	19.4	77.1	100	372
Region					
Midwest	4.8	22.6	72.6	100	3,236
Northeast	4.6	19.6	75.7	100	2,968
Southeast	3.8	23.2	73.0	100	4,301
West	4.1	22.7	73.2	100	2,526
Marital status					
Married/cohabiting	4.8	25.3	69.9	100	8,364
Widowed	1.8	8.9	89.2	100	1,011
Divorced/separated	5.6	20.1	74.3	100	1,446
Never married	2.8	17.7	79.4	100	2,179
Unknown	12.4	27.5	60.1	100	31
Education					
≤11 years	4.9	22.8	72.3	100	2,431
12 years	3.6	20.0	76.5	100	4,872
13–15 years	3.9	22.5	73.6	100	3,118
≥16 years	5.3	26.0	68.7	100	2,610

TABLE 34.—Continued

	Cigar/pipe smoking status				Sample size
	Current user	Former user	Never user	Total	
Household income (dollars per year)					
<10,000	3.1	16.8	80.1	100	1,220
10,000–19,999	4.0	21.2	74.9	100	2,204
20,000–29,999	4.3	23.1	72.6	100	2,853
30,000–39,999	5.0	24.2	70.8	100	1,735
≥40,000	5.5	28.1	66.4	100	2,947
Unknown	3.3	17.1	79.6	100	2,072
Poverty level[a]					
Above	4.7	23.9	71.4	100	9,913
Below	3.0	18.6	78.3	100	1,046
Unknown	3.3	17.1	79.6	100	2,072

[a]Poverty level is based on the definition provided by the U.S. Bureau of the Census.

SOURCE: AUTS 1986 (US DHHS, in press, a).

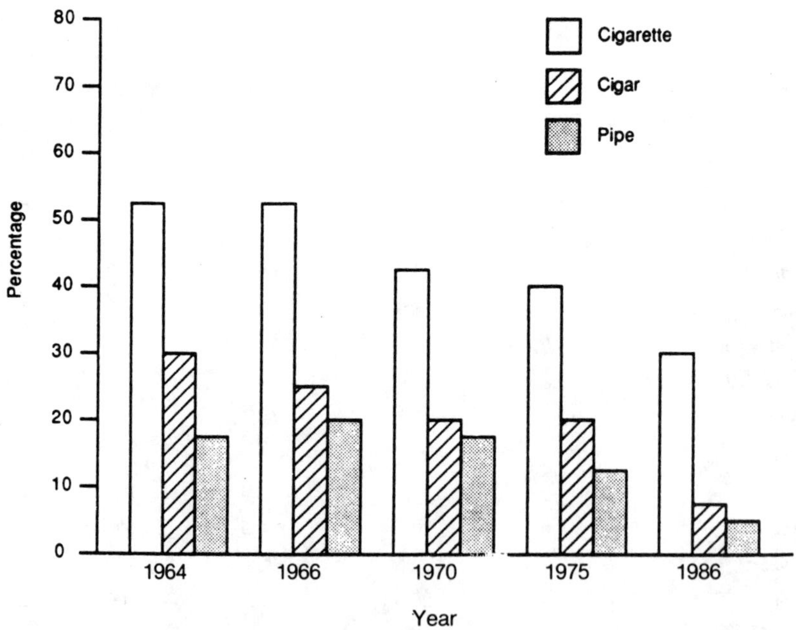

FIGURE 7.—Trends in prevalence of using cigarettes, cigars, and pipes, adult men, United States, 1964–86

SOURCE: AUTSs (US DHHS 1988).

PART II. CHANGES IN KNOWLEDGE ABOUT THE DETERMINANTS OF SMOKING BEHAVIOR

Introduction: Historical and Conceptual Overview

This Section reviews the past 25 years' growth in scientific knowledge of the determinants of smoking. Broad conceptual shifts in understanding smoking are first reviewed by comparing current knowledge, as reflected in the 1988 Surgeon General's Report as well as in more recent investigations, with that reflected in two previous Surgeon General's Reports during the past 25 years: the 1st Report, issued in 1964, and the 15th Anniversary Report, issued in 1979.

1964 Surgeon General's Report

The first Surgeon General's Report devoted a chapter to the psychosocial aspects of smoking and another to the issue of smoking as drug addiction or drug habituation. These topics continue to receive contemporary attention. A third chapter in the 1964 Report discussed morphological characteristics of smokers as important determinants of smoking (e.g., physique, somatotype, and weight). With the exception of body weight, there has been a decline in the attention paid to these variables. The relationship between body weight and smoking cessation, especially among women, has received much recent attention (US DHHS 1988).

The 1964 Report's Chapter on Psychosocial Aspects of Smoking related smoking to a variety of demographic factors including socioeconomic status (smoking being more prevalent among "lower or working classes" but less prevalent among extremely poor, e.g., unemployed groups) and gender (smoking being more prevalent among men). With regard to gender, the Report anticipated contemporary concerns about smoking by women (US DHHS 1980b), noting that "The proportion of women smokers has increased faster than that of men smokers in recent years" (US PHS 1964, p. 363).

The 1964 Report's chapter on psychosocial aspects also linked smoking to such broad personality factors as extraversion and orality. While some research continues to show relationships with extraversion (e.g., Eysenck 1980; Mangan and Golding 1984), most contemporary research focuses on more specific psychological, biological, and social variables and their interactions. The 1964 Report noted that smoking might function to reduce tension but reported little research related to this possibility. In contrast, the 1988 Report on nicotine addiction reviews considerable laboratory and field research on the relationship between smoking and stress and concludes that stress increases cigarette consumption among smokers and is related to initiation of smoking among adolescents and relapse among abstainers (e.g., US DHHS 1988).

The 1964 Report devoted much attention to the role of nicotine in smoking behavior, an issue that continues to be of central interest, as reflected in the 1988 Report. Both reports concluded that nicotine is a critical and substantial determinant of smoking. The focus in 1964, however, centered on whether smoking fit the World Health Organization's (WHO) definition of addiction, which emphasized the importance of physical dependence (WHO 1957). The Report concluded that there was no proof of physical dependence and that smoking was a habit, as was use of cocaine, amphetamines, and other drugs. More recent perspectives (e.g., Pomerleau and Pomerleau 1984), culminating in the 1988 Report, have integrated psychosocial and pharmacologic processes into a single model of addiction or dependence. The 1988 Report demonstrated that there have been substantial data amassed since 1964 that confirm that by the criteria defining addiction, nicotine should be categorized as addicting.

Although the 1964 Report did conclude that "... there is no single cause or explanation of smoking ..." (US PHS 1964, p. 376), its discussion of research reflected an expectation that one or a very few key causes of smoking might be found. Along these lines, the Report emphasized the extent to which evidence demonstrated a cause to be sufficient. For example, in discussing evidence that smoking as a sign of masculinity may motivate many men to smoke, it labeled as "troublesome" the fact that "... some, but not so many others choose this particular means [that is, smoking] of giving evidence of their masculinity" (US PHS 1964, p. 373). Since the 1964 Report, models of causal inference in the behavioral sciences have changed to emphasize multiple causes interacting to bring about complex behavior patterns, and not one cause in itself that is necessary or sufficient.

1979 Surgeon General's Report

The 1979 Report gave much attention to prevention and to the determinants of smoking and smoking cessation, devoting 9 of 23 chapters to these topics. Thus, there was recognition of different stages of smoking behavior and of determinants varying as the stages change. Since the 1979 Report, researchers have continued to elaborate on multiple stages in the development and cessation of smoking.

The 1979 Report also recognized that multiple factors interact to encourage and support smoking. The Chapter "Behavioral Factors in the Establishment, Maintenance and Cessation of Smoking" posited smoking as "... a behavior—a highly complex act ... based on various biochemical and physiological processes ..." (US DHEW 1979a, pp. 16–25). It included research on drug and nondrug factors and called smoking "the prototypical substance-abuse dependency." The Chapter "Smoking in Children and Adolescents: Psychosocial Determinants and Prevention Strategies" explicitly viewed the initiation of smoking as determined by an array of factors. Likewise, the Chapter "Psychosocial Influences on Cigarette Smoking" linked multiple factors to maintenance and cessation of smoking, including personality characteristics, multiple drug use, coexisting chronic disease, price "elasticity" of consumer demand for cigarettes, and differences among cultures in their attitudes toward smoking as personal gratification. The importance of identifying multiple, interacting factors had been enunciated by Schwartz and Dubitzky in 1968 in their research on smoker profiles and the influence of multiple variables on smoking cessation, maintenance of cessation, and relapse (Schwartz and Dubitzky 1968).

The 1979 Report's recognition of an array of determinants was reflected in a recommendation for future research: "There are multiple psychosocial influences on cigarette smoking. Multivariate research is needed ..." (US DHEW 1979a, pp. 18–25). Multiple regression analyses and causal modeling have now become much more common in smoking research (e.g., McAlister, Krosnick, Milburn 1984; Mosbach and Leventhal 1988).

The 1979 Report also was noteworthy in focusing attention on systematic cessation efforts, taking both pharmacologic and psychosocial factors into account. The extensive treatment of cessation research in a separate chapter was a first for the Surgeon General's Report and set a precedent for reviewing the intervention literature in subsequent reports.

Current Views

Current explanations assume that smoking is determined by multiple causes, no one of which is sufficient. The interplay of psychosocial and pharmacologic forces continues to occupy investigators of nicotine addiction as it does investigators of other drug addictions. While the 1964 Report tended to see such factors as mutually exclusive, the 1988 Report (US DHHS 1988) viewed these various pharmacologic, biochemical, and psychosocial processes, such as conditioning, as interacting in the determination of nicotine addiction. In fact, conditioned drug-taking behavior is now thought to be central to the concept of addiction; physical dependence is neither necessary nor sufficient (US DHHS 1988). The biological power of nicotine may make the learned behaviors that form smoking patterns stronger and more resistant to change. At the same time, the plentitude of daily circumstances, activities, and emotions to which smoking is conditioned ties this behavior to numerous rituals of daily life and contributes to the difficulty of breaking this addiction (Fisher, Bishop et al. 1988a; Pomerleau and Pomerleau 1987; Russell, Peto, Patel 1974; US DHHS 1988). This interplay between behavior and the pharmacologic effects of nicotine is mirrored in research on smoking cessation, in which nicotine-containing chewing gum and behavioral interventions have been shown to enhance one another (e.g., Hall et al. 1985; Killen, Maccoby, Taylor 1984; Schneider et al. 1983). In reviewing the evidence for defining smoking as an addiction, the 1988 Report made the important point that the interplay between social, behavioral, and pharmacologic factors that define tobacco addiction is similar to that seen with other drug addictions.

The continuum of smoking behavior can be viewed as occurring in different stages. The 1964 Report identified two stages (or processes): "Taking Up" and "Discontinuation." Current work identifies three major stages—development, maintenance of regular smoking, and cessation. Several investigators have offered descriptions of various smaller stages within smoking development (e.g., Leventhal and Cleary 1980; Flay et al. 1983). These include, for example, preparation, initiation, experimentation, and transition to regular smoking (Flay et al. 1983). Similarly, the process of cessation has been specified in smaller stages (e.g., Marlatt 1985; Prochaska and DiClemente 1983; Rosen and Shipley 1983). These include, for example, precontemplation (not yet considering quitting), contemplation, action, and maintenance or relapse (Prochaska and DiClemente 1983).

Evolution of theoretical models of stages in smoking over the past 25 years is depicted in Figure 8, indicating the stages described around three periods of time, the 1960s,

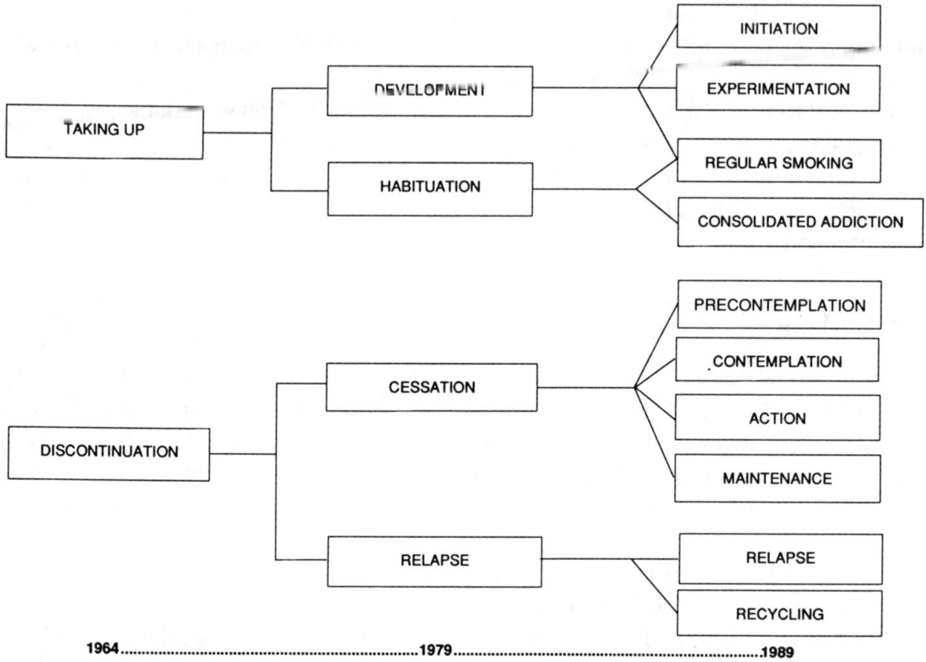

FIGURE 8.—Evolving theoretical concepts of the natural history of smoking, 1964–89

1970s, and 1980s. In 1964, only two broad stages were noted, while in 1989, as many as nine can be observed.

Stages are not explanations of attitudes or behaviors. For example, precontemplation is a description of the attitudes toward smoking and likely responses to antismoking messages of the individual uninterested in stopping. It is not an explanation or a cause of that lack of interest. Neither the sequence of stages nor the boundaries among them are rigid. For example, a young experimenter may stop smoking without ever making the transition to regular smoking. A smoker in the regular smoking stage is, at the same time, a precontemplator or contemplator in the cessation stage. The regular smoking stage is abandoned when the smoker moves into action and stops smoking. Although the boundaries among stages and their sequence may be blurred, the concept serves as a framework for understanding the determinants of smoking behavior. Different determinants are operative to different degrees during each stage.

The three broad stages of smoking and their multiple interacting determinants provide the organization for the remainder of this Chapter. Within the stage framework, historical trends in determinants are discussed primarily within three general domains. The three domains do not constitute a model; they are a useful way to organize the determinants of smoking. The first domain is composed of pharmacologic processes and conditioning, the basic factors that interact to support smoking. The combining of these into one domain reflects present awareness that pharmacologic processes and conditioning interact to produce addiction (US DHHS 1988). The second domain includes cognition and decisionmaking. The stages of smoking reflect appraisals of oneself, of social experiences, and of information, such as that presented in campaigns to deter smoking. The ways in which individuals process such information and make choices about smoking have been the foci of substantial research. The third domain includes personal characteristics (e.g., personality and demographic factors) and social context, which includes the important influences of the social, cultural, and economic environment. Personal characteristics themselves are affected by these environmental influences and mediate their effect rather than independently determine smoking.

Table 35 presents some of the determinants, within each of the domains, that have a strong effect on the indicated stage of smoking. As such, the table provides an outline of the discussion that follows.

Development of Smoking

Pharmacologic Processes and Conditioning

Historically, little attention was paid to the role of pharmacologic effects of nicotine and conditioning in the initial development of smoking behavior. For example, among teenagers, psychosocial determinants have been assumed to play a dominant role (Table 35), as for other dependence-producing substances. Once a smoker starts to inhale, however, it is possible that the pharmacologic properties of nicotine contribute to continued smoking (Kozlowski 1988). A few studies have investigated the potential role of individual-specific psychophysiological responses to nicotine and the development of smoking (Kozlowski and Harford 1976; Silverstein et al. 1982). Reactions to initial cigarettes and the interpretation of these reactions may predispose individuals to continuing or not continuing smoking. Hirschman, Leventhal, and Glynn (1984), for example, found that the initial early physical reaction was predictive of continued smoking. Dizziness was related to a rapid progression to a second cigarette, while coughing and a sore throat were related to discontinuation.

It is not clear how long it takes for the transition from experimental to regular smoking, and there is likely to be much variation (e.g., Hirschman, Leventhal, Glynn 1984). However, results from several recent studies suggest that teenagers become more addicted to smoking than was previously believed. Survey data (Green 1979; Johnson 1986) indicate that teenagers make frequent and often unsuccessful quit attempts. Other studies confirm that teenagers have difficulty stopping and report reasons for the difficulty—social pressure, urges, withdrawal symptoms—similar to those seen with adults (Biglan and Lichtenstein 1984; Hansen et al. 1985; Weissman et al. 1987). Because smoking among children and adolescents is generally confined to relatively few situations, the level of nicotine dependence is limited in this group. Nevertheless, the reports of withdrawal symptoms and relapses among teenage smokers attest to the strength of nicotine dependence even among those still in the early stages of smoking.

More work is needed in this area to facilitate our understanding of the development of smoking addiction. Research on adolescent initiation has not applied the same biobehavioral concepts and measurement tools (e.g., plasma nicotine or cotinine levels) as have been applied to adult smoking. Sensitive human subjects issues related to work-

TABLE 35.—Determinants of smoking within each domain by stage

	Stage		
Domain	Onset/development	Regular use	Cessation
Pharmacologic processes and conditioning	Initial psychopharmacologic effects encourage transition from experimental to regular use	Numerous conditioned associations among smoking, environmental events, and pharmacologic effects of nicotine	Withdrawal symptoms and conditioned and reinforcing effects of nicotine encourage relapse
Cognition and decision-making	Poor awareness of long- and short-term health consequences and addictive nature of smoking	Health consequences are minimized or depersonalized	Increased awareness of smoking-related symptoms or illness
	Positive characteristics are attributed to smokers and smoking	Positive characteristics are attributed to smokers and smoking	Perceived benefits of cessation
			Belief in one's ability to stop
Personal characteristics and social context	Inclination toward problem behaviors	Stress/negative affect are reduced by nicotine	Social norms and support for stopping and maintained abstinence
	Extraversion		
	Peer and family norms and values support smoking	Social acceptability and peer and family norms support continued smoking	Skills for coping with stimuli associated with smoking
	Youth-oriented advertising	Cigarette marketing encourages and legitimizes smoking	Economic, educational, and personal resources to minimize stress and maintain cessation

ing with minors must be resolved; these have slowed understanding of how dependence develops.

Cognition and Decisionmaking

Knowledge of the health effects of smoking is likely to influence initiation for some teenagers. Teenagers reported that one-third of their earliest refusals of cigarettes were based on fear of the effects of smoking on health, attractiveness, or athletic performance (Friedman, Lichtenstein, Biglan 1985). In early adulthood, British medical students' rating of smoking as a "major" or "not major" health risk was associated with their smoking status as reflected by surveys in 1972 and 1981 (Elkind 1982). Heavy smokers among college women evaluated health outcomes of smoking less negatively than did nonsmokers (Loken 1982). The latter two cross-sectional studies, however, may possibly reflect the effect of behavior on cognition rather than the effect of cognition on behavior.

Cognitive appraisals of the attractiveness or desirability of smoking or of smokers are associated with current smoking or intentions to smoke (Barton et al. 1982; McAlister, Krosnick, Milburn 1984), as are beliefs or attributions of the functional role of smoking (Murray and Perry 1984). Tenth graders inclined to smoke indicated greater congruity between the value they place on interest in the opposite sex and the extent to which they ascribe such interest to smokers (Barton et al. 1982). Intentions to smoke were also associated with congruity between the personal value of a characteristic and its attribution to smokers. Murray and Perry's analyses (1984) of the functional meaning of substance use by youth elucidated a variety of attributions correlating with young people's substance use. The report that smoking was useful for relieving boredom was most highly correlated with smoking. Data from England (Charlton 1984) demonstrate that children who smoke compared with nonsmoking children are more likely to agree that "Smoking keeps your weight down." This attribution was especially prominent among older girls.

School health education programs to discourage smoking have traditionally assumed that knowledge of the health consequences of smoking would deter adolescents from smoking (Chapter 6). This assumption has received limited support in the prevention literature (Thompson 1978). Despite school health education programs, children, especially those who smoke, continue to harbor several misconceptions about smoking. These misconceptions include overestimating the prevalence of both peer and adult smoking, underestimating the negative attitudes of their peers, and minimizing the addictive nature of smoking (Leventhal, Glynn, Fleming 1987). The overestimating of prevalence may represent the combined influence of social context and cognitive factors in determining smoking.

Contemporary smoking prevention programs ("psychosocial prevention curricula") emphasize knowledge of short-term consequences of smoking likely to be more pertinent to adolescents who have limited future orientations (Glasgow et al. 1981), and knowledge about the variety of social influences (parental, peer, and media) that affect the development of smoking (Flay 1985; Evans et al. 1978; Chapter 6). Decisionmaking skills (Botvin and Wills 1985) and analysis of cigarette marketing strategies (Evans et al. 1978) also are now taught to help youth make more informed choices.

Personal Characteristics and Social Context

Personal Characteristics

The 1964 Surgeon General's Report described as "one of the best designed studies" (US PHS 1964, p. 365) an investigation in which heavy smokers were found to be more extraverted than were medium smokers, who were in turn more extraverted than were light smokers (Eysenck et al. 1960). The 1964 Report also cited two other papers with similar findings (McArthur, Waldron, Dickinson 1958; Schubert 1960). More recent work by Cherry and Kiernan (1976, 1978) found that neuroticism and extraversion measured at age 16 were positively related to smoking status at age 25, suggesting a causal relationship. Their combined effects showed substantial ability to predict subsequent cigarette use. Eysenck (1980) has argued that the association between smoking and the personality dimensions of extraversion and neuroticism implies a constitutional predisposition for smoking analogous to that seen with other drug addictions (US DHHS 1988). Work on extraversion and smoking does seem to reflect a consistent relationship between them (US DHEW 1979a; Ashton and Stepney 1982).

Studies have linked initiation of smoking with rule breaking in school, general delinquency, age at first intercourse, inadequate contraceptive use, low levels of child compliance within the family, low levels of responsibility, nonconventionality, impulsivity, rebelliousness, and previous use of alcohol and other substances (Brook et al. 1983; Chassin et al. 1984; Jessor and Jessor 1977; Mittelmark et al. 1987; Russell 1971; Zabin 1984). Academic success, as measured by grade point average, is strongly linked to the rate of smoking (Johnson 1986). High school dropouts (Pirie, Murray, Luepker 1988) and high school seniors not planning to go to college (Johnston, O'Malley, Bachman 1987) are much more likely to smoke than are those planning higher education, and this difference has increased over the past 10 years (Table 20). Similar factors are observed with other drug addictions (US DHHS 1988). Jessor (1987) views this covariation as reflecting a problem behavior syndrome. Biglan and Lichtenstein (1984) questioned this interpretation, arguing against the inference of underlying personality factors to explain the acknowledged covariation among smoking and other problem behaviors.

Peer and Family Influences

The influences of peers and parents were considerations in the 1964 Report and remain a major contemporary issue (e.g., Krosnick and Judd 1982). Understanding of the effect of peers has increased since the 1964 Report noted little available evidence of their influence on the onset of smoking. It acknowledged that imitation ". . . may play a role in inducing some, and perhaps many children to take up smoking" (US PHS 1964, p. 372). Studies noted that children of smoking parents were more likely to smoke than children of nonsmoking parents (NIH 1975; Wohlford 1970); and smoking teenagers were more likely to have friends who smoked than were nonsmoking teenagers (Gordon and McAlister 1985; Levitt and Edwards 1970). The chapter on children and adolescents in the 1979 Report (US DHEW 1979a) reviewed the influence of social learning theory on models of the initiation of new behavior. More recent studies have supported the importance of peer models (e.g., Antonuccio and Lichtenstein 1980; Kniskern et al. 1983). The 1988 Report discussed similar factors in the determination of other drug dependence.

The impact of peer smoking on adolescent smoking has been identified in a number of studies (e.g., Chassin et al. 1984; Hundleby and Mercer 1987; McAlister, Krosnick, Milburn 1984; Mittelmark et al. 1987), including their impact on initial smoking episodes (Friedman, Lichtenstein, Biglan 1985) and continuation of smoking among those who already have experimented with cigarettes (Biglan and Lichtenstein 1984). These influences seem to rest on the importance of modeling of smoking, as well as on the setting of norms among subgroups of adolescents. The importance of bidirectional influences in smoking and smoking cessation among young people has been noted by Chassin, Presson, and Sherman (1984). In some cases, a young person's membership in a particular peer group may expose him or her to the example to smoke or to quit; however, in other cases, a young person may actively seek membership in a peer group that represents or is consistent with his or her established intentions about smoking.

More recent research has both reaffirmed the importance of parent and peer influences and attempted to explore the points at which they exert their influence during the process from onset—the initial smoking episode—to regular use (e.g., Friedman et al. 1985; Hirschman, Leventhal, Glynn 1984). The literature has tended to underscore the role of parental example and influence for initiation of smoking by young children and adolescents, and the primacy of peer influences among older youth. In application, this emphasis has often translated into an almost exclusive intervention focus on the social influences of peers for older adolescents (see Chapter 6). Some of the intervention programs include peer leaders chosen by their classmates (Murray et al. 1987). Krosnick and Judd (1982) found no evidence for decreases in parental influences on smoking during adolescence, although they did find that peer influence increases during this period. These studies often include important methodological advances wherein interviews and self-monitoring are used to augment questionnaire data.

A growing body of literature implicates family climate or family interaction patterns in smoking. Family characteristics such as indifference, low levels of trust, parental restrictiveness, and low levels of parental involvement are associated with smoking as well as with marijuana and alcohol use (Hundleby and Mercer 1987). Other research has demonstrated that low levels of adolescent involvement in family decisionmaking predict subsequent experimentation with cigarettes among adolescents (Mittelmark et al. 1987). A variety of characteristics in fathers, including harsh criticism, impulsivity, stereotyped male interests, poor ego integration, and lower levels of interpersonal relatedness has also been demonstrated to be associated with a greater likelihood of sons' smoking (Brook et al. 1983). A decreased likelihood of sons' smoking was associated with paternal affection, emotional support, attentiveness, participation in meaningful conversations, and higher expectations for the sons. It appears that adolescent smoking is more likely in restrictive, punitive, and unempathetic families in which children are uninvolved in decisionmaking. On the other hand, families who provide multiple avenues for identity formation and expression of feelings may obviate the utility of smoking or other problem behaviors as a mode of identity expression (Jessor 1987).

Personal characteristics and attitudes may mediate peer influence on smoking as well as other drug dependencies (US DHHS 1988). Research indicates greater impact of peer smoking among adolescents scoring low on a measure of obedience to parental authority and high on a measure of rebelliousness (McAlister, Krosnick, Milburn 1984). The interactions among social influences, personality, and smoking were highlighted in a study in which seventh and eighth graders described the informal reference or affiliation groups they observed among their schoolmates and identified the group with which they felt the closest affiliation (Mosbach and Leventhal 1988). Two of the four groups that emerged, "hot-shots" (78 percent female, popular leaders in academic and extracurricular activities) and "dirts" (63 percent male, characterized by problem behaviors such as drinking, poor academic performance, and cutting classes), were identified as primary reference groups by only 14.7 percent of respondents but accounted for 55.6 percent of the smokers. In discriminant function analyses, a "macho" dimension was highly associated with one high smoking prevalence group, the "dirts," but not with the "hot-shots." In contrast, academic and social leadership was associated with the "hot-shots" but not with the "dirts." As were the "dirts," the "jocks" were also 63 percent male and high on the macho dimension but low on use of both hard liquor and cigarettes. Adolescent smoking, then, is closely related to individual identification with groups, but these groups differ markedly in their association with other problem behaviors and psychosocial characteristics. Depending on group affiliation, different personality and attitudinal characteristics may be related to smoking.

Social class differences in the onset of smoking continue to be observed as noted in Part I of this Chapter. Racial differences in onset and prevalence and historical shifts in these differences are also well demonstrated in the first part of this Chapter. Sussman and colleagues (1987) in their study of psychosocial predictors of cigarette smoking onset by approximately 1,000 white, black, Hispanic, and Asian adolescents in Southern California demonstrated that different variables predict onset in these different groups. A good predictor for whites but not for other ethnic groups was adult and peer models of smoking behavior, while for blacks, risk-taking preference was a good predictor. These findings possibly reflect unique cultural and social contexts and suggest that tailoring socially relevant treatment components to adolescent subgroups may be beneficial (Sussman et al. 1987).

Cigarette Marketing

Beyond the family and peer group, an important social context determinant of the onset of smoking is the marketing of cigarettes. There have been longstanding concerns about the impact of cigarette advertising on both children and adults as evidenced by the ban on radio and television advertisements, effective in 1971. Yet, "cigarette advertisements continue to appear in publications with large teenage readerships" (Davis 1987, p. 730).

Marketing campaigns seem designed to appeal to specific personality characteristics of groups of potential buyers. In this respect, they exemplify interactions between personal characteristics and the environment. The Marlboro brand was the leading choice of a group of white adolescent male (48 percent) and female (38 percent) smokers surveyed in Louisiana in 1981 (Hunter et al. 1986). In a sample of 306 high school students in Georgia, Marlboro was the preferred brand of 76 percent of smokers who identified a single preferred brand (Goldstein et al. 1987). Similar findings were reported by Glantz (1985). These figures contrast with the overall domestic market share of Marlboro, which was 24 percent in 1987 (Ticer 1988). Given the associations of rebelliousness and behavioral problems with adolescent smoking, as reviewed above, there may be a relationship between the noted disparity of overall brand preference and the emphasis on the tough independence of the "Marlboro Man." In fact, this pattern may be a reflection of extensive market segmentation, in which specific brands are marketed for specific gender or ethnic groups, often with campaign messages and symbols aimed at those groups (Davis 1987). Teenage girls, relative to boys, are more likely to believe that smoking controls weight (Charlton 1984) and are good targets for advertisements that emphasize the desirability of being slender (Gritz 1986).

Some market segmentation appears more subtle, guided by smoker characteristics not as apparent as race and gender. McCarthy and Gritz (1987) surveyed students in grades 6, 9, and 12 regarding their attitudes about cigarette advertisements. Among their findings was the closer relationship, for those youth more likely to be smokers, between personality self-ratings and personality ratings assigned to models in cigarette advertisements. Thus, the way adolescents see themselves appears to be related to their attraction to certain advertisements. This congruity among psychological correlates of teenage smoking, marketing themes, and teenage preferences is especially striking when one considers that the tobacco industry denies that campaigns are aimed at teenagers (Davis 1987).

Summary

The increased understanding of the multiple and interacting determinants of the development of smoking and of the relation of these determinants to the stages of development of smoking is a reflection of progress over the last 25 years. The delineation of stages—from onset to regular use—has been an especially influential development (Figure 2). The development of the addictive processes in teenagers has recently become better appreciated and understood (Biglan and Lichtenstein 1984; Hirschman, Leventhal, Glynn 1984). While information about the long-term disease consequences of smoking has an important role in adolescent smoking initiation, awareness of the short-term health consequences and the influence of peers and advertising are now seen as more critical for adolescent decisionmaking. The effects of peers and family are both supported. Cigarette marketing appears to target teenagers despite the cigarette companies' reported policy efforts to restrict such advertising.

Regular Smoking

Pharmacologic Processes and Conditioning

Pharmacologic processes and conditioning play complementary and major roles in maintaining regular smoking. Early theories of smoking tended to view pharmacologic processes and conditioning as separate explanations of regular smoking (e.g., Hunt 1970; Table 35). They are now viewed as complementary and interacting processes (US DHHS 1988). The 1988 Surgeon General's Report on nicotine addiction affirmed the critical role of nicotine and its varied and powerful pharmacologic effects on the central nervous system (CNS) in the development and maintenance of regular smoking. This acknowledgment and its implications for intervention represent a significant shift in perspective over the 25-year history of the Surgeon General's Reports. Concurrently, increased knowledge of smoking as an addiction has clarified the important role of conditioning in addiction. Conditioning and related processes link the biological effects of nicotine to the many behaviors that make up smoking and to the many concurrent physical and environmental stimuli that guide it.

Nicotine Addiction

The 1964 Report distinguished between drug addiction and drug habituation (US PHS 1964; Table 36) and concluded that smoking is habituation. As noted in the 1988 Report, the addiction/habituation distinction was dropped in 1964 by the WHO shortly after the release of the 1964 Report (US DHHS 1988).

The 1988 Surgeon General's Report on nicotine addiction noted the following three major conclusions: (1) cigarettes and other forms of tobacco are addicting; (2) nicotine is the drug in tobacco that causes addiction; (3) the pharmacologic and behavioral processes that determine tobacco addiction are similar to those that determine addiction to drugs such as heroin and cocaine (US DHHS 1988, p. 9). These conclusions were based on a thorough review of research on addictive aspects of smoking extending over nearly a century.

The criteria that guided the 1988 Report's conclusion that smoking is an addiction are summarized in Table 36. As documented by extensive research cited in the Report, smoking meets all the criteria. Smoking is continued despite a desire to quit and, in many cases, despite clear harm to the individual. A central criterion concerns psychoactive effects of a drug on the CNS. Rapid absorption of nicotine into the bloodstream and consequent delivery to the CNS are features common to all popular forms of tobacco use. Recent evidence confirms that nicotine is absorbed by the brain, which contains receptors specific for this agent (e.g., London et al. 1985; London, Waller, Wamsley 1985); has euphoric effects and perhaps sedative or other anxiolytic effects mediated by neurohormonal processes (e.g., Henningfield, Miyasato, Jasinski 1985); and reinforces behavior, even among animals or human subjects blind to whether they received saline placebo or nicotine (Henningfield, Chait, Griffiths 1983, 1984). As with other addictive drugs, prolonged ingestion of nicotine leads to tolerance, a tendency to consume increasing amounts of a drug, presumably to achieve a desired euphoric or

TABLE 36.—Comparison of characteristics of addiction, habituation, and dependence in 1964 and 1988 Surgeon General's Reports

Characteristics of drug addiction and habituation in 1964 Surgeon General's Report[a]		Characteristics of drug addiction in 1988 Surgeon General's Report[b]
Drug addiction	Drug habituation	Primary Criteria
A state of periodic or chronic intoxication produced by the repeated consumption of a drug (natural or synthetic).	A condition resulting from the repeated consumption of a drug.	Highly controlled or compulsive pattern of drug use.
Its characteristics include:	Its characteristics include:	Psychoactive or mood-altering effects involved in pattern of drug taking.
(1) an overpowering desire or need (compulsion) to continue taking the drug and to obtain it by any means;	(1) a desire (but not a compulsion) to continue taking the drug for the sense of improved well-being it engenders;	Drug functioning as reinforcer to strengthen behavior and lead to further drug ingestion.
(2) a tendency to increase the dose;	(2) little or no tendency to increase the dose;	Additional Criteria
(3) a psychic (psychological) and generally a physical dependence on the effects of the drug; and	(3) some degree of psychic dependence on the effect of the drug, but absence of physical dependence and hence of an abstinence syndrome; and	Tolerance (increased doses either tolerated without discomfort or needed to achieve desired effects).
(4) detrimental effects on the individual and on society.	(4) detrimental effects, if any, primarily on the individual.	Physical dependence (withdrawal syndrome upon termination of drug taking).
		Use despite harmful effects.
		Pleasant (euphoric) effects.
		Stereotypic patterns of drug use.
		Relapse following drug abstinence.
		Recurrent drug cravings.

[a]SOURCE: US PHS (1964, p. 351).
[b]SOURCE: US DHHS (1988, pp. 194, 250–253).

other effect. Prolonged use also leads to physical dependence, as indexed by various psychological and physical withdrawal symptoms following cessation of smoking. The inclusion of tobacco dependence as a disorder in the Diagnostic and Statistical Manual of Mental Disorders III, the official diagnostic reference for the American Psychiatric Association (1980), was another major marker in the shift of scientific opinion about the addictive nature of cigarette smoking.

Central to the 1964 view was the distinction between compulsive use (addiction) and the less compulsive "desire" (habituation). The difference was noted to rest primarily on the source of the desire or compulsion. The 1964 Report emphasized "serious personality defects from underlying psychologic or psychiatric disorders" (US PHS 1964, p. 351) as a defining factor in compulsive use and therefore in addiction. Evidence gathered since the early 1960s contradicts the assumptions that underlying pathology drives the compulsive use seen in addiction. Drugs commonly viewed as addictive, e.g., heroin, may be abandoned with little apparent effort as with many Vietnam veterans addicted to heroin who gave it up after their return to the United States (Robins, Helzer, Davis 1975; US DHHS 1988). On the other hand, the extent to which smoking can be highly compulsive is suggested by its continuance in the face of substantial awareness of its harm, as by cardiac patients (Baile et al. 1982; Burling et al. 1984; Ockene et al. 1985; US DHHS 1984). The generality of nicotine's effects argues against its compulsive use resting on individual psychopathology; the basis for nicotine addiction rests on the interaction of conditioning processes and nicotine action in the brain.

Mechanisms of Nicotine Action

Much research in the 1970s on the behavioral effects of nicotine has been guided by the nicotine regulation (or titration) model put forth over the years by Jarvik (1977), Jarvik, Glick, and Nakamura (1970), Russell (1976), and Schachter, Silverstein and colleagues (1977). According to this model, smokers regulate their smoking to maintain a certain level of blood nicotine within a range of upper and lower limits (Herman and Kozlowski 1979; Kozlowski and Herman 1984). This includes the avoidance of withdrawal symptoms or anticipated withdrawal by maintaining a nicotine level above a lower limit and avoidance of toxicity by maintaining it below an upper limit.

This formulation has been criticized as failing to explain the self-perceived positive effects or benefits of smoking that may promote use (Pomerleau and Pomerleau 1984; Leventhal and Cleary 1980). Interestingly, the 1964 Surgeon General's Report devoted only 1 1/2 pages to such effects. In the last few years, several investigators (e.g., Ockene et al. 1988; Pomerleau and Pomerleau 1984) have proposed that smoking, by virtue of the varied actions of nicotine, provides several positively perceived effects and is employed by many smokers as a responsive and effective coping strategy. This implies that smokers can be reinforced for continued smoking without maintaining a minimum blood nicotine level. The 1988 Report devoted an entire chapter to this topic.

An influential and historically important model of perceived positive effects of smoking stressed the psychological effects of nicotine and other pharmacologic aspects of smoking (Pomerleau and Pomerleau 1984). This model holds that nicotine increases the release of a number of neuroregulatory hormones, conferring on smoking the ability to act as stimulant or sedative depending on level of ingestion, background hormone levels, and the like. Nicotine thus can serve to reduce anxiety or produce euphoria (US DHHS 1988) and enhance vigilance for certain cognitive tasks (e.g., Warburton et al. 1986). The work of Grunberg (1986; US DHHS 1988) also suggests that nicotine may aid smokers in maintaining lower body weight. Although objective judgment indicates that the health effects of smoking are more important than the weight maintenance effects (Abrams et al. 1987), the latter seem to be of particular importance to some women (Klesges and Klesges, in press; US DHHS 1988). This growing recognition that smokers may value several effects of cigarettes can be used not so much to justify the behavior but rather to direct intervention strategies (e.g., physical activity) that might help people meet needs previously served by cigarettes. Interventions also are likely to be seen as more credible to smokers if the coping value of cigarettes is recognized (Ockene et al. 1988).

Conditioning and Smoking

What most distinguishes recent analyses of the conditioning of smoking from earlier views (e.g., Hunt 1970) is their emphasis on the conditioning of the biological effects of nicotine. The occurrence of stimuli previously associated with the effects of nicotine will tend to evoke responses related to those effects or cues for further consumption (e.g., Abrams et al., in press; Herman 1974; Niaura et al. 1988; Rickard-Figueroa and Zeichner 1985). Such conditioned effects may link smoking to aversive states alleviated by nicotine. For example, investigations described earlier (e.g., Schachter, Silverstein et al. 1977) suggested that smoking covaries with stress, which is hypothesized to deplete nicotine. Leventhal and Cleary (1980) suggested that stress as well as other emotions may be alleviated by nicotine and would then come to serve as cues for smoking. Pomerleau and Pomerleau (1984, 1987) identified neurohumoral effects of nicotine as the paths of its impact and elaborated on the ways such effects might be conditioned to circumstances surrounding smoking so as to regulate it in the future.

Two influential theories of addiction emphasize the role of relief of withdrawal or anticipated withdrawal in smoking. As suggested by Wikler's classic work with opioids (Wikler 1973; Wikler and Pescor 1967), withdrawal symptoms may be conditioned to the circumstances in which they occur. This would set the stage for stimuli associated with prior drug taking to elicit withdrawal symptoms and urges. With smoking, greater withdrawal symptoms have been noted when cessation occurs in natural rather than artificial environments, presumably because those natural environments contain numerous cues associated with prior smoking (Hatsukami, Hughes, Pickens 1985). Within this model, return to smoking after brief or extended abstinence is reinforced by the reduction in such conditioned withdrawal symptoms.

Opponent-process theory (Solomon and Corbit 1973) suggests that the reduction of aversive withdrawal symptoms may be the result of the interaction of the immediate response to a drug, called the "A" state, and the delayed response, the "B" state. The B state is "opposed" to or opposite the A—hence "opponent process"; if the A is pleasurable, the B will be aversive. Initially, the A state is stronger. While initial, pleasurable responses to nicotine may encourage increased smoking, regular smoking leads the aversive B state to become stronger, which in turn may be reduced or avoided by the A-state consequences of further smoking. After regular smoking has been established, the A state serves only to avoid or reduce the aversive B state. That is, regular smoking is pursued to reduce displeasure rather than to bring about the pleasure that may have been its initial appeal. It is important to note that there is little evidence on the validity of the Wikler theory or opponent-process theory as applied to smoking.

In contrast to models emphasizing relief of withdrawal, a recent review (Niaura et al. 1988) proposes an "appetitive" model of responses to cues associated with smoking. Evidence indicates that cues surrounding smoking are more strongly conditioned to its positively perceived effects than to withdrawal symptoms. That is, cues associated with intake of nicotine (e.g., holding a cigarette or inhaling) come to elicit conditioned responses similar to the effects of nicotine (e.g., relaxation, heightened arousal). These effects are strong reinforcers and encourage continued efforts to obtain or ingest the drug. These reinforcing effects may be more critical than the reduction of withdrawal symptoms after periods of abstinence.

Critical to understanding the appetitive model is the idea that negative emotions are not necessarily withdrawal symptoms. However, negative emotions previously alleviated by nicotine may serve as cues for seeking repetition of smoking's reinforcing effects (Stewart, DeWit, Eikelboom 1984). For example, social anxiety may be the occasion for smoking, which is then reinforced by nicotine's ability to reduce anxiety. The anxiety, however, is a response to a stressful situation, not a symptom of withdrawal from cigarettes. Smoking is reinforced by the anxiety reduction, not by reduction of withdrawal symptoms.

The many ways smoking is conditioned to circumstances around it may explain "the thorough interweaving of the smoking habit in the fabric of daily life" (Pomerleau and Pomerleau 1987, p. 119). The sheer repetition of smoking also strengthens such interweaving. It is estimated that the average pack-a-day smoker of 20 years' duration has inhaled cigarette smoke over 1 million times (Fisher and Rost 1986; Pomerleau and Pomerleau 1984), each inhalation providing an opportunity for conditioning smoking to numerous circumstances of daily life. Moreover, with years of smoking, the emotional states and daily circumstances conditioned to it may continue to increase, resulting in urges to smoke being conditioned to almost every circumstance encountered and complicating the task of maintaining abstinence.

Cognition and Decisionmaking

Cognitive and decisionmaking processes play a lesser role in the maintenance of regular smoking relative to the other factors discussed here. Smokers have long believed that they derive positive effects from smoking. The "pros" of smoking have been embodied in the instruments used in decisionmaking studies (Mausner and Platt 1971; Velicer et al. 1985) and in the Horn and Waingrow (1966) Reasons-for-Smoking Scale.

As documented in Chapter 4 of this Report, public knowledge of the health consequences of smoking has increased steadily over the past 25 years. Eighty-seven percent of current smokers now report that they understand that smoking is harmful to their health (ALA 1985) and two-thirds of high school seniors report "great risk" being associated with pack-a-day smoking (Johnston, O'Malley, Bachman 1987). Why, then, do so many persist in regular smoking? One reason may be that they do not appreciate just how dangerous smoking is. For example, 75 percent of current smokers agreed that smoking is a cause of lung cancer (ALA 1985), while 94 percent of nonsmokers and 90 percent of former smokers agreed to this. For emphysema, the parallel figures were 75 percent of current smokers compared with 91 percent and 90 percent of former smokers and nonsmokers, respectively (ALA 1985). Surveys indicate a general insensitivity to the relative level of risk associated with smoking. Health professionals rated nonsmoking as the first priority among things Americans can do to protect their health. The public rated nonsmoking as 10th, behind such worthy but, for most Americans, less critical behaviors as consuming adequate vitamins and minerals and drinking water of acceptable quality (Fisher and Rost 1986). As discussed below, the health belief model (Rosenstock 1974) requires that smokers believe they are personally vulnerable to a threat before they will be motivated to attempt change. It has been suggested that personalized acceptance ("Cigarette smoking is dangerous to *my* health") always lags behind general acceptance ("Cigarette smoking is dangerous to health") (Fishbein 1977; Lichtenstein and Bernstein 1980; Shiffman 1987) (See Chapter 4). These considerations suggest that many smokers still find it possible to discount the riskiness of their behavior.

Another possible reason for some smokers' insensitivity to smoking risks is that they have not always been given the full message, or they have been given mixed messages, including prosmoking messages (advertising) from the cigarette industry. Factors that impede public awareness and acceptance of the health hazards of smoking include cigarette advertising and promotion and cigarette companies' public relations and lobbying activities, which are also reviewed in Chapters 6 and 7.

Other issues related to persistence of smoking will be covered in the Section on Quitting and Relapse.

Personal Characteristics and Social Context

Personal Characteristics

The 1964 Surgeon General's Report linked smoking in adulthood and adolescence to extraversion, or as it defined it, a tendency "to live faster and more intensely" (US PHS 1964, p. 366), and this relationship has been confirmed in later studies (e.g., Ashton and Stepney 1982). However, reviews indicate that there is no consistent evidence relating smoking to neuroticism or emotional instability (Smith 1970; US DHEW 1979a). More recent studies have continued to find relationships with smoking and behaviors linked to extraversion: coffee and alcohol consumption (Istvan and Matarazzo 1984); circadian phase differences, being an "evening type" as opposed to a "morning type" (Ishihara et al. 1985); alcohol consumption, driving accidents, divorce, frequent job changes, low levels of vocational success, and impulsivity (Eysenck 1980).

Another personality construct that received a great deal of attention earlier in the smoking literature was Rotter's (1966) internal versus external locus-of-control dimension (e.g., Foss 1973; Best and Steffy 1975; Best 1975; Straits and Sechrest 1963). Two general hypotheses characterized work in this area. The first noted that smokers tended to have a more external locus of control, that is, perceive that things occur because of fate, not because of one's own actions, compared with nonsmokers. The second held that smokers with a greater internal locus of control, that is, a perception that things happen because of one's own actions, would be more successful in quitting. A review of this literature revealed inconsistent support for both hypotheses (Baer and Lichtenstein 1988b).

The multidimensional health locus of control scale (Wallston, Wallston, DeVellis 1978) was an attempt to anchor the locus of control construct specifically to health behavior consistent with the trend away from broad, dispositional traits (Mischel 1973). Most studies using this scale examined the effect of health locus of control on cessation attempts. Three investigations reported small but significant prospective relationships between subscales of the Health Locus of Control Scale and maintenance of abstinence (Kaplan and Cowles 1978; Rosen and Shipley 1983; Shipley 1981).

A popular approach to understanding social or psychological problems has been through typologies. Tomkin's typology of smoking and affect regulation was very influential in the 1960s and early 1970s (Ikard and Tomkins 1973; Tomkins 1966, 1968). Tomkins originally proposed a fourfold typology including positive affect, negative affect, habitual, and addictive smoking. This model gave rise to the Reasons-for-Smoking Scale (Horn and Waingrow 1966), which continues to be used widely in public education and cessation programs despite receiving little empirical support (Shiffman 1988). Validity studies have yielded the most consistent support for the negative affect smoking construct (Ikard and Tomkins 1973; Pomerleau, Adkins, Pertschuk 1978; Joffe, Lowe, Fisher 1981).

The support demonstrated for negative affect smoking is also consistent with recent reviews' emphasis on stress reduction as being among those biological effects of nicotine that maintain regular smoking (e.g., Leventhal and Cleary 1980, Pomerleau and Pomerleau 1987). Much evidence for such effects comes from the retrospective reports of relapsers and smokers attempting to stop, which are reviewed later in this Chapter. However, relatively few data demonstrate that heightened stress leads to greater smoking. Among them are Ikard and Tomkin's observations (1973) of greater incidence among race track spectators during horse races—presumed to be times of stress—than in the periods before and after races, and Silverman's observations of nicotine-induced reductions in aggression among rats (1971). A number of other studies reviewed in the 1988 Surgeon General's Report link smoking and negative affect but, as noted in that review, are not conclusive as to whether reduction of negative affect makes a substantial contribution to regular smoking. Design problems include comparisons of smokers smoking with smokers who are deprived, leaving unclear, for instance, whether smoking reduces negative affect or whether, for regular smokers, *not* smoking merely causes an aversive, deprivation state. As concluded in the 1988 Report, "... caution must be exercised in generalizing about smoking and nicotine's effects on stress and mood ..." (US DHHS 1988, p. 405).

Less direct support for effects of stress on smoking lies in studies of smoking prevalence among groups who are disadvantaged in our society, including psychiatric outpatients (Hughes et al. 1986) and male users of soup kitchens (McDade and Keil 1988). Of the 38 subgroups defined by gender and economic, educational, vocational, or marital status listed in the 1988 Report, divorced or separated men had the highest prevalence of smoking, 48.2 percent (US DHHS 1988). Other social problems such as alcoholism and suicide are also more prevalent in this group (Kaplan and Sadock 1985).

Beyond those groups with significant disadvantages such as psychopathology and very low income, the more general effects of income and education are quite substantial. For instance, preliminary data from the 1987 NHIS indicate a 35-percent smoking prevalence among adults with less than a high school education, more than twice the 16.3 percent prevalence among those with postgraduate college training (see Part I). Prevalence among both women and men declines with increases in income range. Among unemployed men, the prevalence is 44.3 percent (US DHHS 1988). Such trends indicate that the social and economic context affects the relationship of personal characteristics with smoking. Consistent with this, trends presented in Part I of this Chapter indicate that observed differences of race and sex are attributable to effects of income and education (see also Novotny, Warner et al. 1988).

Social Context Influences

The arrival at regular use roughly corresponds to the period of transition from adolescence to adulthood. At least until very recently, the social changes that accompany this passage—entering a university, the military, or the workforce—have been associated with a marked change in the acceptability of smoking. For high school students, smoking is often prohibited on school property, even if the prohibition is poorly enforced. In the workforce, community college, and university setting, smoking has been widely accepted. The military until recently had supported smoking among its men and women, as reflected in low prices for cigarettes at military exchanges and commissaries and by the announcement of breaks with "The smoking lamp is lit." The extent to which smoking is a part of the role of the serviceman was shown in a survey of Navy enlisted men with a mean age of 22.6 years and a mean of 3.9 years' service. Seventy-two percent were self-reported smokers (Burr 1984). That the military has an effect on creating rather than attracting smokers is suggested by a comparison of prevalence among naval recruits, 27.6 percent, and shipboard men, 49.8 percent (Cronan and Conway 1988). The military has recently recognized the enormous costs attendant to the high prevalence of smokers within its ranks and has begun efforts directed at reducing the percentage of smokers among its personnel (See Chapters 6 and 7).

Cigarette marketing, discussed above and in Chapter 7, continues to be an important influence encouraging adult smoking, with several possible direct and indirect influences on smoking patterns (Warner 1985).

Summary

The past 25 years have seen a deepening appreciation of the importance of nicotine in maintaining regular smoking. In contrast to the 1964 Surgeon General's Report, cigarette smoking is now defined as an addiction (US DHHS 1988). Earlier emphasis on the maintenance of blood nicotine levels as a means to avoid withdrawal has been balanced by the awareness that nicotine's varied effects make smoking an efficient coping strategy for affect regulation and perhaps weight regulation. Conditioning models of smoking have become more sophisticated and firmly integrated with the pharmacologic actions of nicotine to explain addiction. While the public is now better informed about the health consequences of smoking, many smokers still minimize their perception of their vulnerability amid extensive marketing of tobacco products. Broad, dispositional traits or motives are now seen to be of limited value in understanding smoking. The role of social settings and social influence in encouraging regular smoking is also better understood.

Cessation and Relapse

A large body of literature on determinants of cessation has evolved, driven by the need to provide empirical and theoretical guidelines for intervention programs. All three sets of determinants—pharmacologic processes and conditioning, cognition and decisionmaking, and personality and social context—play an important role in the cessation stage (Table 39). It is with respect to cessation, especially, that the concept of stages—treating stopping as a process over time—has evolved (Figure 8) and now guides research and interventions (e.g., Marlatt 1985). The influential and well-articulated cessation stage model of Prochaska and DiClemente (1983) defines four stages of cessation. Precontemplation is the stage in which the smoker is neither considering stopping nor actively processing smoking-and-health information. During the contemplation stage, smokers are thinking about stopping and are processing information about the effects of smoking and ways to stop. In the action or cessation stage, the smoker is no longer smoking and has been without cigarettes for less than 6 months. The maintenance phase involves establishment of long-term abstinence, while relapse is the resumption of smoking. When relapse occurs, the smoker recycles to any one of the three previous stages.

Specific cognitive and behavioral processes are employed during the different stages of cessation (Prochaska and DiClemente 1983). Determinants of each stage are also different. Thus, factors that affect an initial decision to stop smoking may not predict success in stopping or sustained maintenance after stopping. Working from a related but different stage model—initial decision, initial control, maintenance—Rosen and Shipley (1983) used health locus of control, desire to stop, and self-esteem to predict self-initiated smoking reduction. Using regression analysis, a different set of predictors was demonstrated at each stage, suggesting the possible need for different intervention techniques at each stage of the smoking reduction process.

An important implication of a stage model is that interventions may need to address cessation's several stages. The precontemplator's tendency to ignore quitting strategies may need to be met with continued personalized information on smoking and health; the contemplator may need social support to attempt cessation; and the abstainer may need help that emphasizes the development of relapse prevention skills. There are as yet no data available to demonstrate the effect of interventions tailored to specific stages of cessation. Thus, a model like the Prochaska and DiClemente stage model is best viewed as a tentative conceptualization, useful for guiding research and interventions. The next section considers changes in our understanding of the determinants of cessation in relation to the stages in the cessation process.

Pharmacologic Processes and Conditioning

Pharmacologic processes and conditioning exert a strong influence on the process of quitting. One indicator of the role of addiction is that heavier, more dependent smokers in intervention programs are less likely to quit than are lighter, less dependent smokers (e.g., Hall et al. 1984; Ockene et al. 1982b), especially when smokers with much variability in baseline smoking are studied, as in the Multiple Risk Factor Intervention Trial (MRFIT) (Hughes et al. 1981). As is noted in the 1988 Surgeon General's Report, "Withdrawal symptoms, whether elicited by acute deprivation or by conditioned stimuli, are hypothesized to be the link between dependence and relapse" (p. 523), although some analyses (e.g., Niaura et al. 1988) place greater emphasis on positive effects of smoking in motivating relapse. Further evidence of the influence of addiction comes from intervention studies evaluating nicotine-containing gum. Several studies have found that nicotine polacrilex gum is more effective when used with nicotine-dependent smokers (as measured by the Fagerstrom (1978) addiction questionnaire) than with less dependent smokers (Hall et al. 1985; Killen et al. 1984; Schneider et al. 1983). Nicotine polacrilex gum most likely is effective because it reduces withdrawal symptoms frequently noticed in the first days and weeks of abstinence (Hughes et al. 1984; West et al. 1984). Recently, more work has focused on nicotine replacement strategies or other pharmacologic treatment adjuncts reflecting the importance of biological factors in smoking and cessation (Grabowski and Hall 1985; US DHHS 1986b; US DHHS 1988).

Conditioning mediates the role of the pharmacologic effects of nicotine in cessation. As noted in the discussion of regular smoking, numerous conditioned environmental stimuli are likely to evoke urges or cues to smoke. Recent work by Abrams and colleagues demonstrates that former smokers manifest psychophysiological reactivity to smoking cues long after they have quit (Abrams et al., in press; Abrams 1986). Conditioned reactivity to environmental cues, then, may be more decisive in the later stage of maintenance after withdrawal symptoms have subsided.

Research on relapse triggers reflects current interest in specific, situational variables. Primary triggers include stress, interpersonal conflict, dysphoria, presence of other smokers, and alcohol consumption (Marlatt and Gordon 1980; Shiffman 1982). Although the data are primarily retrospective reports from relapsed or tempted subjects, there is convincing consistency on the importance of stress and negative affect in determining maintenance or relapse (Baer and Lichtenstein 1988a; Marlatt and Gordon 1980; Ockene et al. 1982a; Shiffman 1982; US DHHS 1988). The mechanism whereby a lapse becomes a full return to smoking has also recently been analyzed as a series of stages (Marlatt 1985). These include a high-risk occasion that triggers a smoking lapse (that is, a brief return to smoking) and a subsequent interpretation of the lapse that may lead to abandoning the cessation effort and a return to regular smoking. Much recent attention has been paid to the importance of coping responses in dealing with both high-risk situations and lapses (e.g., Shiffman 1984; Shiffman and Wills 1985). The available data suggest that the absence of any coping response is predictive of relapse but there are few differences that relate to the use of specific coping strategies used (Shiffman 1984).

Cognition and Decisionmaking

The role of cognitions in smoking cessation is evident in the relapse model noted above (Marlatt 1985). In this model, a lapse diminishes self-efficacy or self-confidence and expectations for long-term success. These diminished efficacy expectations then become the basis for an individual to abandon the effort and return to regular smoking (Marlatt 1985). In fact, lapses are highly predictive of subsequent relapse (Brandon, Tiffany, Baker 1986; Baer et al. 1988).

Researchers have long noted the relationship of knowledge about the health consequences of smoking, beliefs about personal susceptibility, attitudes toward smoking, and expectations about the benefits of quitting to cessation efforts and their long-term success or failure. Cognitive-behavioral models of smoking cessation emphasize the importance of an individual's interpretation of health risks and perceived self-efficacy for refraining from smoking (Pechacek and Danaher 1979), as well as attributions about addiction and lapses during the maintenance stage (Marlatt 1985).

Expectancy-Value Models

Expectancy-value models have guided approaches to smoking cessation for many years (e.g., Kirscht 1983; Mausner and Platt 1971; Sutton 1987). Outcome expectations refer to expected consequences that would occur if one continued smoking or quit smoking (Bandura 1977). Their value refers to the personal importance or weight given to the various possible outcomes and can be extended to perceptions about what significant others wish one to do (Fishbein 1982). Expectations include the positive (e.g., enjoyment) and negative (e.g., disease) consequences of smoking and the positive (e.g., enhanced lung capacity) and negative consequences (e.g., loss of enjoyment, withdrawal symptoms) of quitting. Expectancy-value models tend to assume that human behavior is rationally guided by logical or at least internally consistent thought processes (Henderson, Hall, Linton 1979).

Decisionmaking models represent one variant of the expectancy-value approach and have been (e.g., Mausner and Platt 1971) and continue to be (Velicer et al. 1985) applied to smoking cessation. The more recent applications (Velicer et al. 1985) may prove more useful because they take into account stage of change (Prochaska and DiClemente 1983). Changes in the relative level of pro and con views of smoking, for example, appear related to stages of quitting. Smokers not contemplating quitting report substantially higher levels of pro than con views, while those contemplating quitting report equal pro and con views. For quitters, con views were higher than pro views. These relative pro and con views also predicted subsequent change in smoking (Velicer et al. 1985).

Since the 1960s, the health-belief model (Kirscht 1983; Rosenstock 1974; Swinehart and Kirscht 1966) has been a popular approach to understanding expectancy-value concepts applied to smoking cessation. According to this model, attempting to stop smoking is a function of three factors: beliefs about the health consequences of smoking and perceived susceptibility to the disease consequences, perceptions of available actions that can reduce one's risk, and perceptions of the costs and benefits of accomplishing these actions (Kirscht and Rosenstock 1979). Johnston (1985) and his colleagues (Bachman, Johnston, O'Malley, and Humphrey 1988), for example, have shown that changes in perceived risk have accounted for a considerable reduction in adolescent marijuana use—particularly regular use. They suggest that effects of such beliefs may be more limited in the case of cigarettes because of the addictive properties of nicotine. As described in the next section, some recent models have addressed individuals' belief in their ability to change behaviors, or self-efficacy (Bandura 1977; Eiser 1983; Eiser and Sutton 1977; Sutton and Eiser 1984).

Self-Efficacy and Smoking

Bandura (1977, 1982) defines self-efficacy as an individual's belief in his or her ability to perform a specific behavior and proposes that efficacy beliefs represent a final common pathway mediating behavior change. Information from past behavior, modeling, affective states, and instruction combine to produce a performance expectation, which then predicts future behavior. This behavior would, in turn, influence subsequent efficacy; behavior and efficacy are reciprocally related (Bandura 1982).

The belief in one's ability to stop smoking has been implicated in the health-belief model and in Eiser's (1983) analysis of decisionmaking about stopping smoking. Self-efficacy theory, then, can be viewed as a historical descendant of the health-belief model and recently has had a major impact on models of smoking cessation. It is a major construct in Marlatt's (1985) influential relapse prevention model, which has spawned several intervention studies (e.g., Brown et al. 1984; Curry et al., in press). In Marlatt's model, self-efficacy is the key variable in the stage of maintenance (or relapse). It helps determine how well the individual will deal with high-risk situations or urges and is, in turn, influenced by successful or unsuccessful coping (Marlatt 1985).

Consistent with Marlatt's (1985) model, significant results with self-efficacy primarily pertain to client ratings after intervention, and thus predict smoking during followup periods. When all clients in treatment are considered, posttreatment self-efficacy ratings correlate strongly with short-term maintenance (Condiotte and Lichtenstein 1981; Coelho 1984; McIntyre-Kingsolver, Lichtenstein, Mermelstein 1983). For the most part, efficacy scores seem to correlate with outcome most highly when the followup interval is shorter (e.g., 3 months) and diminish over time (Coelho 1984; McIntyre-Kingsolver, Lichtenstein, Mermelstein 1983).

In order to view efficacy as a determinant of maintenance of cessation, it is necessary to demonstrate that it influences the latter independent of performance (level of smoking) at the time efficacy is assessed. Results using partial correlations suggest that efficacy scores do provide limited information above and beyond that of current smoking behavior (Baer, Holt, Lichtenstein 1986). A second approach is to correlate self-efficacy measured postintervention with subsequent followup status only for those clients who initially quit. Studies using this paradigm have found significant but modest correlation with 3-month followup (McIntyre-Kingsolver, Lichtenstein, Mermelstein 1983; Coelho 1984). Self-efficacy also can be assessed during the maintenance phase, in order to predict longer term followup. Two studies have examined these relationships and both found significant prospective relationships (DiClemente 1981; Baer, Holt, Lichtenstein 1986). While intervention studies have usually found pretreatment efficacy unrelated to outcome, one study of unaided quitters found that baseline efficacy correlated with continuous abstinence at 1 year (Gritz, Carr, Marcus, in press). Another intervention study found that participants' attribution of stopping to their own skill and effort, gathered 3 months after stopping, was correlated with abstinence at 6-month followup (Fisher, Levenkron et al. 1982). National survey data reviewed by Shiffman (1986) suggest that lack of confidence in the ability to stop deters many smokers from attempting cessation.

Outcome Expectations

From a stage perspective, outcome expectations (perceived consequences of smoking or stopping) are more likely to be related to the decision to stop smoking or the initiation of quit attempts than to success in the stopping process. The effects of brief advice from a physician offer indirect support for the role of outcome expectations (Russell et al. 1979). Patients receiving brief advice to stop smoking were more likely to stop relative to control subjects. The physicians'advice probably enhanced the salience of the perceived positive consequences of stopping or the negative consequences of continuing to smoke and thus prompted the decision to attempt to stop. Negative consequences of smoking are potentiated by dramatic illness such as myocardial infarction, which is often the occasion for cessation efforts; however, relapse is often considerable (e.g., Baile et al. 1982), although less than with nondiseased smokers (Ockene et al. 1987). Cognitions concerning the health risks of smoking and the positive benefits of stopping remain very important from a public health perspective (see Chapter 4) and the health-belief model may be useful for guiding interventions aimed at smokers in the precontemplation or contemplation stages of change.

The role of disease in smoking cessation is substantial but not well understood. Certain environmental changes following a serious illness may aid cessation and/or the information and fear arousal provided by serious illness may motivate serious quit attempts, but continued maintenance is problematic (Ockene et al. 1985; Perkins 1988). Approximately one-quarter to one-half of survivors of myocardial infarctions are abstinent from smoking at extended followups (Ockene et al. 1985; Perkins 1988; Rigotti and Tesar 1985). While rates of cessation are impressive in some studies of cardiac and other patients, results of smoking cessation interventions produce inconsistent intervention effects (Perkins 1988; US DHHS 1986b). Research needs to evaluate the impact of diseases and of dimensions of diseases including chronic and acute events, severity, and symptom mitigation following cessation, all of which vary across different diseases.

Information about negative effects on the fetus may trigger cessation among pregnant women, perhaps by potentiating a more general awareness of smoking's dangers. Pregnancy does prompt some cessation or reduction relative to the "natural" population; however, relapse after delivery is high (US DHHS 1980b). Prevalence of smoking among pregnant women and historical shifts are documented in the first part of this Chapter.

Personal Characteristics and Social Context

Personal Characteristics

Less educated smokers who do stop tend to have higher rates of relapse and shorter periods of abstinence than do more educated persons. Stopping smoking is more common among those smokers with greater personal skills or socioeconomic resources (US DHHS 1982). Prospective studies indicate that education level, income, and skills in self-management or personal coping are significantly related to success in self-initiated efforts to stop (Blair et al. 1980; Gritz, Carr, Marcus, in press; Perri, Richards, Schultheis 1977). In a multivariate logistic regression analysis of 1985 NHIS data, blacks were significantly less likely than whites to quit smoking, regardless of SES or demographic factors (Novotny et al. 1988). Currently there are several research projects funded by NCI aimed at better understanding SES and ethnic differences in smoking that may eventually provide information to explain these differences.

The sections on the initiation of smoking and regular smoking discussed the roles of several personality variables such as extraversion and neuroticism. While associations between extraversion and smoking have been replicated over the years (Eysenck 1980), it and other broad personality variables have not shown strong effects in smoking cessation (Lichtenstein 1982). Some evidence indicates that persons high in extraversion and low in neuroticism are more able to stop smoking (US DHEW 1979a). Internal–external locus of control has been hypothesized to be related to cessation (internals more successful) but the evidence is inconclusive (US DHEW 1979a). Research on personal characteristics is now focusing on more situation-specific or interactional variables such as self-efficacy, stress, and social support (Cohen et al. 1988; Condiotte and Lichtenstein 1981; Shiffman 1982).

Stress has been shown to affect initiation of smoking and smoking rate, as well as relapse following smoking cessation (US DHHS 1988). It appears to be a factor especially influencing women's cessation (Abrams et al. 1987; Sorensen and Pechacek 1987), as well as their initiation of smoking (Mitic, McGuire, Neumann 1985). High levels of anxiety (Schwartz and Dubitzky 1968) and self-reported tendencies to smoke to relieve negative affect (Pomerleau, Adkins, and Pertschuk 1978) have been associated with reduced success in stopping. The link of smoking to stress and research demonstrating the role of social support in buffering stress (Cohen and Syme 1985) suggest that women's cessation efforts may benefit from interpersonal support more than those of men (Fisher, Bishop 1986; Gritz 1982).

Gender differences in cessation have been a major focus in recent years (US DHHS 1980b). Sex differences in onset and prevalence and historical shifts in these differences are well documented in the first section of this Chapter. These differences and shifts have prompted a search for physiological (e.g., Silverstein, Feld, Kozlowski 1980) and especially psychosocial variables (US DHHS 1980b) that might account for them. No compelling factors have yet emerged to account for the historical shifts although changes in social acceptability and the women's rights movement seem likely candidates (US DHHS 1980b). It has also been suggested, on the basis of survey data, that women have lower rates of quitting smoking than do men (Remington et al. 1985). This interpretation has been criticized for failing to adjust male quit rates to reflect the proportion of men who switch to other tobacco products (Jarvis 1984).

Women's concern about weight gain associated with smoking cessation has received much recent attention (US DHEW 1980b; US DHHS 1988). The likelihood of women gaining weight following smoking cessation and the role of weight gain in precipitating relapse deserve further investigation (US DHHS 1988) as does the hypothesis that women prefer and are more successful in cessation programs that provide social support (e.g., from a group or counselor) (Fisher and Bishop 1986; Gritz 1982). Studies of sex differences in cigarette cessation programs yield equivocal results, and the issue of gender differences in cessation remains unresolved (US DHHS 1988).

Social Context Influences

Although findings published as early as 1971 indicated the importance of peer smoking in adult smoking and cessation (Eisinger 1971; Graham and Gibson 1971), these factors did not receive the attention they were given in discussions of smoking among adolescents. This difference reflected, perhaps, popular notions that adolescents are especially influenced by social forces such as peer pressure but that adults are more tied to psychological and physiological needs (US DHHS 1988). The popularity of self-management procedures (Fisher 1986) was manifest in smoking cessation programs of the 1970s that stressed the individual's control over smoking by manipulating its triggers or antecedents. Unfortunately, research directed at such procedures failed to yield appreciable improvements in program impacts (Lichtenstein 1982). This led to a search for important variables that had not been well researched. The 1980 and 1982 Surgeon General's Reports (US DHHS 1980b, 1982) identified social support as possibly important in mediating cessation among adults. A number of recent papers have sought to explore empirically the effects of social support on smoking cessation (e.g., Coppotelli and Orleans 1985; Fisher, Lowe et al. 1982; Mermelstein, Lichtenstein, McIntyre 1983; Morgan, Ashenberg, Fisher 1988).

As recently reviewed by Lichtenstein, Glasgow, and Abrams (1986), social support measures have been repeatedly correlated with abstinence, but the addition of social support components to standard behavioral cessation programs has not yielded incremental gains on outcome. For instance, an emphasis on group cohesion to enhance social support led to initial but not long-term advantages over a control group receiving standard intervention (Etringer, Gregory, Lando 1984). Similarly, efforts to mobilize spouse support have been disappointing (McIntyre-Kingsolver, Lichtenstein, Mermelstein 1986).

An understanding of the lack of a relationship between intervention strategies that promote interpersonal support and long-term smoking cessation may be advanced by considering the nature of support and its functions in different stages of smoking cessation (Cohen et al. 1988). Interpersonal emotional support seems especially related to maintained abstinence in the first several months after cessation (Coppotelli and Orleans 1985; Mermelstein, Lichtenstein, McIntyre 1983; Morgan, Ashenberg, Fisher 1988; Ockene et al. 1982a). On the other hand, long-term abstinence of a year or more may be more closely tied to the number of smoking friends and relatives in the social network (Eisinger 1971; Graham and Gibson 1971; Mermelstein et al. 1986; Cohen et al. 1988; Smith 1988).

The parallel between the importance of social network smoking status for long-term abstinence and for development of smoking in adolescence is noteworthy. Just as the adolescent progressing toward regular use will tend to have friends who also are smokers, so the long-term abstainer may benefit from friends who also are nonusers. At the stages of the transition to regular smoking and of long-term maintenance of cessation, the importance of peers' behavior, either smoking or nonsmoking, seems greatest. It may be more effective to intervene to change norms and smoking behavior of networks than to teach supportive strategies to a few significant others.

One way to have an effect on smoking by changing norms and the smoking of social networks is through the workplace, and worksite programs are attracting considerable attention (See Chapters 6 and 7). Worksites differ in smoking prevalence and cessation rates as well as in norms for supporting cessation attempts (Sorensen and Pechacek 1986; Sorensen, Pechacek, Pallonen 1986). Programs aimed at worksite norms and general support for nonsmoking have reported substantial quit rates, even among smokers who did not join cessation clinics. Employees' ratings of management support for such programs were associated with cessation attempts and with ratings of social support for nonsmoking (Fisher, Bishop et al. 1988b; Fisher, Bishop et al. 1988c).

Summary

Cross-sectional data reviewed earlier in this Chapter demonstrate that smokers with lower levels of education are less likely to stop. Stopping smoking seems more common among smokers who have greater personal and socioeconomic resources. Educational level, income, and skills in self-management or personal coping are related to success in self-initiated efforts to quit. Less educated smokers who stop tend to have higher rates of relapse and shorter periods of abstinence than more educated persons. Conditioned responses to smoking cues and alternative coping skills are important in maintenance and avoidance of relapse.

The relationship of cognitive and decisionmaking determinants to smoking cessation has received increasing attention over the past 25 years. Cognitions about outcome expectations—the pros and cons of smoking and quitting—relate primarily to decisions to attempt cessation; efficacy cognitions about perceived ability to manage temptations or urges are related primarily to maintenance or relapse. Prospective studies indicate that the presence of acute disease, which is likely to affect cognitions about the pros and cons of smoking, is related to cessation. Consistent with an overall increasing appreciation of the importance of nicotine in all stages of smoking, more dependent smokers are less likely to succeed in quitting. Interpersonal support helps smokers in the early stages of quitting, but current evidence indicates that a low density of smokers in the social network is decisive for long-term abstinence.

Summary of Changes in Knowledge About Determinants of Smoking Behavior

There has been a dramatic increase in research on the determinants of smoking over the past 25 years. In 1964, there were few studies; by 1979 the number had expanded to a few hundred studies; now there are probably thousands. This increase in research reflects both specific Federal initiatives to support smoking research and larger trends toward recognizing the important relationship of behavioral factors to disease and the effect of preventive strategies in reducing morbidity and mortality.

Several historical trends are predominant in considering all three major stages together—development, regular smoking, and cessation. A strong consensus has evolved on the critical role of nicotine in smoking. The pharmacologic effects of nicotine and the role of conditioning are now understood as integrated processes that combine to produce the addictive nature of cigarette smoking. Cigarette smoking is now recognized to develop over a series of stages with multiple and different determinants at each stage (Figure 8; Table 35). The interaction of determinants (e.g., conditioning and the pharmacologic effects of nicotine with social influences) has become more clearly articulated. Recognition of these stages and their multiple interacting causes currently guides the development of intervention and educational programs.

Smoking onset is associated with social influences, educational and economic disadvantage, alcohol and other drug use, and antisocial behavior.

Our increased knowledge of pharmacologic and psychosocial determinants has facilitated the development of interventions—behavioral or combined behavioral and pharmacologic—to aid cessation of regular smoking. Continued increases in our understanding of the stages of cessation combined with better validated interventions of various levels of intensity or cost will help to offer smokers more choices to meet their needs. There continues to be a gap in our knowledge of how to target intervention programs for the educationally and economically disadvantaged.

As described in the next two chapters, the knowledge gained about the determinants of smoking has guided interventions and campaigns to reduce the prevalence of smoking in adults from 40 percent in 1965 to 29 percent in 1987. It has led to promising prevention and cessation programs, which use existing community channels—media, worksites, schools, physicians' offices, and hospitals—to deliver low-cost but effective interventions (Chapter 6).

CONCLUSIONS

Part I. Changes in Smoking Behavior

1. Prevalence of cigarette smoking has declined substantially among men, slightly among women, and hardly at all among those without a high school diploma. From 1965–87, the prevalence of smoking among men 20 years of age and older decreased from 50.2 to 31.7 percent. Among women, the prevalence of smoking decreased from 31.9 to 26.8 percent. Smoking prevalence among whites fell steadily. Among blacks, the prevalence of smoking changed very little between 1965 and 1974; subsequently, prevalence declined at a rate similar to that of whites during the same period. Smoking prevalence has consistently been higher among blue-collar workers than among white-collar workers.
2. Annual per capita (18 years of age and older) sales of manufactured cigarettes decreased from 4,345 cigarettes in 1963 to 3,196 in 1987, a 26-percent reduction. Total cigarette sales increased gradually to 640 billion cigarettes in 1981 and then fell to 574 billion in 1987.
3. In 1965, 29.6 percent of adults who had ever smoked cigarettes had quit. This proportion (quit ratio) increased to 44.8 percent in 1987. The rate of increase in the quit ratio from 1965–85 was similar for men and women. The rate of change in quitting activity in recent years is similar for whites and blacks. From 1965–85, the quit ratio increased more rapidly among college graduates than among adults without a high school diploma.
4. Of all adults who smoked at any time during the year 1985–86, 70 percent had made at least one serious attempt to quit during their lifetime and one-third stopped smoking for at least 1 day during that year.
5. The age of initiation of smoking has declined over time, particularly among females. Among smokers born since 1935, more than four-fifths started smoking before the age of 21.
6. Trends in prevalence of cigarette smoking among those aged 20 to 24 years are an indicator of trends in initiation. By this measure, initiation has declined between 1965 and 1987 from 47.8 to 29.5 percent. Initiation has fallen four times more rapidly among males than among females. The rate of decline has been similar among whites and blacks. Initiation has decreased three times more rapidly among those with 13 or more years of education than among those with less education.
7. The prevalence of daily cigarette smoking among high school seniors decreased from 29 percent in 1976 to 21 percent in 1980, after which prevalence leveled off at 18 to 21 percent. Prevalence among females has consistently exceeded that among males since 1977. Prevalence was lower for students with plans to pursue higher education than for those without such plans. The difference in prevalence by educational plans widened throughout this period; in 1987, smoking rates were 14 percent and 30 percent in these two groups, respectively.
8. The best sociodemographic predictor of smoking patterns appears to be level of educational attainment. Marked differences in smoking prevalence, quitting, and

initiation have occurred and have increased over time between more and less educated people.

9. The domestic market share of filtered cigarettes increased from 1 percent in 1952 to 94 percent in 1986. The market share of low-tar cigarettes (15 mg or less) increased from 2 percent in 1967 to 56 percent in 1981, after which this proportion fell slightly and then stabilized at 51 to 53 percent. The market share of longer cigarettes (94 to 121 mm) increased from 9 percent in 1967 to 40 percent in 1986.
10. Between 1964 and 1986, use of smokeless tobacco (snuff and chewing tobacco) declined among men and women 21 years of age and older. However, among males aged 17 to 19, snuff use increased fifteenfold and use of chewing tobacco increased more than fourfold from 1970–86.
11. Differences in prevalence of cigarette smoking and smokeless tobacco use between young males and young females suggest that the prevalence of any tobacco use is similar in these two groups.
12. From 1964–86, the prevalence of pipe and cigar smoking declined by 80 percent among men.

Part II. Changes in Knowledge About Determinants of Smoking Behavior

1. Smoking was viewed as a habit in 1964 and is now understood to be an addiction influenced by a wide range of interacting factors, including pharmacologic effects of nicotine; conditioning of those effects to numerous activities, emotions, and settings; socioeconomic factors; personal factors such as coping resources; and social influence factors.
2. Since 1964, there has been a gradual evolution of understanding of the progression of smoking behavior through the broad stages of development, regular use, and cessation. Each of these stages is differentially affected by multiple and interacting determinants.
3. Views of determinants of smoking are affected by the predominating theoretical and methodological perspectives. In smoking, the earlier focus on broad, dispositional variables (e.g., extraversion) has given way to an emphasis on situation-specific and interactional variables; a focus on a search for a single cause has given way to a focus on multiple and interacting causes.

Appendix

Questions Regarding Smoking Status and Quitting from the 1986 AUTS

Smoking status (current, former, never) is decided from responses to the following two questions:

"Have you ever smoked at least 100 cigarettes in your life?"

"Do you smoke cigarettes now?"

Current smokers were then asked:

"Have you ever made a serious attempt to stop smoking cigarettes entirely?"

"Thinking of your last serious attempt to quit, how long did you stay off cigarettes?"

"How long ago did that attempt to quit begin?"

Current smokers who reported that they had never made a serious attempt were asked:

"Have you ever thought about quitting?"

"Would you try to quit if there was an easy way to do so?"

Questions Regarding Smokeless Tobacco Use

1986 AUTS

Ever use:

"Have you ever used (snuff and chewing tobacco asked separately) on a fairly regular basis?"

Current use:

"Do you use (snuff, chewing tobacco) now?"

1964, 1966, 1970, and 1975 AUTS

Ever use:

"Have you ever used snuff at all regularly?"

"Have you ever chewed tobacco regularly?"

Current use:

"Do you now use (snuff, chewing tobacco)?"

1985 NIDA National Household Survey on Drug Abuse

Ever and current use:

"On the average, in the past 12 months, how often, if ever, have you used chewing tobacco or snuff or other smokeless tobacco?" Responses included "never," "almost daily," "less than daily," and "not in past year."

1985 CPS

Current other tobacco use:

"Does (name) presently use any other form of tobacco, such as snuff or chewing tobacco?"

Current smokeless tobacco use:

"What other form(s) of tobacco does (name) presently use?" The categories "snuff," "chewing tobacco," "cigars," "pipe tobacco," or "other" were coded in response to this followup question.

1986, 1987, and 1988 BRFS

Ever use:

"Have you ever used or tried any smokeless tobacco products such as chewing tobacco or snuff?"

Current use:

"Do you currently use any smokeless tobacco products such as chewing tobacco or snuff?"

1987 NHIS

Ever Use:

"Have you ever used chewing tobacco, such as Redman, Levi Garrett, or Beechnut?" "Have you ever used snuff, such as Skoal, Skoal Bandits, or Copenhagen?" In addition, those who answered "yes" to the above questions were asked, "Have you used chewing tobacco at least 20 times?"

Current use:

"Do you use (chewing tobacco, snuff) now?"

1970 NHIS

Current use:

"Do you use any other form of tobacco?" Respondents could answer yes or no to "snuff," "chewing tobacco," or "other."

References

ABRAMS, D.B. Roles of psychosocial stress, smoking cues, and coping in smoking-relapse prevention. *Health Psychology* 5(Supplement):91–92, 1986.

ABRAMS, D.B., MONTI, P.M., CAREY, K.B., PINTO, R.P., JACOBUS, S.I. Reactivity to smoking cues and relapse: Two studies of discriminant validity. *Behaviour Research and Therapy*, in press.

ABRAMS, D.B., MONTI, P.M., PINTO, R.P., ELDER, J.P., BROWN, R.A., JACOBUS, S.I. Psychosocial stress and coping in smokers who relapse or quit. *Health Psychology* 6(4):289–303, 1987.

AMERICAN LUNG ASSOCIATION. *Survey of Attitudes Toward Smoking*. Princeton, New Jersey: Gallup Organization, July 1985.

AMERICAN MEDICAL ASSOCIATION. Citizen petition of the American Medical Association to the Food and Drug Administration. Chicago: American Medical Association, April 25, 1988.

AMERICAN PSYCHIATRIC ASSOCIATION. *Diagnostic and Statistical Manual of Mental Disorders*, Third Edition (DSM-III). Washington, D.C.: American Psychiatric Association, 1980.

ANTONUCCIO, D.O., LICHTENSTEIN, E. Peer modeling influences on smoking behavior of heavy and light smokers. *Addictive Behaviors* 5(4):299–306, 1980.

ASHTON, H., STEPNEY, R. Smoking: Psychology and Pharmacology. London: Tavistock Publications, 1982.

BACHMAN, J.G., JOHNSTON, L.D., O'MALLEY, P.M. *Monitoring the Future. Questionnaire Responses From the Nation's High School Seniors, 1976*. Ann Arbor, Michigan: University of Michigan, 1980a.

BACHMAN, J.G., JOHNSTON, L.D., O'MALLEY, P.M. *Monitoring the Future. Questionnaire Responses From the Nation's High School Seniors, 1978*. Ann Arbor, Michigan: University of Michigan, 1980b.

BACHMAN, J.G., JOHNSTON, L.D., O'MALLEY, P.M. *Monitoring the Future. Questionnaire Responses From the Nation's High School Seniors, 1980*. Ann Arbor, Michigan: University of Michigan, 1981.

BACHMAN, J.G., JOHNSTON, L.D., O'MALLEY, P.M. *Monitoring the Future. Questionnaire Responses From the Nation's High School Seniors, 1982*. Ann Arbor, Michigan: University of Michigan, 1984.

BACHMAN, J.G., JOHNSTON, L.D., O'MALLEY, P.M. *Monitoring the Future. Questionnaire Responses From the Nation's High School Seniors, 1984*. Ann Arbor, Michigan: University of Michigan, 1985.

BACHMAN, J.G., JOHNSTON, L.D., O'MALLEY, P.M. *Monitoring the Future. Questionnaire Responses From the Nation's High School Seniors, 1986*. Ann Arbor, Michigan: University of Michigan, 1987.

BACHMAN, J.G., JOHNSTON, L.D., O'MALLEY, P.M., HUMPHREY, R.H. Explaining the recent decline in marijuana use: Differentiating the effects of perceived risks, disapproval, and general lifestyle factors. *Journal of Health and Social Behavior* 29:92–112, 1988.

BAER, J.S., HOLT, C.S., LICHTENSTEIN, E. Self-efficacy and smoking reexamined: Construct validity and clinical utility. *Journal of Consulting and Clinical Psychology* 54(6):846–852, December 1986.

BAER, J.S., KAMARCK, T.W., LICHTENSTEIN, E., RANSOM, C.R. The prediction of smoking relapse from characteristics of prior temptations and slips. Poster presented at the Wilford Hall Health Promotion Conference, San Antonio, Texas, May 1988.

BAER, J.S., LICHTENSTEIN, E. Classification and prediction of smoking relapse episodes: An exploration of individual differences. *Journal of Consulting and Clinical Psychology* 56(1):104–110, 1988a.

BAER, J.S., LICHTENSTEIN, E. Cognitive assessment. In: Donovan, D.M., Marlatt, G.A. (eds.) *Assessment of Addictive Behaviors.* New York: Guilford Press, 1988b, pp. 189–213.

BAILE, W.F. JR., BIGELOW, G.E., GOTTLIEB, S.H., STITZER, M.L., SACKTOR, J.D. Rapid resumption of cigarette smoking following myocardial infarction: Inverse relation to MI severity. *Addictive Behaviors* 7(4):373–380, 1982.

BANDURA, A. Self-efficacy: Toward a unifying theory of behavioral change. *Psychological Review* 84(2):191–215, 1977.

BANDURA, A. Self-efficacy mechanism in human agency. *American Psychologist* 37(2):122–147, February 1982.

BARTON, J., CHASSIN, L., PRESSON, C.C., SHERMAN, S.J. Social image factors as motivators of smoking initiation in early and middle adolescence. *Child Development* 53(6):1499–1511, December 1982.

BEST, J.A. Tailoring smoking withdrawal procedures to personality and motivational differences. *Journal of Consulting and Clinical Psychology* 43(1):1–8, 1975.

BEST, J.A., STEFFY, R.A. Smoking modification procedures for internal and external locus of control clients. *Canadian Journal of Behavioural Science* 7(2):155–165, 1975.

BIGLAN, A., LICHTENSTEIN, E. A behavior-analytic approach to smoking acquisition: Some recent findings. *Journal of Applied Social Psychology* 14(3):207–223, 1984.

BLAIR, A., BLAIR, S.N., HOWE, H.G., PATE, R.R., ROSENBERG, M., PARKER, G.M., PICKLE, L.W. Physical, psychological, and sociodemographic differences among smokers, exsmokers, and nonsmokers in a working population. *Preventive Medicine* 9(6):747–759, November 1980.

BLAKE, G.H. Smoking and the military. *New York State Journal of Medicine* 85(7):354–356, 1985.

BOTVIN, G.J., WILLS, T.A. Personal and social skills training: Cognitive-behavioral approaches to substance abuse prevention. In: Bell, C.S., Battjes, R. (eds.) *Prevention Research: Deterring Drug Abuse Among Children and Adolescents*, NIDA Research Monograph 63. U.S. Department of Health and Human Services, Public Health Service, Alcohol, Drug Abuse, and Mental Health Administration, National Institute on Drug Abuse. DHHS Publication No. (ADM) 85-1334, 1985, pp. 8–49.

BOYD, G., AND ASSOCIATES. Use of smokeless tobacco among children and adolescents in the United States. *Preventive Medicine* 16(3):402–421, May 1987.

BRANDON, T.H., TIFFANY, S.T., BAKER, T.B. The process of smoking relapse. In: Tims, F.M., Leukefeld, C.G. (eds.) *Relapse and Recovery in Drug Abuse*, NIDA Research Monograph 72. U.S. Department of Health and Human Services, Public Health Service, Alcohol, Drug Abuse, and Mental Health Administration, National Institute on Drug Abuse. DHHS Publication No. (ADM) 86-1473, 1986, pp. 104–117.

BROOK, J.S., WHITEMAN, M., GORDON, A.S., BROOK, D.W. Fathers and sons: Their relationship and personality characteristics associated with the son's smoking behavior. *Journal of Genetic Psychology* 142(2):271–281, 1983.

BROWN, R.A., LICHTENSTEIN, E., MCINTYRE, K.O., HARRINGTON-KOSTUR, J. Effects of nicotine fading and relapse prevention on smoking cessation. *Journal of Consulting and Clinical Psychology* 52(2):307–308, 1984.

BURLING, T.A., SINGLETON, E.G., BIGELOW, G.E., BAILE, W.F., GOTTLIEB, S.H. Smoking following myocardial infarction: A critical review of the literature. *Health Psychology* 3(1):83–96, 1984.

BURR, R.G. Smoking among U.S. Navy enlisted men: Some contributing factors. *Psychological Reports* 54(1):287–294, February 1984.

CENTERS FOR DISEASE CONTROL. Behavioral Risk Factor Surveillance—Selected States, 1984. *Morbidity and Mortality Weekly Report* 35:253–254, 1986a.

CENTERS FOR DISEASE CONTROL. Behavioral Risk Factor Surveillance in selected States—1985. *Morbidity and Mortality Weekly Report* 35:441–444, 1986b.

CENTERS FOR DISEASE CONTROL. Cigarette smoking in the United States, 1986. *Morbidity and Mortality Weekly Report* 36(35):581–585, September 11, 1987a.

CENTERS FOR DISEASE CONTROL. Indian Health Service facilities become smoke-free. *Morbidity and Mortality Weekly Report* 36(22):348–350, June 12, 1987b.

CENTERS FOR DISEASE CONTROL. Smokeless tobacco use in rural Alaska. *Morbidity and Mortality Weekly Report* 36(10):140–143, March 20, 1987c.

CENTERS FOR DISEASE CONTROL. Smokeless tobacco use in the United States—Behavioral Risk Factor Surveillance System, 1986. *Morbidity and Mortality Weekly Report* 36(22):337–340, June 12, 1987d.

CENTERS FOR DISEASE CONTROL. Regional variation in smoking prevalence and cessation: Behavioral Risk Factor Surveillance, 1986. *Morbidity and Mortality Weekly Report* 36:751–754, 1987e.

CENTERS FOR DISEASE CONTROL. Behavioral Risk Factor Surveillance—Selected States, 1986. *Morbidity and Mortality Weekly Report* 36(16):252–254, May 1, 1987f.

CENTERS FOR DISEASE CONTROL. Prevalence of oral lesions and smokeless tobacco use in Northern Plains Indians. *Morbidity and Mortality Weekly Report* 37(39):608–611, October 7, 1988.

CHARLTON, A. Smoking and weight control in teenagers. *Public Health* (London) 98:277–281, 1984.

CHASSIN, L., PRESSON, C., SHERMAN, S.J. Cognitive and social influence factors in adolescent smoking cessation. *Addictive Behaviors* 9:383–390, 1984.

CHASSIN, L., PRESSON, C.C., SHERMAN, S.J., CORTY, E., OLSHAVSKY, R.W. Predicting the onset of cigarette smoking in adolescents: A longitudinal study. *Journal of Applied Social Psychology* 14(3):224–243, 1984.

CHERRY, N., KIERNAN, K.E. Personality scores and smoking behaviour. A longitudinal study. *British Journal of Preventive and Social Medicine* 30(2):123–131, June 1976.

CHERRY, N., KIERNAN, K.E. A longitudinal study of smoking and personality. In: Thornton, R.E. (ed.) *Smoking Behaviour. Physiological and Psychological Influences*. Edinburgh: Churchill Livingstone, 1978.

CHUNG, C.S. A Report on the Hawaii Behavioral Risk Factor Surveillance System for 1986. Unpublished manuscript. School of Public Health, University of Hawaii, 1986.

COALITION ON SMOKING OR HEALTH. Petition to classify R.J. Reynolds new alternative nicotine delivery product to be subject to the jurisdiction of the Food and Drug Administration as a drug, April 25, 1988.

COELHO, R.J. Self-efficacy and cessation of smoking. *Psychological Reports* 54(1):309–310, February 1984.

COHEN, S., LICHTENSTEIN, E., MERMELSTEIN, R., KINGSOLVER, K., BAER, J., KAMARCK, T. Social support interventions for smoking cessation. In: Gottlieb, B.H. (ed.) *Marshalling Social Support: Formats, Processes and Effects*. New York: Sage, 1988, pp. 211–240.

COHEN, S., SYME, S.L. *Social Support and Health*. Orlando: Academic Press, 1985.

CONDIOTTE, M.M., LICHTENSTEIN, E. Self-efficacy and relapse in smoking cessation programs. *Journal of Consulting and Clinical Psychology* 49(5):648–658, October 1981.

COPPOTELLI, H.C., ORLEANS, C.T. Partner support and other determinants of smoking cessation maintenance among women. *Journal of Consulting and Clinical Psychology* 53(4): 455–460, August 1985.

COULTAS, D.B., HOWARD, C.A., PEAKE, G.T., SKIPPER, B.J., SAMET, J.M. Discrepancies between self-reported and validated cigarette smoking in a community survey of New Mexico Hispanics. *American Review of Respiratory Disease* 137:810–814, 1988.

CRONAN, T.A., CONWAY, T.L. *Is the Navy Attracting or Creating Smokers?* Smoking Behavior and Policy Discussion Paper Series. Cambridge, Massachusetts: Institute for the Study of Smoking Behavior and Policy, John F. Kennedy School of Government, Harvard University, November 1987.

CRONAN, T.A., CONWAY, T.L. Is the Navy attracting or creating smokers? *Military Medicine* 153(4):175–178, April 1988.

CUMMINGS, K.M., GIOVINO, G., MENDICINO, A.J. Cigarette advertising and black–white differences in brand preference. *Public Health Reports* 102(6):698–701, November–December 1987.

CURRY, S., MARLATT, G.A., GORDON, J., BAER, J.S. A comparison of alternative theoretical approaches to smoking cessation and relapse. *Health Psychology*, in press.

CURRY, S.J. A comparison of alternative theoretical approaches to smoking cessation and relapse. *Health Psychology*, in press.

DAVIS, R.M. Current trends in cigarette advertising and marketing. *New England Journal of Medicine* 316(12):725–732, March 19, 1987.

DICLEMENTE, C.C. Self-efficacy and smoking cessation maintenance: A preliminary report. *Cognitive Therapy and Research* 5(2):175–187, June 1981.

EISER, J.R. Smoking, addiction and decision-making. *International Review of Applied Psychology* 32:11–28, 1983.

EISER, J.R., SUTTON, S.R. Smoking as a subjectively rational choice. *Addictive Behaviors* 2:129–134, 1977.

EISINGER, R.A. Psychosocial predictors of smoking recidivism. *Journal of Health and Social Behavior* 12:355–362, December 1971.

ELKIND, A.K. Changes in the smoking behaviour, knowledge and opinion of medical students, 1972–1981. *Social Science and Medicine* 16(24):2137–2143, 1982.

ESCOBEDO, L.G., REMINGTON, P.L. Birth cohort analysis of prevalence of cigarette smoking among Hispanics in the United States. *Journal of the American Medical Association* 261(1):66–69, January 6, 1989.

ETRINGER, B.D., GREGORY, V.R., LANDO, H.A. Influence of group cohesion on the behavioral treatment of smoking. *Journal of Consulting and Clinical Psychology* 52(6):1080–1086, 1984.

EVANS, R.I., ROZELLE, R.M., MITTLEMARK, M.B., HANSEN, W.B., BANE, A.L., HAVIS, J. Deterring the onset of smoking in children: Knowledge of immediate physiological effects and coping with peer pressure, media pressure, and parent modeling. *Journal of Applied Social Psychology* 8(2):126–135, 1978.

EYSENCK, H.J. *The Causes and Effects of Smoking*. Beverly Hills, California: Sage Publications, 1980.

EYSENCK, H.J., TARRANT, M., WOOLF, M., ENGLAND, L. Smoking and personality. *British Medical Journal* 1:1456–1460, 1960.

FAGERSTROM, K. Measuring degree of physical dependence to tobacco smoking with reference to individualization of treatment. *Addictive Behaviors* 3(3/4):235–241, 1978.

FEDERAL TRADE COMMISSION. *"Tar," Nicotine and Carbon Monoxide of the Smoke of 207 Varieties of Domestic Cigarettes*. Federal Trade Commission, January 1985.

FEDERAL TRADE COMMISSION. *Report to Congress Pursuant to the Federal Cigarette Labeling and Advertising Act, 1986*. Federal Trade Commission, May 1988.

FIORE, M.C., NOVOTNY, T.E., PIERCE, J.P., HATZIANDREU, E.J., PATEL, K.M., DAVIS, R.M. Trends in cigarette smoking in the United States. The changing influence of gender and race. *Journal of the American Medical Association* 261(1):49–55, January 6, 1989.

FISHBEIN, M. Consumer beliefs and behavior with respect to cigarette smoking: A critical analysis of the public literature. In: *Federal Trade Commission, Report to Congress: Pursuant to the Public Health Cigarette Smoking Act, For the Year 1976*. Federal Trade Commission, May 1977.

FISHBEIN, M. Social psychological analysis of smoking behavior. In: Eiser, J.R. (ed.) *Social Psychology and Behavioral Medicine*. New York: John Wiley and Sons, 1982, pp. 179–197.

FISHER, E.B. JR. A skeptical perspective: The importance of behavior and environment. In: Holroyd, K.A., Creer, T.L. (eds.) *Self-Management of Chronic Disease*. Orlando: Academic Press, 1986.

FISHER, E.B. JR., BISHOP, D.B. Sex-roles, social support, and smoking cessation. Paper presented at Society of Behavioral Medicine, San Francisco, March 1986.

FISHER, E.B. JR., BISHOP, D.B., GOLDMUNTZ, J., JACOBS, A. Implications for the practicing physician of the psychosocial dimensions of smoking. *Chest* 93(2, Supplement):69S–78S, February 1988a.

FISHER, E.B. JR., BISHOP, D.B., LEVITT-GILMOUR, T., NEWMAN, E., LANKESTER, L., TORMEY, B. Impacts on smoking prevalence of organizational and social support in worksite smoking cessation. Paper presented at Society of Behavioral Medicine, Boston, April 1988b.

FISHER, E.B. JR., BISHOP, D.B., MAYER, J., BROWN, T., WHITE-COOK, T. The physician's contribution to smoking cessation in the workplace. *Chest* 93(2, Supplement):56S–65S, February 1988c.

FISHER, E.B. JR., LEVENKRON, J.C., LOWE, M.R., LORO, A.D. JR., GREEN, L. Self-initiated self-control in risk reduction. In: R.B. Stuart (ed.) *Adherence, Compliance, and Generalization in Behavioral Medicine*. New York: Brunner/Mazel, 1982, pp. 169–191.

FISHER, E.B. JR., LOWE, M.R., LEVENKRON, J.C., NEWMAN, A. Reinforcement and structural support of maintained risk reduction. In: Stuart, R.B. (ed.) *Adherence, Compliance, and Generalization in Behavioral Medicine*. New York: Brunner/Mazel, 1982, pp. 145–168.

FISHER, E.B. JR., ROST, K. Smoking cessation: A practical guide for the physician. *Clinics in Chest Medicine* 7(4):551–565, December 1986.

FLAY, B.R. Psychosocial approaches to smoking prevention: A review of findings. *Health Psychology* 4(5):449–488, 1985.

FLAY, B.R., D'AVERNAS, J.R., BEST, J.A., KERSELL, M.W., RYAN, K.B. Cigarette smoking: Why young people do it and ways of preventing it. In: McGrath, P., Firestone, P. (eds.) *Pediatric and Adolescent Behavioral Medicine*, Volume 10. New York: Springer Publishing, 1983, pp. 132–183.

FORTMANN, S.P., ROGERS, T., VRANIZAN, K., HASKELL, W.L., SOLOMON, D.S., FARQUHAR, J.W. Indirect measures of cigarette use: Expired-air carbon monoxide versus plasma thiocyanate. *Preventive Medicine* 13(1):127–135, January 1984.

FOSS, R. Personality, social influence and cigarette smoking. *Journal of Health and Social Behavior* 14(3):279–286, September 1973.

FRIEDMAN, G.D., SIEGELAUB, A.B., DALES, L.G., SELTZER, C.C. Characteristics predictive of coronary heart disease in ex-smokers before they stopped smoking: Comparison with persistent smokers and nonsmokers. *Journal of Chronic Diseases* 32:175–190, 1979.

FRIEDMAN, L.S., LICHTENSTEIN, E., BIGLAN, A. Smoking onset among teens: An empirical analysis of initial situations. *Addictive Behaviors* 10:1–13, 1985.

GLANTZ, S.A. Death in the West Curriculum Project. (Letter.) *New York State Journal of Medicine* 85(7):470–471, July 1985.

GLASGOW, R.E., MCCAUL, K.D., FREEBORN, V.B., O'NEILL, H.K. Immediate and long term health consequences information in the prevention of adolescent smoking. *Behavior Therapist* 4(5):15–16, 1981.

GOLDSTEIN, A.O., FISCHER, P.M., RICHARDS, J.W. JR., CRETEN, D. Relationship between high school student smoking and recognition of cigarette advertisements. *Journal of Pediatrics* 110(3):488–491, March 1987.

GORDON, N.P., MCALISTER, A.L. A prospective text of a social learning risk factor model of smoking onset and cessation among junior high school students. *Health Psychology*, 1985.

GRABOWSKI, J., HALL, S.M. (eds.) *Pharmacological Adjuncts in Smoking Cessation*, NIDA Research Monograph 53. U.S. Department of Health and Human Services, Public Health Service, Alcohol, Drug Abuse, and Mental Health Administration, National Institue on Drug Abuse. DHHS Publication No. 85-1333, 1985.

GRAHAM, S., GIBSON, R.W. Cessation of patterned behavior: Withdrawal from smoking. *Social Science and Medicine* 5(4):319–337, August 1971.

GREEN, D.E. *Teenage Smoking: Immediate and Long-Term Patterns*. U.S. Department of Health, Education, and Welfare, National Institute of Education, November 1979.

GRITZ, E., CARR, C.R., MARCUS, A.C. Unaided smoking cessation: Great American Smokeout and New Year's Day quitters. *Journal of Psychosocial Oncology*, in press.

GRITZ, E.R. The female smoker: Research and intervention targets. In: Cohen, J., Cullen, J.W., Martin, L.R. (eds.) *Psychosocial Aspects of Cancer*. New York: Raven Press, 1982, pp. 39–49.

GRITZ, E.R. Gender and the teenage smoker. In: Ray, B.A., Braude, M.C. (eds.) *Women and Drugs: A New Era for Research*, NIDA Research Monograph 65. U.S. Department of Health and Human Services, Public Health Service, Alcohol, Drug Abuse, and Mental Health Administration, National Institute on Drug Abuse. DHHS Publication No. 83-1268, 1986, pp. 70–79.

GRUNBERG, N.E. Behavioral and biological factors in the relationship between tobacco use and body weight. In: Katkin, E.S., Manuck, S.B. (eds.) *Advances in Behavioral Medicine* 2:97–129, 1986.

HALL, R.L., DEXTER, D. Smokeless tobacco use and attitudes toward smokeless tobacco among Native Americans and other adolescents in the Northwest. *American Journal of Public Health* 78(12):1586–1588, December 1988.

HALL, S.M., HERNING, R.I., JONES, R.T., BENOWITZ, N.L., JACOB, P. III. Blood cotinine levels as indicators of smoking treatment outcome. *Clinical Pharmacology and Therapeutics* 35(6):810–814, June 1984.

HALL, S.M., TUNSTALL, C., RUGG, D., JONES, R.T., BENOWITZ, N. Nicotine gum and behavioral treatment in smoking cessation. *Journal of Consulting and Clinical Psychology* 53(2):256–258, 1985.

HANSEN, W.B., COLLINS, L.M., JOHNSON, C.A., GRAHAM, J.W. Self-initiated smoking cessation among high school students. *Addictive Behaviors* 10:265–271, 1985.

HARRIS, J.E. Cigarette smoking among successive birth cohorts of men and women in the United States during 1900–80. *Journal of the National Cancer Institute* 71(3):473–479, September 1983.

HATSUKAMI, D.K., HUGHES, J.R., PICKENS, R.W. Blood nicotine, smoke exposure and tobacco withdrawal symptoms. *Addictive Behaviors* 10:413–417, 1985.

HATZIANDREU, E., PIERCE, J.P., FIORE, M., GRISE, V., NOVOTNY, T.E., DAVIS, R.M. Trends in estimates of cigarette consumption in the United States from tax data and from self-reported survey data. *American Journal of Public Health*, in press.

HAWAII STATE DEPARTMENT OF HEALTH. *Hawaii's Health: A Report on the Prevalence of Behavioral Risk Factors in Hawaii—1984*. Hawaii State Department of Health, Health Promotion and Education Office, 1984.

HAYNES, S. Statement. In: *The Impact of Cigarette Smoking on Minority Populations. Proceedings of the Federal Interagency Committee on Smoking and Health.* U.S. Department of Health and Human Services, Public Health Service, Centers for Disease Control, Center for Health Promotion and Education, Office on Smoking and Health. Publication No. HHS/PHS/CDC-87-8403, March 31, 1987, pp. 129–131.

HENDERSON, J.B., HALL, S.M., LINTON, H.L. Changing self-destructive behaviors. In: Stone, G.C., Cohen, F., Adler, N.E., et al. (eds.) *Health Psychology: A Handbook*. San Francisco: Jossey-Bass, 1979, pp. 141–160.

HENNINGFIELD, J.E., CHAIT, L.D., GRIFFITHS, R.R. Cigarette smoking and subjective response in alcoholics: Effects of pentobarbital. *Clinical Pharmacology and Therapeutics* 33(6):806–812, June 1983.

HENNINGFIELD, J.E., CHAIT, L.D., GRIFFITHS, R.R. Effects of ethanol on cigarette smoking by volunteers without history of alcoholism. *Psychopharmacology* 82(1/2):1–5, 1984.

HENNINGFIELD, J.E., MIYASATO, K., JASINSKI, D.R. Abuse liability and pharmacodynamic characteristics of intravenous and inhaled nicotine. *Journal of Pharmacology and Experimental Therapeutics* 234(1):1–12, July 1985.

HERBOLD, J.R. Smoking habits of U.S. military personnel. *Military Medicine* 152(4):194–195, April 1987.

HERMAN, C.P. External and internal cues as determinants of the smoking behavior of light and heavy smokers. *Journal of Personality and Social Psychology* 30(5):664–672, 1974.

HERMAN, C.P., KOZLOWSKI, L.T. Indulgence, excess, and restraint: Perspectives on consummatory behavior in everyday life. *Journal of Drug Issues* 9(2):185–196, Spring 1979.

HIRSCHMAN, R.S., LEVENTHAL, H., GLYNN, K. The development of smoking behavior: Conceptualization and supportive cross-sectional survey data. *Journal of Applied Social Psychology* 14(3):184–206, 1984.

HORN, D., WAINGROW, S. Behavior and attitudes. Questionnaire, April 1966.

HUGHES, J.R., HATSUKAMI, D.K., MITCHELL, J.E., DAHLGREN, L.A. Prevalence of smoking among psychiatric outpatients. *American Journal of Psychiatry* 143(8):993–997, August 1986.

HUGHES, G.H., HYMOWITZ, N., OCKENE, J.K., SIMON, N., VOGT, T.M. The Multiple Risk Factor Intervention Trial (MRFIT). *Preventive Medicine* 10(4):476–500, July 1981.

HUNDLEBY, J.D., MERCER, G.W. Family and friends as social environments and their relationship to young adolescents' use of alcohol, tobacco, and marijuana. *Journal of Marriage and the Family* 49:151–164, February 1987.

HUNT, W.A. (ed.) *Learning Mechanisms in Smoking*. Chicago: Aldine, 1970.

HUNTER, S.M., CROFT, J.B., BURKE, G.L., PARKER, F.C., WEBBER, L.S., BERENSON, G.S. Longitudinal patterns of cigarette smoking and smokeless tobacco use in youth: The Bogalusa Heart Study. *American Journal of Public Health* 76(2):193–195, February 1986.

IKARD, F.F., TOMKINS, S. The experience of affect as a determinant of smoking behavior: A series of validity studies. *Journal of Abnormal Psychology* 81(2):172–181, 1973.

ISHIHARA, K., MIYASITA, A., INUGAMI, M., FUKUDA, K., YAMAZAKI, K., MIYATA, Y. Differences in the time or frequency of meals, alcohol and caffeine ingestion, and smoking found between 'morning' and 'evening' types. *Psychological Reports* 57(2):391–396, October 1985.

ISTVAN, J., MATARAZZO, J.D. Tobacco, alcohol, and caffeine use: A review of their interrelationships. *Psychological Bulletin* 95(2):301–326, March 1984.

JARVIK, M.E. Biological factors underlying the smoking habit. In: Jarvik, M.E., Cullen, J.W., Gritz, E.R., Vogt, T.M., West, L.J. (eds.) *Research on Smoking Behavior*, NIDA Research Monograph 17. U.S. Department of Health, Education, and Welfare, Public Health Service, Alcohol, Drug Abuse, and Mental Health Administration, National Institute on Drug Abuse. DHEW Publication No. (ADM) 78-581, December 1977, pp. 122–148.

JARVIK, M.E., GLICK, S.D., NAKAMURA, R.K. Inhibition of cigarette smoking by orally administered nicotine. *Clinical Pharmacology and Therapeutics* 11(4):574–576, July–August 1970.

JARVIS, M. Gender and smoking: Do women really find it harder to give up? *British Journal of Addiction* 79(4):383–387, December 1984.

JESSOR, R. Problem-behavior theory, psychosocial development, and adolescent problem drinking. *British Journal of Addiction* 82:331–342, 1987.

JESSOR, R.R., JESSOR, S.L. *Problem Behavior and Psychosocial Development*. New York: Academic Press, 1977.

JOFFE, R., LOWE, M.R., FISHER, E.B. JR. A validity test of the Reasons For Smoking Scale. *Addictive Behaviors* 6(1):41–45, 1981.

JOHNSTON, L.D. The etiology and prevention of substance use: What can we learn from recent historical change? In: Jones, C.L., Battjes, R.J. (eds.) *Etiology for Drug Abuse: Implications for Prevention*, NIDA Research Monograph 56. National Institute on Drug Abuse, 1985.

JOHNSTON, L.D., BACHMAN, J.G. *Monitoring the Future. Questionnaire Responses From the Nation's High School Seniors, 1975*. Ann Arbor, Michigan: University of Michigan, 1980.

JOHNSTON, L.D., BACHMAN, J.G., O'MALLEY, P.M. *Monitoring the Future. Questionnaire Responses From the Nation's High School Seniors, 1977*. Ann Arbor, Michigan: University of Michigan, 1980a.

JOHNSTON, L.D., BACHMAN, J.G., O'MALLEY, P.M. *Monitoring the Future. Questionnaire Responses From the Nation's High School Seniors, 1979*. Ann Arbor, Michigan: University of Michigan, 1980b.

JOHNSTON, L.D., BACHMAN, J.G., O'MALLEY, P.M. *Monitoring the Future. Questionnaire Responses From the Nation's High School Seniors, 1981*. Ann Arbor, Michigan: University of Michigan, 1982.

JOHNSTON, L.D., BACHMAN, J.G., O'MALLEY, P.M. *Monitoring the Future. Questionnaire Responses From the Nation's High School Seniors, 1983*. Ann Arbor, Michigan: University of Michigan, 1984.

JOHNSTON, L.D., BACHMAN, J.G., O'MALLEY, P.M. *Monitoring the Future. Questionnaire Responses From the Nation's High School Seniors, 1985*. Ann Arbor, Michigan: University of Michigan, 1986.

JOHNSTON, L.D., O'MALLEY, P.M., BACHMAN, J.G. *National Trends in Drug Use and Related Factors Among High School Students and Young Adults, 1975–1986*. U.S. Department of Health and Human Services, Public Health Service, Alcohol, Drug Abuse, and Mental Health Administration, National Institute on Drug Abuse. DHHS Publication No. (ADM) 87-1535, 1987.

KAPLAN, G.D., COWLES, A. Health locus of control and health value in the prediction of smoking reduction. *Health Education Monographs* 6(2):129–137, Spring 1978.

KAPLAN, H.I., SADOCK, B.J. (eds.) *Comprehensive Textbook of Psychiatry*, Fourth Edition. Baltimore: Williams and Wilkins, 1985.

KILLEN, J.D., MACCOBY, N., TAYLOR, C.B. Nicotine gum and self-regulation training in smoking relapse prevention. *Behavior Therapy* 15(3):234–248, 1984.

KIRSCHT, J.P. Preventive health behavior: A review of research and issues. *Health Psychology* 2(3):277–301, 1983.

KIRSCHT, J.P., ROSENSTOCK, I.M. Patients' problems in following recommendations of health experts. In: Stone, G.C., Cohen, F., Adler, N.E. et al. (eds.) *Health Psychology: A Handbook.* San Francisco: Jossey-Bass, 1979, pp. 189–215.

KLEINMAN, J.C., KOPSTEIN, A. Smoking during pregnancy, 1967–80. *American Journal of Public Health* 77(7):823–825, 1987.

KLESGES, R.C., KLESGES, L.M. Cigarette smoking as a dieting strategy in a university population. *International Journal of Eating Disorders*, in press.

KNISKERN, J., BIGLAN, A., LICHTENSTEIN, E., ARY, D., BAVRY, J. Peer modeling effects in the smoking behavior of teenagers. *Addictive Behaviors* 8:129–132, 1983.

KOZLOWSKI, L.T. Pack size, reported smoking rates and public health. *American Journal of Public Health* 76(11):1337–1338, November 1986.

KOZLOWSKI, L.T. Less hazardous smoking and the pursuit of satisfaction. *American Journal of Public Health* 77(5):539–541, May 1987.

KOZLOWSKI, L.T. Evidence for limits on acceptability of lowest-tar cigarettes. *American Journal of Public Health* 79(2):198–199, February 1989.

KOZLOWSKI, L.T., HARFORD, M.R. On the significance of never using a drug: An example from cigarette smoking. *Journal of Abnormal Psychology* 85(4):433–434, August 1976.

KOZLOWSKI, L.T., HERMAN, C.P. The interaction of psychosocial and biological determinants of tobacco use: More on the boundary model. *Journal of Applied Social Psychology* 14(3):244–256, 1984.

KROSNICK, J.A., JUDD, C.M. Transitions in social influences at adolescence: Who induces cigarette smoking? *Developmental Psychology 18(3):359–368, 1982.*

LAZARUS, G. Cigar makers can't snuff out sales drop. *Chicago Tribune*, June 3, 1979, Section 5, p. 6.

LEVENTHAL, H., CLEARY, P.D. The smoking problem: A review of the research and theory in behavioral risk modification. *Psychological Bulletin* 88(2):370–405, 1980.

LEVENTHAL, H., GLYNN, K., FLEMING, R. Is the smoking decision an 'informed choice'? Effect of smoking risk factors on smoking beliefs. *Journal of the American Medical Association* 257(24):3373–3376, June 26, 1987.

LEVITT, E.E., EDWARDS, J.A. A multivariate study of correlative factors in youthful cigarette smoking. *Developmental Psychology* 2(1):5–11, 1970.

LICHTENSTEIN, E. The smoking problem: A behavioral perspective. *Journal of Consulting and Clinical Psychology* 50(6):804–819, 1982.

LICHTENSTEIN, E., BERNSTEIN, D.A. Cigarette smoking as indirect self-destructive behavior. In: Farberow, N.L. (ed.) *The Many Faces of Suicide. Indirect Self-Destructive Behavior.* New York: McGraw Hill, 1980, pp. 243–253.

LICHTENSTEIN, E., GLASGOW, R.E., ABRAMS, D.B. Social support in smoking cessation: In search of effective interventions. *Behavior Therapy* 17:607–619, 1986.

LOKEN, B. Heavy smokers', light smokers', and nonsmokers' beliefs about cigarette smoking. *Journal of Applied Psychology* 67(5):616–622, October 1982.

LONDON, E.D., CONNOLLY, R.J., SZIKSZAY, M., WAMSLEY, J.K. Distribution of cerebral metabolic effects of nicotine in the rat. *European Journal of Pharmacology* 110(3):391–392, April 15, 1985.

LONDON, E.D., WALLER, S.B., WAMSLEY, J.K. Autographic localization of (^{3}H) nicotine binding sites in rat brains. *Neuroscience Letters* 53(2):179–184, January 1985.

MANGAN, J.L., GOLDING, J.F. *The Psychopharmacology of Smoking.* Cambridge, England: Cambridge University Press, 1984.

MARCUS, A.C., CRANE, L.A. Smoking behavior among US Latinos: An emerging challenge for public health. *American Journal of Public Health* 75(2):169–172, February 1985.

MARCUS, A.C., CRANE, L.A. Current estimates of adult cigarette smoking by race/ethnicity. In. *The Impact of Cigarette Smoking on Minority Populations. Proceedings of the Federal Interagency Committee on Smoking and Health.* U.S. Department of Health and Human Services, Centers for Disease Control, Center for Health Promotion and Education, Office on Smoking and Health. Publication No. HHS/PHS/CDC-87-8403, March 31, 1987, pp. 3–20.

MARCUS, A.C., CRANE, L.A., SHOPLAND, D.R., LYNN, W.R. Use of smokeless tobacco in the United States: Recent estimates from the Current Population Survey. In: NCI Monograph. National Cancer Institute, in press.

MARLATT, G.A. Relapse prevention: Theoretical rationale and overview of the model. In: Marlatt, G.A., Gordon, J.R. (eds.) *Relapse Prevention: Maintenance Strategies in the Treatment of Addictive Behaviors.* New York: Guilford Press, 1985.

MARLATT, G.A., GORDON, J.R. Determinants of relapse: Implications for the maintenance of behavior change. In: Davidson, P.O., Davidson, S.M. (eds.) *Behavioral Medicine: Changing Health Lifestyles.* New York: Brunner/Mazel, 1980, pp. 410–452.

MARLATT, G.A., GORDON, J.R. (eds.) *Relapse Prevention: Maintainance Strategies in the Treatment of Addictive Behaviors.* New York: Guilford Press, 1985.

MAUSNER, B., PLATT, E.S. *Smoking: A Behavioral Analysis.* New York: Pergamon Press, 1971.

MCALISTER, A.L., KROSNICK, J.A., MILBURN, M.A. Causes of adolescent cigarette smoking: Tests of a structural equation model. *Social Psychology Quarterly* 47(1):24–36, 1984.

MCARTHUR, C., WALDRON, E., DICKINSON, J. The psychology of smoking. *Journal of Abnormal and Social Psychology* 56:267–275, 1958.

MCCARTHY, W.J., GRITZ, E.R. Teenagers' responses to cigarette advertising. Paper presented at the meeting of the American Psychological Association, New York, August 28–September 1, 1987.

MCDADE, E.A., KEIL, J.E. Characterization of a soup kitchen population. In: *Proceedings of the American Heart Association Conference on Epidemiology.* Santa Fe, New Mexico, March 1988.

MCGINNIS, J.M., SHOPLAND, D., BROWN, C. Tobacco and health: Trends in smoking and smokeless tobacco consumption in the United States. *Annual Review of Public Health,* Volume 8. Palo Alto, California: Annual Reviews, 1987, pp. 441–467.

MCINTYRE-KINGSOLVER, K., LICHTENSTEIN, E., MERMELSTEIN, R.J. Spouse training in a multicomponent smoking-cessation program. *Behavior Therapy* 17:67–74, 1986.

MCINTYRE-KINGSOLVER, K.O., LICHTENSTEIN, E., MERMELSTEIN, R.J. Selfefficacy and relapse in smoking cessation: A replication and extension. *Journal of Consulting and Clinical Psychology* 51(4):632–633, 1983.

MERMELSTEIN, R., COHEN, S., LICHTENSTEIN, E., BAER, J.S., KAMARCK, T. Social support and smoking cessation and maintenance. *Journal of Consulting and Clinical Psychology* 54(4):447–453, 1986.

MERMELSTEIN, R., LICHTENSTEIN, E., MCINTYRE, K. Partner support and relapse in smoking-cessation programs. *Journal of Consulting and Clinical Psychology* 51:465–466, June 1983.

MILLAR, W.J. Smoking prevalence among Canadian adolescents: A comparison of survey estimates. *Canadian Journal of Public Health* 76(1):33–37, January–February 1985.

MISCHEL, W. Toward a cognitive social learning reconceptualization of personality. *Psychological Review* 80(4):252–283, 1973.

MITIC, W.R., MCGUIRE, D.P., NEUMANN, B. Perceived stress and adolescents' cigarette use. *Psychological Reports* 57(3, Part 2):1043–1048, December 1985.

MITTELMARK, M.B., MURRAY, D.M., LUEPKER, R.V., PECHACEK, T.F., PIRIE, P.L., PALLONEN, U.E. Predicting experimentation with cigarettes: The Childhood Antecedents of Smoking Study (CASS). *American Journal of Public Health* 77(2):206–208, February 1987.

MORGAN, G.D., ASHENBERG, Z.S., FISHER, E.B. JR. Abstinence from smoking and the social environment. *Journal of Consulting and Clinical Psychology* 56(2):298–301, 1988.

MOSBACH, P., LEVENTHAL, H. Peer group identification and smoking: Implications for intervention. *Journal of Abnormal Psychology* 97(2):238–245, 1988.

MURRAY, D.M., PERRY, C.L. The functional meaning of adolescent drug use. Paper presented at the 92d annual meeting of the American Psychological Association, Toronto, Canada, August 24–28, 1984.

MURRAY, D.M., RICHARDS, P.S., LUEPKER, R.V., JOHNSON, C.A. The prevention of cigarette smoking in children: Two- and three-year follow-up comparisons of four prevention strategies. *Journal of Behavioral Medicine* 10(6):595–611, 1987.

NATIONAL CENTER FOR HEALTH STATISTICS, KOVAR, M.G., POE, G.S. The National Health Interview Survey design, 1973–84, and procedures, 1975–83. *Vital and Health Statistics*, Series 1, No. 18. Public Health Service. DHHS Publication No. (HHS) 85-1320, 1985.

NATIONAL CENTER FOR HEALTH STATISTICS, THORNBERRY, O. An experimental comparison of telephone and personal health interview surveys. *Vital and Health Statistics*, Series 2, No. 106. U.S. Department of Health and Human Services, Public Health Service. DHHS Publication No. (PHS) 87-1380, August 1987.

NATIONAL CENTER FOR HEALTH STATISTICS, MOSHER, W.D., PRATT, W.F. Fecundity, infertility, and reproductive health in the United States, 1982. *Vital and Health Statistics*, Series 2, No. 106, Public Health Service. DHHS Publication No. (PHS) 88-1591, 1988a.

NATIONAL CENTER FOR HEALTH STATISTICS, SCHOENBORN, C.A. Health promotion and disease prevention: United States, 1985. *Vital and Health Statistics*, Series 10, No. 163. Public Health Service. DHHS Publication No. (PHS) 88-1591, February 1988b.

NATIONAL CENTER FOR HEALTH STATISTICS. *Health, United States, 1987*. U.S. Department of Health and Human Services, Public Health Service. DHHS Publication No. (PHS) 88-1232, March 1988c.

NATIONAL INSTITUTES OF HEALTH. *Teenage Smoking, National Patterns of Cigarette Smoking, Ages 12 Through 18, in 1972 and 1974*. U.S. Department of Health, Education, and Welfare, Public Health Service, National Institutes of Health. DHEW Publication No. (NIH) 76-931, 1975.

NATIONAL RESEARCH COUNCIL. *Environmental Tobacco Smoke. Measuring Exposures and Assessing Health Effects*. Washington, D.C.: National Academy Press, 1986.

NIAURA, R.S., ROHSENOW, D.J., BINKOFF, J.A., MONTI, P.M., PEDRAZA, M., ABRAMS, D.B. Relevance of cue reactivity to understanding alcohol and smoking relapse. *Journal of Abnormal Psychology* 97(2):133–152, 1988.

NISWANDER, K.R., GORDON, M. *The Women and Their Pregnancies. The Collaborative Perinatal Study of the National Institute of Neurological Diseases and Stroke*. U.S. Department of Health, Education, and Welfare, Public Health Service, National Institutes of Health, DHEW Publication No. (NIH) 73-379, 1972.

NOVOTNY, T., LYNN, W.R., MAKLAN, D. Smokeless tobacco use in the United States, 1986: What have we learned? In: Aoki, M., Hisamichi, S., Tominaga, S. (eds.) *Smoking and Health 1987*. Proceedings of the 6th World Conference on Smoking and Health, November 9–12, 1987. Amsterdam: Excerpta Medica, 1988, pp. 879–881.

NOVOTNY, T.E., PIERCE, J.P., FIORE, M.C., HATZIANDREU, E., DAVIS, R.M. *Smokeless Tobacco Use in the United States: The Adult Use of Tobacco Surveys*, NCI Monograph. National Cancer Institute, in press.

NOVOTNY, T.E., WARNER, K.E., KENDRICK, J.S., REMINGTON, P.L. Smoking by blacks and whites: Socioeconomic and demographic differences. *American Journal of Public Health* 78(9):1187–1189, September 1988.

O'MALLEY, P.M., BACHMAN, J.G., JOHNSTON, L.D. Period, age, and cohort effects on substance use among young Americans: A decade of change, 1976–86. *American Journal of Public Health* 78(10):1315–1321, October 1988.

OCKENE, J.K., BENFARI, R.C., NUTTALL, R.L., HURWITZ, I., OCKENE, I.S. Relationship of psychosocial factors to smoking behavior change in an intervention program. *Preventive Medicine* 11(1):13–28, January 1982a.

OCKENE, J.K., HYMOWITZ, N., SEXTON, M., BROSTE, S.K. Comparison of patterns of smoking behavior change among smokers in the Multiple Risk Factor Intervention Trial (MRFIT). *Preventive Medicine* 11:621–638, 1982b.

OCKENE, J.K., HOSMER, D., RIPPE, J., WILLIAMS, J., GOLDBERG, R.J., DECOSIMO, D., MAHER, P.M., DALEN, J.E. Factors affecting cigarette smoking status in patients with ischemic heart disease. *Journal of Chronic Disease* 38(12):985–994, 1985.

OCKENE, J.K., HOSMER, D.W., WILLIAMS, J.W., GOLDBERG, R.J., OCKENE, I.S., RAIA, T.J. III. Factors related to patient smoking status. *American Journal of Public Health* 77(3):356–357, March 1987.

OCKENE, J.K., SORENSEN, G., KABAT-ZINN, J., OCKENE, I.S., DONNELLY, G. Benefits and costs of lifestyle change to reduce risk of chronic disease. *Preventive Medicine* 17(2):224–234, March 1988.

PECHACEK, T.F., DANAHER, B.G. How and why people quit smoking: A cognitive-behavioral analysis. In: Kendall, P.C., Hollon, S.D. (eds.) *Cognitive-Behavioral Interventions: Theory, Research and Procedures*, Volume 21. New York: Academic Press, 1979, pp. 389–422.

PERKINS, K.A. Maintaining smoking abstinence after myocardial infarction. *Journal of Substance Abuse* 1(1):91–107, 1988.

PERRI, M.G., RICHARDS, C.S., SCHULTHEIS, K.R. Behavioral self-control and smoking reduction: A study of self-initiated attempts to reduce smoking. *Behavior Therapy* 8:360–365, 1977.

PETITTI, D.B., FRIEDMAN, G.D., KAHN, W. Accuracy of information on smoking habits provided on self-administered research questionnaires. *American Journal of Public Health* 71(3):308–311, March 1981.

PHILLIP MORRIS. *Military Smoker* 1(1), September 1988.

PIERCE, J.P., ALDRICH, R.N., HANRATTY, S., DWYER, T., HILL, D. Uptake and quitting smoking trends in Australia 1974–1984. *Preventive Medicine* 16(2):252–260, March 1987a.

PIERCE, J.P., DWYER, T., DIGIUSTO, E., CARPENTER, T., HANNAM, C., AMIN, A., YONG, C., SARFATY, G., SHAW, J., BURKE, N., QUIT FOR LIFE STEERING COMMITTEE. Cotinine validation of self-reported smoking in commercially run community surveys. *Journal of Chronic Diseases* 40(7):689–695, 1987b.

PIERCE, J.P., FIORE, M.C., NOVOTNY, T.E., HATZIANDREU, E.J., DAVIS, R.M. Trends in cigarette smoking in the United States. Projections to the year 2000. *Journal of the American Medical Association* 261(1):61–65, January 6, 1989a.

PIERCE, J.P., FIORE, M.C., NOVOTNY, T.E., HATZIANDREU, E.J., DAVIS, R.M. Trends in cigarette smoking in the United States. Educational differences are increasing. *Journal of the American Medical Association* 261(1):56–60, January 6, 1989b.

PILLSBURY, H.C., BRIGHT, C.C., O'CONNOR, K.J., IRISH, F.W. Tar and nicotine in cigarette smoke. *Journal of the Association of Official Analytical Chemists* 52(3):458–462, May 1969.

PIRIE, P.L., MURRAY, D.M., LUEPKER, R.V. Smoking prevalence in a cohort of adolescents, including absentees, dropouts, and transfers. *American Journal of Public Health* 78(2): 176–178, 1988.

POJER, R., WHITFIELD, J.B., POULOS, V., ECKHARDT, I.F., RICHMOND, R., HENSLEY, W.J. Carboxyhemoglobin, cotinine, and thiocyanate assay compared for distinguishing smokers from non-smokers. *Clinical Chemistry* 30(8):1377–1380, August 1984.

POMERLEAU, O., ADKINS, D., PERTSCHUK, M. Predictors of outcome and recidivism in smoking cessation treatment. *Addictive Behaviors* 3:65–70, 1978.

POMERLEAU, O.F., POMERLEAU, C.S. Neuroregulators and the reinforcement of smoking: Towards a biobehavioral explanation. *Neuroscience and Biobehavioral Review* 8(4):503–513, 1984.

POMERLEAU, O.F., POMERLEAU, C.S. A biobehavioral view of substance abuse and addiction. *Journal of Drug Issues* 17:111–131, Spring 1987.

PROCHASKA, J.O., DICLEMENTE, C.C. Stages and processes of self-change of smoking: Toward an integrative model of change. *Journal of Consulting and Clinical Psychology* 51(3):390–395, 1983.

R.J. REYNOLDS TOBACCO COMPANY. R.J. Reynolds Tobacco Co. developing new cigarette. Press release. Winston-Salem, North Carolina: R.J. Reynolds Tobacco Company, September 14, 1987.

REMINGTON, P.L., FORMAN, M.R., GENTRY, E.M., MARKS, J.S., HOGELIN, G.S., TROWBRIDGE, F.L. Current smoking trends in the United States. The 1981–1983 Behavioral Risk Factor Surveys. *Journal of the American Medical Association* 253(20):2975–2978, May 24–31, 1985.

RICKARD-FIGUEROA, K., ZEICHNER, A. Assessment of smoking urge and its concomitants under an environmental smoking cue manipulation. *Addictive Behaviors* 10:249–256, 1985.

RIGOTTI, N.A., TESAR, G.E. Smoking cessation in the prevention of cardiovascular disease. *Cardiology Clinics* 3(2):245–257, May 1985.

ROBINS, L.N., HELZER, J.E., DAVIS, D.H. Narcotic use in Southeast Asia and afterward. An interview study of 898 Vietnam returnees. *Archives of General Psychiatry* 32:955–961, August 1975.

ROGERS, R.G., CRANK, J. Ethnic differences in smoking patterns: Findings from NHIS. *Public Health Reports* 103(4):387–393, July–August 1988.

ROGOT, E., REID, D.D. The validity of data from next-of-kin in studies of mortality among migrants. *International Journal of Epidemiology* 4(1):51–54, March 1975.

ROSEN, T.J., SHIPLEY, R.H. A stage analysis of self-initiated smoking reductions. *Addictive Behaviors* 8(3):263–272, 1983.

ROSENSTOCK, I.M. The health belief model and preventive health behavior. *Health Education Monographs* 2:354–386, 1974.

ROTTER, J.B. Generalized expectancies for internal versus external control of reinforcement. *Psychological Monographs: General and Applied* 80(1), 1966.

ROUSE, B. *Epidemiology of Smokeless Tobacco Use: A National Study*, NCI Monograph. National Cancer Institute, in press.

RUSSELL, M.A.H. Cigarette smoking: Natural history of a dependence disorder. *British Journal of Medical Psychology* 44(1):1–16, May 1971.

RUSSELL, M.A.H. Tobacco smoking and nicotine dependence. In: Gibbons, R.J., Israel, Y., Kalant, H., Popham, R.E., Schmidt, W., Smart, R.G. (eds.) *Research Advances in Alcohol and Drug Problems*, Volume 3. New York: John Wiley and Sons, 1976, pp. 1–47.

RUSSELL, M.A.H., PETO, S., PATEL, U.A. The classification of smoking by factorial structure of motives. *Journal of the Royal Statistical Society* 137(3):313–346, 1974.

RUSSELL, M.A.H., WILSON, C., TAYLOR, C., BAKER, C.D. Effect of general practitioners' advice against smoking. *British Medical Journal* 2(6184):231–235, July 28, 1979.

SCHACHTER, S., KOZLOWSKI, L.T., SILVERSTEIN, B. Studies on the interaction of psychological and pharmacological determinants of smoking. 2. Effects of urinary pH on cigarette smoking. *Journal of Experimental Psychology* 106(1):13–19, 1977.

SCHACHTER, S., SILVERSTEIN, B., KOZLOWSKI, L.T., PERLICK, D., HERMAN, C.P., LIEBLING, B. Studies of the interaction of psychological and pharmacological determinants of smoking. *Journal of Experimental Psychology: General* 106(1):3–4, 1977.

SCHINKE, S.P., GILCHRIST, L.D., SCHILLING, R.F. II., WALKER, R.D., LOCKLEAR, V.S., KITAJIMA, E. Smokeless tobacco use among Native American adolescents. (Letter.) *New England Journal of Medicine* 314(16):1051–1052, April 17, 1986.

SCHINKE, S.P., SCHILLING, R.F., GILCHRIST, L.D., ASHBY, M.R., KITAJIMA, E. Pacific Northwest Native American youth and smokeless tobacco use. *International Journal of Addictions* 22(9):881–884, 1987.

SCHNEIDER, N.G., JARVIK, M.E., FORSYTHE, A.B., READ, L.L., ELLIOTT, M.L., SCHWEIGER, A. Nicotine gum in smoking cessation: A placebo-controlled, double-blind trial. *Addictive Behaviors* 8(3):253–261, 1983.

SCHUBERT, D.S.P. Volunteering as arousal seeking. (Abstract.) *American Psychologist* 15:413, 1960.

SCHWARTZ, J.L., DUBITZKY, M. *Psycho-social Factors Involved in Cigarette Smoking Cessation. Final Report of the Smoking Control Research Project.* Berkeley, California: Institute for Health Research, Permanente Medical Group, Kaiser Foundation Health Plan, September 1968.

SHIFFMAN, S. Relapse following smoking cessation: A situational analysis. *Journal of Consulting and Clinical Psychology* 50(1):71–86, February 1982.

SHIFFMAN, S. Coping with temptations to smoke. *Journal of Consulting and Clinical Psychology* 52:261–267, 1984.

SHIFFMAN, S. A cluster-analytic classification of smoking relapse episodes. *Addictive Behaviors* 11(3):295–307, 1986.

SHIFFMAN, S. Psychosocial factors in smoking and quitting: Health beliefs, self-efficacy, and stress. In: Ockene, J.K. (ed.) *The Pharmacological Treatment of Nicotine Dependence.* Cambridge, Massachusetts: Institute for the Study of Smoking Behavior and Policy, John F. Kennedy School of Government, Harvard University, 1987, pp. 48–62.

SHIFFMAN, S. Behavioral assessment for smoking cessation. In: Donovan, D.M., Marlatt, G.A. (eds.) *Assessment of Addictive Behaviors: Behavioral, Cognitive, and Physiological Procedures.* New York: Guilford Press, 1988.

SHIFFMAN, S., WILLS, T.A. *Coping and Substance Use.* Orlando, Florida: Academic Press, 1985.

SHIPLEY, R.H. Maintenance of smoking cessation: Effect of follow-up letters, smoking motivation, muscle tension, and health locus of control. *Journal of Consulting and Clinical Psychology* 49(6):982–984, December 1981.

SILVERMAN, A.P. Behaviour of rats given a 'smoking dose' of nicotine. *Animal Behaviour* 19:67–74, 1971.

SILVERSTEIN, B., FELD, S., KOZLOWSKI, L.T. The availability of low-nicotine cigarettes as a cause of cigarette smoking among teenage females. *Journal of Health and Social Behavior* 21(4):383–388, December 1980.

SILVERSTEIN, B., KELLY, E., SWAN, J., KOZLOWSKI, L.T. Physiological predisposition toward becoming a cigarette smoker: Experimental evidence for a sex difference. *Addictive Behaviors* 7(1):83–86, 1982.

SMITH, G.M. Personality and smoking: A review of the empirical literature. In: Hunt, W.A. (ed.) *Learning Mechanisms in Smoking*. Chicago: Aldine Publishing, 1970, pp. 42–61.

SMITH, J.W. Long term outcome of clients treated in a commercial stop smoking program. *Journal of Substance Abuse Treatment* 5:33–36, 1988.

SOLOMON, R.L., CORBIT, J.D. An opponent-process theory of motivation: II. Cigarette addiction. *Journal of Abnormal Psychology* 81(2):158–171, 1973.

SORENSEN, G., PECHACEK, T. Occupational and sex differences in smoking and smoking cessation. *Journal of Occupational Medicine* 28(5):360–364, May 1986.

SORENSEN, G., PECHACEK, T., PALLONEN, U. Occupational and worksite norms and attitudes about smoking cessation. *American Journal of Public Health* 76(5):544–549, May 1986.

SORENSEN, G., PECHACEK, T.F. Attitudes toward smoking cessation among men and women. *Journal of Behavioral Medicine* 10(2):129–137, April 1987.

STEWART, J., DEWIT, H., EIKELBOOM, R. The role of unconditioned and conditioned drug effects in the self-administration of opiates and stimulants. *Psychology Review* 91(2):251–268, 1984.

STRAITS, B., SECHREST, L. Further support of some findings about the characteristics of smokers and nonsmokers. *Journal of Consulting and Clinical Psychology* 27:282, 1963.

SUSSMAN, S., DENT, C.W., FLAY, B.R., HANSEN, W.B., JOHNSON, C.A. Psychosocial predictors of cigarette smoking onset by white, black, Hispanic, and Asian adolescents in southern California. *Morbidity and Mortality Weekly Report* 36(4S):115–165, September 4, 1987.

SUTTON, S. Social-psychological approaches to understanding addictive behaviours: Attitude–behaviour and decision-making models. *British Journal of Addiction* 82:355–370, 1987.

SUTTON, S.R., EISER, J.R. The effect of fear-arousing communications on cigarette smoking: An expectancy-value approach. *Journal of Behavioral Medicine* 7(1):13–33, March 1984.

SWINEHART, J.W., KIRSCHT, J.P. Smoking: A panel study of beliefs and behavior following the PHS report. *Psychological Reports* 18:519–528, 1966.

THOMPSON, E.L. Smoking education programs 1960–1976. *American Journal of Public Health* 68(3):250–257, March 1978.

TICER, S. Where there's smoke, there's trouble. Slower sales have cigarette makers trying promotions, 'Smokeless' brands—and price hikes. *Business Week*, January 18, 1988.

TOMKINS, S. A modified model of smoking behavior. In: Borgatta, E.F., Evans, R.R. (eds.) *Smoking, Health, and Behavior*. Chicago: Aldine, 1968.

TOMKINS, S.S. Psychological model for smoking behavior. *American Journal of Public Health* 56(12):17–20, December 1966.

U.S. DEPARTMENT OF AGRICULTURE. *Tobacco Situation and Outlook Report*. U.S. Department of Agriculture, Economic Research Service, National Economics Division, TS-199, June 1987.

U.S. DEPARTMENT OF DEFENSE. *The 1985 Worldwide Survey of Alcohol and Nonmedical Drug Use Among Military Personnel*. Report of the Research Triangle Institute to the Office of the Assistant Secretary of Defense (Health Affairs), Department of Defense, June 1986.

U.S. DEPARTMENT OF DEFENSE. *Updated Report on Smoking and Health in the Military*. U.S. Department of Defense, Office of the Assistant Secretary of Defense (Health Affairs), Office of the Assistant Secretary of Defense (Force Management and Personnel), June 1987.

U.S. DEPARTMENT OF DEFENSE. *The 1988 Worldwide Survey of Substance Abuse and Health Behavior Among Military Personnel.* Report of the Research Triangle Institute to the Office of the Assistant Secretary of Defense (Public Affairs), Department of Defense, 1988.

U.S. DEPARTMENT OF HEALTH AND HUMAN SERVICES. *Promoting Health/Preventing Disease: Objectives for the Nation.* U.S. Department of Health and Human Services, Public Health Service, 1980a.

U.S. DEPARTMENT OF HEALTH AND HUMAN SERVICES. *The Health Consequences of Smoking for Women. A Report of the Surgeon General.* U.S. Department of Health and Human Services, Public Health Service, Office of the Assistant Secretary for Health, Office on Smoking and Health, 1980b.

U.S. DEPARTMENT OF HEALTH AND HUMAN SERVICES. *The Health Consequences of Smoking. The Changing Cigarette: A Report of the Surgeon General.* U.S. Department of Health and Human Services, Public Health Service, Office of the Assistant Secretary for Health, Office on Smoking and Health. DHHS Publication No. (PHS) 81-50156, 1981.

U.S. DEPARTMENT OF HEALTH AND HUMAN SERVICES. *The Health Consequences of Smoking: Cancer. A Report of the Surgeon General.* U.S. Department of Health and Human Services, Public Health Service, Office on Smoking and Health. DHHS Publication No. (PHS) 82-50179, 1982.

U.S. DEPARTMENT OF HEALTH AND HUMAN SERVICES. *The Health Consequences of Smoking: Cardiovascular Disease. A Report of the Surgeon General.* U.S. Department of Health and Human Services, Public Health Service, Office on Smoking and Health. DHHS Publication No. (PHS) 84-50204, 1983.

U.S DEPARTMENT OF HEALTH AND HUMAN SERVICES. *The Health Consequences of Smoking: Chronic Obstructive Lung Disease. A Report of the Surgeon General.* U.S. Department of Health and Human Services, Public Health Service, Office on Smoking and Health. DHHS Publication No. (PHS) 84-50205, 1984.

U.S DEPARTMENT OF HEALTH AND HUMAN SERVICES. *The Health Consequences of Smoking: Cancer and Chronic Lung Disease in the Workplace. A Report of the Surgeon General.* U.S. Department of Health and Human Services, Public Health Service, Office on Smoking and Health. DHHS Publication No. (PHS) 85-50207, 1985.

U.S. DEPARTMENT OF HEALTH AND HUMAN SERVICES. *The Health Consequences of Using Smokeless Tobacco. A Report of the Advisory Committee to the Surgeon General, 1986.* U.S. Department of Health and Human Services, Public Health Service. NIH Publication No. 86-2874, April 1986a.

U.S. DEPARTMENT OF HEALTH AND HUMAN SERVICES. *Smoking and Health. A National Status Report. A Report to Congress.* U.S. Department of Health and Human Services, Public Health Service, Centers for Disease Control, Center for Health Promotion and Education, Office on Smoking and Health. DHHS Publication No. (CDC) 87-8396, 1986b.

U.S. DEPARTMENT OF HEALTH AND HUMAN SERVICES. *The 1990 Health Objectives for the Nation: A Midcourse Review.* U.S. Department of Health and Human Services, Public Health Service, Office of Disease Prevention and Health Promotion, November 1986c.

U.S. DEPARTMENT OF HEALTH AND HUMAN SERVICES. *The Health Consequences of Smoking: Nicotine Addiction. A Report of the Surgeon General, 1988.* U.S. Department of Health and Human Services, Public Health Service, Centers for Disease Control, Center for Health Promotion and Education, Office on Smoking and Health. DHHS Publication No. (CDC) 88-8406, 1988.

U.S. DEPARTMENT OF HEALTH AND HUMAN SERVICES. *Adult Use of Tobacco, 1986.* U.S. Department of Health and Human Services, Public Health Service, Centers for Disease Control, Office on Smoking and Health, in press,a.

U.S. DEPARTMENT OF HEALTH AND HUMAN SERVICES. *The 1987 National Adolescent Student Health Survey*. U.S. Department of Health and Human Services, Public Health Service, Office of Disease Prevention and Health Promotion, in press,b.

U.S. DEPARTMENT OF HEALTH, EDUCATION, AND WELFARE. *Use of Tobacco: Practices, Attitudes, Knowledge, and Beliefs, United States—Fall 1964 and Spring 1966*. U.S. Department of Health, Education, and Welfare, Public Health Service, National Clearinghouse for Smoking and Health, July 1969.

U.S. DEPARTMENT OF HEALTH, EDUCATION, AND WELFARE. *Adult Use of Tobacco, 1970*. U.S. Department of Health, Education, and Welfare, Public Health Service, Center for Disease Control, Health Services and Mental Health Administration, National Clearinghouse for Smoking and Health, June 1973a.

U.S. DEPARTMENT OF HEALTH, EDUCATION, AND WELFARE. *The Health Consequences of Smoking*. U.S. Department of Health, Education, and Welfare, Public Health Service, Health Services and Mental Health Administration. DHEW Publication No. (HSM) 73-8704, 1973b.

U.S. DEPARTMENT OF HEALTH, EDUCATION, AND WELFARE. *Adult Use of Tobacco—1975*. U.S. Department of Health, Education, and Welfare, Public Health Service, Center for Disease Control, 1976.

U.S. DEPARTMENT OF HEALTH, EDUCATION, AND WELFARE. *Smoking and Health. A Report of the Surgeon General*. U.S. Department of Health, Education, and Welfare, Public Health Service, Office of the Assistant Secretary for Health, Office on Smoking and Health. DHEW Publication No. (PHS)79-50066, 1979a.

U.S. DEPARTMENT OF HEALTH, EDUCATION, AND WELFARE. *Teenage Smoking: Intermediate and Long-Term Patterns*. U.S. Department of Health, Education, and Welfare, National Institute of Education, 1979b.

U.S. PUBLIC HEALTH SERVICE. *Smoking and Health. Report of Advisory Committee to the Surgeon General of the Public Health Service*. U.S. Department of Health, Education, and Welfare, Public Health Service, Center for Disease Control. PHS Publication No. 1103, 1964.

VELICER, W.F., DICLEMENTE, C.C., PROCHASKA, J.O., BRANDENBURG, N. Decisional balance measure for assessing and predicting smoking status. *Journal of Personality and Social Psychology* 48(5):1279–1289, May 1985.

WALLSTON, K.A., WALLSTON, B.S., DEVELLIS, R. Development of the Multidimensional Health Locus of Control (MHLC) scales. *Health Education Monographs* 6(2):160–170, Spring 1978.

WARBURTON, D.M., WESNES, K., SHERGOLD, K., JAMES, M. Facilitation of learning and state dependency with nicotine. *Psychopharmacology* 89(1):55–59, May 1986.

WARNER, K.E. Possible increases in the underreporting of cigarette consumption. *Journal of the American Statistical Association* 73(362):314–318, June 1978.

WARNER, K.E. Cigarette advertising and media coverage of smoking and health. *New England Journal of Medicine* 312:384–388, February 7, 1985.

WARNER, K.E., MURT, H.A. Impact of the antismoking campaign on smoking prevalence: A cohort analysis. *Journal of Public Health Policy* 3(4):374–390, December 1982.

WEINKAM, J.J., STERLING, T.D. Changes in smoking characteristics by type of employment from 1970 to 1979/1980. *American Journal of Industrial Medicine* 11:539–561, 1987.

WEISSMAN, W., GLASGOW, R., BIGLAN, A., LICHTENSTEIN, E. Development and preliminary evaluation of a cessation program for adolescent smokers. *Psychology of Addictive Behaviors* 1(2):84–91, 1987.

WEST, R.J., JARVIS, M.J., RUSSELL, M.A.H., CARRUTHERS, M.E., FEYERABEND, C. Effect of nicotine replacement on the cigarette withdrawal syndrome. *British Journal of Addiction* 79:215–219, 1984.

WIKLER, A. Requirements for extinction of relapse-facilitating variables and for rehabilitation in a narcotic-antagonist program. *Advances in Biochemistry and Psychopharmacology* 8: 399–414, 1973.

WIKLER, A., PESCOR, F.T. Classical conditioning of a morphine abstinence phenomenon, reinforcement of opioid-drinking behavior and "relapse" in morphine-addicted rats. *Psychopharmacologia* (Berlin) 10:255–284, 1967.

WILLIAMSON, D.F., SERDULA, M.K., KENDRICK, J.S., BINKIN, N.J. Comparing the prevalence of smoking in pregnant and nonpregnant women, 1985 to 1986. *Journal of the American Medical Association* 261(1):70–74, January 6, 1989.

WOHLFORD, P. Initiation of cigarette smoking: Is it related to parental smoking behavior? *Journal of Consulting and Clinical Psychology* 34(2):148–151, April 1970.

WORLD HEALTH ORGANIZATION. *Expert Committee on Addiction-Producing Drugs.* Seventh Report, Technical Report Series No. 116. Geneva: World Health Organization, 1957.

WORLD HEALTH ORGANIZATION. *Tobacco or Health. Report by the Director-General.* Forty-First World Health Assembly, provisional agenda item 22. Geneva: World Health Organization, March 23, 1988.

YATES, G.L., MACKENZIE, R., PENNBRIDGE, J., COHEN, E. A risk profile comparison of runaway and non-runaway youth. *American Journal of Public Health* 78(7):820–821, July 1988.

ZABIN, L.S. The association between smoking and sexual behavior among teens in US contraceptive clinics. *American Journal of Public Health* 74(3):261–263, March 1984.

CHAPTER 6

SMOKING PREVENTION, CESSATION, AND ADVOCACY ACTIVITIES

CONTENTS

INTRODUCTION

The tobacco control movement in the United States has involved the efforts of many diverse groups. Voluntary health agencies, State and local health departments, the Federal Government, medical organizations, private industry, and grassroots organizations have all contributed. This Chapter reviews the nonpolicy activities of these groups in the areas of smoking prevention and cessation, and advocacy over the past 25 years. It will not provide a complete review of the efficacy of different prevention and cessation methods; this has been done by others (e.g., Lichtenstein and Brown 1980; Pechacek 1979; Schwartz 1969, 1987; Schwartz and Rider 1978; Flay 1985a,b; Best et al. 1988; Biglan and Ary 1985; McCaul and Glasgow 1985; Snow, Gilchrist, and Schinke 1985; US DHEW 1979b; US DHHS 1986a). A selective review of the broader trends in these activities will provide a basis for understanding the current status of the smoking control movement and its possible future directions. A review of advocacy activities intended to lead to changes in smoking control policies over the last 25 years will serve as a bridge between this Chapter and Chapter 7, Smoking Control Policies.

The smoking prevention and cessation activities discussed in this Chapter were designed as direct antismoking messages incorporating advice and instruction on how to remain or become a nonsmoker. Smoking prevention programs include school curricula, both those specific to smoking and those integrated within a multicomponent health education approach; media-based efforts; and an array of other materials, events, and campaigns. Smoking cessation programs include a broad variety of activities ranging from self-help cessation materials to special smoking groups to the use of medication. The programs occur in various channels in the community including worksites, physician offices, hospitals, schools, and media.

Integrating Educational and Behavioral Interventions With Policy Initiatives

The integration of educational and behavioral programs with policy initiatives, including those that affect the price of cigarettes, the information printed on the packaging, the manner in which cigarettes can be advertised, the conditions of their sale, and the circumstances under which they may be smoked, has been one of the most important recent trends in smoking prevention, as well as in cessation-oriented interventions. Projects such as "Tobacco-Free America Project" (Bailey 1987) work on both fronts, advocating nonsmoking policies in schools along with providing more traditional smoking prevention materials and programs to reduce the number of new smokers. Advocacy activities and lobbying leading to policy changes were almost nonexistent at the time of the 1964 Surgeon General's Report, but became progressively more evident during the 1970s and expanded significantly during the 1980s, setting the stage for many of the changes in prevention and cessation policies and activities.

Even when explicit policy components are lacking in prevention or cessation programs, the content and impact of these programs should be considered in the context of the social and policy climate prevailing at the time of their design and implementation (see Best et al. 1988; Chassin, Presson, Sherman 1985; Chassin et al. 1987; Perry and Murray 1982). For example, the effects of a prevention or cessation activity might be moderated by whether it was conducted during the era of television cigarette commercials alone (pre-1967), the era of both commercials and antismoking public service announcements (PSAs) mandated by the Government (1967–70) (see Chapter 7), or during the subsequent era of no televised cigarette commercials and the end of the mandated PSAs (post-1970). Other potentially relevant policy contexts include school regulation of student smoking and the level of public debate and restrictions on smoking in other settings at the time of the smoking prevention or cessation program. Both the smoking prevention and cessation programs and the public policy context remain in a continuous process of evolution and interaction.

PART I. SMOKING PREVENTION ACTIVITIES

Overview of Major Approaches to Smoking Prevention

In the years since the release of the first Surgeon General's Report (US PHS 1964), both the basic design of prevention efforts and their designated targets have changed. Generally, there has been a shift in the target group from high school and college students (US PHS 1964) to middle school and junior high school students, and a shift away from information-oriented antismoking education to psychosocial curricula designed not only to address youth's motivations to smoke but also to impart skills for resisting influences to smoke (Botvin, Eng, Williams 1980; Flay 1985a; McAlister, Perry, Maccoby 1979).

The changes in focus and design and the proliferation of prevention programs since the early 1960s have resulted in such a variety of approaches that they are now rarely considered together in reviews of smoking prevention programs. These differing approaches include (1) media-based prevention programs and resources, (2) smoking prevention as a component of multicomponent school health education curricula, and (3) smoking prevention through the psychosocial approaches of social influence and generic life skills curricula. Other smoking prevention resources and activities such as physician presentations to school assemblies, brochures, community campaigns, and educational resources have been sponsored by voluntary, professional, and community groups.

While the prevention approaches overlap considerably, both in form and content, this differentiation of program types can serve as a framework for tracing the prevention initiatives and directions taken by various organizations, as well as for highlighting the evolution of smoking prevention programs over the years. The following outline of the major prevention approaches will be expanded upon in a later section.

Media-based messages and campaigns were part of the earliest smoking prevention activities. The National Clearinghouse for Smoking and Health (later reorganized as the Office on Smoking and Health (OSH)) and the voluntary health organizations were among the early and continuing sponsors of newspaper and broadcast antismoking campaigns. These smoking prevention campaigns have continued with varying intensity over the decades, continuing into the present era of controlled research in the development and evaluation of media-based smoking prevention programs (e.g., Bauman et al. 1988; Flay et al. 1988; NCI 1986a; Ramirez and McAlister 1988; Sussman et al. 1986; Worden et al. 1988).

The integration of smoking prevention curricula into comprehensive and multicomponent school health education curricula was one response to the findings of limited impact from early smoking-specific prevention efforts (see Davis 1977). The development of psychosocial approaches including social-influence and life skills programs in the 1970s was another response to the limited impact of early prevention efforts (Evans 1976; US DHEW 1979b). The integration of smoking prevention into general health education represented an important shift in the vehicle for antismoking messages, and the psychosocial approaches were based on a fundamental revision of the model underlying prevention strategies for smoking by youth.

The psychosocial approaches deviated from traditional antismoking education models by deemphasizing communication of the long-term health risks of smoking. Instead, these new curricula focused on young people's susceptibility to social pressures to smoke—influences inferred from consistent findings relating smoking by youth to smoking by their parents, siblings, and peers (Flay et al. 1983; US DHEW 1979c; US PHS 1964). In their various forms, social influence and life skills curricula have been designed to raise young people's awareness of the influences to smoke; to highlight the more immediate, and especially socially based, negative effects of smoking; and to "inoculate" youth against the effects of continued pressure and examples of others who smoke. The new approaches were bolstered by the literature on communication theory and on the psychosocial development of adolescents (US DHEW 1979b).

This Section covers the course of smoking prevention activities over the past 25 years. The first part presents a model of developmental stages of smoking acquisition as a framework for describing trends and options for prevention programs. This is followed by further description of the three major categories of current prevention programs and of cessation programs for youth. The next part describes in more detail the history of prevention activities of the major national voluntary health agencies, Federal support with emphasis on their early responses in the campaign to prevent smoking, and the activities of State and other organizations and agencies with emphasis on their recent activities. Considered next are problems in program dissemination and the gaps that frequently exist between the scientific literature and widespread program application in the field. Problems in program evaluation are reviewed in the next section. The review closes with a consideration of population factors such as changing attitudes toward smoking and secular trends in smoking prevalence as they relate to program diversification.

Prevention Opportunities Associated With Stages in the Acquisition of Smoking

As noted in the preceding chapter, several researchers (e.g., Flay et al. 1983; Leventhal and Cleary 1980) have proposed models of developmental stages in the acquisition of smoking. These models provide one dimension for describing and evaluating prevention opportunities and trends. The stages—for example, "preparation and anticipation," "initiation," "experimentation," "transition (becoming)," and "regular smoking" (Flay et al. 1983)—suggest a continuum of associated prevention opportunities. Spanning this developmental continuum are approaches to keep children from experimenting with tobacco, efforts to disrupt the evolution from experimentation to regular smoking, and early interventions aimed at influencing the young smoker to stop before the behavior and nicotine dependence become more firmly entrenched.

Stage models of smoking acquisition posit that different influences are at play at various ages; for instance, parents have a greater influence than peers in determining smoking intentions and behavior among young adolescents, while peers are more important for older adolescents. Social factors are viewed as more influential for beginning smokers, and physiological dependence and coping patterns as more important for the older, more established smokers (Flay et al. 1983; Leventhal and Cleary 1980; Chassin, Presson, Sherman 1985). (See Chapter 5, Part II.)

Prevention programs designed to reduce the number of young adolescents who initiate smoking reflect the dominant model for current smoking prevention. However, early antismoking education efforts addressed smoking by high school and college students (US PHS 1964), age groups encompassing several stages in smoking acquisition. The majority of current prevention programs focus on adolescents in grades 6 through 8, the age groups now at maximal risk for cigarette experimentation (Flay et al. 1983; Flay 1985a; Chapter 5). The shift of interest to smoking prevention programs aimed at younger adolescents is related to four considerations: (1) the findings of greater program impact among younger children (Jason, Mollica, Ferrone 1982; Johnson et al. 1986; Merki et al. 1968), (2) the general ineffectiveness of previous prevention approaches (Thompson 1978), (3) the recognition of secular trends toward earlier initiation of smoking (Evans et al. 1979; Flay et al. 1983; Chapter 5), and (4) the appeal of prevention versus the challenge of adult cessation (Evans et al. 1979).

A stage model of smoking acquisition and associated prevention opportunities suggests the potential for prevention programs aimed at even younger children in the preparation stage of smoking acquisition, the period during which early attitudes toward smoking are formed. The stage model also suggests cessation programs among older adolescents at the other end of the prevention continuum. Thus, some smoking prevention programs are directed at very young children in preschool or early elementary grades (ACS described in US DHHS 1986a; Peterson described in NCI 1986a; Pigg et al. 1985), and there are cessation programs directed at adolescents (e.g., ACS 1980, 1986; Weissmann et al. 1987). A call for continued development of programs addressing "pre-onset" issues and youth cessation was included in the National Cancer Institute (NCI) expert advisory panel's recommendations (Glynn, in press). Youth smoking cessation approaches are described in a later section in this Chapter.

Prevention Program Approaches

As outlined above, the evolution of prevention programs since the 1960s can be classified into three major approaches: media-based programs, smoking prevention in the context of multicomponent school health education, and psychosocial curricula. The three major approaches will be more fully described in this Section. Other resources and activities in the field will be described in a subsequent section.

Media-Based Prevention Programs

Media-based prevention approaches have included antismoking messages delivered through newspapers and television and radio broadcasts. Most often these have taken the form of brief announcements, but more extended special programs and curricula have also been developed and distributed. The American Lung Association (ALA), American Heart Association (AHA), American Cancer Society (ACS), and National Heart, Lung, and Blood Institute (NHLBI) sponsored one such extended prevention program, first aired in November 1984, a 1-hr Public Broadcasting System special, "Breathing Easy," aimed at young people (Bailey 1985; US DHHS 1986a).

Mass-media-based messages and programs were included among the earliest smoking prevention efforts of the Federal agencies and voluntary health associations. Flay (1986 and 1987b) has provided comprehensive reviews of these and later media-based smoking control efforts.

Early evaluations of mass media in health promotion were not encouraging, leading to Flay's (l986) appraisal that mass media programs alone are not effective. Reviewing studies of media campaigns that were used either as the sole intervention or in conjunction with other material and programming, Flay concluded that the most effective use of mass media in substance abuse prevention lies in furthering the dissemination of other prevention resources, such as school-based programs. Parents, for example, may become more supportive of the efforts of school-based prevention programs brought to their attention through the mass media (Flay 1986). In reviews of mass media campaigns specifically focused on smoking, Flay (l987a,b) found some basis for optimism about their potential impact on adult smoking cessation. He recommended, however, further evaluation of mass media campaigns for the prevention of adolescent smoking; only 3 of the 56 evaluations reviewed included specific reference to smoking by children (Flay 1987b).

There have been several controlled studies of mass-media-based prevention programs in recent years (Bauman et al. 1988; Sussman et al. 1986; Flay et al. 1988; Worden et al. 1988; Ramirez and McAlister 1988). A University of Southern California study demonstrated that effects on student smoking correlated with amount of attention to the television segments and amount of discussion of the program with others (Sussman et al. 1986; Flay 1987b; Flay and Sobel 1983; Flay, Hansen et al. 1987). The program, which parents were encouraged to watch with their children, also had a cessation effect on the adults' smoking (Flay 1986).

Mass media interventions can also augment other prevention programs, generating prevention effects that occur more broadly, acting over time in the aggregate to affect the level of public awareness and the social acceptability of smoking. The potential for this level of public health impact is described by Leventhal and Cleary (1980) and Warner and Murt (1982) in their consideration of factors inhibiting the rise of smoking rates in the late 1960s and 1970s.

Even small program effects can have a large public health impact, given the very large audiences of mass media (Flay 1987b), making the actual distribution and broadcasting of these programs critical. Dissemination of media materials has been dependent on the good will and interest of publishers and broadcast managers, or on funds for purchase of air time and print space. In recent years, video news releases (essentially press releases on videotape) have been used increasingly by private health organizations and Federal agencies (including the Office on Smoking and Health) to motivate television news coverage of tobacco-related "events" (Davis 1988a).

Smoking Prevention Programs in the Context of Multicomponent School Health Education Curricula

Smoking prevention components have long been incorporated in more general school health programs. This represents an alternative approach to programs focused exclusively on smoking prevention. The development and evaluation of the 8- to 10-week curriculum of "Growing Healthy" have involved a partnership between Federal agencies and national voluntary organizations spanning three decades, with ALA serving as a lead agency in these endeavors. "Growing Healthy" is the combined Primary Grades Health Curriculum Project aimed at students in kindergarten through grade 3, and the School Health Curriculum Project (SHCP) aimed at students in grades 4 through 7. Both are designed to integrate smoking and health into a comprehensive school health education curriculum. An evaluation of the original SHCP component between 1982 and 1985 demonstrated a delay in onset of smoking among the seventh grade students who had been in the program. Among the intervention students, 7.7 percent had started smoking by grade 7, compared with 12.7 percent among the control group (US DHHS 1986a).

The School Health Education Evaluation Project (Connell and Turner 1985; Connell, Turner, Mason 1985) also included a review of "Growing Healthy," as well as of three other school health programs with various dimensions of program implementation and impact. "Growing Healthy" has been validated by the Department of Education and included in the National Diffusion Network (NDN), an organization that includes data on the extent of diffusion of curricula that have been evaluated and validated by the Department of Education (US DHHS 1986a). As part of NDN, dissemination of "Growing Healthy" is facilitated and monitored.

The Teenage Health Teaching Modules, a comprehensive health education program for junior and senior high school students, were developed by the Centers for Disease Control (CDC) Center for Chronic Disease Prevention and Health Promotion through a contract with Education Development Center, Inc., and are also currently being evaluated (US DHHS 1986a). They are also now being promoted as part of ALA's "Growing Healthy" activities. The American Health Foundation "Know Your Body" program is a multicomponent school health education curriculum aimed at reducing smoking and risk factors for coronary heart disease. A recent study of program impact after 6 years of intervention found significantly lower rates of initiation of smoking among subjects in the intervention schools (Walter, Vaughan, Wynder 1988). Another study comparing the effectiveness of this program's smoking prevention component when offered alone or as part of the multicomponent package is currently under way.

Although many substance abuse prevention programs have adopted social influence and life skills training approaches (Bell and Battjes 1985; Polich et al. 1984), prevention of tobacco use is not consistently part of, let alone prominent in, the derivative programs. One rationale for integrating tobacco use prevention with prevention programs for other forms of substance abuse is provided by the recently increasing appreciation of the common nature of licit and illicit drug addictions (US DHHS 1988).

In addition to comprehensive school health education curricula developed and evaluated by Federal agencies and national voluntary organizations, curriculum guidelines designed by individual school systems and commercial textbook writers sometimes include antismoking components. No systematic review of this category of smoking prevention programs in comprehensive health education curricula exists.

The degree of emphasis on and implementation of smoking-specific prevention curricula can be obscured within more general health education curricula. Evaluation of the impact of these programs on smoking behavior has been far less detailed than in smoking-specific curricula. In addition, the integration of tobacco prevention programs into a basic health education curricula presents substantive questions of program impact: Will the same basic prevention material be more effective if presented independently, as a special program? Will its impact be augmented or decreased by an ongoing context of basic health education? Drawing on the currently available research and on preliminary findings from ongoing studies, an expert advisory panel convened by NCI in December 1987 concluded that school-based smoking prevention conducted within a multicomponent health focus appeared as effective as programs with an exclusive emphasis on smoking, provided the smoking component received a minimum level of attention. One criterion for this minimum level of attention was five classroom sessions in each of 2 years (Glynn, in press). More focused evaluations of smoking prevention in the context of school health education are needed to answer these questions.

While a unified multicomponent health education curriculum may be attractive to schools faced with a multitude of health education requirements, this approach to smoking prevention depends on the state of health education at the State and national levels and faces all the obstacles and challenges experienced by such larger enterprises (Iverson and Kolbe 1983; Kolbe and Gilbert 1984; Kolbe and Iverson 1984; Lohrmann, Gold, Jubb 1987).

Psychosocial Curricula

Increased funding of smoking prevention research in the 1980s (Bell and Levy 1984; NCI 1984, 1986a; Stone 1985), as well as the advocacy of using psychosocial approaches developed for smoking prevention for other substance abuse prevention efforts (Bell and Battjes 1985; Polich et al. 1984), has brought psychosocial approaches to the forefront of attention. From a research perspective, they represent the dominant strategy in smoking prevention, the culmination of the preceding 25 years of investigation.

Reviewing the literature on the psychosocial prevention curricula, Bell and Battjes (1985) identified two main types of programs: (1) the social influence curricula that foster youths' awareness of and ability to resist peer and other social pressures and influences to smoke (Dielman et al. 1985; Flay et al. 1985; Hurd et al. 1980; Johnson et al. 1986; Killen 1985; Luepker et al. 1983; Perry, Killen, Telch et al. 1980; Shaffer,

Beck, Boothroyd 1983), and (2) those more broadly structured to also strengthen more general social skills and competencies underlying initial vulnerability to these pressures to smoke, referred to as life skills training approaches or generic life skills approaches (Botvin, Eng, Williams 1980; Botvin and Wills 1985; Gilchrist and Schinke 1985; Schinke et al. 1985). Both varieties include programs that have been originally designed or expanded to include substance abuse prevention of other kinds. Components of psychosocial approaches have also been integrated into the more general health education curricula. The social influence approach growing out of work by Evans and his colleagues (Evans 1976; Evans et al. 1981) shifted the smoking prevention agenda from issues in the development and dissemination of antismoking educational messages to questions about ways to affect the psychosocial processes underlying children's responses to social influences to smoke.

The social influence and generic life skills curricula for smoking prevention are the best documented and most thoroughly evaluated among the smoking prevention programs. The field has reached the point that some general statements can be made concerning components of programs and the general extent of their effect (e.g. Glynn, in press).

Common features of programs that have been found to have positive prevention effects include a focus on students in the middle and junior high grades; multiple sessions; intervention components designed to correct young people's misimpressions of the social significance and prevalence of smoking among peers; emphasis on the short-term reasons not to smoke (both physiological and social); education regarding the variety of social factors (parental, peer, and media) influencing smoking; practice with skills used to resist offers to smoke and examples of smoking; involvement of peers, either as peer leaders or as videotaped role models; and public commitment procedures (Flay 1985a,b). In addition, life skills training curricula are likely to include program components to enhance decisionmaking, self-esteem, and social competencies (Botvin and Wills 1985).

Three minimum program components were recommended by the 1987 NCI expert advisory panel: information about the social consequences and short-term physiological effects of tobacco use; information about social influences on tobacco use, especially peer, parent, and media influences; and training in refusal skills, including modeling and practice of resistance skills (Glynn, in press). The panel added the caveat that the quality of the delivery of these components would be critical to their success. Teacher training and adoption of existing smoking prevention programs, as designed, were recommended as two assurances of better quality program delivery.

Although use of peer leaders or models has been a frequent component of these programs, evaluations comparing the role of peer versus adult leaders have been mixed regarding the importance of peer leaders to program success (Arkin et al. 1981; Clarke et al. 1986; Murray et al. 1984; Perry, Killen, Slinkard et al. 1980; Perry et al. 1983). The logistic challenges entailed in implementing a peer-led program also must be considered. Arkin and colleagues (1981) found, for instance, that "Teachers, principals and students generally had more trouble adjusting to peer-led programs than to the health educator led programs" (p. 614). The recent NCI panel concluded that the most effective use of peer leaders was as assistants to a trained teacher, with responsiblity for carrying out specified program components (Glynn, in press). The findings of Perry and colleagues (1983) suggest that peer leaders may be most effective in delivering curricula focused on social pressures, as opposed to more traditional health effects curricula.

Within social influence and life skills curricula there has been a marked refinement of research methods and a better scientific and theoretical basis for program design and evaluation. Flay (1985a,b) described in detail the evolution of psychosocial smoking prevention programs and their evaluations, in which methodological progress has been made. This progress includes greater numbers of schools per condition, use of randomization, and greater emphasis on internal validity of programs. The use of procedures to validate reports of smoking status (Evans 1976) has also reflected the increasing methodological rigor of the psychosocial curricula research. Validated behavioral outcomes of prevention programs have progressively replaced earlier reliance on changes in measures of attitudes and intentions and on self-reported smoking, thus providing a firmer ground for comparison of program impact.

After more than one decade of this research, however, the findings are characterized as tentative and subject to further evidence. No single study unequivocally establishes the effectiveness of the psychosocial approaches, but reviewers, taking the sum of the research, see support for the potential of these programs. The social influence and life skills training approaches programs have been characterized as capable of a 50-percent reduction of smoking onset that has been shown to persist for up to 2 years (Flay 1985a; Botvin, Renick, Baker 1983). The promise of these programs is tempered by such factors as the complexity of the natural history of smoking acquisition (Cleary et al. 1988) and the continued need for long-term followup. (See subsequent sections for further discussion of these factors.)

Two other variations in smoking prevention programs also have been considered and, pending their further development, are best classified along with the social influence approaches. One is the parent-oriented approach to social influences, whereby parents and their communication skills and influences are the direct object of intervention (Worden et al. 1987; Oei and Fea 1987). Parental support and involvement in school-based smoking prevention programs, especially for pre- to grade 6 programs, is recommended in Glynn (in press). Worden and colleagues (1987) tested the smoking prevention effects of communication skills workshops for parents. While not presented to parents as a smoking prevention program, smoking was a focal topic and example throughout. Six months after the program was offered, significantly lower levels of self-reports of smoking among the fifth and sixth grade students in the communities that received high-intensity workshop coverage were demonstrated. Based on Oei and Fea's (1987) review of data and rationale from studies bearing on youth smoking and on parents as educators, they recommend further utilization of parents in smoking prevention programs with young children.

Another variation of smoking prevention programs using a cognitive development approach also builds on a developmental perspective on smoking acquisition. However, it considers social influences as but one set of factors bearing on the initiation of smoking among the young. Understanding processes of addiction, mechanisms for controlling emotions, and the relationship between smoking-induced sensations and health threats is also seen as bearing on smoking by youth (Glynn, Leventhal, Hirschman 1985). A prevention program based on this model has been developed for students in the early stages of contemplating *and* experimenting with smoking. This cognitive development program significantly deviates from the social influence curricula in its inclusion of both young nonsmokers and smokers and in its examination of nonsocial influences on their experience of smoking. However, the age groups targeted are the same, social influences are also part of the curricula, and, more fundamentally, the program shares with the social influence curricula a theory-based approach to directly intervening in the processes and needs thought to underlie the development of smoking among young people. An 18-month followup of program and control students in grades 6 through 8 revealed significant differences in attitudes toward smoking and in students' self-reports of smoking (Glynn, Leventhal, Hirschman 1985).

Youth Smoking Cessation Programs

Youth smoking cessation programs are properly viewed as part of smoking prevention efforts to the extent that their ultimate goal is the prevention of the establishment of dependent, regular smoking. The limited research in this area cannot yet suggest the optimal balance of traditional "prevention" and cessation strategies for programs targeting young smokers. Some young smokers may exhibit much variability in their smoking; others show a pattern of consumption very closely resembling older, addicted smokers. (See Chapter 5.)

Recent interest in teenage cessation has been heightened by increasing social disapproval of smoking and acceptance of its restriction on the part of adolescents and society more broadly (Johnston, O'Malley, Bachman 1987; US DHHS 1986b), as well as voluntary health association and public health agency commitments to promoting nonsmoking environments in the schools (National School Boards Association 1987; US DHHS 1986a).

Data on naturally occurring rates of quit attempts and cessation among young smokers support interest in teenage cessation. These rates range from 18 to over 50 percent cessation with varying followup periods and suggest considerable flux in the natural history of smoking, as well as opportunities for intervention with young smokers after they begin experimenting with cigarettes (Alexander et al. 1983; Chassin, Presson, Sherman 1984; Ershler et al., in press; Hansen 1983; Hansen et al. 1985; O'Rourke, Nolte, Smith 1985; Skinner et al. 1985; US DHHS 1982).

Many of the early antismoking education programs incorporated cessation functions by virtue of their inclusion of older youth. Description of these early teenage smoking cessation programs, including those among the prototypes of antismoking education for youth, is included in the 1979 Surgeon General's Report (US DHEW 1979b) and in Seffrin and Bailey (1985). Smoking cessation programs specifically for youth have been developed by researchers (Weissman et al. 1987; St. Pierre, Shute, Jaycox 1983), voluntary associations (ACS 1980, 1986; Bennett, Austin, Janizewski 1986), and school personnel (Hulbert 1978). Program effects on cessation rates among young smokers have also been examined in studies that emphasize prevention of initiation (Best et al. 1984; Botvin, Renick, Baker 1983; Johnson et al. 1986; Perry, Killen, Telch et al. 1980). Cessation programs addressing young people's use of smokeless tobacco have also been designed (e.g., Glover 1986; Severson et al. 1987). NCI is currently funding research on both prevention and cessation interventions for smokeless tobacco use, though no outcomes have been reported as yet (NIH 1986).

Teenage cessation programs have met with mixed success, in terms of both recruitment and retention of program participants, and of program impact. Study of teenage cessation programs has also generally suffered from very small numbers of participants (in part, a reflection of difficulty in recruitment) and from a dearth of formal outcome evaluations. Subject characteristics, including baseline smoking levels, vary greatly from study to study, as do length of followup periods and outcome criteria considered. Although these limitations to the research are substantial and restrict conclusions that can be made concerning the efficacy of teen smoking cessation programs, the emergence of new demands for and research on such programs warrants the following review in comparatively more detail than for other larger and more controlled smoking prevention studies.

St. Pierre, Shute, and Jaycox (1983) found reductions in self-reported rates of consumption among 10 of the 11 teen smokers who regularly participated in their program of peer-designed and peer-led "stop smoking" clinics. In evaluating AHA's "Save a Sweet Heart" program's no-smoking pledge day component, Bennett, Austin, and Janizewski (1986) found that the pledging was related to cessation at a 1-year posttest in their sample of 194 10th-grade male smokers only, but not in the sample of 315 10th-grade female smokers. Overall, female students, including nonsmokers and smokers, were more apt than males to participate in the pledge component of the program.

Weissman and colleagues' teen cessation program (1987) used a contingency-based system of monetary rewards for reduction of expired carbon monoxide levels. The study suggested some promise among the males; four of the six male participants maintained abstinence during the 5-month followup period, with only limited "slips." However, all of the five females dropped out of the program before completion.

Perry, Killen, Telch, and colleagues (1980) compared the effects of a four-session program emphasizing the immediate physiological effects of smoking and the role of social influences with outcomes from a more traditional curriculum emphasizing the long-term health effects of smoking. Statistically significant differences in self-reports of smoking 5 months later were found within the treatment group of 498 10th-grade students, pre-and posttest for daily and monthly smoking; and between treatment and control (399 10th-grade students) groups posttest only for weekly and monthly smoking. Significant differences in corresponding measures of expired carbon monoxide were also found.

Taken in sum, there is some evidence that adolescent smoking cessation programs are efficacious, although the data and analyses are limited and difficult to interpret, and results are, therefore, far from conclusive. Further research and continued program development in this area are greatly needed.

History of Agency and Organizational Prevention Activities

Although the concept of disease prevention did not gain its widest currency and impact in antismoking efforts or in health promotion and medicine as a whole until the late 1970s (US DHEW 1979a), young smokers always have been an important focus of antismoking efforts. Prevention activities were under way during the 1950s and early 1960s, even as the data on the health consequences of smoking were being reviewed by the scientific community (US DHEW 1979b). This Section on the history of prevention programs covers the national organizations' initial antismoking efforts and State departments' more current responses to the smoking problem, and the activities of a range of other organizations and agencies. The emphasis is on the major directions of their efforts, as opposed to comprehensive cataloging of all programs and initiatives.

National Voluntary Health Organizations

The three major national voluntary health organizations involved in the antismoking campaign, ACS, AHA, and ALA (previously called the National Tuberculosis Association and later the National Tuberculosis and Respiratory Diseases Association), developed their own curricular materials and resources for use in schools, as well as mass-distributed brochures, posters, films, and PSAs. In addition, they have funded smoking prevention research conducted by outside investigators (Bell and Levy 1984) and have contributed to the development of comprehensive school health education curricula that include smoking.

In the late 1960s, in conjunction with CDC and other agencies, ALA began funding the development of the School Health Curriculum Project and the Primary Grades Health Curriculum Project, now jointly referred to as "Growing Healthy" (see description in earlier section). In addition to promoting the adoption of "Growing Healthy" in schools nationwide, ALA has developed smoking education modules and curriculum materials, and a variety of films and posters.

More recently, ALA developed the Biofeedback Smoking Education Project (BIOSEP) for students in grades 7 through 12, using student smokers and laboratory equipment, as a firsthand demonstration of the immediate negative physiological effects of smoking (Mitchell 1978; Young, Chen, Cernada 1982). Two studies have evaluated the effect of BIOSEP on the smoking behavior of adolescents, Mitchell (1978) and Young, Chen, and Cernada (1982). However, the outcomes from these two studies are not consistent and offer only modest support for BIOSEP's effects on smoking behavior.

An alternative approach for younger students aged 9 to 13 years is ALA's "Smoking Deserves a Smart Answer" (Bailey 1985). This kit uses a social influence approach centered on specific responses to direct peer pressure to smoke and includes humorous posters, stickers, a teacher resource guide, student worksheets, and sample role-playing situations.

Having issued a policy statement in 1963 to discourage smoking among both children and adults, AHA in 1967 developed sets of materials including a kit with a brochure for children to help their parents quit, a program that again may have had both cessation *and* prevention impact. Similarly, AHA's "Like Father, Like Son" campaign tapped both cessation and prevention themes.

AHA also has developed educational modules to prevent smoking among youth. Both the "Save a Sweet Heart" program and "Let's Talk About Smoking" are based on social influence approaches, the former involving parodies of cigarette advertisements and the use of a pledging procedure, the latter teaching skills to resist peer pressure to smoke (US DHHS 1986a). Brochures have also been aimed at smoking in the context of the family (*Children and Smoking: Message to Parents* (AHA 1987)).

In 1964, a National Conference on Cigarette Smoking and Youth was held under the auspices of ACS. Forty-four national organizations with a mission concerning young people participated. ACS developed numerous antismoking PSAs with prevention messages, including a 1967 television spot focused on the influence of parental smoking on children's acquisition of smoking. Other early campaigns used popular cartoon and children's story characters such as "The Three Little Pigs" to convey antismoking messages.

ACS has developed a series of health and smoking prevention programs for students in kindergarten through the intermediate grades. "An Early Start to Good Health," "ACS Health Network," "Healthy Decisions," and "Health Myself" are among the most widely disseminated ACS youth health education programs (US DHHS 1986a). The last of these programs, geared to students in the intermediate grades, emphasizes the role of societal influences on smoking. Referred to earlier in this Section, ACS has also developed teen cessation programs (ACS 1980, 1986).

In 1987, ACS, AHA, and ALA began a collaborative campaign for a "Tobacco-Free America." The project involves multiple goals and strategies, including smoke-free schools, mass media and advertising campaigns, a smoke-free class of 2000 promotion, and legislative initiatives (Bailey 1987). State-level coalitions of the three voluntary organizations also have developed programs of their own in support of this effort (US DHHS 1986a).

The prevention program efforts of the voluntary associations were fairly quick responses to the accumulating data on the health risks of smoking. Their materials have used several channels of potential influence on young people's smoking, primarily including family, media, and the school system. Compared with other prevention approaches, the family and parental influences have been emphasized—specifically, the influence of parental smoking on the initiation of smoking by children. Antismoking messages in the context of the family thus could have both prevention and cessation effects; parental nonsmoking was advocated as a powerful preventive influence. Wide distribution of materials was possible. The comprehensive school health education curricula were evaluated while the other programs incorporated only limited evaluation. The extent of actual utilization and impact of the specific distributed materials is not known.

National Interagency Council on Smoking and Health

The National Interagency Council on Smoking and Health, created shortly after the first Surgeon General's Report, fostered the early development of a variety of innovative smoking prevention programs, many of which went on to receive continued major support from other Federal agencies. The "Youth Leadership in Smoking Controls Program," begun in 1976 with funds from CDC and renewed through 1979, was not intended as a study of adolescent smoking education programs per se. Rather, its primary goal was "to identify new approaches for involving youth in smoking control activities" (National Interagency Council on Smoking and Health 1979, p. 12.). Anticipating later prevention programs' orientation to the psychosocial factors affecting youth smoking, the program required that projects "show sensitivity to the needs, lifestyles and feelings of the 12–18-year-old adolescent," and involve youth in the design and delivery of the material (p. 12). Thirteen smoking prevention projects were supported through these contract funds, none receiving more than 10,000 dollars in any one award. Extent of program evaluation varied greatly. Projects resulting from this program were described in the program's final report (National Interagency Council on Smoking and Health 1979) and in *Cookbook for a Smokeless Diet*, a humorous manual written for teachers and community members (National Interagency Council on Smoking and Health 1977). (See next section for further discussion of the National Interagency Council.)

Federal Government Prevention Support

The late 1970s were a key time for Federal Government involvement in and funding of prevention programs. Until that time, federally funded research emphasized biomedical mechanisms of smoking-related disease, as opposed to research on smoking behavior and interventions to reduce its prevalence (Bell and Levy 1984). Secretary of Health, Education, and Welfare Joseph A. Califano's 1978 initiative to combat smoking led to appropriations for Federal agencies to support biobehavioral research into the factors affecting smoking and for the development of prevention and cessation programs (Bell and Levy 1984). Each of the Federal agencies developed initiatives for such research.

Depending on the agency, smoking was the sole behavior targeted or, in other cases, one of a set of behaviors the agency sought to prevent. For instance, the National Institute on Drug Abuse (NIDA) was concerned with substance use more broadly, NHLBI with cardiovascular risk factors. The agencies within the Department of Health and Human Services (successor to the Department of Health, Education, and Welfare (DHEW)) with initiatives most directly bearing on the prevention of tobacco use among children and adolescents included NCI, the National Institute for Child Health and Human Development (NICHD), NIDA, NHLBI, and CDC. In addition, OSH (Bell and Levy 1984) (OSH is now part of CDC) developed such initiatives. Federal health agency and OSH prevention initiatives included both research support leading to the development of prevention programs and the production of prevention resources and programs for direct use by schools and other organizations. In addition, guides of existing resources are periodically produced by Federal agencies, including *Smoking Programs for Youth* (US DHHS 1980a) and *Smokescreen: Guidelines for Helping Teenagers Become Nonsmokers* (American Institutes for Research 1980), contracted by CDC.

Office on Smoking and Health

The U.S. Public Health Service first officially became engaged in an appraisal of the available data on smoking and health in June 1956 when, under the direction of Surgeon General Leroy Burney, a scientific study group was established (Burney 1959). In 1957, the Public Health Service adopted the position that "excessive smoking is one of the causative factors in lung cancer" (Burney 1959). In 1964, DHEW became actively involved in efforts to discourage smoking.

The seminal smoking-and-health event in this evolution of Federal involvement was the 1964 release of the Surgeon General's Report on Smoking and Health. At that time, Surgeon General Luther Terry established an office within the Public Health Service Chronic Disease Control Program (US DHHS 1986a) to help collect, organize, and analyze information on smoking and health. This office later became the National Clearinghouse for Smoking and Health and still later (March 1978), OSH. (See Chapter 7.)

In the early years of the Clearinghouse, a number of innovative smoking control initiatives were supported, some of which are continued today by CDC, Center for Chronic Disease Prevention and Health Promotion (which now includes OSH), and by the Department of Education (US DHHS 1986a). Initially, the Clearinghouse developed curricula and teaching materials to educate young people about the hazards of tobacco use (US DHHS 1986a). Many of these materials are now being used in schools across the country. The Clearinghouse pioneered an effort to place PSAs in high school newspapers. It was also involved with mass distribution of pamphlets, program materials, and television PSAs. Between 1966 and 1971, the Clearinghouse conducted the first study of a communitywide smoking control intervention in San Diego County, CA (US DHEW 1976). This project involved interventions aimed at schoolchildren, health professionals, and adult smokers.

The San Diego project developed curriculum guides for students in grades 1 through 12, as well as newsletters to support the efforts of teachers and other health professionals involved in the project. A "Youth-to-Youth" program, precursor to peer-led programs, was also included. Although evaluation of the project was limited, the data collected suggested that the intervention had been successful. Survey results show significant reductions between 1966 and 1975 in the percentage of teenage and adult smokers in San Diego compared with national samples (US DHEW 1976). The programs of the San Diego Community Laboratory led to the development of other comprehensive health curriculum projects such as the School Health Curriculum Project.

Today, OSH continues its efforts for smoking prevention through the development and distribution of educational materials. It currently has a program of disseminating print PSAs through high school and college newspapers, as well as televised PSAs aimed at teenagers (US DHHS 1986a).

OSH has been the only Federal office devoted solely to the smoking issue. Now part of CDC, the Office continues to perform the same functions that were established for the Clearinghouse in the 1960s (US DHHS 1986a). OSH continues to serve as a repository for information on smoking and health and responds to thousands of public inquiries for information each year. As part of its technical information service, it publishes a bimonthly bulletin of abstracts of published literature on smoking and health and periodically compiles a directory of ongoing research in smoking and health. OSH also periodically conducts surveys to estimate the prevalence of tobacco use among adults and adolescents and to determine the Nation's attitudes, knowledge, and beliefs concerning smoking, tobacco use, and their health effects. OSH continues to plan, coordinate, and produce public and professional information and education programs on smoking and health that are distributed either directly or through other institutions such as voluntary health organizations and State and local health departments. It is the responsibility of OSH to prepare and disseminate the annual Surgeon General's Report to Congress on the Health Consequences of Smoking, as required by Federal law (Public Law 91-222). Finally, OSH has new responsibilities under the Comprehensive Smoking Education Act of 1984 (Public Law 98-474) to collect information from the cigarette industry on cigarette additives, to transmit to Congress a biennial status report on smoking and health (US DHHS 1986a), and to provide staff support to the newly created Federal Interagency Committee on Smoking and Health (see Chapter 7).

National Cancer Institute

In the 1950s, scientists working at the NCI were among those who helped identify cigarettes as a cause of illness and premature death (Burney 1959). In 1955, NCI, in cooperation with the U.S. Bureau of the Census, sponsored the first large-scale national survey of smoking patterns in the United States (Burney 1959). It was not until 1968, however, with the appointment of the Lung Cancer Task Force, that NCI established a formal research program to address the smoking issue. The Lung Cancer Task Force and a subcommittee of the Task Force, the Tobacco Working Group, established three objectives for the program: (1) production of a less hazardous cigarette, (2) identification of persons at increased risk of tobacco-related disease, and (3) development of pharmaceutical interventions to control smoking behavior. Development of a less hazardous cigarette was given a high priority until 1978, when this aspect of the program was abandoned.

Prior to 1977, NCI funded little research on behavioral interventions for smoking. A major shift occurred in 1980, when prevention was identified as an NCI priority (NCI 1984). In 1982, NCI reorganized its smoking research program, establishing the Smoking, Tobacco, and Cancer Program (STCP) within the Division of Cancer Control (Cullen 1986; Cullen, McKenna, Massey 1986; Glynn, in press). Included in STCP funding was research to prevent adolescent tobacco use. In fiscal year 1985, STCP funded 14 grants on adolescent tobacco use and its prevention, with budgets totaling over 5.5 million dollars for the year. The studies were designed to include approximately 170,000 students in grades 6 through 12 (NCI 1984, 1986a). Twenty-three adolescent smoking intervention trials, involving approximately 1 million youth, were under way by early 1988 (Glynn, in press). In response to increased use of smokeless tobacco among young males in the 1970s and 1980s (US DHHS 1986c), NCI also took the lead in funding smokeless tobacco prevention programs. Seven of the 23 NCI-funded trials focus on the prevention of adolescent use of smokeless tobacco.

The prevention and control of smoking and other forms of tobacco use have become top priorities for cancer prevention within NCI (Fanning 1988). In 1987, 80 percent of the 37 million dollars spent on smoking research was allocated to studies of smoking behavior. Smoking research accounted for approximately 2.7 percent of NCI's total budget in 1987.

After funding intensive research for several years in the development and evaluation of smoking prevention programs, NCI has begun to emphasize the need for widespread dissemination of these and other smoking intervention programs (NCI 1986b) and has so far funded two new studies of the integration of tobacco education in the schools.

National Heart, Lung, and Blood Institute

NHLBI began funding smoking prevention efforts in 1974 through the Vermont Lung Center; NHLBI had received an expanded mandate (for research on the prevention of behavioral risk factors) legislated by the National Heart, Blood Vessel, Lung and Blood Act of 1972. Continuing through 1983, the Vermont Lung Center's activities included a smoking prevention program aimed at youth aged 10 to 15 years (Stone 1985).

During the mid-1970s, NHLBI supported the paradigm-setting work of Evans and his colleagues in the development of socially and psychologically based prevention programs (Evans 1976; Evans et al. 1981), and the development of the peer-taught smoking and substance abuse prevention program of McAlister and colleagues (McAlister et al. 1980; Stone 1985). The majority of the smoking prevention programs sponsored by NHLBI in the years to follow were part of more comprehensive, and often communitywide, approaches to cardiovascular risk reduction. In the early 1980s NHLBI was sponsoring 15 school-based cardiovascular risk studies, 10 with explicit smoking prevention components—in all but 2 of the 10 studies, other risk factors such as nutrition and physical activity were also targeted (Stone 1985).

National Institute on Drug Abuse

In the mid-1970s, NIDA addressed the behavioral factors of cigarette smoking and the addictive properties of nicotine by supporting research and issuing a series of monographs on cigarette smoking by Jarvik and colleagues (1977) and Krasnegor (1979a,b). In addition to sponsoring research on nicotine dependence and treatment in their own right, NIDA has approached cigarette smoking as another form of substance abuse and as a possible "gateway drug" that could lead to the use of other substances (US DHHS 1986a). The new smoking prevention programs were used as a prototype for the prevention of other forms of substance abuse (Bell and Battjes 1985).

National Institute for Child Health and Human Development

NICHD began funding of research on smoking and health in the early seventies. During the mid-1970s, this effort was intensified as part of a program initiated by Secretary of Health, Education, and Welfare Joseph A. Califano. At that time the Institute identified two primary research areas: (1) factors related to risk-taking behavior by children and the initiation of smoking, and (2) the effect of maternal smoking on the developing fetus. Emphasis on these two areas continues to the present. NICHD is working with the American College of Obstetricians and Gynecologists to develop a smoking cessation program for pregnant women,to be used in private obstetricians' practices.

Office of Disease Prevention and Health Promotion

The Office of Disease Prevention and Health Promotion (ODPHP) coordinates all prevention activities in the Public Health Service. ODPHP has sponsored evaluation of school health curricula's effects on smoking behavior (US DHHS 1986a) and supported a national survey of 8th and 10th graders' health knowledge, attitudes, and practices, including their smoking behaviors (US DHHS, in press; see Chapter 5).

Surgeon General's Reports

The Surgeon General's Reports and the media coverage surrounding them are among the primary ways that the Federal Government informs the public about the health consequences of tobacco use. The themes, emphases, and detailed reviews of these reports reflect the knowledge and interests of a large group of scientists in the United States and abroad. (Chapter 1 provides a list of the major topics covered in each of the Surgeon General's Reports since 1964.)

While not including a description of or specific recommendations for prevention programs, a section entitled "Taking Up Smoking" was included in the 1964 Report's Chapter entitled "Psychosocial Aspects of Smoking." The changing relationship of the child's smoking to parental and peer smoking as the child grows older was noted in the 1964 Surgeon General's Report: "As children grow older, they themselves, as well as their relationship to the home, change. With approaching adulthood and its associated new social patterns, other influences supplant those of the parents" (US PHS 1964, p. 369). As a further indication of prevention programs' roots in a stage approach to smoking acquisition, the 1964 Report continued, "It is quite possible that parents' influence affects the age at which children start smoking much more than it affects the ultimate taking or not taking up of the habit" (p. 370). (See Chapter 5 regarding determinants of smoking behavior.)

Consideration of young people and smoking in the Surgeon General's Reports after 1964 was initially restricted to documenting the extent of health effects among young smokers. Then in the 1977–78 Report, under the heading "Implications for Action," it was concluded that "dissuading young nonsmokers from starting to smoke" would result in the "greatest long-term benefits" compared with modifying the content of cigarettes or getting adult smokers to quit (US DHEW 1978, pp. 48–49). As for specific prevention approaches, the Report concluded that "health education of the young" was one of several antismoking efforts affected by "lack of knowledge on smoking behavior ...Although much is known about some of the principles contributing to effective health education of the young, these have not yet been incorporated into programmes, which could provide convincing evidence of their ability to reduce smoking" (US DHEW 1978, p. 54).

The 1979 Surgeon General's Report was a watershed for smoking prevention, as well as other smoking issues. Two chapters were devoted exclusively to smoking among young people and its prevention, Chapter 17 ("Smoking in Children and Adolescents: Psychosocial Determinants and Prevention Strategies") and Chapter 20 ("Youth Education") (US DHEW 1979b). In merging considerations of psychosocial smoking determinants among youth with considerations of more traditionally phrased "educational" programs, the 1979 Report reflected a critical transition in the development of prevention approaches and in their treatment in the Surgeon General's Reports. The introduction to Chapter 17 began with "It is possible that prevention programs directed at children and adolescents have generally placed too much confidence in merely communicating knowledge about the dangers of smoking" (p. 17-5). The Chapter then reviewed the range of psychosocial influences on youths' decisions to smoke, and called for including developmental and social psychological theory in the conceptual basis of prevention programs.

Demographic and psychosocial correlates of smoking among adolescents and smoking prevention approaches, with special reference to young girls and gender differences, were reviewed in the 1980 Surgeon General's Report on the health consequences of smoking for women (US DHHS 1980b). The 1981 Report on the changing cigarette (US DHHS 1981) did not consider smoking prevention per se, but briefly reviewed data on preferences among young smokers for cigarettes with various tar and nicotine levels. The natural history and prevention of smoking among adolescents were considered again in the 1982 Report on cancer (US DHHS 1982). Consensus was reached in this Report: the newly developed prevention programs based on social psychological theory were capable of a 50-percent reduction in smoking onset. The 1982 Report also included data on smoking cessation among adolescents. Prevention programs were not considered in the 1983 Report on cardiovascular disease (US DHHS 1983a), the 1985 Report on cancer and chronic lung disease in the workplace (US DHHS 1985a), or, with the exception of its review of nonsmoking policies in the schools, in the 1986 Report on involuntary smoking (US DHHS 1986b). While several smoking prevention programs were reviewed in the 1984 Report's review of community studies of smoking control, it was noted that, for the most part, community studies focused on smoking cessation among adults, rather than on prevention (US DHHS 1984). Most recently, the 1988 Surgeon General's Report on nicotine addiction concluded that smoking prevention should be integrated into substance abuse prevention programs for youth (US DHHS 1988), though the specific program options available were not reviewed.

State Health Departments

State health department initiatives to curb tobacco use have increased in the past decade (US DHHS 1986d). Many State health departments have established smoking education programs (US DHHS 1986a). State departments of education and departments of health often serve as clearinghouses, compiling guides to existing prevention resources (e.g., University of the State of New York 1979). Several State health departments have organized special committees to develop comprehensive smoking control plans (Coye 1988; Minnesota Department of Health 1987; US DHHS 1986a), with most focusing on prevention rather than cessation. Several of these plans are cited in Chapter 7 (Table 20). Most notable among the plans is Minnesota's, which, in addition to a broad range of other prevention program and policy components, earmarks a portion of the State cigarette excise tax to support smoking control initiatives (Minnesota Department of Health 1987).

The 1986 inventory of State and local programs (US DHHS 1986d) described prevention programs operating through 20 State departments of health, State interagency coalitions on smoking and health, and State departments of education. These prevention initiatives include a variety of approaches: implementation of existing health curricula, the development of specific new resources and guidelines, teacher training programs, promotion of resource centers, and community and parent programs. In an additional nine States, county organizations, including departments of health and interagency coalitions, were listed as undertaking specific smoking prevention projects that were most often curriculum based.

Other Organizations and Agencies

Although tobacco control is not their central mission, other institutions, agencies, and medical societies integrate smoking prevention programs into materials for distribution through schools and other settings. The program materials include the March of Dimes' for (often) young, expectant mothers; National Institute on Alcohol Abuse and Alcoholism materials on substance abuse (US DHHS 1986a); and the American Dental Association materials on tobacco use, especially the use of smokeless tobacco and oral disease.

Through their professional organizations and as individuals, physicians and other health researchers have designed materials and presentations, primarily for school assemblies. The American Medical Association (AMA) (1987), the American Medical Women's Association, and Doctors Ought to Care (DOC) are among those organizations that have designed smoking prevention materials and currently promote their delivery through school assemblies. Volunteers for Health Awareness, a society of health researchers and health care providers in the Boston area, have delivered antismoking assemblies to junior high school students each year since 1969 (Reif 1976; US DHEW 1979b).

In collaboration with ALA and researchers at Lawrence Hall of Science at the University of California, Berkeley, the American Nonsmokers' Rights Foundation (formerly California Nonsmokers' Rights Foundation) has also developed smoking prevention curricula centered around a television documentary, "Death in the West" (Bailey 1985) and a film entitled "Second Hand Smoke" (American Nonsmokers' Rights Foundation 1986). Addiction and tobacco industry tactics are highlighted in the curricula (California Nonsmokers' Rights Foundation 1983). The foundation has also developed an adjunct peer-led program called "Teens as Teachers" to complement use of the films.

By 1979, it was estimated that there were thousands of smoking prevention activities independently undertaken by schools and community groups, programs largely neither formally described nor evaluated (Evans et al. 1979; US DHEW 1979b). While there is increasing documentation of programs on the national and State level (US DHHS 1986a, 1986b), program development and implementation by schools and communities, as special events or as part of existing health education curricula, are far less likely to be systematically recorded and evaluated.

Problems in Dissemination of Smoking Prevention Programs

Evaluation of the development and progress of prevention programs must include both controlled, scientific examination of program efficacy and study of the factors characterizing actual and potential widespread use of programs and their public health impact. This represents a merger of perspectives only recently formally considered in the field of smoking prevention programs (NCI 1986b; Best et al. 1988; Cleary et al. 1988; Flay 1985b).

The current state of smoking prevention programs and resources reveals a gap between these two approaches. The research-driven smoking prevention curricula have most often been developed without a mechanism for widespread application and use. In turn, many of the materials likely to be used in the field by public health professionals, educators, and other policymakers responsible for young people's health have had limited evaluation, except for the comprehensive health education curricula, and the extent and process of their dissemination have generally not been systematically documented.

Once research-based programs are developed and initially found to have potential impact, there have not typically been mechanisms to encourage their active distribution to school systems and other organizations. Most at best can only respond to specific requests for information about their program or dissemination of their materials. Recognizing this research gap, NCI (1986b) has initiated research to determine the most effective method to integrate tobacco education programs that have been proven to be efficacious into school programs. It is encouraging research that is focused more on application and dissemination than on the development of new curricula and interventions.

Some of the issues bearing on program dissemination are reviewed in the smoking prevention literature (Best et al. 1988; Cleary et al. 1988); others are considered in broader literature on health education, program adoption, and the diffusion of innovation (Basch, Eveland, Portnoy 1986; Basch and Sliepcevich 1983; Murray 1986). Barriers specific to widespread institutionalization of smoking-specific programs within schools include demands on teacher time, cost of materials for specific programs and teacher training, and the variety of competing educational and health priorities found within a school system. (See also Kolbe and Gilbert (1984) for a discussion of obstacles to school implementation and maintenance of new health education programs.) Ideally, the likelihood of distribution and use of prevention programs in the field should be considered throughout the course of program design and evaluation and not restricted to end-stage discussions of the feasibility of disseminating already developed and evaluated programs.

The availability of funding to bolster dissemination of existing programs has varied over time. Federal funding for implementation and demonstration of health education programs was provided by the 1979 Health Education Risk Reduction Grant Program (Kolbe and Iverson 1984). Additional funds were appropriated in 1980 for grants to deter smoking and use of alcohol by adolescents. The reorganization of such categorical grant programs into a block grant structure in 1981 resulted in a shift of Federal funds to the State level. However, the reduction of total available funds and the restructuring of the funding mechanism created competition within States for these funds and eliminated smoking-specific demonstration grants. It also made for less secure support of health education in general (Kolbe and Iverson 1984). Although a variety of organizational, social, and political factors can affect the likelihood of adoption and use of a particular prevention program, the effect of availability of funds for teacher training, purchase of materials, and even the simplest of evaluations must be considered in any analysis of the history and prospects of prevention efforts.

Dissemination mechanisms also include providing information about programs. Federally funded databases and programs with potential for aiding the dissemination of smoking prevention programs are available. The Combined Health Information Database includes information on State and local programs listed in the National Status Report on Smoking and Health (US DHHS 1986a), as well as information on programs funded under the 1979–81 smoking and alcohol grant program (US DHHS 1986a).

The NDN of the National Institute on Education includes data on extent of diffusion of evaluated and validated curricula. While health education is not its primary focus, NDN does include five comprehensive health education and substance abuse prevention programs into which smoking prevention has been integrated, including "Growing Healthy" (NDN 1988b). Other promising programs, such as "Know Your Body," are currently under review. By providing information on the programs, awarding grants to further the dissemination of selected curricula, and maintaining annual records on program dissemination among participants (NDN 1988a), NDN functions both in the active dissemination of programs and in monitoring the extent of use of various curricula nationwide.

Complementing the need to get research-derived programs into the hands of schools and other organizations, continued program evaluation is needed once they are out in the field. These data are needed to address questions concerning the applicability of programs, the extent and quality of implementation, and their effectiveness once outside of controlled research settings. Additionally, through inquiry into factors affecting actual distribution and use of programs, these evaluations could also contribute to the development of guidelines supporting effective dissemination of smoking prevention programs.

In these evaluations of the dissemination process, statistics need to go beyond data such as number of sets of program materials distributed, to include surveys of actual use and degree of implementation as well as program impact. The evaluation of two ACS elementary school health education programs, for example, included data on teacher use of materials (Pigg et al. 1985). There was considerable variation in the percentage of teachers reported to have used materials in those schools that had kits available. The ACS "Usage Report Card," a record-keeping system for use by teachers to document numbers of children exposed to the materials, was not always completed and mailed as requested, according to 75 percent of schools surveyed. Variability in extent of use and in documenting such use contributes to the difficulty of interpreting levels of implementation even when, in the case of this study, approximately 80,000 copies of the programs had been distributed to schools.

Best and colleagues (1988) have outlined research needs on the diffusion of smoking prevention programs—research the authors consider at least as vital as that evaluating effectiveness of program content. Diffusion studies, they conclude, should entail consideration of five sets of factors: planned diffusion strategies, program packaging, provider training, implementation monitoring, and costing (both cost of materials and cost-effectiveness of the program).

Problems in Evaluation of Smoking Prevention Programs

Prevention efforts within the psychosocial, more general health education, and media approaches have operated with very different goals, intended mechanisms for effect, and standards for evaluation. As reviewed above, the psychosocial influence smoking prevention curricula have been subjected to years of research development and evaluation (e.g., Best et al. 1988; Biglan and Ary 1985; Flay 1985b; McCaul and Glasgow 1985; Snow, Gilchrist, Schinke 1985). The literature contains much detail about their effects in university-administered research projects. However, far fewer data are available on the extent of their adoption and use by others in the field and on their impact when implemented in less-controlled settings (Best et al. 1988; Cleary et al. 1988). In most cases, active mechanisms for dissemination of the research products are lacking. These programs are most often not part of a system to ensure their dissemination once the typical 3- to 5-year development and evaluation phase of the research is complete. (See Prevention Section, Problems in Dissemination of Prevention Programs.)

Prevention programs based on PSAs, posters, brochures, and other curriculum resources sponsored by Federal agencies and professional and voluntary organizations have been widely distributed through the tremendous efforts of these agencies and organizations. However, their effectiveness has generally been less thoroughly evaluated than that of the psychosocial smoking prevention curricula. Reflecting the priority of using their limited resources for dissemination, the programs and their outcomes rarely receive a level of evaluation comparable to that found in the peer-reviewed research literature on smoking prevention.

Continuing methodological problems in prevention research include variations in criteria for measuring smoking outcomes in different studies, problems of attrition (Biglan et al. 1987; McAlister and Gordon 1986), limitation to white middle-class subjects (Gilchrist and Schinke 1985; Glynn in press), differences in level of analysis of effects and level of assignment to treatment or control group (Flay 1985a), and limited long-term followup.

Need for Long-Term Followup

The need for long-term perspectives and followup of the effects of smoking prevention programs has been noted in the 1979 Surgeon General's Report (US DHEW 1979b) and by Chassin and colleagues (1985), Evans (1984), and others. Prevention effects need to be maintained and monitored throughout the high school years to ensure that youth pass through this risk period without becoming smokers. Although long-term evaluation of prevention programs is frequently included in review article recommendations for future research (Biglan and Ary 1985; McAlister, Perry, Maccoby 1979), reports of 2-year or, less frequently, 3-year impact (for study subjects most often originally in junior high) constitute the most common long-term followups (Telch et al. 1982; Johnson et al. 1986; Chassin et al. 1985). A recent report by Flay, Thompson, and colleagues (1987) included results for a 6-year followup of students in the Waterloo Smoking Prevention trial. While prevention of onset of experimental smoking persisted through the end of grade 8, at the next assessment, during grade 12, no significant effect remained. Another NCI-funded smoking prevention project is currently tracing subjects through the important transition beyond high school (Murray, described in Glynn, in press).

There are data suggesting that *delay* in initiation can constitute a desirable prevention outcome: delayed onset has been found to be associated with decreased mortality (US DHHS 1986a) and increased likelihood of quit attempts and cessation during the school years (Ershler et al., in press). However, variations in age of onset considered in these studies were naturally occurring and not the result of a specific prevention program. Thus, it remains to be confirmed that program-induced delays in onset among contemporary youth have the same relationship to later smoking behavior and health outcomes as do the naturally occurring variations.

Construct Validity

Another major methodological challenge posed in the evaluation of prevention programs is the problem of construct validity (Flay 1985a; McCaul and Glasgow 1985). With even the most highly developed programs, given their use of a multiple component format, it has been difficult to determine the key elements responsible for a prevention effect. Best and colleagues (1984, 1988), among others, express the more general need to study the factors mediating program impact in order to understand what program components work for whom. Given the current gender differential in smoking prevalence among young people (Chapter 5), and the possibility of gender differences in effectiveness of intervention strategies, further attention should, for example, be given to gender differences relevant to prevention programs (Gilchrist, Schinke, Nurius, in press; Gritz, 1986).

The studies of Hops and colleagues (1986), Murray and associates (1984), Perry and colleagues (1983), and Botvin, Renick, and Baker (1983) are among efforts to pursue construct validity and develop data on the efficacy and necessity of the specific program components. Hops and colleagues (1986) focused on refusal skills training and assessment of program impact through audiotaped test situations (offers to smoke). While this study of seventh grade students did not include a sufficient number of smokers to test for program impact in preventing smoking, analysis of student responses to the test situations found that students who received a smoking prevention program involving refusal skills training took less time to respond to the taped offer to smoke, and gave longer responses than did the control subjects, thus confirming several measures of behavioral impact of the program.

The studies of Murray and associates (1984) and Perry and colleagues (1983) compared program conditions varying instructors (adult or peer) and program content (long-term health consequences, social consequences, and immediate health effects). Murray and colleagues found the short-term-influences material, both social and physiological, to be most effective in preventing onset of smoking. Delivery of short-term-influence messages material by same-age peer leaders was more effective than by adult leaders. Perry and colleagues found a similar instructor by material interaction. In this study of 10th grade students, college-age peer leaders were more effective in delivering material on social pressures; adult classroom teachers were more effective with the traditional health effects curriculum. In this study, however, no differences were found overall between the effectiveness of the different curriculum programs. The curriculum emphasizing long-term health effects was as effective as those emphasizing more immediate social and physical effects.

In their study of the impact of characteristics of program delivery of the Life Skills Training material, Botvin, Renick and Baker (1983) found that an intensive "mini-course" format had comparable preventive effects at 1 year as the same material offered one classroom session per week. By the end of the second year, however, the more intensive format had greater impact on several measures of student smoking. The addition of "booster" sessions also added to the program's effectiveness.

Failure to Reach Dropouts and Other Youth at Higher Risk for Smoking

An intrinsic limitation of school-based prevention programs includes failure to reach truants and dropouts who are at higher risk for smoking (Flay, Thompson et al. 1987; Pirie, Murray, Luepker 1988). Numerous studies have suggested that those adolescents who skip classes and have lower grades and educational aspirations are more likely to smoke (Flay et al. 1983; Johnston, O'Malley, Bachman 1987). The recent studies by Pirie, Murray, and Luepker (1988) and Flay, Thompson, and coworkers (1987) confirmed that high school dropouts are more likely to be smokers. This limitation has implications both for the effectiveness of the intervention efforts and their evaluations. The need for more attention to high-risk youth, those young people apt to smoke and, more generally, to be involved in multiple risk behaviors (e.g., other forms of substance use, early sexual activity, and pregnancy) is particularly acute. Groups of youth who are at especially high risk of smoking are likely to receive more attention in new research (Glynn,in press), paralleling trends in the field of adult cessation, where interest has turned to heavy smokers who appeared to experience the most difficulty in smoking cessation (NCI 1984, 1986a). Gilchrist and Schinke (1985) have called attention to the need for broader strategies for high-risk youth. Sussman and colleagues (1987) have noted ethnic group differences in rates of smoking and in psychosocial predictors of smoking among seventh and eighth grade students in southern California, differences bearing on the effectiveness of various prevention strategies. (See Chapter 5.)

Differences in likelihood of smoking among subgroups of youth led Best and colleagues (1988) to raise a question of strategy for young smokers: Should efforts be focused on groups at high smoking risk, or should prevention programs seeking full population coverage be continued? The need to address high-risk youth, and in particular those from blue-collar socioeconomic backgrounds, is apparent in the face of the continuing marked differences in the likelihood of smoking among youth who drop out of school (Pirie, Murray, Luepker 1988; Flay, Thompson, et al. 1987), those who stay in high school but without plans for further education, and those who go on for postsecondary education (Johnston, O'Malley, Bachman 1987). (See Chapter 5.) Marked occupational differences in smoking prevalence further reinforce socioeconomic differences in smoking when young people enter the workplace (US DHHS 1985a).

Population Factors Related to Diversification of Smoking Prevention Programs

The evidence so far does not support the hypothesis that a single program has been or can be developed to prevent adolescent smoking across the board. Rather, successful smoking prevention may result from the aggregate of multiple types of programs and avenues of delivery, thus supporting continued diversification of program approaches. (See Glynn, in press; Perry et al. 1983.) Consideration of secular trends of smoking attitudes and behavior as well as other characteristics of the population also supports the need for program change and diversification over time.

Shifts in the effectiveness of prevention or intervention strategies may reflect as much the target population and the historical era as the inherent quality of their design. As Green and Green (1977) stated, any health education effort, any diffusion of a new program or behavior must consist of a series of "time-dependent strategies." Approaches effective with the early cohorts—for instance, the approaches that showed promise in influencing the first cohorts of young people to avoid smoking—may not be effective with later cohorts or with the remainder of the first cohort that was not affected by the initial intervention. Flay (1987a,b), for example, with regard to media-based adult smoking cessation programs, suggested that there are differential potentials for program impact as the level of knowledge about the health risks of smoking changes. Best and associates (1988) and Chassin and others (1987) have also considered the changes in optimal prevention target populations that can occur with either differential prior program impact or changes in secular trends in knowledge and behavior.

The effectiveness of different prevention programs has also been influenced historically by the social and demographic shifts of age and gender in smoking among young people that occurred over the last 25 years (Chapter 5). The young smokers of the early 1960s started at more advanced ages than contemporary youth; smoking was more prevalent among males than females. In the mid-1970s through the 1980s, the rate of smoking by girls first matched and then exceeded the rapidly declining rate of smoking by boys. (See Chapter 5). Many schools used to grant students smoking privileges. Now schools have revoked or seem increasingly likely to revoke student smoking privileges and to strengthen and enforce existing nonsmoking policies. Society, as a whole, is in a new period of increased disapproval and regulation of smoking (Chapters 4 and 7).

The relationship between these larger social trends in smoking behavior and attitudes and the impact of prevention programs on the prevalence of smoking by youth should also be considered. The increasing social disapproval of smoking by both adults and young people (Johnston, O'Malley, Bachman 1987) may reinforce prevention program effects. Prevention programs implemented during the time when smoking behavior was increasing among youth were swimming against the secular stream of increasing pressures and examples to smoke; later programs could, on the other hand, benefit from the growing attitudinal and behavioral momentum against smoking. Moskowitz (1983, p. 239) observed that "The current social climate regarding cigarette smoking may be essential to the success of recent programs in preventing cigarette smoking." In contrast, the generally unsuccessful smoking prevention programs of the 1950s, 1960s, and early 1970s were conducted during a period of increasing acceptance of smoking by youth, the creation of new school-sanctioned smoking privileges, and rising rates of smoking by young females. The prevalence of smoking by American youth did not begin to decrease until the mid- to late 1970s, precisely the time that research on the more successful social influence curricula began (Evans 1976). The sharpest decrease in the smoking prevalence among youth occurred during the late 1970s.

As presented in Chapter 5, the rate of smoking among high school seniors failed to decline in the 1980s. Should this plateau of smoking prevalence by high school seniors persist, further shifts in prevention approaches may be needed. This could include changes in the content balance of program and policy approaches and in increased efforts to ensure wider dissemination of existing programs. More broadly, it highlights the need for continued adjustment of prevention strategies and the importance of diversified approaches upon which to draw.

PART II. SMOKING EDUCATION AND CESSATION ACTIVITIES

Changes in Cessation Activities Over Time

As medical research has increasingly related smoking to disease, efforts to aid smoking cessation have proliferated. Organized efforts to assist smokers in stopping actually began in the late 1950s with the "Five-Day Plan to Stop Smoking," developed by the Seventh Day Adventist Church (McFarland 1986). This program emphasized both the physical and psychological aspects of addiction to cigarettes. Components of the Five-Day Plan, such as a buddy system, a public pledge to stop smoking, increased physical activity, and changes in diet, are important elements of many of today's cessation programs.

Smoking cessation treatments have been available since before 1900 (Dillow 1981). Many different methods have been advocated as effective treatments for stopping smoking. These have included drug treatments such as amphetamines, tranquilizers, lobeline, and nicotine gum, hypnosis, acupuncture, professional counseling, aversive conditioning procedures such as rapid smoking and satiation smoking, and a wide range of behavioral self-management strategies. Different types of treatments have been emphasized during different time periods: conditioning-based approaches were emphasized in the 1960s, cognitively based self-management procedures were emphasized in the 1970s, and relapse prevention and pharmacologic interventions were emphasized in the 1980s. The new generation of strategies concerned with relapse prevention focus attention on weight gain, high-risk situations, and cognitive and behavioral coping behaviors.

While the emphasis given to different cessation treatments has varied over time and certain relapse prevention strategies and pharmacologic approaches have been added, other specific methods for helping people stop smoking have not changed much over the past 25 years (Schwartz 1969, 1987; Schwartz and Rider 1978). The packaging and marketing of cessation aids and services have become more sophisticated, with increasing emphasis on tailoring approaches to special groups (e.g., worksites, pregnant women, and black and Hispanic smokers).

In addition, the last decade has seen a rapid increase in the accessibility of smoking intervention activities in community channels such as physicians' offices, worksites, and the media (Ockene 1987). This increasing availability of activities in the smoker's natural setting has in large part been a response to smoking as a public health issue and the recognition that about 90 percent of former smokers report stopping without the use of a special program (Fiore et al. 1988).

Smoking cessation researchers have long recognized smoking to be a complex behavior influenced by physiological, psychological, cognitive, and social factors. (See Chapter 5.) In recent years there has been a trend toward combining elements of different cessation methods into programs that respond to the multifactorial nature of smoking (Pechacek 1979; Schwartz 1987; US DHHS 1988). Research on multicomponent cessation programs has been encouraging, generally producing the best results, although evidence suggests that even with such methods the majority of smokers return to smoking within 1 year (Schwartz 1987; US DHHS 1988). In general, most cessation treatments yield 1-year quit rates (based on all original participants) between 10 and 40 percent (Danaher 1980; Glasgow and Lichtenstein 1987; Schwartz 1987; US DHHS 1986a; US DHHS 1988). Variation in cessation rates among treatment methods is probably due more to differences in smoker selection of the various programs than to the treatment methods themselves (Schwartz 1987). (Table 1 provides a summary of 6- and 12-month outcomes for different cessation methods.)

Over the decades, studies of long-term outcomes in smoking cessation programs have consistently demonstrated that abstinence maintenance rates fall as time passes, making maintenance procedures an important adjunct to cessation (Hunt and Bespalec 1973; Lichtenstein and Danaher 1976; US DHHS 1986a). Thus, more recent smoking cessation research has focused on ways to prevent relapse and facilitate abstinence maintenance (Hall, Rugg et al. 1984; Lichtenstein and Brown 1983; Marlatt and Gordon 1985). Relapse prevention strategies have included: (1) efforts to teach smokers how to recognize cues to smoke and use behavioral strategies for dealing with urges to smoke (Hall, Rugg et al. 1984; Emmons et al. 1988); (2) interventions to enhance support for not smoking (e.g., extra group sessions, telephone contacts, use of spouses and

TABLE 1.—Summary of followup quit rates (percentages) of 416 smoking cessation trials, by method, reported 1959–85

Intervention method	Quit rate (at least 6-mo followup)				Quit rate (at least 1-yr followup)			
	Number of trials	Range	Median[a]	Percent 33%[b]	Number of trials	Range	Median[a]	Percent 33%[b]
Self-help	11	0–33	17	18	7	12–33	18	14
Educational	7	13–50	36	71	12	15–55	25	25
Five-day plan	4	11–23	15	0	14	16–40	26	21
Group[c]	15	0–54	24	20	31	5–71	28	39
Medication	7	0–47	18	14	12	6–50	18.5	17
Nicotine chewing gum	3	17–33	23	33	9	8–38	11	11
Nicotine chewing gum and behavioral treatment or therapy	3	23–50	35	67	11	12–49	29	36
Hypnosis, individual	11	0–60	25	36	8	13–68	19.5	38
Hypnosis, group	10	8–68	34	50	2	14–88		50
Acupuncture	7	5–61	18	29	6	8–32	27	0
Physician advice or counseling	3	5–12	5	0	12	3–13	6	0
Physician intervention, more than counseling	3	23–40	29	33	10	13–38	22.5	20
Physician intervention, pulmonary patients	10	10–51	24	20	6	25–76	31.5	50

TABLE 1.—Continued

Intervention method	Quit rate (at least 6-mo followup)				Quit rate (at least 1-yr followup)			
	Number of trials	Range	Median[a]	Percent 33%[b]	Number of trials	Range	Median[a]	Percent 33%[b]
Physician intervention, cardiac patients	5	21–69	44	80	16	11–73	43	63
Risk factor					7	12–46	31	43
Rapid smoking	12	7–62	25.5	33	6	6–40	21	17
Rapid smoking and other procedures	21	8–67	38	57	10	7–52	30.5	50
Satiation smoking[d]	11	14–76	38	64	12	18–63	34.5	58
Regular-paced aversive smoking[d]	13	0–56	29	31	3	20–39	26	33
Nicotine fading[d]	7	26–46	27	29	16	7–46	25	44
Contingency contracting[d]	9	25–76	46	89	4	14–38	27	25
Multiple programs[d]	13	18–52	32	38	17	6–76	40	65

NOTE: Quit rates provided suggest overall trends. Most quit rates were based on self-reports. Some quit rates were recalculated to include all subjects, but most quit rates were based on reports by investigators. Some quit rates omitted subjects who did not complete treatment or persons who did not reply to followups. Definitions of followup may vary between trials.

[a]Median not calculated for fewer than three trials.

[b]Percentage of trials with quit rates of at least 33 percent.

[c]Three group trials had 5-month followups.

[d]Other procedures may have been used, and some trials may be included in more than one method.

SOURCE: Schwartz (1987).

coworkers) (Lichtenstein, Glasgow, Abrams 1986; Ockene et al. 1982); and (3) cognitive interventions to facilitate changes in self-perception, attitudes, and cognitions (Lichtenstein and Brown 1983; Marlatt and Gordon 1985). In general, findings in studies using relapse prevention strategies as part of a cessation program have been inconsistent (US DHHS 1986a).

Providers and researchers also have become more responsive to the idea that smoking cessation involves a process of change rather than a discrete act. (See Chapter 5 for a discussion of stages of cessation.) The process of cessation has been characterized, for example, as occurring in four stages: precontemplation, contemplation, action, and maintenance or relapse (Prochaska and DiClemente 1983). The stage model of cessation posits that separate influences are at play at different stages and that differing interventions may need to be tailored to these stages of smoking behavior change. This stage approach to cessation intervention has evolved over the last decade and is still in an early phase of development with no data available to test its effect.

Although the number and sophistication of cessation programs have grown over the past several decades, this does not fully account for the decreasing rate of smoking, because about 90 percent of former smokers report stopping without the benefit of any program or device (Fiore et al. 1988). During this same period, a separate but related development can be traced: the growing recognition of smoking as a socially mediated practice susceptible to change in its social environment (Bailey 1986; Iglehart 1986; Nuehring and Markle 1974; Slade 1985; Warner 1986a). Although most health agencies continue to sponsor programs to assist individual smokers in stopping, these organizations also are increasingly advocating policies addressing the environmental factors that support or discourage smoking (e.g., smoking control regulations) (ACS 1976, 1978; Blum 1986; US DOD 1986, 1987; Lundberg 1985; Lundberg and Knoll 1986; Warner et al. 1986; Whelan 1984; see Chapter 7).

As noted above, the evaluation of cessation programs and techniques has been adequately covered in numerous past and recent reviews and is not the subject of this Section. (For recent extensive reviews of cessation activities, see reviews by Schwartz (1987) or US DHHS (1986a).) The remainder of this review will be devoted to a historical perspective of the efforts of the many diverse groups involved in promoting cessation activities.

National Voluntary Health Organizations

The three major national voluntary health organizations, ACS, ALA, and AHA, have played an important role over the last 25 years in disseminating information about the hazards of smoking and in providing assistance to those who want to stop. Introduced in Part I, these efforts have included such interventions as the production and distribution of print and broadcast materials, including pamphlets, posters, and television and radio public service advertising; public educational programs; direct provision of services to smokers who want to stop smoking, including self-help materials and clinics; and training and materials for such intermediaries as educators and health care providers who influence smokers to stop. While the resources devoted to the antismoking effort have varied over time and among agencies, it was estimated that the sum total of financial resources available from the major voluntary organizations has never exceeded 1 or 2 percent of tobacco industry expenditures for the promotion of cigarettes (ACS 1978). It is also true that these voluntary agencies receive support in the form of donated public service time and space and contributed effort. However, even with this support, the level of resources devoted to antismoking efforts represents a small fraction of tobacco industry expenditures to promote smoking.

In 1965, ACS initiated its "The Time to Stop Is Now" campaign based on recent epidemiologic studies showing that smokers can ameliorate the ill effects of cigarettes by quitting. ACS followed this with a series of television commercial campaigns focusing on the negative aspects of smoking. In 1968, ACS issued a posthumous PSA featuring television actor William Talman, a smoker who died of lung cancer. At the same time, ACS was producing films (one nominated for an Academy Award) and pamphlets providing advice on quitting (Patterson 1987) and was initiating a small-group public education campaign that by the late 1980s had reached more than 60 million people.

In 1964, AHA issued the pamphlet *Where There's Smoke There's Danger from Heart Disease* and in 1966 distributed to affiliates a kit containing broadcast media materials, posters, pamphlets, and newspaper features. In 1967 and 1968, AHA issued television spots highlighting nonhealth advantages of not smoking (e.g., saving money, no bad breath). In 1968, AHA produced the film "Smoking and Heart Disease" and in 1969 issued the pamphlet *How to Stop Smoking*, which was its first effort to develop material to assist smokers in stopping. Since then, AHA has produced other pamphlets and films; however, a primary focus of its smoking control efforts has been prevention of smoking by youth.

ALA, in 1965, produced a public education campaign against smoking, "New Viewpoint on Smoking," based on the 1964 Surgeon General's Report. ALA again produced significant public education antismoking materials in the late 1960s, when the Federal Communications Commission (FCC) ruled that broadcasters must present antismoking public service messages to balance prosmoking advertisements (Patterson 1987). As part of this campaign, ALA produced two pamphlets, *Me Quit Smoking? Why?* and *Me Quit Smoking? How?* These booklets present the health effects of smoking and describe cigarette use as a socially learned behavior to be broken either through quitting cold turkey or by gradual withdrawal.

As noted in the previous section, in 1964 the major national voluntary and Government agencies had joined to form the National Interagency Council on Smoking and Health to coordinate antismoking activities. In general, the voluntary organizations during the late 1960s and the 1970s stressed the public health education approach to disease control rather than the legislative approach.

In 1967, attorney John Banzhaf obtained a ruling from the FCC applying the Fairness Doctrine to cigarette advertising and requiring broadcasters to provide a significant amount of time to antismoking messages to balance the prosmoking message of cigarette advertisements (Patterson 1987). In 1968, Banzhaf formed a new organization, Action on Smoking and Health (ASH), with the immediate goal of legally defending application of the FCC Doctrine to cigarettes and monitoring broadcaster compliance. (See Section on Advocacy, this Chapter).

The FCC's ruling was ultimately upheld by the Supreme Court in 1969. Beginning in mid-1967, the ruling opened the airwaves to an unprecedented barrage of antismoking messages produced by the major national voluntary agencies (Warner 1986). At its peak in 1970, the donated television and radio time constituted a subsidy of approximately 200 million dollars (in 1985 dollars) (Warner 1986). These messages probably helped contribute to changing public opinion on smoking, not only because they provided information about its health effects, but also because their mere presence on television reflected, and may have contributed to, a normative change in attitudes toward the entire issue (Warner 1978, 1986). In 1971, cigarette advertising disappeared from broadcasting, and the frequency of antismoking messages fell dramatically (Warner 1977). (See Chapter 7.)

During the 1970s, the efforts of the voluntary agencies continued to focus on educating the public about the dangers of smoking, as exemplified by the title of a film produced by ALA in 1970: "Is It Worth Your Life?" ACS sponsored a series of programs on smoking cessation on the Public Broadcasting System and recruited actor Tony Curtis as its first national IQ (I Quit) Chairman. As early as 1964, ACS had used athletes and show business personalities in poster campaigns, both to draw attention to antismoking messages and to provide social validation of the messages. This trend continued through the 1980s.

In 1973, ALA was the first major voluntary organization to explicitly recognize the importance of fostering norms supportive of nonsmoking (ASH 1978). ALA had already begun addressing the issue of environmental tobacco smoke (ETS) in 1971 with a television public service campaign and a jingle, "Mind Very Much If They Smoke." This campaign and those that followed almost every year thereafter portrayed smoking as antisocial behavior and were intended both to inform smokers that their behavior offended others and to reinforce nonsmokers' rights to object to ETS.

In addressing the ETS issue, ALA had an advantage over ACS and AHA, whose activities were restricted by their mandates to control cancer and cardiovascular disease, which in the early 1970s had not yet been related to ETS. The 1972 Surgeon General's Report, the first to review the evidence that ETS harms nonsmokers, provided ALA with sufficient justification to initiate action (US DHEW 1972). In 1973, ALA established protection of nonsmokers as a major program priority and in 1975 became the first major agency to retain a full-time staff member dedicated to promoting smoking restrictions.

The nonsmokers' rights movement continued to build through the 1970s (see next section on advocacy and Chapter 7), but for the most part it was a local, grassroots campaign. In a report prepared for the Tobacco Institute, the Roper Organization (1978) called this movement "the most dangerous development to the viability of the tobacco industry that has yet occurred." The movement undercut the image of smoking as a socially acceptable and even socially necessary behavior, and it motivated many more people to join in the antismoking movement out of self-interest. However, the major voluntary organizations involved in smoking activities for the most part continued to focus their efforts on a public education approach to the smoking problem.

In 1976, ACS announced a new initiative against smoking entitled "Target 5." Among other goals, it aimed to persuade 25 percent of smokers to quit and to reduce cigarette tar and nicotine levels by half (ACS 1976). Toward attaining the former goal, ACS in 1977 issued the "I Quit Kit," a sophisticated package of materials including booklets, posters, buttons, a calendar, stickers, and a phonograph record. The basic cessation techniques included: self-monitoring of smoking pattern, deliberate changes in daily routine, gradual reduction in the number of cigarettes smoked, and suggestions for nonsmoking maintenance. Two years later, ALA issued its "Freedom From Smoking"® program, similarly a handsomely packaged kit that has been experimentally evaluated (Davis, Faust, Ordentlich 1984).

The effort to educate smokers about the possible reduction in danger from low-tar and -nicotine cigarettes and to encourage the marketing of lower tar cigarettes culminated in the late 1970s when NCI scientist Dr. Gio Gori and a colleague published a paper speculating that some low-tar cigarettes, smoked in moderate amounts, might present little health risk (Gori and Lynch 1978). The voluntary and Government agencies responded with intense criticism. However, the perception existed among many smokers that some cigarettes are less hazardous than others (see Table 3, Chapter 4). This was probably related, at least in part, to efforts by the voluntary agencies and Government agencies suggesting that smokers could lower their risk with steps short of quitting (ACS 1978). This perception of the safe cigarette changed as evidence gathered that the use of lower yield cigarettes has almost no health benefit except for lung cancer (US DHHS 1981) and may even increase the health risk due to compensation (US DHHS 1988) (See Chapter 5).

In 1972, a no-smoking day was sponsored in Oklahoma by ALA and in 1974 in Minnesota by ALA, ACS, and AHA. In 1977, ACS adopted the Minnesota program and rechristened it "The Great American Smokeout" (GASO) (Smith 1977). The program can now be seen as a forerunner of contemporary programs to help smokers quit by fostering social support for cessation. A nationally publicized event held on the Thursday before Thanksgiving, GASO encourages antismoking activities in the community and provides materials to those wishing to conduct antismoking activities in places such as schools, worksites, and health care facilities.

Every year since 1978, ACS has commissioned a Gallup poll of public awareness and participation in GASO. Awareness has always been high; in 1978, 82 percent of adults polled were aware of GASO, a figure that reached 90 percent by 1987. Reported participation by smokers has grown over time also. In 1978, 6.7 percent of smokers interviewed reported abstaining from smoking on GASO day, with another 19.9 percent reporting they cut down. In the peak year, 1986, 12.8 percent reported that they did not smoke and 30.9 percent cut down (Figure 1).

Only two published studies provide data on how many people maintain cessation long term after GASO. In 1979, Dawley and Finkel (1981) followed 125 smokers at the New Orleans Veterans Administration Hospital who registered to quit on GASO day. Two months after GASO day, 66 percent reported that they had attempted to reduce or quit smoking on GASO day. Of those who attempted to stop smoking on GASO day, 13 percent (9 percent of the 125 smokers in the study) reported not smoking 2 months later. In 1984, Gritz, Carr, and Marcus (1988) followed a group of 240 smokers who

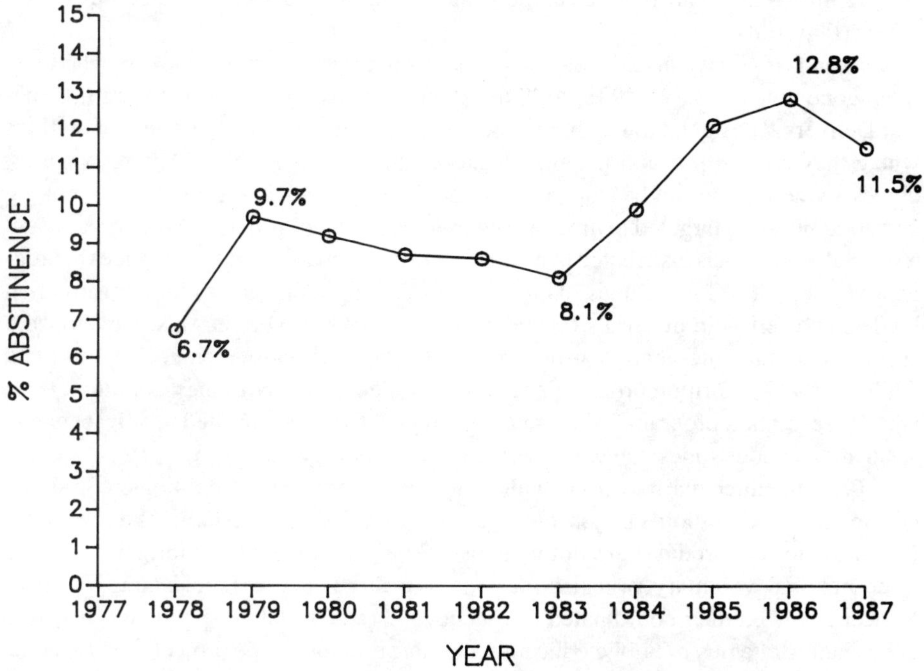

FIGURE 1.—Reported abstinence during Great American Smokeout

SOURCE: The Impact of the Great American Smokeout (1978–87), conducted by the Gallup Organization, analyzed by Lieberman Research, Inc.

pledged to quit smoking on GASO day. At 1-year followup, 25 percent reported not smoking and 13 percent had continuously quit for the entire year.

The voluntary agencies increased antismoking efforts in the early 1980s. By then, three of the five television spots ALA produced every year were antismoking messages. These, as many voluntary agency spots had done, used celebrities to call attention to the health consequences of smoking. In addition to vigorously promoting GASO, ACS released a series of attention-getting PSAs, including a simulated "Smoking Fetus" spot and Yul Brynner in a posthumous plea to smokers to quit.

Building on the nonsmokers' rights movement and the trend toward health promotion at worksites, the voluntary organizations have begun actively marketing smoking policy and cessation services to businesses. ACS, with a national policy prohibiting it from charging for any services, has been limited in its activities in this area, but both ALA and AHA have developed self-supporting intervention programs ("Freedom From Smoking® at Work" and "Heart at Work," respectively). Both include consultation on the development and implementation of smoking policies and provision of cessation clinics and self-help materials.

In 1985, ALA worked with a local television news show in Chicago to produce a stop-smoking series that aired during 4:30 p.m. or 10:00 p.m. news broadcasts (Flay 1987b). The series, based on the ALA "Freedom From Smoking"® self-help guide, has been replicated in about 10 cities in the United States and has been planned for several others (Flay 1987b).

ALA and ACS have also developed programs to target pregnant smokers who have often gone unnoticed. In 1988, ACS developed a smoking cessation program, "Special Delivery," designed to reach low-income pregnant women in a variety of settings where they receive prenatal health, education, and social services. The package includes a video, slides, and a stop-smoking book. In 1986, ALA developed a smoking cessation program targeted at pregnant women, "Freedom From Smoking for You and Your Baby," which is distributed to health care professionals providing services to pregnant women. The kit includes instructions to the provider, posters, and information leaflets and self-help materials for the pregnant woman. ALA has also developed a special smoking intervention program for the Los Angeles Women, Infants, and Children (WIC) nutrition program's Healthy Mothers, Healthy Babies Coalition. This smoking cessation program for low-income pregnant women enrolled in WIC began in 1986 and includes slides, handouts, and reminder messages.

In 1982, the three major national voluntary bodies formed the Coalition on Smoking OR Health. The Coalition's major roles are to monitor Federal legislative and regulatory issues and to support those promoting nonsmoking (see the next Section). In 1986 the three national voluntary organizations, through the Tobacco-Free Young America Project, extended their coordinated efforts beyond the legislative sphere and began to coordinate strategies in public education and information. This project developed an educational approach, referred to in the preceding section, intended to produce a tobacco-free high school graduating class in the year 2000 (US DHHS 1986a).

Health Professional Associations

Medical and public health groups have played an important leadership role in directing efforts to curtail smoking and its promotion (Lundberg 1985). In terms of their own smoking behavior, physicians and other health professionals were among the first groups to respond to the evidence relating smoking and disease. In the early 1950s, 53 percent of U.S. physicians were cigarette smokers (Garfinkel and Stellman 1986). Subsequently, smoking rates fell steadily (US DHHS 1985a), and today, 9 percent smoke (Harvey and Shubat 1987).

Although in the early years many health professionals spoke out against tobacco, many did not fully accept the epidemiologic evidence (Patterson 1987; Rosenberg 1983). Officially, the American Medical Association (AMA) and most other medical and public health groups supported the position that research was needed to deal with the cigarette problem (Patterson 1987; Rosenberg 1983). It was assumed that smokers would stop smoking if the medical evidence linking smoking and disease was sound. With regard to public education efforts, AMA and specialty groups urged their members to persuade others to cut down or give up smoking (Cohen 1978; Rosenberg 1983) but did not otherwise extensively support public education efforts. Even today, data suggest that many physicians are not advising cessation to patients who smoke (Anda et al. 1988; Ockene et al. 1987). According to a 1986 national survey of 13,031 adults aged 17 years and older, only 45 percent of smokers reported that a physician had ever advised them to stop smoking (Davis 1988b). In other studies it was determined that the presence of disease is positively related to whether physicians advised cessation (Anda et al. 1988; Ockene et al. 1987).

In 1964, AMA officially called smoking ". . .a serious health hazard" and recommended that health education programs on smoking be developed by AMA and be made available to the public through the media (Iglehart 1986; Lundberg 1985; Rosenberg 1983). However, no funds were appropriated to support the antismoking campaign. AMA opposed the addition of warning labels to cigarette packages, stating in a 1964 letter to the FTC that "The health hazards of excessive smoking have been well publicized for more than 10 years. . .they are common knowledge" (Rosenberg 1983). When warning labels were mandated by Congress in 1965, AMA reversed its position on the labeling issue. In 1969, AMA passed a resolution to discourage smoking through pronouncements and education programs (Rosenberg 1983).

In 1978, AMA published a report, *Tobacco and Health*, summarizing the results of a tobacco research program sponsored by the AMA Education and Research Foundation (AMA 1978) that included financial support from the tobacco industry. This report, which received wide media coverage, concluded that cigarette smoking was an important cause of cancer and chronic obstructive pulmonary disease and constituted a danger to persons with preexisting coronary disease. The preamble to the report stated that the findings from the project had not altered the conclusions of the 1964 Surgeon General's Report. Following issuance of the report, AMA allocated 45,000 dollars to support a public service antismoking campaign emphasizing smoking cessation and research (Rosenberg 1983).

Frustrated by the reluctance of medical organizations to take a stronger stand against smoking, a family physician, Dr. Alan Blum, in 1977 founded the organization Doctors Ought to Care (DOC), a group of health professionals who direct their attention at tobacco advertising (Blum 1979, 1980). (See Advocacy Section, this Chapter.) Other medical and public health organizations have recently taken strengthened stands against the tobacco industry.

In 1986, AMA accepted a proposal for a public awareness campaign that called for a localized public health initiative designed for implementation by local medical societies or individual physicians (Lundberg and Knoll 1986). The result of this proposal was the development of the "Physicians Leadership Kit" (AMA 1987). The kit contains information on developing smoke-free health care facilities, material to lobby legislators and other public health officials to enact antismoking laws, and information for presentation to school groups to encourage a tobacco-free lifestyle. The kit presents sample materials that have been used successfully in various locations around the country and includes camera-ready copies of materials that can be easily reproduced. A total of 3,000 kits was produced in 1987, with copies sent to 1,000 local medical societies and auxiliaries.

In addition to AMA, several other medical and public health groups have been active in promoting smoking control measures. As long ago as 1968, the American College of Chest Physicians (ACCP), in conjunction with the National Clearinghouse for Smoking and Health, cosponsored a national forum on office management of smoking problems (Soffer 1988). The proceedings of the conference were published in ACCP's official journal, *Chest* (ACCP 1968). Beginning with the convocation at the 1979 Scientific Assembly and repeated at every convocation since, new ACCP fellows pledge to make their offices and clinics centers of smoking cessation (Soffer 1980). In 1982, ACCP prepared work kits for physicians to use as teaching aids in instructing patients about the dangers of smoking and techniques for smoking cessation (ACCP 1982).

In 1987, the American Academy of Family Physicians (AAFP) developed a stop-smoking kit for use by family physicians in their offices (AAFP 1987). The kit includes a physician and office staff manual, stickers to identify the charts of patients who smoke, a smoking history form, and cessation materials for patients. The American Society of Internal Medicine has produced three antismoking kits for its members, one with material for physician offices (e.g., posters, tent cards, lapel pins), another with material for lobbying, and a third with material to stimulate media coverage on smoking and health (Davis 1988b). The American Academy of Pediatrics (AAP) is a sponsor of the Tobacco-Free Young America Project (AAP 1987). The American Dental Association (ADA) in 1987 published a pamphlet describing the hazards of smokeless tobacco use. ADA has produced similar pamphlets on smoking and oral cancer.

Available evidence indicates that physicians can have a significant impact on the smoking behavior of their patients and that cessation outcomes increase as interventions such as self-help materials, development of a cessation plan, and groups are added (Kottke et al. 1988; Ockene et al. 1988; Russell et al. 1979; Russell et al. 1983). Medical organizations such as AAFP, the American Society of Internal Medicine, and the American Medical Women's Association are therefore supporting programs at their national and regional meetings to train physicians to be more effective in helping smokers to stop smoking.

Through funding in 1984 from NCI's Smoking, Tobacco, and Cancer Program, investigators involved in physician training have demonstrated that smoking intervention training programs can have a significant impact on physician skills (e.g., Ockene et al. 1988; Wilson et al. 1988). These investigators have produced their own training packages. Other NCI-funded investigators have demonstrated the importance of office management materials that are needed to provide systematic identification of smokers, who are then given advice to stop smoking (Cohen et al. 1987; Solberg 1988). With the use of office procedures such as chart stickers and a system to monitor smokers, significantly more smokers are identified and available for physician advice. These programs indicate that physician smoking intervention skills and office practices can be improved with relatively brief training programs. Concern has been expressed, though, about the lack of coordination among the many private medical organizations and public health agencies producing materials for use by physicians to encourage smoking cessation by patients (Davis 1988b).

The contemporary efforts of medical and public health groups to curb tobacco use have recognized that smoking control efforts must not only attempt to persuade individual smokers to stop, but also must help change the social environment that supports smoking (Iglehart 1986; Lundberg and Knoll 1986; Kottke et al. 1988). This is discussed later in this Chapter.

Federal Government Cessation Support

Office on Smoking and Health

In January 1968, the National Clearinghouse for Smoking and Health worked closely with ACS and the Public Broadcasting Service (PBS) to produce the "National Smoking Test," which was aired over the CBS television network during prime time. This 1-hr program was designed to give cigarette smokers suggestions on how to stop smoking (ASH 1978).

The Clearinghouse implemented the first study of a communitywide smoking control intervention in San Diego County, CA, between 1966 and 1971 (US DHEW 1976) (see Part I). This study included interventions aimed at schoolchildren, health professionals, and adult smokers. Although evaluation of the project was limited, the data collected suggested that the intervention had been successful. Survey results showed significant reductions between 1966 and 1975 in the percentage of adult smokers in San Diego compared with those in national samples (US DHEW 1976).

The first Government antismoking poster was produced by the Clearinghouse in 1968. The poster, carrying the message "100,000 Doctors Have Quit Smoking Cigarettes. Maybe They Know Something You Don't," appeared on U.S. Post Office trucks (Davis 1988b). Between 1967 and 1971, the Clearinghouse worked with ACS, ALA, and AHA to produce antismoking messages to be aired as a result of the FCC Fairness Doctrine ruling (Patterson 1987). Over the years, OSH has planned and produced several award-winning public education and information campaigns on smoking and health (US DHHS 1986a).

National Cancer Institute: Smoking, Tobacco, and Cancer Program

As discussed in the preceding section, the primary thrust of the Smoking, Tobacco, and Cancer Program (STCP) has been to study smoking behavior and to test intervention strategies for reducing tobacco use. Research programs have been supported in the areas of adolescent smoking prevention, self-help smoking cessation, mass media approaches to smoking control, and the use of physicians and dentists as interveners, as well as in special populations including blacks, Hispanics, women, and smokeless tobacco chewers (Fanning 1988; NCI 1986a). In 1986, STCP launched a multicenter study to evaluate the impact of a communitywide intervention effort to reduce smoking prevalence, particularly among heavy smokers. Costing 42.5 million dollars over 8 years, the effort is funding 11 institutions and involves 2 million people in 22 communities in North America; 11 of these 22 communities receive support to develop and promote cessation interventions. Interventions range from communitywide approaches including mass media and environmental change to those focused on groups of individuals, such as physician counseling, worksite programs, and self-help strategies. The campaigns will be linked with the existing programs of major voluntary and civic organizations in an effort to widely disseminate intervention components (Hamm 1988; Pechacek 1988).

Although research has always been the primary mission of NCI, in the mid-1970s, it began developing broad public and professional information programs on smoking through its Office of Cancer Communications (OCC) (US DHHS 1986a). In 1977, OCC published *Clearing the Air*, a self-help smoking cessation booklet. An updated version of the booklet was produced in 1987. This booklet is among the most popular NCI publications. It has been promoted through print and television announcements produced by OSH and through the OCC supermarket distribution program. Since the booklet was first produced, approximately 7 million copies have been distributed.

In 1978, OCC, in collaboration with AAFP and ALA, produced a speaker's kit for use by physicians and local organizations to present a community-based smoking education program. The kit, entitled "Everyone Can Do Something About Smoking," consisted of a slide–tape presentation narrated by Dick Cavett, "Smoking Digest," a planner's guide, physician guidelines, *Clearing the Air*, and a community action pamphlet. It was promoted initially through AAFP and ALA chapters, which resulted in about 250 orders for the kit. In 1979, the kit was duplicated for distribution through the National Audio/Visual Center.

OCC has been active in trying to increase the involvement of health professionals in counseling patients about cessation of tobacco use (NCI 1982). In 1978, OCC produced "Helping Smokers Quit," a cessation kit for use by physicians to help their patients stop smoking. The kit emphasized the "how-to" rather than the "why" of smoking cessation and contained a physician guide, followup note, memo to the nurse, waiting room posters, and a set of materials for 50 patients (including a repackaged version of *Clearing the Air*). The kit was promoted beginning in 1978 through two national mailings of a flier to 175,000 primary care physicians, several targeted direct mailings, special activities by outside organizations, and print advertisements and editorial placements in professional journals. About 150,000 kits were distributed over a 4-year period. A qualitative assessment of the kit showed that physicians were generally positive about using the materials (NCI 1982). However, a key finding was the failure of physicians to use the followup mail piece, emphasizing the need to develop practical ways to reinforce and maintain the smoking cessation effort begun in the physician's office.

In 1979, the "Helping Smokers Quit" program for physicians was adapted for use by dentists and dental professionals (NCI 1982). The program was called "Let's Help Smokers Quit." Beginning in 1980, this program was promoted by direct mail to 137,000 dentists, 37,000 dental hygienists, and 25,000 dental assistants; by a targeted mailing to specialized dental groups; through print advertisements and editorial placements in journals; and through exhibits at dental meetings and conferences. About 50,000 kits were distributed. User evaluation of the kit in 1981 found that the majority of dentists used the kit's guidelines to counsel 25 percent or fewer of their smoking patients. Most dentists found the kit materials to be useful and practical. The waiting room posters and followup postcards were the least-used components of the kit (NCI 1982).

"Quit for Good," developed in 1982, is a combined and streamlined version of the "Helping Smokers Quit" and "Let's Help Smokers Quit" kits and is based on the evaluation results of the earlier kits (NCI 1982). It features a health professional guide, waiting room materials, and 50 sets of two patient booklets, *Quit It*, a redesigned version of *Clearing the Air*, and a new piece, *For Good*, which focuses on maintenance of nonsmoking rather than initial cessation. The "Quit for Good" kit was promoted beginning in 1984 by direct mail to 120,000 dentists, cardiologists, chest physicians, community health physicians, and black physicians, and through print advertisements, editorial mention in professional journals, and exhibits at major medical meetings. About 60,000 kits have been distributed to date. In collaboration with ACS, the kit is currently being revised in response to user feedback and an official protocol that NCI recently developed for physician stop-smoking programs.

The "Pharmacist's Helping Smokers Quit" kit program was developed in collaboration with the American Pharmaceutical Association and is similar to the physician and dentist kits (NCI 1982). The distinctive feature of this program is its focus on drug interactions in smoking. The kit contains a pharmacist's guide, counter cards, posters, and sets of take-home materials for 25 patients. In addition, OCC and the American Pharmacological Association worked with a private vendor to produce a special patient education label for containers that warn of possible adverse smoking–drug interactions. The program was launched officially in June 1986 at a national news conference at the American Pharmaceutical Association headquarters. The kit was promoted in succeeding months by direct mail to 25,000 members of the Association, a special mailing to chain drugstore owners, and print advertisements and editorial mention in pharmaceutical journals. A second wave of direct mail promotions was conducted during summer 1987 targeting the Nation's 67,000 retail and hospital pharmacies. Response to these direct mail promotions has been about 15 percent, with about 15,000 kits distributed.

In 1976, NCI established the Cancer Information Service (CIS), a toll-free telephone public inquiry system providing information about cancer (US DHHS 1986a). CIS offices are located near major cancer research centers across the United States. In addition to providing telephone assistance, CIS offers free printed materials on subjects ranging from types of cancer and treatments to smoking cessation. Many of the materials developed by OCC are distributed through the CIS network. CIS receives approximately 80,000 calls from smokers annually. In summer 1986, OCC collaborated with the NCI Division of Cancer Prevention and Control to develop a slide training program for CIS staff to help them better counsel patients who smoke on how to stop. This represented the first formal training effort for CIS staff on the topic of smoking since the service was launched.

National Heart, Lung, and Blood Institute

Like NCI, over the years, the National Heart, Lung, and Blood Institute (NHLBI) has devoted the majority of its smoking control dollars to biomedical research documenting the health hazards associated with tobacco use. Smoking has long been identified as one of the major risk factors for cardiovascular disease and the major risk factor for chronic obstructive pulmonary disease (e.g., Doyle et al. 1964; Hammond and Horn 1958; US DHHS 1983a, 1984) (See Chapter 2.). In the mid-1970s, NHLBI undertook a number of major clinical studies to evaluate whether risk factor intervention for cardiovascular disease could influence disease rates. The best known of these studies was the Multiple Risk Factor Intervention Trial (MRFIT), a randomized controlled trial to investigate the effect of reducing cardiovascular risk factors in a group of asymptomatic men at high risk for cardiovascular disease (MRFIT Research Group 1982). A total of 12,866 men were randomized into two groups, special intervention (SI) and usual care (UC), with similar baseline characteristics. Those in the SI group received an intensive intervention program aimed at facilitating cessation of smoking, reduction in serum cholesterol by dietary changes, and reduction of blood pressure levels for hypertensives. Men in the UC group received annual medical checkups but no special program to modify smoking or other risk factors. The smoking intervention consisted initially of 10 weekly group classes that included smoking intervention and individual cessation counseling by health counselors and physicians (Hughes et al. 1981). After 6 years, the SI group reduced its prevalence of smoking 18 percentage points more than the UC group.

More recently, NHLBI has supported cardiovascular risk reduction studies involving entire communities (US DHHS 1984, 1986a). Smoking control has been a prominent element of these clinical research studies. Currently, NHLBI is funding several research projects on the topic of relapse prevention and cessation interventions aimed at special patient populations (e.g., post-myocardial-infarction patients) (NHLBI 1988). In 1984, NHLBI began a multicenter study of early intervention for chronic obstructive pulmonary disease, the Lung Health Study (NHLBI 1986). The objective of this study is to determine whether or not an intervention program of vigorous smoking cessation and use of an inhaled bronchodilator can slow the decline of lung function over the course of the 5-year period of followup. Approximately 6,000 men and women aged 35 to 59 years who are at high risk for chronic obstructive pulmonary disease based on lung function level have been entered into the study. Followup for the study will be completed in 1993.

In 1985, NHLBI initiated the Smoking Education Program (SEP), modeled after the highly successful National High Blood Pressure Education Program (NHLBI 1988). This program seeks to identify and implement strategies to reach critical target audiences that can serve as intermediaries in reaching smokers. For example, health care professionals have frequent opportunities to advise smokers to quit and are therefore identified as key targets of SEP. SEP also is developing materials for use in worksites where employee health programs provide an effective means of risk-factor reduction.

NHLBI efforts to develop and disseminate information to health providers on smoking control initiatives began in 1983 with the publication of the physician guide *How To Help Your Hypertensive Patient Stop Smoking* (US DHHS 1983b). This 24-page color booklet presented four simple smoking cessation procedures that emphasize patient commitment and physician followup. The guide was disseminated through print advertisements, and over 30,000 copies were distributed.

In 1983, NHLBI produced "We Can't Go On Like This," a series of seven video vignettes developed as part of MRFIT. From 3 to 7 min long, they provide a humorous approach to the subject of helping people stop smoking permanently. Each segment of this program helps workshop participants share and express their feelings and frustrations about their decision to stop smoking (US DHHS 1986a).

In 1986, SEP produced *Clinical Opportunities for Smoking Intervention: A Guide for the Busy Physician* (US DHHS 1986e). This physician guide represented an update of the material presented in the guide for *Counseling Hypertensive Patients To Stop Smoking*. The guide describes a variety of methods for smoking intervention, including what can be done in a waiting room and what can be done during a physical exam, and how the briefest of interventions can have an impact on patients. Support material was also developed for the guide, including a slide kit that can be used as part of a medical training program to alert health professionals to methods they can use to have an impact on their smoking patients. In addition, the program distributes outreach materials, including reproducible print advertisements and guides to State and local programs designed to reduce smoking.

In 1986, SEP produced a guide for smoking policies at the worksite. This guide, *It's Your Business: Smoking Policies for the Workplace*, includes practical information about implementing smoking policies in the workplace. Facts are provided about smoking in the workplace and the effects of involuntary smoking. Short passages about companies that have successfully implemented smoking policies are included along with a resource section. SEP is continuing to plan and develop approaches to provide practical how-to information for worksites that plan to establish smoke-free or limited smoking environments. Future SEP initiatives will focus on reaching special populations, including patients with chronic heart or lung disease, minorities, and blue-collar workers (NHLBI 1988).

A joint conference on "Smoking Policies in the Workplace: Research Needs and Potential Applications" was convened in 1987 by NHLBI, and cosponsored by NCI and the Harvard Institute for the Study of Smoking Behavior and Policy. Proceedings of this conference are forthcoming in the *New York State Journal of Medicine* (Parker and Warner 1989).

Office of Disease Prevention and Health Promotion

ODPHP conducted a survey of worksite health promotion programs that included information on smoking cessation, education, and corporate policies (US DHHS 1987). It collaborated with OSH to produce "A Decision-Maker's Guide to Reducing Smoking at the Worksite" (US DHHS 1985b). Between 1984 and 1988, the Office managed the Department's "Healthy Older People" public education program, which targeted smoking cessation as one of six health promotion subjects of importance for people over 55 years of age. The U.S. Preventive Services Task Force, created and staffed by the Office, has published recommendations for clinical settings on smoking cessation counseling, together with a supporting scientific review (U.S. Preventive Services 1988). ODPHP staffed smoking and health workshops and participated in symposia organized by the International Union Against Cancer and delivered in Bolivia and Columbia (1983), Brazil, Paraguay, Ecuador, and Panama (1984), Costa Rica (1986), and Hong Kong and China (1987).

Department of Defense

There is a strong historical link between tobacco use and the military. Until 1975, cigarettes were part of the K- and C-rations provided to soldiers and sailors. In many military commissaries, cigarettes sell for approximately 35 percent less than in civilian stores (Blake 1985). A 1985 survey of active duty military personnel found that nearly one-half smoked cigarettes, one quarter smoked cigars or a pipe, and almost one-fifth used chewing tobacco, snuff, or other smokeless tobacco (Bray et al. 1986; Herbold 1987). Cigarette use was more common among nonofficers and varied by pay grades, with those at the lower end of the pay scale exhibiting a higher prevalence of smoking. A 1986 Department of Defense (DOD) report estimated that smoking-related health care costs to the military were 209 million dollars in 1984 (DOD 1986).

In March 1986, prompted by the medical evidence linking smoking with disease and the high prevalence of smoking among military personnel, the Secretary of Defense initiated an intensive antismoking campaign to be conducted at all levels of all services (DOD 1987). In April 1986, a DOD smoking reduction framework defined three smoking reduction goals for the military: (1) to reduce active duty smoking and other tobacco use by 10 percent per year, (2) to provide smoking reduction information and motivation and cessation assistance to DOD personnel, and (3) to specify designated places and times where smoking can occur to minimize effects of smoking on nonsmokers (DOD 1987).

Print and audiovisual materials for the campaign were obtained from voluntary and Federal agencies. In addition, in 1986, DOD allocated 97,000 dollars for publications and 324,000 dollars for antismoking on military radio and television PSAs (DOD 1987).

Each branch of the service developed its own smoking control plan consistent with the overall goals of DOD (DOD 1987). The U.S. Air Force (USAF) modified the curricula at the Basic Military Training School, the USAF Officer Training School, the USAF Academy, and the Air Force Reserve Officers' Training Corps to include mandatory classes on the hazards of using tobacco products. Similar course material was included in all professional military education for all officers and enlisted personnel.

In June 1986, the Air Force Surgeon General directed that there be on-base smoking cessation classes at every medical treatment facility in the Air Force. Nicotine-containing chewing gum was made available in all pharmacies, and tobacco sales were discontinued at all Air Force medical treatment facilities. Smoking was banned in all hospital and clinic facilities. Smoking was also prohibited on aeromedical evacuation flights, and the Officer Training School banned smoking during duty hours.

In July 1986, the Army banned the use of tobacco products in basic training and restricted smoking in other military courses. Army training centers and service schools incorporated antitobacco information into the curriculum. Smoking cessation courses were offered to soldiers, retirees, and family members. In November 1986, the Army participated in GASO.

In March 1987, the Navy Medical Commander directed that all naval hospitals offer group smoking cessation programs and prohibited the sale of tobacco in medical and dental facilities. Curricula for all Navy personnel include information on the health risks of tobacco use. Naval hospitals stock nicotine-containing gum for members in formal cessation classes. The Navy participated in the 1986 GASO.

The Marine Corps smoking control program is similar to that offered by the Navy. Guidance and smoking cessation materials are disseminated at all accession training commands and formal schools. Family Service Centers and Alcohol Counseling

Centers provide cessation programs. Smoking is prohibited in all medical and dental facilities.

To monitor the impact of the smoking control program, DOD conducts annual tobacco use surveys of military personnel (DOD 1987). Comparison of the 1982 and 1985 DOD worldwide surveys on alcohol and nonmedical drug use among military personnel revealed that the percentage of active duty smokers has dropped significantly from 53 percent in 1982 to 46 percent in 1985 (DOD 1987) (see Chapter 5). Between November 1986 and March 1987, the monthly dollar sales of tobacco products in military commissaries dropped by 18 percent (DOD 1987). The evidence available to date suggests that the DOD antismoking campaign has been successful (DOD 1987; Institute for the Study of Smoking Behavior and Policy 1988). The impact of the campaign is still being monitored, and the issue of tobacco sales pricing policies is being reassessed.

State Health Departments

A 1987 survey of State and territorial health agencies found that 33 of 52 (61 percent) reported having sponsored smoking cessation programs (CDC 1987). Most State plans focus on prevention rather than smoking cessation.

Several States have established programs to encourage cessation by pregnant women. New Jersey, Maryland, and Pennsylvania have developed protocols for use in State-supported maternity clinics (Coye 1988; US DHHS 1986a). New York has conducted a mass media education initiative, "Healthy Mothers, Healthy Babies," to encourage pregnant women to refrain from alcohol and tobacco use (US DHHS 1986a). Many local health departments also have established programs that provide cessation activities although these are not consistently cataloged.

Three State health departments, Colorado, Maryland, and Missouri, in collaboration with the Division of Reproductive Health of CDC, are developing and implementing a Smoking Cessation in Pregnancy (SCIP) Project to be used in public prenatal clinics. The purpose of the project is to reduce the incidence of low birthweight among women using publicly funded prenatal care services. One of the interventions used will be directed at helping the women to stop smoking. It is anticipated that approximately 4,000 women will be involved in the project and that 2,000 smokers will be exposed to the smoking cessation intervention.

Commercial Ventures in Smoking Control

As the number of smokers attempting to stop has increased, so have commercial ventures to develop and market cessation aids and services. Today, for-profit stop-smoking programs can be found in almost all major cities in the United States (Schwartz 1987). This Section provides a brief review of commercial ventures in smoking cessation, focusing first on the development and marketing of pharmacologic aids, followed by a discussion of nonpharmacologic aids and behavioral and motivational programs. Pharmacologic aids have been reviewed in the 1988 Surgeon General's Report on nicotine addiction (US DHHS 1988). The description of commercial ventures in smoking control is selective. Those nonpharmacologic programs described were chosen because they provide a historical perspective and have well-used national networks.

Pharmacologic Cessation Aids

Smoking deterrent drug products have been available since the early part of this century. Early drug treatments included herbs and spices and mouthwashes that altered the taste of tobacco so that smoking was less pleasant (Schwartz 1969). In 1936, Dorsey (1936) developed lobeline sulfate capsules to minimize the craving for tobacco. Lobeline sulfate is the active ingredient in Nikoban and Bantron, two popular nonprescription cessation aids available in most drugstores today. In 1982, a Food and Drug Administration (FDA) panel that reviewed smoking deterrent drug products concluded that the data were insufficient to demonstrate the effectiveness of lobeline as a smoking cessation aid (FDA 1982). A similar conclusion was reached regarding the effectiveness of drug products such as chewing gums, mouthsprays, and tablets containing silver acetate (FDA 1982). In its proposed monograph for over-the-counter (OTC) smoking deterrent drugs (FDA 1985), FDA tentatively adopted this panel's conclusions, but FDA has not yet issued a final rule. Silver acetate when combined with tobacco creates an unpleasant metallic taste in the mouth that presumably serves to discourage smoking.

Clonidine, a drug used to treat high blood pressure, currently is being investigated as an aid to help people stop smoking (Glassman et al. 1988). Interest in clonidine as a smoking cessation aid was stimulated by Glassman and colleagues (1984), who demonstrated a reduction in cigarette urges associated with its use. It is speculated that clonidine may relieve nicotine withdrawal symptoms through its effect on the central nervous system's adrenergic mechanism (Glassman et al. 1984, 1988; US DHHS 1988). Boehringer Ingelheim Pharmaceuticals, Inc., currently is conducting studies to evaluate the effectiveness of a clonidine transdermal patch as a smoking cessation aid. Clonidine is not currently approved for marketing as a smoking cessation aid by FDA.

To date, the most successful and effective drug product developed to assist smokers in stopping is nicotine polacrilex gum, a nicotine-containing chewing gum (US DHHS 1988). It is marketed by Lakeside Pharmaceuticals, a Division of Merrell Dow. Nicotine-containing gum was developed on the premise that nicotine is the primary reinforcer of smoking. It was reasoned that a product that could deliver nicotine into the body in a form with lower potential to produce dependence could aid smokers in stopping (Fernoe, Lichtneckert, Lundgren 1973).

Nicotine-containing gum was first developed and manufactured by A.B. Leo in Sweden in 1971. Early studies with the gum showed poor results. However, a carbonate buffer added to improve absorption of nicotine improved cessation rates (Axelsson and Brantmark 1977). The main benefit associated with gum use is the alleviation of withdrawal symptoms. Several studies have demonstrated the effect of nicotine-containing gum in relieving irritability, anxiety, problems in concentrating, restlessness, and hunger (Hughes and Miller 1984; Schneider, Jarvik, Forsythe 1984; US DHHS 1988). Studies suggest that the gum does not fully replace the nicotine provided by cigarette smoke. Benowitz, Jacob, and Savanapridic (1987) reported that chewing 2-

mg nicotine gum on an hourly schedule for 10 hr yielded blood nicotine levels comparable to one-third that achieved while smoking. Use of a 4-mg nicotine gum causes a greater increase in blood nicotine levels and may increase cessation rates (Tonnesen et al. 1988). However, only the 2-mg dose is approved for use in the United States (US DHHS 1988).

Numerous studies have reported on the efficacy of nicotine polacrilex gum in achieving smoking cessation (Schwartz 1987; US DHHS 1988). Many of these studies are well-controlled double-blind investigations comparing nicotine-containing gum with a placebo gum (British Thoracic Society 1983; Campbell, Lyons, Prescott 1987; Fagerstrom 1982; Fee and Stewart 1982; Hall et al. 1987; Hjalmarson 1984; Jamrozik et al. 1984; Jarvis et al. 1982; Puska, Bjorkqvist, Koskela 1979; Schneider et al. 1983; Tonnesen et al. 1988). No studies to date have compared nicotine-containing gum with other cessation drug products, such as those containing lobeline or clonidine (US DHHS 1988). Not all studies have shown nicotine polacrilex gum to be effective (British Thoracic Society 1983; Campbell, Lyons, Prescott 1987; Fee and Stewart 1982; Jamrozik et al. 1984). Long-term cessation rates (over 1-year followup) vary widely from 3 to 49 percent (US DHHS 1988). Nicotine-containing gum has become an increasingly popular adjunct to behaviorally based cessation programs. Studies suggest that behaviorally based treatment in conjunction with nicotine polacrilex gum tends to be more effective than the same program without gum, or compared with gum alone (Fagerstrom 1982; Hall et al. 1987; Killen, Maccoby, Taylor 1984).

FDA approved the marketing of nicotine-containing gum in the United States as a prescription smoking cessation aid in January 1984 (IMS 1984). The product became available to the public in mid-March of that year. It retails for about 18 dollars for a box of 96 pieces. A mailing piece introducing the gum was circulated to 77,000 physicians (IMS 1984). In the 4 months after FDA approval of nicotine polacrilex gum, Merrell Dow spent more than 4 million dollars to launch the product (IMS 1984). Over 80 percent of promotion dollars was used for in-person promotion in physicians' offices and other health care settings. The result of this massive promotional campaign was one of the fastest selling prescription products ever introduced (IMS 1984). Sales were 42 million dollars in 1984, 46 million dollars in 1985, 54 million dollars in 1986, and 60 million dollars in 1987.

As part of its promotional campaign, Merrell Dow has supported many medical symposia on smoking, underwritten the cost of a newsletter on smoking cessation sent to over 40,000 physicians annually, and helped support the development and distribution of training materials on smoking cessation for health professionals.

Since the gum was introduced in March 1984, an estimated 4 to 6 million smokers (approximately one-tenth) have used it. Surveys of gum users show that two-thirds of prescriptions are generated by the patient rather than the physician. Lakeside advertising in public media (which does not mention the product or brand name) encourages smokers to ask their physicians for help in stopping smoking. The commercial success of nicotine polacrilex gum is likely to encourage other pharmaceutical companies to consider developing and marketing cessation drug products. Several nicotine-containing products are under investigation as cessation aids, including nasal nicotine solutions, nicotine dermal patches, and nicotine aerosols (US DHHS 1988).

Nonpharmacologic Cessation Aids

A variety of nonpharmacologic aids have been produced over the years to assist smokers in reducing or stopping smoking, including filter systems, smokeless cigarettes, self-help books, audiotapes, and more recently, videos (Schwartz 1987). Evidence regarding the effectiveness of these cessation aids is extremely limited or nonexistent. Many companies have developed cigarette filter systems to help people stop smoking. The basic idea behind a filter system as a cessation aid is to reduce the amount of nicotine taken in, allowing smokers to wean themselves from the chemical addiction (Schwartz 1987). One of the most popular filter systems available, One Step at a Time, manufactured by Teledyne Water Pik, was first marketed in 1977 and is sold primarily through chain drugstores and advertised in conjunction with local retailers. The filter system consists of four reusable filters, each of which further reduces the amount of tar, nicotine, and carbon monoxide from cigarette smoke. Each of the filters is to be used for 2 weeks. The One Step at a Time filter system sells for about 10 dollars. Teledyne Water Pik also markets a single filter system called Step Four, which is the fourth filter in the filter system and sells for about 5 dollars. In the FDA's 1980 response to a petition filed by Action on Smoking and Health for the regulation of cigarette filters as medical devices (FDA 1980), the agency concluded that some of the labeling and advertising for detached cigarette filters established intended therapeutic uses for One Step at a Time and certain other products. Thus, One Step at a Time and certain other detached cigarette filters were considered as medical devices within the agency's jurisdiction.

Smokeless cigarettes that simulate the taste of tobacco smoke are another popular cessation aid. E-Z Quit, a smokeless cigarette sold through a mail order company, consists of a plastic cigarette with three menthol flavor capsules. The product sells for about 10 dollars and is widely advertised in popular magazines and newspapers. E-Z Quit was designed to deliver flavoring ingredients through inhalation, and was intended and labeled for use as a smoking deterrent. Products so formulated and labeled are regarded by the FDA as drugs and have been included in the agency's ongoing OTC drug review. Under this review, in 1982 an Advisory Review Panel (FDA 1982) concluded that the data are insufficient to demonstrate the effectiveness of such products as smoking deterrents. In 1985 the FDA tentatively concurred with this conclusion in its proposed monograph (FDA 1985). A final rule has not yet been issued.

Dozens of different how-to-quit-smoking books have been produced. Many of the books are written by former smokers and psychologists who provide a wide range of suggestions on how to stop smoking. Studies evaluating the efficacy of quit-smoking books have reported mixed results (Cummings et al. 1988; Davis, Faust, Ordentlich 1984; Glasgow and Lichtenstein 1987; Glasgow and Rosen 1978; FDA 1982). In general, the findings of studies comparing the effectiveness of different quit-smoking books suggest that no one book appears to be better than any other. The addition of a personal contact to the provision of written materials appears to enhance quitting behavior (Flay 1987b; Kottke et al. 1988). Many bookstores also sell audiotapes on how to stop smoking. In 1985, ALA produced "In Control,"® a smoking cessation video program that smokers can use at home on a videocassette recorder. "In Control" runs for 2 hr and consists of 13 segments that viewers are encouraged to see on different days. Users also receive a 124-page viewer guide and a 20-min audiotape with motivational and relaxation messages. The package sells for 60 dollars. A recent evaluation of the program, which did not use a control group, involved 100 smokers and found that 53 completed the program, with 31 verified abstinent by carbon monoxide testing 1 month after completion. Twenty-one of the 100 smokers who started the program were not smoking 1 year after completing it and 16 of these reported total abstinence during the 1-year followup period (Marston and Bettencourt 1988). ACS recently produced the ACS Freshstart video, a 21-day program that focuses on maintaining cessation (i.e., quit day is day 1). The video sells for about 20 dollars.

Recently, Health Innovations, Inc., developed and began marketing a computer-assisted smoking cessation program called "LifeSign." "LifeSign" consists of a credit-card-sized microcomputer and self-help booklet. The microcomputer is used to assist smokers in designing a tailored, gradual cutdown program that helps the smoker withdraw from the nicotine in cigarettes. Two studies of "LifeSign" show validated 6-month cessation rates of 18 and 28 percent (Frederiksen et al. 1988). However, both of these studies were based on small samples of self-selected smokers and did not involve comparisons with other cessation interventions.

Stop-Smoking Programs

Hypnosis has long been advocated as an effective treatment for stopping smoking (Schwartz 1987). A review of smoking cessation treatments listed in the telephone yellow pages of 47 U.S. cities found that hypnosis was the most frequently advertised service (Schwartz 1987). Hypnotists accounted for 31 percent of all services listed. The intent of hypnosis as a smoking cessation treatment is often to increase personal motivation to stop smoking (Spiegel 1970). This is usually done by posthypnotically suggesting a link between smoking and unpleasant experiences (e.g., "smoking is a poison"). Many hypnosis techniques are similar to behavioral therapy methods (e.g., relaxation training, increased awareness of smoking cues), making it difficult to distinguish the specific effects of hypnosis. Spiegel (1970) suggests that hypnosis alone does not make a person stop smoking, but when combined with motivation, helps the subject concentrate on changing his or her smoking behavior. Schwartz's review of 31 hypnosis trials concluded that hypnosis, when used as the only cessation method, is ineffective (Schwartz 1987).

More recently, acupuncture has been touted as an effective treatment for smoking cessation (Schwartz 1987). Acupuncture involves the use of needles or staplelike attachments placed in the nose or ear (Schwartz 1987). The mechanism by which acupuncture may help a person stop smoking is not clear. Several investigators suggest that acupuncture relieves smoking withdrawal symptoms, although there is little evidence to support this claim (Fuller 1982; Schneideman 1981). Others suggest that the effect of acupuncture is psychological and depends on personal motivation to stop smoking (Machovec and Man 1978; Martin and Waite 1981). Studies that evaluate acupuncture as a smoking deterrent vary widely in the methods used and in the cessation rates reported (Schwartz 1987).

One of the oldest and most successful commercial cessation programs is SmokEnders, which was started by a former smoker, Jacquelyn Rogers, in 1969. Headquartered in New Jersey, SmokEnders has chapters or franchises in many U.S. cities and in several foreign countries (Schwartz 1987). The program consists of six 2-hr sessions held over a 6-week period. Classes are conducted by former smokers who are graduates of the SmokEnders program. The program emphasizes motivation for stopping and brand switching, as well as behavioral and cognitive skills for gradually reducing the amount smoked. In 1985, Comprehensive Care Corporation purchased the license to operate SmokEnders. However, the program is basically the same as the one developed by Rogers in 1969. The cost of the program varies by location, ranging from 225 to 300 dollars. Since SmokEnders was established in 1969, an estimated 600,000 smokers have completed the program.

The Schick Stop Smoking program, started in 1971, was the first well-known commercial program to use counterconditioning techniques to help people stop smoking (Smith 1988). The Schick Stop Smoking program includes three phases: a 1-week preparation phase, a 1-week counterconditioning phase, and a support phase (Smith 1988). In the preparation phase, smokers are instructed to keep a record of each cigarette smoked. The counterconditioning phase of the program consists of five 1-hr treatment sessions held on consecutive days. Two counterconditioning techniques—mild electric shock to the wrist and quick puffing on a cigarette—are used to attach negative experiences to common cues for smoking. In the support phase, clients return to the center for group counseling, receive weekly telephone contacts, and have one additional counterconditioning session. The program is run by trained nonmedical personnel and treats about 2,000 smokers annually. The cost of the program is 595 dollars.

Worksite and Hospital Wellness Programs

Stimulated by both public and private initiatives, an increasing number of businesses have adopted policies that either limit or ban smoking at work (Bureau of National Affairs 1987; Orlandi 1986; US DHHS 1986b; Martin, Fehrenbach, Rosner 1986) (see Chapter 7). This trend has resulted in an increased demand for smoking control programs offered at worksites. Worksite programs have the advantage of having an available defined population that can potentially be reached. Many organizations have attempted to capitalize on the demand by developing and marketing smoking control programs specifically for worksites (Newsweek, August 29, 1988). The efficacy of worksite smoking programs was reviewed in the 1985 Surgeon General's Report (US DHHS 1985a), which presented somewhat disappointing results. Since that review, other outcomes have been somewhat more encouraging (e.g., Omenn et al. 1988).

In 1980, Control Data Corporation began marketing "Stay Well," a health promotion program designed for businesses (Anderson and Jose 1987). The smoking control component of the "Stay Well" program is called "How to Quit Smoking" and consists of eight 1-hr group sessions conducted over 7 weeks. The program emphasizes nicotine fading and behavioral coping skills. When the program was first introduced in 1980, classes were conducted by staff from Control Data. However, this proved to be costly and limited the geographical reach of the program. In 1982, the "Stay Well" program began licensing hospitals to deliver and market the program. Today, there are 50 licensed distributors located in most major population centers. More than 600 corporations have used the "How to Quit Smoking" program. The cost of the program varies by distributor, ranging from 35 to 80 dollars per smoker.

Johnson and Johnson, Inc., has recently begun marketing "Live for Life" (LFL), a wellness program designed for the workplace (Wilbur 1983). The smoking cessation component of LFL includes an annual health screen with medical advice on smoking, environmental changes to support nonsmoking, and regularly scheduled stop-smoking classes. Classes consist of 14 1-hr sessions held over a 3-week period. Smoke holding, group support, relaxation training, and behavioral coping skills are the primary elements of the program (Shipley et al. 1988). A recent report on the effectiveness of the

LFL stop-smoking program showed that in four companies exposed to the program, 23 percent of smokers were not smoking 2 years later compared with 17 percent in three matched comparison companies (Shipley et al. 1988). Among smokers in the LFL companies, 21 percent enrolled in the stop-smoking classes and 32 percent of these were not smoking after 2 years (Shipley et al. 1988).

In 1976 the American Institute for Preventive Medicine began marketing a stop-smoking program called "Smokeless." The program includes five 1-hr sessions held on consecutive days, plus three maintenance classes spread over 2 weeks (Powell and McCann 1981). The program instructs smokers in a wide range of behavioral and cognitive coping skills and includes some mild counterconditioning procedures (e.g., "pinky puffing" (puffing a cigarette while holding it between the pinky and ring finger)), loud white noise, filters dipped in anti-nail-biting solution). "Smokeless" has recently been adapted into a self-help format that sells for 39 dollars. The self-help program is packaged in an attractive kit with six booklets and a relaxation audiotape. The Institute also markets a guide for establishing a smoking policy in the workplace. "Smokeless" is licensed to hospitals or businesses to use and market program materials. Hospitals in turn will offer the program to people in the community. Corporate affiliates offer the program solely to their own employees. Each hospital affiliate is responsible for marketing the program in a defined geographic region. Since 1983, 250 hospitals and several large corporations have been licensed to conduct "Smokeless," although this does not mean that they actually run the program. The Institute conducts a 3-day training seminar on how to run the program and provides each trainee with a set of materials. The Institute also assists hospital affiliates in marketing the program. Program materials are sold to the affiliate hospital or corporation for 30 dollars per person. The fee for "Smokeless" varies by affiliate, ranging from 75 to 225 dollars per smoker.

Smoke Stoppers is another commercial stop-smoking program that licenses hospitals and other outlets to use its materials. The program is marketed by the National Center for Health Promotion in Ann Arbor, MI. The format of Smoke Stoppers is similar to that of "Smokeless," with five classes in the first week, followed by three maintenance sessions. Outlets certified to conduct Smoke Stoppers programs are given exclusive rights to market the program in a defined geographical region. All Smoke Stoppers instructors are required to be former smokers and must attend a 40-hr training program. Program materials are sold to affiliates at a cost of 39 dollars per person. The fee charged to smokers varies by outlet, averaging about 150 dollars per person. Smoke Stoppers was established in 1977 and has licensed over 300 outlets to conduct programs.

One of the 1990 Health Objectives for the Nation calls for at least 35 percent of all workers to be offered employer/employee-sponsored or -supported smoking cessation programs either at the worksite or in the community. While there are no national data available to measure the percentage of all workers who have access to such a program, a 1985 survey, the National Survey of Worksite Health Promotion Activities, gathered data on smoking cessation programs in worksites with 50 or more employees, which is reflective of approximately 58 percent of the U.S. workforce (US DHHS 1987). Preliminary analyses indicate that approximately 36 percent offer some kind of smoking cessation program. Due to the incompleteness of the data, evaluation of progress toward achievement of the objective cannot be adequately accomplished.

In addition to offering cessation programs, businesses are increasingly providing incentives to employees to encourage them to stop smoking (Orleans and Shipley 1982). A small ambulance company in Oregon offered a 5 dollar monthly bonus to any employee who did not smoke during work hours. As an added incentive, the accumulated bonuses for the year were matched at Christmastime. After 1 year, 4 of the 16 smokers claimed abstinence from smoking at work (Rosen and Lichtenstein 1977). Smokers employed at a hospital in upstate New York were offered the chance to win a 250 dollar cash prize if they stopped smoking for 1 month. Of all smokers, 14 percent enrolled in the contest, and 36 percent of these enrollees were not smoking 3 months after the contest ended (Cummings, Hellmann, Emont 1988). A common type of incentive is the offer to pay part or all of the cost to attend a cessation program. Campbell Soup Company splits the cost for employees to attend an onsite smoking cessation program (Schwartz 1987). General Motors absorbed 75 percent of the fee for a smoking cessation program offered to employees (Schwartz 1987). The evidence available does suggest that incentives can serve as a useful adjunct to other cessation services in the workplace (Klesges, Vasey, Glasgow 1986; US DHHS 1985b).

Summary

The Chapter 8 Appendix includes a chronology of key events that have influenced smoking education and cessation activities over the past 25 years. The antismoking campaign of the 1960s focused primarily on educating the public about the health hazards of tobacco use (Warner 1986). An assumption underlying the early antismoking efforts was that an informed public would discontinue smoking. This assumption was not without merit in that cigarette consumption did fall significantly in response to information about the dangers of cigarette use (Hamilton 1972; Warner 1977, 1981, 1986). However, the assumption that smokers merely needed to be motivated to stop ignored the addictive nature of smoking and the fact that many found it extremely difficult to stop smoking (US DHHS 1988).

The 1970s saw an increased emphasis on devising methods to assist smokers in stopping and staying off cigarettes (Schwartz 1987), with special attention to cognitively based self-management approaches.

The 1980s have seen a renewed emphasis on educating the public about the hazards of tobacco use and increased efforts to recruit smokers to attempt cessation. Such an emphasis seems appropriate given the fact that the vast majority of smokers need first to be persuaded to stop before efforts are directed at offering assistance in stopping.

The national voluntary agencies, especially ACS, ALA, and AHA, have played a significant role in educating the public about the hazards of tobacco use. This has been achieved through a wide variety of interventions including the distribution of educational materials, sponsorship of cessation programs, and production and dissemination of PSAs that carry an antismoking message. Although the smoking education efforts of the national voluntary health agencies have been the most visible of any group, some critics note that more might have been accomplished if a higher level of interagency collaboration had existed. In 1978, a blue ribbon panel of experts commissioned by ACS to study the problem of smoking and the effectiveness of antismoking activities concluded that the major voluntary health organizations should actively pursue increased coordination of their efforts and resources in producing materials to assist smokers in quitting (ACS 1978).

Until the 1980s, the voluntary health agencies focused their efforts on educating the public about the facts on smoking and health and did little to initiate political and legal challenges to the tobacco industry (Patterson 1987). The formation of the Tri-Agency Coalition on Smoking OR Health in 1982 represented a major shift in the smoking control focus of the voluntary health agencies. The Coalition was formed primarily to promote cooperation in obtaining legislation on smoking control issues.

Government smoking control efforts have been characterized by some observers as modest (ACS 1978). OSH, the only Federal agency devoted exclusively to the smoking issue, today has a budget that, in real dollars, is roughly one-half of the budget in 1966 when its predecessor, the National Clearinghouse, was established. (See Chapter 7.) Federal spending on smoking control has increased over the years, with the majority of funds supporting research rather than interventions. In recent years, there has been a shift away from supporting biomedical research on the hazards of tobacco to supporting studies on the behavioral aspects of smoking, including smoking cessation. However, there is little evidence of transfer of research findings to community settings, and some observers have questioned whether limited public health resources should be disproportionately expended on treating smokers individually or in small groups, to the exclusion of mass media and public relations efforts aimed at changing the social, economic, and political environment that supports smoking (Chapman 1985). NCI now emphasizes support of studies that investigate effective application and dissemination of smoking programs (Fanning 1988; NCI 1986b) and NHLBI is supporting large community programs of applied research that include smoking (US DHHS 1984, 1986a).

The opportunity to develop and market cessation aids and programs has expanded in the past decade as more smokers have attempted to stop. The use of pharmacologic therapies to aid cessation increased markedly with the introduction of nicotine polacrilex gum in 1984. Alternative methods of nicotine replacement are currently under investigation along with other pharmacologic cessation approaches (e.g., clonidine) (US DHHS 1988). In addition to pharmacologic aids, behaviorally oriented cessation programs, particularly those targeting worksites, have increased in the past decade. Likewise, greater efforts are now being made to increase involvement of physicians and other health care professionals in smoking intervention.

In general, different types of smoking cessation strategies (e.g., condition- or cognition-based) have been emphasized during different time periods, new strategies have been added, and some specific behaviorally oriented smoking cessation strategies appear to have changed relatively little in the past 25 years. The packaging and marketing of these programs have also become more sophisticated, with an increased emphasis on targeting specific groups of smokers (e.g., pregnant women, Hispanics, blacks). There has been a gradual shift in the way cessation interventions are promoted from approaches that largely require smokers to seek assistance on their own to more aggressive strategies that actively recruit smokers to seek help and stop. Examples of active recruitment strategies include televised stop-smoking clinics (Flay 1987b) and contests and competitions to promote abstinence behavior (Cummings, Hellmann, Emont 1988;

King et al. 1987; Klesges, Vasey, Glasgow 1986). The level of smoking cessation activity has increased in recent years, spurred by regulatory decisions restricting smoking (Chapter 7) and changing public perceptions and attitudes regarding tobacco use (Chapter 4).

A significant event in terms of promoting smoking cessation activities of the national organizations was the 1967 FCC ruling applying the Fairness Doctrine to broadcast cigarette advertising. This policy prompted organizations to become involved in activities such as production of PSAs. The next chapter will cover this and other policy activities. Evidence indicates that the resulting increase in the volume of antismoking messages helped contribute to a substantial decline in cigarette consumption (Hamilton 1972; Warner 1977, 1981, 1986).

The last 25 years have seen an increase in smoking cessation research and the implementation of numerous public health approaches designed to help people stop smoking. Working toward an integrated approach of policies and programs in the available community networks seems to be a direction in which the smoking-and-health campaign is moving (US DHHS 1986b).

PART III. ANTISMOKING ADVOCACY AND LOBBYING

Nature and Objectives of Advocacy and Lobbying

Individual citizens and organized groups have played an active role in the development of public and private policies affecting smoking and the cigarette product. Their activities range from efforts to inform and educate individuals and the public at large about the health consequences of smoking to advocacy and lobbying to influence policies and legislation to prevent or reduce smoking. The latter are considered in this concluding part of the present chapter as a bridge between voluntary antismoking activities and mandated activities (Chapter 7). Advocacy and lobbying are undertaken voluntarily by private citizens and organizations, but with the intent of influencing smoking-related laws and regulations.

Development and implementation of health information and education strategies are oriented toward providing or imparting information to teach or instruct, often with a view toward influencing thought and behavior. Earlier parts of this Chapter and other sections of this Report address information and education activity as a component of health education efforts designed to provide antismoking messages. As discussed in this Chapter, several such efforts incorporate advice and instruction on how to remain or become a nonsmoker.

Advocacy encompasses efforts to shape opinion in support of public policy. Lobbying, in its strictest sense, means directly attempting to influence legislators, especially in favor of a special interest. Frequently, lobbying also is used to mean directly trying to influence officials to take desired action, or to influence the political process toward a specific outcome. Despite these definitions, advocacy and lobbying activities often overlap and their distinction is not always clear.

A primary purpose of these pursuits is to shift perceptions and attitudes about smoking: to change from viewing smoking as a matter of personal choice toward viewing smoking as a significant public health problem requiring adoption of public health policy interventions. Antismoking advocacy and lobbying both recognize and act on the fact that smoking is a political as well as a health, social, and economic issue.

Few antismoking advocacy and lobbying efforts have been studied systematically, making it difficult to attribute changes in policy or public opinion to a specific group or activity. Furthermore, little exists in the published literature on smoking that describes the advocacy and lobbying activities of groups or individuals or evaluates the impact of those activities on public awareness or public and private policies regarding smoking. For example, the available data show that public support for restrictions on smoking in public and at work has increased substantially in recent years (Chapter 4). A temporal relationship can be demonstrated between this increasing support and the growth of antismoking advocacy and lobbying activities targeted at these same issues. It is not clear, however, to what extent changing public attitudes led to or followed advocacy efforts.

Analyses of the relationship between legislative lobbying activities and the enactment of legislation have been predominantly qualitative. For example, an analysis of lobbying efforts for the introduction and subsequent passage of the Comprehensive Smoking Education Act of 1984 (Public Law 98-424) concluded that the Coalition on Smoking OR Health, a group representing ACS, AHA, and ALA, significantly influenced passage of the Act. The analysis also concluded that the "woeful miscalculations of the tobacco lobbyists" made a significant contribution to the outcome (Pertschuk 1986).

Objectives

Smoking-and-health advocacy and lobbying efforts during the 25 years since the first Surgeon General's Report have centered on a number of specific objectives, including: broader and more effective dissemination of information on the hazards of smoking; provision of increased resources for research, public education, and prevention; reduction in consumption and encouragement of cessation by smokers; prevention of uptake by children and adolescents; creation of public support for policies to restrict or prevent smoking; protection of nonsmokers from exposure to environmental tobacco smoke; regulation of the contents and emissions of the cigarette; regulation of the marketing, promotion, and advertising practices related to tobacco products; limitation on access through restriction of the sale and distribution of cigarettes (e.g., through vending machines and free samples); increase in the price of smoking through taxation of cigarettes; and stimulation or creation of public demand for political action on a specific policy or issue. Many of the advocacy and lobbying groups active since 1964 have pursued a variety of these objectives with varying degrees of activism and political involvement.

The origin and objectives of the National Interagency Council on Smoking and Health, the first major organization created in response to the 1964 Surgeon General's Report, provide an illustration of the variety of purposes diverse groups may want to achieve, individually or jointly.

Following the release of the Report, Surgeon General Luther Terry called together representatives from the major national voluntary health agencies to discuss what actions might be taken in response to the Report. One result of this meeting was the creation of the National Interagency Council on Smoking and Health, which included among its members the voluntary health agencies, a variety of medical and health professions groups, organizations such as the National Congress of Parents and Teachers, and Federal agencies such as the Public Health Service and the Veterans Administration. By 1969, the Council's membership included 25 national organizations and 3 Government agencies.

The purpose of the Council was "(1) to use its professional talents to bring to the nation—particularly to the young—an increasing awareness of the harmfulness of cigarette smoking; (2) to encourage, support and assist national,State,and local smoking and health programs; and (3) to generate and coordinate public interest and action related to this area of health" (Diehl 1969). The Council's statement of purpose reflects an early perception that stimulating some form of public interest and action would be necessary to achieve other Council purposes related to smoking and health.

The Council did not initiate its own programs of education or intervention, however, and operated on a very small budget contributed by the member organizations. Its activities in the area of advocacy were extremely limited, although it spawned much activity at the State and local levels that has carried over into the present. The Interagency Council became the principal national forum for the exchange of information and coordination of efforts among the many groups concerned about smoking.

In addition to the National Interagency Council, there were 40 State and many city interagency councils in operation with the primary function of coordinating and stimulating action by member groups (Diehl 1969). These State and local interagency councils consisted, in large part, of the State and local affiliates of the national groups represented in the National Interagency Council.

Troyer and Markel (1983) analyzed the announcements and proposed actions of health groups regarding smoking as reported in the press during the period 1954–78. They found that through 1973, the overwhelming majority of announcements and actions (26 of 29) were targeted toward education and persuasion, while during the period 1974–78, almost all (9 of 10) were focused on laws and regulations restricting smoking. The reasons for the initial apparent prioritization of information and education activities are not known, but it is clear that during the early period of antismoking efforts, the major groups considered their primary contributions to be made by informing the public and testifying before legislative groups, not by lobbying for specific regulations or motivating the public to political action. For example, AHA stated in 1967 that "its 'proper responsibility' involved testimony on the health hazards of smoking, not legal action" (Troyer and Markel 1983).

Over the years, the national voluntary agencies and other significant organizations have continued their critical information and education activities, as described in Parts I and II of this Chapter. More recently, many of these organizations have begun to supplement their more traditional educational campaigns with more active efforts in support of specific heath policy outcomes. Accordingly, they have emerged as strong advocates in support of antismoking policies. In addition, as part of a health strategy, some have developed specific components within their organizations, and sometimes have fostered special coalitions to advocate or lobby for specific purposes on behalf of their organizations.

A significant example is the Coalition on SmokingORHealth, an organization formed in 1982 to initiate and coordinate antismoking lobbying activity on behalf of ACS, AHA, and ALA, and to supplement the more traditional information and education approaches of these three organizations. The Coalition's statement of purpose reflects its emphasis on political action in support of smoking and health issues:

> To more effectively bring tobacco and health issues to the attention of federal legislators, administrators and other public officials; . . . to work with legislators and other government officials to enact policies which will discourage tobacco use, further educate the public about the hazards of tobacco use, and limit the demand for and marketing of this deadly product in the future (ACS 1988).

Organizational Characteristics

Five relatively distinct types of groups operating at the national, State, or local level carry out smoking control advocacy and lobbying activities. The first group, and perhaps the largest and most visible, is composed of the three major national voluntary health agencies (ACS, ALA, and AHA) and their State and local affiliates. Each of the three agencies concentrates primarily on research and public education related to the diseases of interest to the agencies, and delivery of services to those affected by such diseases. In addition to forming the Coalition on Smoking OR Health, each also has become more focused on leadership in health policy development, and has increased its level of interest and participation in advocacy and lobbying. Much of what the voluntary health agencies are allowed to do in this regard may be affected by both their Internal Revenue Code status as nonprofit agencies and the Tax Reform Act of 1976, which specifies permissible lobbying activites by nonprofit groups.

The second group is made up of special focus or special population organizations that have targeted their efforts on a particular aspect of the smoking problem or a specific approach. This group includes such organizations as Action on Smoking and Health (ASH), which has pursued a legal action campaign to force legislators and regulatory bodies to address a variety of aspects of the smoking problem; Stop Teenage Addiction to Tobacco (STAT), which focuses on teenage tobacco issues; the Tobacco Products Liability Project (TPLP), which, as a public health strategy, supports efforts to bring product liability lawsuits against cigarette manufacturers; and Doctors Ought to Care (DOC), founded to provide physicians with a rallying point for health promotion and antismoking advocacy, especially through counteradvertising. These groups are more involved in advocacy than in lobbying.

The third group is composed of health and health professions organizations such as the American Medical Association, American Public Health Association, American Dental Association, American Academy of Pediatrics, American College of Chest Physicians, American Medical Women's Association, American Academy of Family Physicians, American Society of Internal Medicine, American College of Obstetricians and Gynecologists, and American Association for Respiratory Care. These groups increasingly have promoted a role for their members as advocates for smoking control in their respective communities, in addition to engaging, as organizations, in advocacy and lobbying activities at the Federal level.

Organizations devoted to the rights of and protections for nonsmokers make up the fourth group. This would include organizations such as Americans for Nonsmokers' Rights, the only national antismoking group devoted solely to clean indoor air legislation. Other examples would be the numerous State and local groups that have formed independent chapters of Group Against Smoking Pollution (GASP) or that focus on nonsmoker protection and nonsmokers' rights. There are approximately 85 such groups at the State and local level (unpublished data, OSH).

The fifth group is made up of antismoking coalitions (groups of organizations) operating at the national, State, and local levels. Such coalitions have formed increasingly as the voluntary health agencies and other organizations have become more active in advocacy and lobbying and have found common interests. The National Interagency Council on Smoking and Health, referred to earlier, was the first major antismoking coalition formed, but, as discussed, it did not engage in advocacy or lobbying. The National Interagency Council no longer is active, but a number of State interagency councils remain active (US DHHS 1986d).

The most prominent coalition today is the Coalition on Smoking OR Health, also discussed earlier. The apparent successes of this Coalition and the growth of the "nonsmokers' rights" movement have led to an increasing number of State-level coalitions formed to undertake a variety of public education and advocacy activities and to pass specific antismoking legislation. In addition, goals such as the achievement of a smoke-free society by the year 2000 have spurred the formation of additional coalitions aimed at advocacy and lobbying activity in support of these broad goals.

The resources represented by and available to these five groupings are difficult to estimate. The large voluntary and professional organizations have many thousands of members, but no data are available to determine what number are involved actively in advocacy or lobbying or what resources may be directed to those purposes. The smaller groups, such as ASH, have modest budgets and staffs, but collectively represent a significant number of volunteers and dues-paying supporters.

The Tobacco Lobby

In discussing the nature and scope of antismoking lobbying, it is important to consider the nature of the political environment in which this takes place. An influential component of this environment has been the "tobacco lobby." The lobbying activities of the tobacco lobby do not vary greatly from the activities of other groups on behalf of other interests or causes, groups with vested economic or political interests using a variety of approaches to influence the outcome of legislation (Pertschuk 1986).

The term "tobacco lobby" has been used throughout the past 25 years as a generic description of those interest groups whose political activities have been directed toward protecting tobacco and cigarette interests from adverse policies. The groups included most often in this description are: the cigarette manufacturers and other commercial firms involved in the manufacture, marketing, and sale of cigarettes; the Tobacco Institute, the trade association representing the cigarette manufacturers; the tobacco farmers and those commercial firms involved in the trading of unmanufactured tobacco; and the registered lobbyists representing these various interests.

As in the case of antismoking advocacy and lobbying, there is little in the published literature on which to base a detailed analysis of the activities or impact of the tobacco lobby. It is difficult to determine the precise composition of the lobby at any point in time, and particularly at those points during which efforts of the lobby have been alleged to have had significant impact on the outcome of legislative or regulatory efforts to control smoking or the cigarette product. The available data indicate that since 1964, the cigarette manufacturers and the Tobacco Institute often have played the lead role in developing strategies and initiating lobbying against antismoking legislation and regulation.

The available historical record indicates that, unlike the voluntary health agencies, the tobacco lobby and its constituent members have engaged in active lobbying throughout the years. Among the legislative outcomes purportedly influenced by the tobacco lobby at the national level are the following: negotiating provisions of the Cigarette Labeling and Advertising Act of 1965 to ensure that the Federal Trade Commission would be precluded from regulating cigarette advertising for 3 1/2 years (1965); negotiating provisions of the Public Health Cigarette Smoking Act of 1969 to include preemption of State regulation of cigarette advertising (see Chapters 7 and 8; see also Friedman 1975; Fritschler 1975); and precluding the Consumer Product Safety Commission from exercising jurisdiction over cigarettes (1972). At the State level, influences attributed to the tobacco lobby relate to defeat of statewide nonsmokers' rights legislation in California on two separate occasions (1978, 1980; Whelan 1984). There are numerous anecdotal reports of tobacco lobby opposition to efforts to pass other State and local ordinances restricting smoking. It is difficult to establish the extent of the tobacco lobby's influence on these events, or to determine what combination of interest groups and individuals was involved.

Antismoking Advocacy and Lobbying: 1964 to the Present

Early Efforts

A succession of legislative and regulatory actions aimed at labeling the cigarette as dangerous and restricting the advertising and marketing practices of the cigarette manufacturers marked the period following the 1964 Surgeon General's Report. (See next chapter.) Throughout the period from 1964–69, the major national voluntary agencies provided extensive expert medical testimony in support of these initiatives but did not lobby actively for their passage. While the expert testimony contributed to the decision process, more aggressive advocacy and direct lobbying that supplemented these efforts undoubtedly influenced the process as well. One important example is the citizen petition that John F. Banzhaf III filed, as an individual, with the Federal Communications Commission (FCC) contending that smoking should be subject to the Fairness Doctrine. This action led to the FCC ruling that the Fairness Doctrine applied to cigarette advertising. As a result, stations broadcasting cigarette commercials were required to donate time to antismoking messages (see Chapter 7).

In the process of pursuing this legal course, Banzhaf founded ASH as a legal action arm for the antismoking community and launched an ongoing series of legal challenges to advance smoking control policies. ASH played a major role in establishing the legal concept of the right of nonsmokers to be free from exposure to tobacco smoke. A major component of that effort was pressure brought to bear on the Federal Aviation Administration to require separate smoking and nonsmoking areas on commercial flights. Through these and other initiatives, which other organizations also supported, ASH introduced the principle of private legal activism to influence legislation and other decisions on smoking and health issues.

Nonsmokers' Rights

The specific origin of concerns about the health hazards to nonsmokers of exposure to environmental tobacco smoke is difficult to date. In 1971, ASH already had targeted restrictions on smoking on airliners and in public as major regulatory initiatives. Dr. Jesse Steinfeld, U.S. Surgeon General from 1969–73, called official attention to the hazards of ETS for the first time in the 1972 Surgeon General's Report (US DHEW 1972) and was outspoken throughout his public career on the need to protect nonsmokers.

During the mid-1970s, groups concerned about nonsmokers' exposure to environmental tobacco smoke began to appear around the United States. One of the largest, California GASP, was the forerunner of Americans for Nonsmokers' Rights, the principal national antismoking group devoted solely to clean indoor air legislation. California GASP was founded in 1976 as a nonprofit public interest group and became Californians for Nonsmokers' Rights (CNR) in 1978. That year, CNR succeeded in placing a statewide proposition on the California ballot seeking restrictions on smoking in public. Although defeated in a vote preceded by a well-funded campaign by the tobacco lobby (Wong 1978), this initiative set the stage for repeated and increasingly successful smoking ordinances at the community level in California and in other States and cities. As Americans for Nonsmokers' Rights, the group reports having assisted in the passage of scores of city and county ordinances (Americans for Nonsmokers' Rights 1988).

ALA also has played an important role in public education and advocacy on the issue of protecting nonsmokers. Due in large part to its strong interest in promoting clean air, ALA was the first of the three national voluntary health organizations to become involved in the nonsmokers' rights issue. In fact, ALA did so early in the 1970s with a campaign stressing the concept that nonsmokers objected to involuntary exposure to tobacco smoke.

As it evolved, the nonsmokers' rights issue introduced a new element in the growth of antismoking advocacy and lobbying: a basis for involving nonsmokers in activities other than encouraging smokers to quit or discouraging initiation among teenagers.

Resulting initiatives provided a new rallying point outside the traditional focus of the voluntary health agencies and at the same time appealed to and prompted greater activity among those groups.

The effect of this element in the smoking control movement has yet to be fully evaluated. Surveys of public attitudes about smoking and the need to restrict it to protect nonsmokers show a widespread acceptance of these principles and an increasing consensus that the social acceptability of smoking is declining (Chapter 4).

Coalition Building and the Growth of Advocacy

As mentioned previously, ACS, AHA, and ALA in 1982 formed a tripartite Coalition on Smoking OR Health, primarily to coordinate their Federal legislative activities related to smoking control. The creation of the Coalition came at the end of a long period of gradual expansion in the public policy activities of the three voluntary organizations. The National Commission on Smoking and Public Policy, a study group ACS established in 1976, added impetus to the concept of the Coalition by recommending the three voluntary health agencies do more to support public policy initiatives to control smoking (ACS 1978). The Coalition has served as a mechanism for coordinating and implementing lobbying efforts of the three agencies. At the time the Coalition was established, ACS, AHA, and ALA also increased the staffs and resources of their individual public policy components.

Through the Coalition, the three voluntary health agencies have worked with other organizations and coalitions with common interests in support of smoking control policies, relating to health warning labels, tobacco advertising, smoking on airlines, the tobacco excise tax, and the price support program. Successful antismoking efforts the Coalition supported have included: passage of the Comprehensive Smoking Education Act of 1984, which requires four rotating warning labels on cigarette packages and advertisements, as well as disclosure to the Secretary of Health and Human Services of additives used in the manufacture of cigarettes; passage of the Comprehensive Smokeless Tobacco Health Education Act of 1986, banning advertising for smokeless tobacco in the electronic media and requiring warning labels on packages and advertisements; permanent extension of the Federal excise tax at 16 cents per pack as a provision of the Consolidated Omnibus Budget Reconciliation Act of 1985 (Public Law 99-272); and banning of smoking on commercial domestic airline flights scheduled for flight time of 2 hr or less as part of the fiscal year 1988 Department of Transportation appropriations bill (see Chapter 7). One analyst has concluded that the Coalition has enabled the three national voluntary health agencies to take the initiative in a variety of areas, placing the tobacco lobby in a reactive posture (Pertschuk 1986).

Other factors that have accompanied the Coalition's efforts are believed to have contributed to the Coalition's success and to an apparent steady increase in the level of antismoking advocacy and lobbying throughout the United States. One of these factors is the recruitment of new allies and the energizing of old ones. In addition to the Coalition, other groups and organizations have taken more aggressive positions. For example, the American Council on Science and Health has been an aggressive advocate on all aspects of smoking control. Another example is the American Medical Association, which has become involved in a major effort to mobilize its members at the State and local levels, in addition to using its considerable influence in Washington, in support of antismoking legislation (Lundberg 1985; AMA Council on Scientific Affairs 1984; American Medical Association 1987).

Another important factor is the growth in knowledge and sophistication of the advocates and lobbyists themselves. Drawing on the experience and expertise of other public interest groups, the antismoking interests have become significantly more proficient at employing their resources. In addition, through its Smoking Control Advocacy Resource Center, the Advocacy Institute, a public interest advocacy strategy and skills training resource, has contributed new thinking and coordination to the effort to counter the influence of the tobacco lobby (Advocacy Institute 1987a, 1987b).

One of the most important aspects of the growth of antismoking advocacy and lobbying has been the increase in State and local activity. The creation of coalitions and the success of local antismoking ordinances appear to have encouraged more groups and individuals to become politically active. Surveys and studies of trends in local and State smoking control ordinances (US DHHS 1986d) indicate that the restrictiveness of those ordinances is increasing, as is public support. (See also Chapter 7.)

CONCLUSIONS

Part I. Smoking Prevention Activities

1. Diverse program approaches to the prevention of smoking among youth grew out of antismoking education efforts in the 1960s. These approaches include media-based programs and resources; smoking prevention as part of multicomponent school health education; psychosocial prevention curricula; and a variety of other resources developed and sponsored by professional and voluntary health organizations, Federal and State agencies, and schools and community groups.
2. Psychosocial curricula addressing youths' motivations for smoking and the skills they need to resist influences to smoke have emerged as the program approach with the most positive outcomes. Evolution in program content has been accompanied by a shift since the 1960s in prevention program focus from youths in high school and college to adolescents in grades 6 through 8.
3. Existing prevention programs vary greatly in the extent to which they have been evaluated and used. Psychosocial prevention curricula have been intensively developed over the last decade and have been the most thoroughly evaluated and best documented; however, they are generally not part of a dissemination system. More widely disseminated smoking prevention materials and programs, such as those using mass media and brochures, have not always been as thoroughly evaluated; however, they have achieved wider use in the field.
4. The model of stages of smoking behavior acquisition underlies current smoking prevention programs and suggests new intervention opportunities, ranging from prevention activities aimed at young children to cessation programs for adolescent smokers.

5. There has been and continues to be a lack of smoking prevention programs that target youth at higher risk for smoking, such as those from lower socioeconomic backgrounds or school dropouts.

Part II. Smoking Education and Cessation Activities

1. During the past 25 years, national voluntary health agencies, especially the American Cancer Society, the American Heart Association, and the American Lung Association, have played a significant role in educating the public about the hazards of tobacco use.
2. Individual and group smoking cessation programs evolved from an emphasis on conditioning-based approaches in the 1960s, to the cognitively based self-management procedures of the 1970s, to the relapse prevention and pharmacologically based components of the 1980s.
3. There has recently been an increased emphasis on targeting specific groups of smokers for cessation activities (e.g., pregnant women, Hispanics, blacks).
4. Packaging and marketing of self-help smoking cessation materials have become more sophisticated and there is more of an emphasis on relapse prevention, while much of the content has changed relatively little over the years.
5. Mass-mediated quit-smoking programs have become an increasingly popular strategy for influencing the smoking behavior of a large number of smokers.
6. The 1980s have seen an increase in the promotion of smoking control efforts in the workplace in response to increasing demand and opportunity for worksite wellness programs and smoking control policies.
7. In the last decade there has been an increasing interest in involving physicians and other health care professionals in smoking control efforts. Medical organizations have played a more prominent role in smoking and health during the 1980s than they had in the past.

Part III. Antismoking Advocacy and Lobbying

1. Lobbying and advocacy efforts have expanded through the increasing commitment of the national voluntary health agencies to political action and the formation of coalitions at the local, State, and national levels.
2. Antismoking advocacy and lobbying have evolved over the past 25 years and now focus on a growing number of local, State, and national legislative and regulatory initiatives designed to reduce smoking, regulate the cigarette product, and prevent the uptake of smoking by children and adolescents.

References

ACTION ON SMOKING AND HEALTH. *History of the War Against Smoking. 1964–1978.* Washington, D.C.: Action on Smoking and Health, 1978.

ADVOCACY INSTITUTE. *Smoke Fighting. A Smoking Control Movement Building Guide.* New York: American Cancer Society, 1987a.

ADVOCACY INSTITUTE. *Smoke Signals. The Smoking Control Media Handbook.* New York: American Cancer Society, 1987b.

ALEXANDER, H.M., CALLCOTT, R., DOBSON, A.J., HARDES, G.R., LLOYD, D.M., O'CONNELL, D.L., LEEDER, S.R. Cigarette smoking and drug use in schoolchildren: IV—Factors associated with changes in smoking behaviour. *International Journal of Epidemiology* 12(1):59–66, 1983.

AMERICAN ACADEMY OF FAMILY PHYSICIANS. *AAFP Stop Smoking Program. Patient Stop Smoking Guide.* Kansas City, Kansas: American Academy of Family Physicians, 1987.

AMERICAN ACADEMY OF PEDIATRICS. Tobacco use by children and adolescents. *Pediatrics* 79(3):479–481, March 1987.

AMERICAN CANCER SOCIETY. *Task Force on Tobacco and Cancer: Target 5.* Report to the Board of Directors of the American Cancer Society. New York: American Cancer Society, October 1976.

AMERICAN CANCER SOCIETY. *A National Dilemma: Cigarette Smoking or the Health of Americans.* Report of the National Commission on Smoking and Public Policy to the Board of Directors. New York: American Cancer Society, January 31, 1978.

AMERICAN CANCER SOCIETY. *Facilitator's Guide: Youth Smoking Cessation Clinic.* New York: American Cancer Society, 1980.

AMERICAN CANCER SOCIETY. *Breaking Free. Discussion Guide.* New York: American Cancer Society, 1986.

AMERICAN CANCER SOCIETY. *Summary of Federal Legislative Activities.* New York: American Cancer Society, 1988.

AMERICAN COLLEGE OF CHEST PHYSICIANS. Proceedings of the national forum on office management of smoking problems. *Chest* 54:169, 1968.

AMERICAN COLLEGE OF CHEST PHYSICIANS. The management of smoking in the physician's "workshop." *Chest* 82:359–361, September 1982.

AMERICAN HEART ASSOCIATION. *Children and Smoking: A Message to Parents.* Dallas: American Heart Association, 1987.

AMERICAN INSTITUTES FOR RESEARCH. *Smokescreen. Guidelines for Helping Teenagers Become Nonsmokers.* Prepared for the Bureau of Health Education, Centers for Disease Control. Palo Alto, California: American Institutes for Research, 1980.

AMERICAN MEDICAL ASSOCIATION. *Tobacco and Health.* Report compiled by the AMA-ERF Committee for Research on Tobacco and Health. Chicago: American Medical Association and Research Foundation, 1978.

AMERICAN MEDICAL ASSOCIATION. *Creating a Tobacco-Free Society: A Physician Leadership Kit.* Chicago: American Medical Association, 1987.

AMERICAN MEDICAL ASSOCIATION BOARD OF TRUSTEES. Media advertising for tobacco products. *Journal of the American Medical Association* 255(8):1033, February 28, 1986.

AMERICAN MEDICAL ASSOCIATION COUNCIL ON SCIENTIFIC AFFAIRS. Nonsmoking in hospitals. *Connecticut Medicine* 48(5):297–305, May 1984.

AMERICAN NONSMOKERS' RIGHTS FOUNDATION. *A Curriculum for Secondhand Smoke.* Berkeley, California: American Nonsmokers' Rights Foundation, 1986.

ANDA, R.F., REMINGTON, P.L., SIENKO, D.G., DAVIS, R.M. Are physicians advising smokers to quit? The patient's perspective. *Journal of the American Medical Association* 257(14):1916–1919, April 10, 1987.

ANDERSON, D.R., JOSE, W.S. II. Employee lifestyle and the bottom line: Results from the StayWell evaluation. *Fitness in Business*, December 1987, pp. 86–91.

ARKIN, R.M., ROEMHILD, H.F., JOHNSON, C.A., LUEPKER, R.V., MURRAY, D.M. The Minnesota Smoking Prevention Program: A seventh-grade health curriculum supplement. *Journal of School Health* 51(9):611–616, November 1981.

AXELSSON, A., BRANTMARK, B. The antismoking effect of chewing gum with nicotine of high and low bioavailability. In: Steinfeld, J., Griffiths, W., Ball, K., Taylor, R.M. (eds.) *Smoking and Health. II. Health Consequences, Education, Cessation Activities, and Governmental Action.* Proceedings of the 3rd World Conference on Smoking and Health. U.S. Department of Health, Education, and Welfare, Public Health Service, National Institutes of Health, National Cancer Institute. DHEW Publication No. (NIH) 77-1413, 1977, pp. 549–559.

BAILEY, B.J. Tobaccoism is the disease—Cancer is the sequela. *Journal of the American Medical Association* 255(14):1923, April 11, 1986.

BAILEY, W.J. Ten smoking education programs for schools. *Journal of School Health* 55(1):33–34, January 1985.

BAILEY, W.J. Minneapolis workshop kicks-off national campaign for a tobacco-free young America by the year 2000. *Tobacco-Free Young America Reporter* 4(2):1, 1987.

BASCH, C.E., EVELAND, J.D., PORTNOY, B. Diffusion systems for education and learning about health. *Family and Community Health* 9(2):1–26, 1986.

BASCH, C.E., SLIEPCEVICH, E.M. Innovators, innovations and implementation: A framework for curricular research in school health education. *Health Education* 14(2):20–24, March–April 1983.

BAUMAN, K.E., BROWN, J.D., BRYAN, E.S., FISHER, L.A., PADGETT, C.A., SWEENEY, J.M. Three mass media campaigns to prevent adolescent cigarette smoking. *Preventive Medicine* 17:510–530, 1988.

BELL, C.S., BATTJES, R. (eds.) *Prevention Research: Deterring Drug Abuse Among Children and Adolescents*, NIDA Research Monograph 63. U.S. Department of Health and Human Services, Public Health Service, Alcohol, Drug Abuse, and Mental Health Administration, National Institute on Drug Abuse. DHHS Publication No. (ADM) 85-1334, 1985.

BELL, C.S., LEVY, S.M. Public policy and smoking prevention: Implications for research. In: Matarazzo, J.D., Weiss, S.M., Herd, J.A., Miller, N.E., Weiss, S.M. (eds.) *Behavioral Health. A Handbook of Health Enhancement and Disease Prevention.* New York: John Wiley and Sons, 1984, pp. 775–785.

BENNETT, G., AUSTIN, D., JANIZEWSKI, R. Save a sweet heart: A smoking intervention in senior high school. Paper presented at 114th annual meeting of American Public Health Association, Las Vegas, September 29, 1986.

BENOWITZ, N.L., JACOB, P. III., SAVANAPRIDI, C. Determinants of nicotine intakes while chewing nicotine polacrilex gum. *Clinical Pharmacology and Therapeutics* 41:467–473, 1987.

BEST, J.A., FLAY, B.R., TOWSON, S.M.J., RYAN, K.B., PERRY, C.L., BROWN, K.S., KERSELL, M.W., D'AVERNAS, J.R. Smoking prevention and the concept of risk. *Journal of Applied Social Psychology* 14(3):257–273, 1984.

BEST, J.A., THOMSON, S.J., SANTI, S.M., SMITH, E.A., BROWN, K.S. Preventing cigarette smoking among school children. *Annual Review of Public Health* 9:161–201, 1988.

BIGLAN, A., ARY, D.V. Methodological issues in research on smoking prevention. In: Bell, C.S., Battjes, R. (eds.) *Prevention Research: Deterring Drug Abuse Among Children and*

Adolescents, NIDA Research Monograph 63. U.S. Department of Health and Human Services, Public Health Service, Alcohol, Drug Abuse, and Mental Health Administration, National Institute on Drug Abuse. DHHS Publication No. (ADM) 85-1334, 1985, pp. 170–195.

BIGLAN, A., SEVERSON, H., ARY, D., FALLER, C., GALLISON, C., THOMPSON, R., GLASGOW, R., LICHTENSTEIN, E. Do smoking prevention programs really work? Attrition and the internal and external validity of an evaluation of a refusal skills training program. *Journal of Behavioral Medicine* 10(2):159–171, 1987.

BLAKE, G.H. Smoking and the military. *New York State Journal of Medicine* 85(7):354–355, 1985.

BLUM, A. DOC—Counter advertising has impact. Physicians group launches innovative prevention campaign. *Focus on Alcohol and Drug Issues* 2:22–24, 1979.

BLUM, A. Medicine vs. Madison Avenue. Fighting smoke with smoke. *Journal of the American Medical Association* 243(8):739–740, February 22–29, 1980.

BLUM, A. Strategies to reduce cigarette sales. Excise taxes and beyond. *Journal of the American Medical Association* 255(8):1049–1050, February 28, 1986.

BOTVIN, G.J., ENG, A., WILLIAMS, C.L. Preventing the onset of cigarette smoking through life skills training. *Preventive Medicine* 9:135–143, 1980.

BOTVIN, G.J., RENICK, N.L., BAKER, E. The effects of scheduling format and booster sessions on a broad-spectrum psychosocial approach to smoking prevention. *Journal of Behavioral Medicine* 6(4):359–379, 1983.

BOTVIN, G.J., WILLS, T.A. Personal and social skills training: Cognitive-behavioral approaches to substance abuse prevention. In: Bell, C.S., Battjes, R. (eds.) *Prevention Research: Deterring Drug Abuse Among Children and Adolescents*, NIDA Research Monograph 63. U.S. Department of Health and Human Services, Public Health Service, Alcohol, Drug Abuse, and Mental Health Administration, National Institute on Drug Abuse. DHHS Publication No. (ADM) 85-1334, 1985, pp. 8–49.

BRAY, R.M., MARSDEN, M.E., GUESS, L.L., WHEELESS, S.C., PATE, D., DUNTEMAN, G.H., IANNACCHIONE, V.G. *1985 Worldwide Survey of Alcohol and Nonmedical Drug Use Among Military Personnel.* North Carolina: Research Triangle Institute, June 1986.

BRITISH THORACIC SOCIETY. Comparison of four methods of smoking withdrawal in patients with smoking related diseases. *British Medical Journal* 286(6366):595–597, February 19, 1983.

BUREAU OF NATIONAL AFFAIRS. *Where There's Smoke: Problems and Policies Concerning Smoking in the Workplace*, Second Edition. Washington, D.C.: Bureau of National Affairs, 1987.

BURNEY, L.E. Smoking and lung cancer. A statement of the Public Health Service. *Journal of the American Medical Association* 171(13):1829–1837, November 28, 1959.

CALIFORNIA NONSMOKERS' RIGHTS FOUNDATION. *A Curriculum for Death in the West.* Berkeley, California: California Nonsmokers' Rights Foundation, 1983.

CAMPBELL, I.A., LYONS, E., PRESCOTT, R.J. Stopping smoking. Do nicotine chewing-gum and postal encouragement add to doctors' advice. *Practitioner* 231:114–117, January 8, 1987.

CENTERS FOR DISEASE CONTROL. Survey of chronic disease activities in State and territorial health agencies. *Morbidity and Mortality Weekly Report* 36(34):565–568, September 4, 1987.

CHAPMAN, S. Stop smoking clinics: A case for their abandonment. *Lancet* 1(8434):918–920, April 20, 1985.

CHASSIN, L., PRESSON, C.C., SHERMAN, S.J. Cognitive and social influence factors in adolescent smoking cessation. *Addictive Behaviors* 9:383–390, 1984.

CHASSIN, L., PRESSON, C.C., SHERMAN, S.J., MCGREW, J. The changing smoking environment for middle and high school students: 1980–1983. *Journal of Behavioral Medicine* 10(6):581–593, 1987.

CHASSIN, L.A., PRESSON, C.C., SHERMAN, S.J. Stepping backward in order to step forward: An acquisition-oriented approach to primary prevention. *Journal of Consulting and Clinical Psychology* 53(5):612–622, 1985.

CLARKE, J.H., MACPHERSON, B., HOLMES, D.R., JONES, R. Reducing adolescent smoking: A comparison of peer-led, teacher-led, and expert interventions. *Journal of School Health* 56(3):102–106, March 1986.

CLEARY, P.D., HITCHCOCK, J.L., SEMMER, N., FLINCHBAUGH, L.J., PINNEY, J.M. Adolescent smoking: Research and health policy. *Milbank Quarterly* 66(1):137–171, 1988.

COHEN, S.B. Should medical associations discourage smoking? *Journal of the American Medical Association* 239(29):2158, May 19, 1978.

COHEN, S.J., CHRISTEN, A.G., KATZ, B.P., DROOK, C.A., DAVIS, B.J., SMITH, D.M., STOOKEY, G.K. Counseling medical and dental patients about cigarette smoking: The impact of nicotine gum and chart reminders. *American Journal of Public Health* 77(3):313–316, 1987.

CONNELL, D.B., TURNER, R.R. The impact of instructional experience and the effects of cumulative instruction. *Journal of School Health* 55(8):324–331, 1985.

CONNELL, D.B., TURNER, R.R., MASON, E.F. Summary of findings of the School Health Education Evaluation: Health promotion effectiveness, implementation and costs. *Journal of School Health* 55(8):316–321, 1985a.

COYE, M.J. Preventing tobacco dependence: The New Jersey Commission on Smoking or Health. *New Jersey Medicine* 85(2):151–155, February 1988.

CULLEN, J.W. Design of cancer prevention studies. *Cancer Detection and Prevention* 9:125–138, 1986.

CULLEN, J.W., MCKENNA, J.W., MASSEY, M.M. International control of smoking and the US experience. *Chest* 89(4, Supplement):206S–218S, April 1986.

CUMMINGS, K.M., EMONT, S.L., JAEN, C., SCIANDRA, R. Format and quitting instructions as factors influencing the impact of a self-administered quit smoking program. *Health Education Quarterly* 15(2):199–216, Summer 1988.

CUMMINGS, K.M., HELLMANN, R., EMONT, S.L. Correlates of participation in a worksite stop-smoking contest. *Journal of Behavioral Medicine* 11(3):267–277, 1988.

DANAHER, B.G. Smoking cessation programs in occupational settings. *Public Health Reports* 95(2):149–157, March–April, 1980.

DAVIS, A.L., FAUST, R., ORDENTLICH, M. Self-help smoking cessation and maintenance programs: A comparative study with 12-month follow-up by the American Lung Association. *American Journal of Public Health* 74:1212–1217, 1984.

DAVIS, R.L. Positive smoking education programs for the school-age child. In: Steinfeld, J., Griffiths, W., Ball. K., Taylor, R.M. (eds.) *Smoking and Health. II. Health Consequences, Education, Cessation Activities, and Governmental Action.* Proceedings of the 3rd World Conference on Smoking and Health. U.S. Department of Health, Education, and Welfare, Public Health Service, National Institutes of Health, National Cancer Institute. DHEW Publication No. (NIH) 77-1413, 1977, pp. 237–244.

DAVIS, R.M. Health education on the six-o'clock news: Motivating television coverage of news in medicine. *Journal of the American Medical Association* 259(7):1036–1038, February 19, 1988a.

DAVIS, R.M. Uniting physicians against smoking: The need for a coordinated national strategy. *Journal of the American Medical Association* 259(19):2900–2901, May 20, 1988b.

DAWLEY, H.H. JR., FINKEL, C. The Great American Smokeout: A follow-up report. *Addictive Behaviors* 6(2):153–154, 1981.

DIEHL, H.S. *Tobacco and Your Health: The Smoking Controversy.* New York: McGraw-Hill, 1969.

DIELMAN, T.E., LORENGER, A.T., LEECH, S.L., LYONS, A.L., KLOS, D.M., HORVATH, W.J. Fifteen-month follow-up results of an elementary school based smoking prevention project. *Hygiene* 4(4):28–35, 1985.

DILLOW, G.L. The hundred-year war against the cigarette. *American Heritage*, February–March, 1981, pp. 3–15.

DORSEY, J.L. Control of the tobacco habit. *Annals of Internal Medicine* 10:628–631, 1936.

DOYLE, J.T., DAWBER, T.R., KANNEL, W.B., KINCH, S.H., KAHN, H.A. The relationship of cigarette smoking to coronary heart disease. *Journal of the American Medical Association* 190(10):108–112, December 7, 1964.

EMMONS, K.M., EMONT, S.L., COLLINS, R.L., WEIDNER, G. Relapse prevention versus broad spectrum treatment for smoking cessation: A comparison of efficacy. *Journal of Substance Abuse* 1(1):79–89, 1988.

ERSHLER, J., LEVENTHAL, H., FLEMING, R., GLYNN, K. The quitting experience for smokers in sixth through twelfth grade. *Addictive Behaviors*, in press.

EVANS, R.I. Smoking in children: Developing a social psychological strategy of deterrence. *Preventive Medicine* 5:122–127, 1976.

EVANS, R.I. A social inoculation strategy to deter smoking in adolescents. In: Matarazzo, J.D., Weiss, S.M., Herd, J.A., Miller, N.E., Weiss, S.M. (eds.) *Behavioral Health: Handbook of Health Enhancement and Disease Prevention.* New York: John Wiley and Sons, 1984, pp. 765–774.

EVANS, R.I., HENDERSON, A.H., HILL, P.C., RAINES, B.E. Current psychological, social, and educational programs in the control and prevention of smoking: A critical methodological review. *Atherosclerosis Review* 6:203–245, 1979.

EVANS, R.I., ROZELLE, R.M., MAXWELL, S.E., RAINES, B.E., DILL, C.A., GUTHRIE, T.J., HENDERSON, A.H., HILL, P.C. Social modeling films to deter smoking in adolescents: Results of a three-year field investigation. *Journal of Applied Psychology* 66(4):399–414, 1981.

FAGERSTROM, K.-O. A comparison of psychological and pharmacological treatment in smoking cessation. *Journal of Behavioral Medicine* 5(3):343–351, 1982.

FANNING, O. Prevention efforts shift from passive to active. *Oncology and Biotechnology News* 2(4):2, 1988.

FEE, W.M., STEWART, M.J. A controlled trial of nicotine chewing gum in a smoking withdrawal clinic. *Practitioner* 226(1363):148, 151, January 1982.

FERNOE, O., LICHTNECKERT, S.J.A., LUNDGREN, C.E.G. A substitute for tobacco smoking. *Psychopharmacologia* 31(3):201–204, 1973.

FIORE, M., NOVOTNY, T., LYNN, W., MAKLAN, D., DAVIS, R. Smoking cessation: Data from the 1986 Adult Use of Tobacco Survey. In: Aoki, M., Hisamichi, S., Tominaga, S. (eds.) *Smoking and Health 1987.* Proceedings of the 6th World Conference on Smoking and Health, Tokyo, November 9–12, 1987. Amsterdam: Excerpta Medica, 1988, pp. 189–194.

FLAY, B.R. Psychosocial approaches to smoking prevention: A review of findings. *Health Psychology* 4(5):449–488, 1985a.

FLAY, B.R. What we know about the social influences approach to smoking prevention: Review and recommendations. In: Bell, C.S., Battjes, R. (eds.) *Prevention Research: Deterring Drug Abuse Among Children and Adolescents*, NIDA Research Monograph 63. U.S. Department of Health and Human Services, Public Health Service, Alcohol, Drug Abuse, and

Mental Health Administration, National Institute on Drug Abuse. DHHS Publication No. (ADM) 85-1334, 1985b, pp. 67–112.

FLAY, B.R. Mass media linkages with school-based programs for drug abuse prevention. *Journal of School Health* 56(9):402–406, November 1986.

FLAY, B.R. Mass media and smoking cessation: A critical review. *American Journal of Public Health* 77(2):153–160, February 1987a.

FLAY, B.R. *Selling the Smokeless Society: 56 Evaluated Mass Media Programs and Campaigns Worldwide*. Washington, D.C.: American Public Health Association, 1987b.

FLAY, B.R., BRANNON, B.R., JOHNSON, C.A., HANSEN, W.B., ULENE, A.L., WHITNEY-SALTIEL, D.A., GLEASON, L.R., SUSSMAN, S., GAVIN, M.D., GLOWACZ, K.M., SOBOL, D.F., SPIEGEL, D.C. The Television School and Family Smoking Prevention and Cessation Project. I. Theoretical basis and program development. *Preventive Medicine* 17:585–607, 1988.

FLAY, B.R., D'AVERNAS, J.R., BEST, J.A., KERSELL, M.W., RYAN, K.B. Cigarette smoking: Why young people do it and ways of preventing it. In: McGrath, P., Firestone, P. (eds.) *Pediatric and Adolescent Behavioral Medicine*, Volume 10. New York: Springer Publishing, 1983, pp. 132–183.

FLAY, B.R., HANSEN, W.B., JOHNSON, C.A., COLLINS, L.M., DENT, C.W., DWYER, K.M., GROSSMAN, L., HOCKSTEIN, G., RAUCH, J., SOBEL, J.L., SOBOL, D.F., SUSSMAN, S., ULENE, A. Implementation effectiveness trial of a social influences smoking prevention program using schools and television. *Health Education Research* 2(4):385–400, 1987.

FLAY, B.R., RYAN, K.B., BEST, J.A., BROWN, K.S., KERSELL, M.W., D'AVERNAS, J.R., ZANNA, M.P. Are social-psychological smoking prevention programs effective? The Waterloo Study. *Journal of Behavioral Medicine* 8(1):37–59, March 1985.

FLAY, B.R., SOBEL, J.L. The role of mass media in preventing adolescent substance abuse. In: Glynn, T.J., Leukefeld, C.G., Ludford, J.P. (eds.) *Preventing Adolescent Drug Abuse: Intervention Strategies*, NIDA Research Monograph 47. U.S. Department of Health and Human Services, Public Health Service, Alcohol, Drug Abuse, and Mental Health Administration, National Institute on Drug Abuse. DHHS Publication No. (ADM) 85-1280, 1983, pp. 5–35.

FLAY, B.R., THOMPSON, S., SANTI, S., BEST, J.A., BROWN, S.K. Long-term follow-up of the Waterloo Smoking Prevention Trial. Paper presented at the 6th World Conference on Smoking and Health, Tokyo, November 9–12, 1987.

FOOD AND DRUG ADMINISTRATION. Letter from Mark Novitch for Jere E. Glyan, Commissioner of Food and Drugs, to John F. Banzhaf III and Peter N. Georgiades, Action on Smoking and Health, November 25, 1980 (Docket Nos. 77P-0185 and 78P-0338/CP).

FOOD AND DRUG ADMINISTRATION. Smoking deterrent drug products for over-the-counter human use; establishment of a monograph. *Federal Register* 47:490–500, January 5, 1982.

FOOD AND DRUG ADMINISTRATION. Smoking deterrent drug products for over-the-counter human use; tentative final monograph. *Federal Register* 50:27552–27557, July 3, 1985.

FREDERIKSEN, L.W., PRUE, D.M., ORLANDI, M.A., EDELMAN, B.R., WYNDER, E.L. *Development of a Computer Assisted Smoking Treatment Program: A Preliminary Report.* Cambridge, Massachusetts: Institute for the Study of Smoking Behavior and Policy, John F. Kennedy School of Government, Harvard University, February 1988.

FRIEDMAN, K.M. *Public Policy and the Smoking–Health Controversy. A Comparative Study.* Lexington, Massachusetts: D.C. Heath, 1975.

FRITSCHLER, A.L. *Smoking and Politics: Policymaking and the Federal Bureaucracy*, Second Edition. Englewood Cliffs, New Jersey; Prentice-Hall, 1975.

FULLER, J.A Smoking withdrawal and acupuncture. *Medical Journal of Australia* 1:28–29, 1982.

GARDNER, J.W. *In Common Cause*. New York: W.W. Norton, 1973.

GARFINKEL, L., STELLMAN, S.D. Cigarette smoking among physicians, dentists, and nurses. *CA—A Cancer Journal for Clinicians* 36(1):2–8, January–February 1986.

GILCHRIST, L.D., SCHINKE, S.P. Improving smoking prevention programs. *Journal of Psychosocial Oncology* 3(1):67–78, Spring 1985.

GILCHRIST, L.D., SCHINKE, S.P., NURIUS, P. Reducing initiation of habitual smoking among women. *Preventive Medicine*, in press.

GLASGOW, R.E., LICHTENSTEIN, E. Long-term effects of behavioral smoking cessation interventions. *Behavior Therapy* 18:297–324, 1987.

GLASGOW, R.E., ROSEN, G.M. Behavioral bibliotherapy: A review of self-help behavior therapy manuals. *Psychological Bulletin* 85(1):1–23, January 1978.

GLASSMAN, A.H., JACKSON, W.K., WALSH, B.T., ROOSE, S.P., ROSENFELD, B. Cigarette craving, smoking withdrawal, and clonidine. *Science* 226:864–866, November 16, 1984.

GLASSMAN, A.H., STETNER, F., WALSH, T., RAIZMAN, P.S., FLEISS, J.L., COOPER, T.B., COVEY, L.S. Heavy smokers, smoking cessation, and clonidine: Results of a double-blind, randomized trial. *Journal of the American Medical Association* 259(19):2863–2866, May 20, 1988.

GLOVER, E.D. Conducting smokeless tobacco cessation clinics. *American Journal of Public Health* 76(2):207, 1986.

GLYNN, K., LEVENTHAL, H., HIRSCHMAN, R. A cognitive developmental approach to smoking prevention. In: Bell, C.S., Battjes, R. (eds.) *Prevention Research: Deterring Drug Abuse Among Children and Adolescents*, NIDA Research Monograph 63. U.S. Department of Health and Human Services, Public Health Service, Alcohol, Drug Abuse, and Mental Health Administration, National Institute on Drug Abuse. DHHS Publication No. (ADM) 85-1334, 1985, pp. 130–152.

GLYNN, T.J. Essential elements of school-based smoking prevention programs: Research results. *Journal of School Health*, in press.

GORI, G.B., LYNCH, C.J. Toward less hazardous cigarettes. *Journal of the American Medical Association* 240(12):1255–1259, September 15, 1978.

GREEN, L.W., GREEN, P.F. Intervening in social systems to make smoking education more effective. In: Steinfeld, J., Griffiths, W., Ball, K., Taylor, R.M. (eds.) *Smoking and Health. II. Health Consequences, Education, Cessation Activities, and Governmental Action.* Proceedings of the 3rd World Conference on Smoking and Health. U.S. Department of Health, Education, and Welfare, Public Health Service, National Institutes of Health, National Cancer Institute. DHEW Publication No. (NIH) 77-1413, 1977, pp. 393–401.

GRITZ E., CARR, C.R., MARCUS, A.C. Unaided smoking cessation: Great American Smokeout and New Year's Day quitters. *Journal of Psychosocial Oncology*, in press.

GRITZ, E.R. Gender and the teenage smoker. In: Ray, B.A., Braude, M.C. (eds.) *Women and Drugs: A New Era for Research*, NIDA Research Monograph 65. U.S. Department of Health and Human Services, Public Health Service, Alcohol, Drug Abuse, and Mental Health Administration, National Institute on Drug Abuse. DHHS Publication No. (ADM) 86-1447, 1986, pp. 70–79.

HALL, R.G., SACHS, D.P.L., HALL, S.M., BENOWITZ, N.L. Two-year efficacy and safety of rapid smoking therapy in patients with cardiac and pulmonary disease. *Journal of Consulting and Clinical Psychology* 52(4):574–581, 1984a.

HALL, S.M., RUGG, D., TUNSTALL, C., JONES, R.T. Preventing relapse to cigarette smoking by behavioral skill training. *Journal of Consulting and Clinical Psychology* 52:373–382, 1984b.

HALL, S.M., TUNSTALL, C.D., GINSBERG, D., BENOWITZ, N.L., JONES, R.T. Nicotine gum and behavioral treatment: A placebo controlled trial. *Journal of Consulting and Clinical Psychology* 55(4):603–605, 1987.

HAMILTON, J.L. The demand for cigarettes: Advertising, the health scare, and the cigarette advertising ban. *Review of Economics and Statistics* 54:401–411, November 1972.

HAMM, A.C. Massive antismoking intervention trial to begin in the fall. *Journal of the National Cancer Institute* 80(10):717–718, July 20, 1988.

HAMMOND, E.C., HORN, D. Smoking and death rates—Report on forty-four months of follow-up of 187,783 men. I. Total mortality. *Journal of the American Medical Association* 166(10):1159–1172, March 8, 1958.

HANSEN, W.B. Behavioral predictors of abstinence: Early indicators of a dependence on tobacco among adolescents. *International Journal of the Addictions* 18(7):913–920, 1983.

HANSEN, W.B., COLLINS, L.M., JOHNSON, C.A., GRAHAM, J.W. Self-initiated smoking cessation among high school students. *Addictive Behaviors* 10:265–271, 1985.

HARVEY, L., SHUBAT, S. Public opinion on health issues. In: *AMA Surveys of Physician and Public Opinion on Health Care Issues, 1987*. Chicago: American Medical Association, April 1987.

HERBOLD, J.R. Smoking habits of U.S. military personnel. *Military Medicine* 152(4):194–195, April 1987.

HJALMARSON, A.I.M. Effect of nicotine gum in smoking cessation. A randomized, placebo-controlled, double-blind study. *Journal of the American Medical Association* 252(20):2835–2838, November 23–30, 1984.

HOPS, H., WEISSMAN, W., BIGLAN, A., THOMPSON, R., FALLER, C., SEVERSON, H.H. A taped situation test of cigarette refusal skill among adolescents. *Behavioral Assessment* 8:145–154, 1986.

HUGHES, G.H., HYMOWITZ, N., OCKENE, J.K., SIMON, N., VOGT, T.M. The Multiple Risk Factor Intervention Trial (MRFIT). V. Intervention on smoking. *Preventive Medicine* 10(4):476–500, July 1981.

HUGHES, J.R., MILLER, S.A. Nicotine gum to help stop smoking. *Journal of the American Medical Association* 252(20):2855–2858, November 23–30, 1984.

HULBERT, J. Cessation among youth: Experiences in selected secondary schools in Iowa. In: Schwartz, J.L. (ed.) *Proceedings of International Conference on Smoking Cessation*. New York: American Cancer Society, 1978, pp. 335–337.

HUNT, W.A., BESPALEC, D.A. An evaluation of current methods of modifying smoking behavior. *Journal of Clinical Psychology* 30:431–438, 1973.

HURD, P.D., JOHNSON, C.A., PECHACEK, T., BAST, L.P., JACOBS, D.R., LUEPKER, R.V. Prevention of cigarette smoking in seventh grade students. *Journal of Behavioral Medicine* 3(1):15–28, 1980.

IGLEHART, J.K. The campaign against smoking gains momentum. *New England Journal of Medicine* 314(16):1059–1064, April 17, 1986.

IMS. Nicorette. *New Products Digest*, August 1984.

INSTITUTE FOR THE STUDY OF SMOKING BEHAVIOR AND POLICY. *The Policy Implications of the 1986 Surgeon General's Report on Involuntary Smoking*. Cambridge, Massachusetts: Institute for the Study of Smoking Behavior and Policy, John F. Kennedy School of Government, Harvard University, 1988.

IVERSON, D.C., KOLBE, L.J. Evolution of the national disease prevention and health promotion strategy: Establishing a role for the schools. *Journal of School Health* 53(5):294–302, May 1983.

JAMROZIK, K., FOWLER, G., VESSEY, M., WALD, N. Placebo controlled trial of nicotine chewing gum in general practice. *British Medical Journal* 289(6448):794–797, 1984.

JARVIK, M.E., CULLEN, J.W., GRITZ, E.R., VOGT, T.M., WEST, L.J. (eds.) *Research on Smoking Behavior*, NIDA Research Monograph 17. U.S. Department of Health, Education, and Welfare, Public Health Service, Alcohol, Drug Abuse, and Mental Health Administration, National Institute on Drug Abuse. DHEW Publication No. (ADM) 78-581, December 1977.

JARVIS, M.J., RAW, M., RUSSELL, M.A.H., FEYERABEND, C. Randomised controlled trial of nicotine chewing-gum. *British Medical Journal* 285(6341):537–540, December 21, 1982.

JASON, L.A., MOLLICA, M., FERRONE, L. Evaluating an early secondary smoking prevention intervention. *Preventive Medicine* 11:96–102, 1982.

JOHNSON, C.A., HANSEN, W.B., COLLINS, L.M., GRAHAM, J.W. High-school smoking prevention: Results of a three-year longitudinal study. *Journal of Behavioral Medicine* 9(5): 439–452, 1986.

JOHNSTON, L.D., O'MALLEY, P.M., BACHMAN, J.G. *National Trends in Drug Use and Related Factors Among American High School Students and Young Adults, 1975–1986*. U.S. Department of Health and Human Services, Public Health Service, Alcohol, Drug Abuse, and Mental Health Administration, National Institute on Drug Abuse. DHHS Publication No. (ADM) 87-1535, 1987.

KILLEN, J.D. Prevention of adolescent tobacco smoking: The social pressure resistance training approach. *Journal of Child Psychology and Psychiatry* 26(1):7–15, 1985.

KILLEN, J.D., MACCOBY, N., TAYLOR, C.B. Nicotine gum and self-regulation training in smoking relapse prevention. *Behavior Therapy* 15(3):234–248, 1984.

KING, A.C., FLORA, J.A., FORTMANN, S.P., TAYLOR, C.B. Smokers' challenge: Immediate and long-term findings of a community smoking cessation contest. *American Journal of Public Health* 77(10):1340–1341, October 1987.

KLESGES, R.C., VASEY, M.M., GLASGOW, R.E. A worksite smoking modification competition: Potential for public health impact. *American Journal of Public Health* 76(2):198–200, February 1986.

KOLBE, L.J., GILBERT, G.G. Involving the schools in the national strategy to improve the health of Americans. In: *Proceedings of Prospects for a Healthier America: Achieving the Nation's Health Promotion Objectives.* U.S. Department of Health and Human Services, Public Health Service, Office of Disease Prevention and Health Promotion, 1984, pp. 57–69.

KOLBE, L.J., IVERSON, D.C. Comprehensive school health education programs. In: Matarazzo, J.D., Weiss, S.M., Herd, J.A., Miller, N.E., Weiss, S.M. (eds.) *Behavioral Health: A Handbook of Health Enhancement and Disease Prevention.* New York: John Wiley and Sons, 1984, pp. 1094–1116.

KOTTKE, T.E., BATTISTA, R.N., DEFRIESE, G.H., BREKKE, M.L. Attributes of successful smoking cessation interventions in medical practice. A meta-analysis of 39 controlled trials. *Journal of the American Medical Association* 259:2883–2889, May 20, 1988.

KRASNEGOR, N.A. (ed.) *Cigarette Smoking as a Dependence Process*, NIDA Research Monograph 23. U.S. Department of Health, Education, and Welfare, Public Health Service, Alcohol, Drug Abuse, and Mental Health Administration, National Institute on Drug Abuse. DHEW Publication No. (ADM) 79-800, 1979a.

KRASNEGOR, N.A. (ed.) *The Behavioral Aspects of Smoking*, NIDA Research Monograph 26. U.S. Department of Health, Education, and Welfare, Public Health Service, Alcohol, Drug

Abuse, and Mental Health Administration, National Institute on Drug Abuse. DHEW Publication No. (ADM) 79-882, 1979b.
LEVENTHAL, H., CLEARY, P.D. The smoking problem: A review of the research and theory in behavioral risk modification. *Psychological Bulletin* 88(2):370–405, 1980.
LICHTENSTEIN, E., BROWN, R.A. Smoking cessation methods: Review and recommendations. In: Miller, W.R. (ed.) *The Addictive Behaviors: Treatment of Alcoholism, Drug Abuse, Smoking, and Obesity*. Oxford: Pergamon Press, 1980.
LICHTENSTEIN, E., BROWN, R.A. Current trends in the modification of cigarette dependence. In: Bellach, A., Hersen, M., Kazdig, A.E. (eds.) *International Handbook of Behavior Modification*, Volume 2. New York: Plenum Press, 1983.
LICHTENSTEIN, E., DANAHER, B.G. Modification of smoking behavior: A critical analysis of theory, research, and practice. In: Hersen, M., Eisler, R., Miller, P.M. (eds.) *Progress in Behavioral Modification*, Volume 3. New York: Academic Press, 1976.
LICHTENSTEIN, E., GLASGOW, R.E., ABRAMS, D.B. Social support in smoking cessation: In search of effective interventions. *Behavior Therapy* 17:607–619, 1986.
LOHRMANN, D.K., GOLD, R.S., JUBB, W.H. School health education: A foundation for school health programs. *Journal of School Health* 57(10):420–425, December 1987.
LUEPKER, R.V., JOHNSON, C.A., MURRAY, D.M., PECHACEK, T.F. Prevention of cigarette smoking: Three-year follow-up of an education program for youth. *Journal of Behavioral Medicine* 6(1):53–62, 1983.
LUNDBERG, G.D. The AMA, policy follows science: A case history of tobacco. *Journal of the American Medical Assocation* 253(20):3001–3003, May 24–31, 1985.
LUNDBERG, G.D., KNOLL, E. Tobacco: For consenting adults in private only. *Journal of the American Medical Association* 255(8):1051–1053, February 1986.
MACHOVEC, F.J., MAN, S.C. Acupuncture and hypnosis compared: Fifty-eight cases. *American Journal of Clinical Hypnosis* 21(1):45–47, July 1978.
MARLATT, G.A., GORDON, J.R. *Relapse Prevention: Maintenance Strategies in the Treatment of Addictive Behaviors*. New York: Guilford Press, 1985.
MARSTON, A.R., BETTENCOURT, A. An evaluation of the American Lung Association's home video smoking cessation program. *American Journal of Public Health* 78(9):1226–1227, 1988.
MARTIN, G.P., WAITE, P.M.E. The efficacy of acupuncture as an aid to stopping smoking. *New Zealand Medical Journal* 93:421–423, June 24, 1981.
MARTIN, M.J., FEHRENBACH, A., ROSNER, R. Ban on smoking in industry. (Letter.) *New England Journal of Medicine* 315(10):647–648, September 4, 1986.
MCALISTER, A., GORDON, N.P. Attrition bias in a cohort study of substance abuse onset and prevention. *Evaluation Review* 10(6):853–859, December 1986.
MCALISTER, A.L., PERRY, C., KILLEN, J., SLINKARD, L.A., MACCOBY, N. Pilot study of smoking, alcohol and drug abuse prevention. *American Journal of Public Health* 70(7): 719–721, July 1980.
MCALISTER, A.L., PERRY, C., MACCOBY, N. Adolescent smoking: Onset and prevention. *Pediatrics* 63:650–658, 1979.
MCCAUL, K.D., GLASGOW, R.E. Preventing adolescent smoking: What have we learned about treatment construct validity? *Health Psychology* 4(4):361–387, 1985.
MCFARLAND, M.I. When five became twenty-five. A silver anniversary of the five-day plan to stop smoking. *Adventist Heritage* 11(1):57–64, 1986.
MERKI, D.J., CRESWELL, W.H., STONE, D.B., HUFFMAN, W., NEWMAN, I. The effects of two educational methods and message themes on rural youth smoking behavior. *Journal of School Health* 38:448–454, 1968.

MINNESOTA DEPARTMENT OF HEALTH. *The Minnesota Nonsmoking Initiative. June, 1985–December 1986. A Report to the 1987 Legislature*, Minnesota Department of Health, Center for Nonsmoking and Health, 1987.

MITCHELL, V. Instant answers for students on what smoking does to the body. *American Lung Association Bulletin* 64(8):6–9, October 1978.

MOSKOWITZ, J.M. Preventing adolescent substance abuse through drug education. In: Glynn, T.J., Leukefeld, C.G., Ludford, J.P. (eds.) *Preventing Adolescent Drug Abuse*, NIDA Research Monograph 47. U.S. Department of Health and Human Services, Public Health Service, Alcohol, Drug Abuse, and Mental Health Administration, National Institute on Drug Abuse. DHHS Publication No. (ADM) 85-1280, 1983, pp. 233–249.

MULTIPLE RISK FACTOR INTERVENTION TRIAL RESEARCH GROUP. Multiple Risk Factor Intervention Trial: Risk factor changes and mortality results. *Journal of the American Medical Association* 248(12):1465–1477, September 24, 1982.

MURRAY, D.M. Dissemination of community health promotion programs: The Fargo-Moorhead Heart Health Program. *Journal of School Health* 56(9):375–381, November 1986.

MURRAY, D.M., JOHNSON, C.A., LUEPKER, R.V., MITTELMARK, M.B. The prevention of cigarette smoking in children: A comparison of four strategies. *Journal of Applied Social Psychology* 14(3):274–288, 1984.

NATIONAL CANCER INSTITUTE. *Utilizing Physicians, Dentists, and Pharmacists as Health Exemplars to Help Smokers Quit—A Case Study*. National Cancer Institute, Office of Cancer Communications, April 1982.

NATIONAL CANCER INSTITUTE. *Smoking, Tobacco, and Cancer Program. Annual Report 1983*. U.S. Department of Health and Human Services, National Cancer Institute. NIH Publication No. 84-2687, September 1984.

NATIONAL CANCER INSTITUTE. *Smoking, Tobacco, and Cancer Program. 1985 Report*. National Cancer Institute, U.S. Department of Health and Human Services, Public Health Service, National Institutes of Health. NIH Publication No. 86-2687, April 1986a.

NATIONAL CANCER INSTITUTE. Integrating tobacco education into the school system. Request for research grant applications: NIH-NCI-DCPC-HPSB-CA. U.S. Department of Health and Human Services, Public Health Service, National Institutes of Health, National Cancer Institute, 1986b.

NATIONAL DIFFUSION NETWORK. *Final Report: Adoption Data*. Hampton, New Hampshire: National Diffusion Network Technical Assistance, April 1988a.

NATIONAL DIFFUSION NETWORK. *Educational Programs That Work. A Collection of Proven Exemplary Educational Programs and Practices*, Fourteenth Edition. Longmont, Colorado: Sophis West, 1988b.

NATIONAL HEART, LUNG, AND BLOOD INSTITUTE. *Smoking Education Program Overview*. National Heart, Lung, and Blood Institute, Office of Prevention, Education, and Control, 1988.

NATIONAL HEART, LUNG, AND BLOOD INSTITUTE, NATIONAL INSTITUTES OF HEALTH. *Protocol for the Study of Early Intervention for Chronic Obstructive Pulmonary Disease*. National Heart, Lung, and Blood Institute, Division of Lung Diseases, 1986.

NATIONAL INSTITUTES OF HEALTH. Announcement. Prevention and cessation of use of smokeless tobacco. *NIH Guide for Grants and Contracts* 15(3):38–41, February 28, 1986.

NATIONAL INTERAGENCY COUNCIL ON SMOKING AND HEALTH. *Cookbook for a Smokeless Diet*. U.S. Department of Health, Education, and Welfare, Public Health Service, Centers for Disease Control, Bureau of Health Education, National Clearinghouse for Smoking and Health, 1977.

NATIONAL INTERAGENCY COUNCIL ON SMOKING AND HEALTH. *Final Report: Youth Leadership in Smoking Controls Program.* CDC 200-78-0815. National Interagency Council on Smoking and Health, September 30, 1979.

NATIONAL SCHOOL BOARDS ASSOCIATION. *No Smoking: A Board Member's Guide to Nonsmoking Policies for the Schools.* Alexandria, Virginia: National School Boards Association, June 1987.

NEWSWEEK. The kick-the-habit business: Corporations pay big money to help smokers quit. *Newsweek,* August 29, 1988, pp. 42–43.

NUEHRING, E., MARKLE, G.E. Nicotine and norms: The re-emergence of a deviant behavior. *Social Problems* 21:513–526, 1974.

O'ROURKE, T., NOLTE, A.E., SMITH, B.J. Improving anti-smoking education: Profiling the ex-smoker. *Journal of Drug Education* 15(1):7–22, 1985.

OCKENE, J.K. Physician-delivered interventions for smoking cessation: Strategies for increasing effectiveness. *Preventive Medicine* 16:723–737, 1987.

OCKENE, J.K., HOSMER, D.W., WILLIAMS, J.W., GOLDBERG, R.J., OCKENE, I.S., BILIOURIS, T., DALEN, J.E. The relationship of patient characteristics to physician delivered smoking cessation advice. *Journal of General Internal Medicine* 2:337–340, 1987.

OCKENE, J.K., HYMOWITZ, N., SEXTON, M., BROSTE, S.K. Comparison of patterns of smoking behavior change among smokers in the Multiple Risk Factor Intervention Trial (MRFIT). *Preventive Medicine* 11:621–638, 1982.

OCKENE, J.K., QUIRK, M.E., GOLDBERG, R.J., KRISTELLER, J.L., DONNELLY, G., KALAN, K.L., GOULD, B., GREENE, H.L., HARRISON-ATLAS, R., PREASE, J., PICKENS, S., WILLIAMS, J.W. A residents' training program for the development of smoking intervention skills. *Archives of Internal Medicine* 148:1039–1045, May 1988.

OEI, T.P.S., FEA, A. Smoking prevention program for children: A review. *Journal of Drug Education* 17(1):11–42, 1987.

OMENN, G.S., THOMPSON, B., SEXTON, M., HESSOL, N., BREITENSTEIN, B., CURRY, S., MICHNICH, M., PETERSEN, A. A randomized comparison of worksite-sponsored smoking cessation programs. *American Journal of Preventive Medicine* 4(5):261–267, 1988.

ORLANDI, M.A. The diffusion and adoption of worksite health promotion innovations: An analysis of barriers. *Preventive Medicine* 15:522–536, 1986.

ORLEANS, C.S., SHIPLEY, R.H. Worksite smoking cessation initiatives: Review and recommendations. *Addictive Behaviors* 7:1–16, 1982.

PARKER, S., WARNER, K.E. Smoking policies in the workplace: Research needs and potential applications. *New York State Journal of Medicine 89(1):2–4,* January 1989.

PATTERSON, J.T. *The Dread Disease. Cancer and Modern American Culture.* Cambridge, Massachusetts: Harvard University Press, 1987.

PECHACEK, T. A randomized community trial for smoking cessation. In: Aoki, M., Hisamichi, S., Tominaga, S. (eds.) *Smoking and Health, 1987.* Proceedings of the 6th World Conference on Smoking and Health, Tokyo, November 9–12, 1987. Amsterdam: Excerpta Medica, 1988. pp. 241–243.

PECHACEK, T.F. Modification of smoking behavior. In: Krasnegor, N.A. (ed.) *The Behavioral Aspects of Smoking,* NIDA Research Monograph 26. U.S. Department of Health, Education, and Welfare, Public Health Service, Alcohol, Drug Abuse, and Mental Health Administration, National Institute on Drug Abuse. DHEW Publication No. 79-882, August 1979, pp. 127–188.

PERRY, C.L., KILLEN, J., SLINKARD, L.A., MCALISTER, A.L. Peer teaching and smoking prevention among junior high students. *Adolescence* 15(58):277–281, 1980.

PERRY, C.L., KILLEN, J., TELCH, M., SLINKARD, L.A., DANAHER, B.G. Modifying smoking behavior of teenagers: A school-based intervention. *American Journal of Public Health* 70(7):722–725, 1980.

PERRY, C.L., MURRAY, D.M. Enhancing the transition years: The challenge of adolescent health promotion. *The Journal of School Health* 52(5):307–311, 1982.

PERRY, C.L., TELCH, M.J., KILLEN, J., BURKE, A., MACCOBY, N. High school smoking prevention: The relative efficacy of varied treatments and instructors. *Adolescence* 18(71): 561–566, 1983.

PERTSCHUK, M. *Giant Killers.* New York: Norton, 1986.

PIGG, R.M. JR., BAILEY, W.J., SEFFRIN, J.R., TORABI, M.R., LAVE, J.S. Evaluation of American Cancer Society elementary school public education programs. *Journal of School Health* 55(4):157–160, 1985.

PIRIE, P.L., MURRAY, D.M., LUEPKER, R.V. Smoking prevalence in a cohort of adolescents, including absentees, dropouts, and transfers. *American Journal of Public Health* 78(2):176–178, 1988.

POLICH, J.M., ELLICKSON, P.L., REUTER, P., KAHAN, J.P. *Strategies for Controlling Adolescent Drug Use.* Santa Monica, California: Rand Corporation, 1984.

POWELL, D.R., MCCANN, B.S. The effects of a multiple treatment program and maintenance procedures on smoking cessation. *Preventive Medicine* 10:94–104, 1981.

PROCHASKA, J.O., DICLEMENTE, C.C. Stages and processes of self-change of smoking: Toward an integrative model of change. *Journal of Consulting and Clinical Psychology* 51(3): 390–395, 1983.

PUSKA, P., BJORKQVIST, S., KOSKELA, K. Nicotine-containing chewing gum in smoking cessation: A double blind trial with half year follow-up. *Addictive Behaviors* 4:141–146, 1979.

RAMIREZ, A.G., MCALISTER, A.L. Mass media campaign—A Su Salad. *Preventive Medicine* 17(5):608–621, September 1988.

REIF, A.E. Public information on smoking. An urgent responsibility for cancer research workers. *Journal of the National Cancer Institute* 57(6):1207–1210, December 1976.

ROPER. *A Study of Public Attitudes Toward Cigarette Smoking and the Tobacco Industry in 1978*, Volume 1. Roper Organization, May 1978.

ROSEN, G.M., LICHTENSTEIN, E. An employee incentive program to reduce cigarette smoking. *Journal of Consulting and Clinical Psychology* 45(5):957, 1977.

ROSENBERG, J. The AMA tackles smoking: "A Strong Stand." *New York State Journal of Medicine* 83(13):1363–1365, December 1983.

RUSSELL, M.A.H., MERRIMAN, R., STAPLETON, J., TAYLOR, W. Effect of nicotine gum as an adjunct to general practitioners' advice against smoking. *British Medical Journal* 287(6407):1782–1785, December 10, 1983.

RUSSELL, M.A.H., WILSON, C., TAYLOR, C., BAKER, C.D. Effect of general practitioners' advice against smoking. *British Medical Journal* 2(6184):231–235, July 28, 1979.

ST. PIERRE, R.W., SHUTE, R.E., JAYCOX, S. Youth helping youth: A behavioral approach to the self-control of smoking. *Health Education* 14(1):28–31, January–February1983.

SCHINKE, S.P., GILCHRIST, L.D., SNOW, W.H., SCHILLING, R.F. Skills-building methods to prevent smoking by adolescents. *Journal of Adolescent Health Care* 6:439–444, 1985.

SCHNEIDEMAN, I. Acupuncture and smoking. (Letter.) *New Zealand Medical Journal* 94(693):276, October 14, 1981.

SCHNEIDER, N.G., JARVIK, M.E., FORSYTHE, A.B. Nicotine vs. placebo gum in the alleviation of withdrawal during smoking cessation. *Addictive Behaviors* 9(2):149–156, 1984.

SCHNEIDER, N.G., JARVIK, M.E., FORSYTHE, A.B., READ, L.L., ELLIOTT, M.L., SCHWEIGER, A. Nicotine gum in smoking cessation: A placebo-controlled, double-blind trial. *Addictive Behaviors* 8(3):253–261, 1983.

SCHWARTZ, J.L. A critical review and evaluation of smoking control methods. *Public Health Reports* 84(6):483–506, June 1969.

SCHWARTZ, J.L. *Review and Evaluation of Smoking Cessation Methods: United States and Canada, 1978–1985.* U.S. Department of Health and Human Services, Public Health Service, National Institutes of Health. NIH Publication No. 87-2940, April 1987.

SCHWARTZ, J.L., RIDER, G. *Review and Evaluation of Smoking Control Methods: The United States and Canada, 1969–1977.* U.S. Department of Health, Education, and Welfare, Public Health Service, Center for Disease Control, Bureau of Health Education. HEW Publication No. (CDC) 79-8369, 1978.

SEFFRIN, J.R., BAILEY, W.J. Approaches to adolescent smoking cessation and education. *Special Services in the Schools* 1(3):25–38, 1985.

SEVERSON, H., JAMES, L.E., LACHANCE, P.-A., EAKIN, E. *Up to Snuff. A Handbook on Smokeless Tobacco.* Eugene, Oregon: Independent Video Services, 1987.

SHAFFER, H., BECK, J.C., BOOTHROYD, P. The primary prevention of smoking onset: An inoculation approach. *Journal of Psychoactive Drugs* 15(3):177–184, July–September 1983.

SHIPLEY, R.H., ORLEANS, C.T., WILBUR, C.S., PISERCHIA, P.V., MCFADDEN, D.W. Effect of the Johnson and Johnson LIVE FOR LIFE Program on employee smoking. *Preventive Medicine* 17(1):25–34, January 1988.

SKINNER, W.F., MASSEY, J.L., KROHN, M.D., LAUER, R.M. Social influences and constraints on the initiation and cessation of adolescent tobacco use. *Journal of Behavioral Medicine* 8(4):353–376, December 1985.

SLADE, J.D. A disease model of cigarette use. *New York State Journal of Medicine* 85(7):294–297, July 1985.

SMITH, J.W. Long term outcome of clients treated in a commercial stop smoking program. *Journal of Substance Abuse Treatment* 5:33–36, 1988.

SMITH, L. The D-Day story. In: Steinfeld, J., Griffiths, W., Ball, K., Taylor, R.M. (eds.) *Smoking and Health. II. Health Consequences, Education, Cessation Activities, and Governmental Action.* Proceedings of the 3rd World Conference on Smoking and Health. U.S. Department of Health, Education, and Welfare, Public Health Service, National Institutes of Health, National Cancer Institute. DHEW Publication No. (NIH) 77-1413, 1977, pp. 409–413.

SNOW, W.H., GILCHRIST, L.D., SCHINKE, S.P. A critique of progress in adolescent smoking prevention. *Children and Youth Services Review* 7:1–19, 1985.

SOFFER, A. Smoking, the new ACCP fellowship pledge, and preventive medicine. *Chest* 77(4):459–460, April 1980.

SOFFER, A. Introduction. *Chest* 93(2, Supplement):33S, February 1988.

SOLBERG, L.I. Implementing a tobacco cessation program in clinical practice. *Medical Times* 116(4):119–124, April 1988.

SPIEGEL, H. A single-treatment method to stop smoking using ancillary self-hypnosis. *International Journal of Clinical and Experimental Hypnosis* 18(4):235–250, 1970.

STONE, E.J. School-based health research funded by the National Heart, Lung, and Blood Institute. *Journal of School Health* 55(5):168–174, May 1985.

SUSSMAN, S., BRANNON, B.R., FLAY, B.R., GLEASON, L., SENOR, S., SOBOL, D.F., HANSEN, W.B., JOHNSON, C.A. The television, school and family smoking prevention/cessation project. II. Formative evaluation of television segments by teenagers and parents—Implications for parental involvement in drug education. *Health Education Research* 1(3):185–194, 1986.

SUSSMAN, S., DENT, C.W., FLAY, B.R., HANSEN, W.B., JOHNSON, C.A. Psychosocial predictors of cigarette smoking onset by white, black, Hispanic, and Asian adolescents in southern California. *Morbidity and Mortality Weekly Report* 36(4S):11S–16S, September 4, 1987.

TAYLOR, P. *The Smoke Ring. Tobacco, Money, and Multinational Politics.* New York: Pantheon Books, 1984.

TELCH, M.J., KILLEN, J.D., MCALISTER, A.L., PERRY, C.L., MACCOBY, N. Long-term follow-up of a pilot project on smoking prevention with adolescents. *Journal of Behavioral Medicine* 5(1):1–8, 1982.

THOMPSON, E.L. Smoking education programs 1960–1976. *American Journal of Public Health* 68(3):250–257, March 1978.

TONNESEN, P., HANSEN, M., HELSTED, J., GUNNERSEN, A.B., FORCHAMMER, H., STOCKNER, M. Effect of nicotine chewing gum in combination with group counseling on the cessation of smoking. *New England Journal of Medicine* 318(1):15–18, 1988.

TROYER, R.J., MARKEL, G.E. *Cigarettes, the Battle Over Smoking.* New Brunswick, New Jersey: Rutgers University Press, 1983.

U.S. DEPARTMENT OF DEFENSE. *Report on Smoking and Health in the Military.* U.S. Department of Defense, Office of the Assistant Secretary of Defense (Health Affairs), Office of the Assistant Secretary of Defense (Force Management and Personnel), March 1986.

U.S. DEPARTMENT OF DEFENSE. *Updated Report on Smoking and Health in the Military.* U.S. Department of Defense, Office of the Assistant Secretary of Defense (Health Affairs), Office of the Assistant Secretary of Defense (Force Management and Personnel), June 1987.

U.S. DEPARTMENT OF HEALTH AND HUMAN SERVICES. *Smoking Programs for Youth.* U.S. Department of Health and Human Services, Public Health Service, National Institutes of Health, National Cancer Institute. NIH Publication No. 80-2156, June 1980a.

U.S. DEPARTMENT OF HEALTH AND HUMAN SERVICES. *The Health Consequences of Smoking for Women. A Report of the Surgeon General.* U.S. Department of Health and Human Services, Public Health Service, Office of the Assistant Secretary for Health, Office on Smoking and Health, 1980b.

U.S. DEPARTMENT OF HEALTH AND HUMAN SERVICES. *The Health Consequences of Smoking. The Changing Cigarette: A Report of the Surgeon General.* U.S. Department of Health and Human Services, Public Health Service, Office of the Assistant Secretary for Health, Office on Smoking and Health. DHHS Publication No. (PHS) 81-50156, 1981.

U.S. DEPARTMENT OF HEALTH AND HUMAN SERVICES. *The Health Consequences of Smoking: Cancer. A Report of the Surgeon General.* U.S. Department of Health and Human Services, Public Health Service, Office on Smoking and Health. DHHS Publication No. (PHS) 82-50179, 1982.

U.S. DEPARTMENT OF HEALTH AND HUMAN SERVICES. *The Health Consequences of Smoking: Cardiovascular Disease. A Report of the Surgeon General.* U.S. Department of Health and Human Services, Public Health Service, Office on Smoking and Health. DHHS Publication No. (PHS) 84-50204, 1983a.

U.S. DEPARTMENT OF HEALTH AND HUMAN SERVICES. *The Physician's Guide. How to Help Your Hypertensive Patients Stop Smoking.* U.S. Department of Health and Human Services, Public Health Service, National Institutes of Health. DHHS Publication No. (NIH) 83-1271, April 1983b.

U.S. DEPARTMENT OF HEALTH AND HUMAN SERVICES. *The Health Consequences of Smoking: Chronic Obstructive Lung Disease. A Report of the Surgeon General.* U.S. Department of Health and Human Services, Public Health Service, Office on Smoking and Health. DHHS Publication No. (PHS) 84-50205, 1984.

U.S. DEPARTMENT OF HEALTH AND HUMAN SERVICES. *The Health Consequences of Smoking: Cancer and Chronic Lung Disease in the Workplace. A Report of the Surgeon General.* U.S. Department of Health and Human Services, Public Health Service, Office on Smoking and Health. DHHS Publication No. (PHS) 85-50207, 1985a.

U.S. DEPARTMENT OF HEALTH AND HUMAN SERVICES. *A Decision Maker's Guide to Reducing Smoking at the Worksite.* U.S. Department of Health and Human Services, Public Health Service, Office on Smoking and Health, Office of Disease Prevention and Health Promotion, 1985b.

U.S. DEPARTMENT OF HEALTH AND HUMAN SERVICES. *Smoking and Health. A National Status Report. A Report to Congress.* U.S. Department of Health and Human Services, Public Health Service, Centers for Disease Control, Center for Health Promotion and Education, Office on Smoking and Health. DHHS Publication No. (CDC) 87-8396, 1986a.

U.S. DEPARTMENT OF HEALTH AND HUMAN SERVICES. *The Health Consequences of Involuntary Smoking. A Report of the Surgeon General.* U.S. Department of Health and Human Services, Public Health Service, Centers for Disease Control. DHHS Publication No. (CDC) 87-8398, 1986b.

U.S. DEPARTMENT OF HEALTH AND HUMAN SERVICES. *The Health Consequences of Using Smokeless Tobacco. A Report of the Advisory Committee to the Surgeon General.* U.S. Department of Health and Human Services, Public Health Service, National Institutes of Health. NIH Publication No. 86-2874, 1986c.

U.S. DEPARTMENT OF HEALTH AND HUMAN SERVICES. *State and Local Programs on Smoking and Health.* U.S. Department of Health and Human Services, Public Health Service, Office of the Assistant Secretary for Health, Office on Smoking and Health. DHHS Publication No. (PHS) 86-50190, 1986d.

U.S. DEPARTMENT OF HEALTH AND HUMAN SERVICES. *Clinical Opportunities for Smoking Intervention. A Guide for the Busy Physician.* U.S. Department of Health and Human Services, Public Health Service, National Institutes of Health. NIH Publication No. 86-2178, August 1986e.

U.S. DEPARTMENT OF HEALTH AND HUMAN SERVICES. *National Survey of Worksite Health Promotion Activities: A Summary.* U.S. Department of Health and Human Services, Public Health Service, Office of Disease Prevention and Health Promotion. Monograph series, Summer 1987.

U.S. DEPARTMENT OF HEALTH AND HUMAN SERVICES. *The Health Consequences of Smoking: Nicotine Addiction. A Report of the Surgeon General, 1988.* U.S. Department of Health and Human Services, Public Health Service, Centers for Disease Control, Center for Health Promotion and Education, Office on Smoking and Health. DHHS Publication No. (CDC) 88-8406, 1988.

U.S. DEPARTMENT OF HEALTH AND HUMAN SERVICES. *The 1987 National Adolescent Student Health Survey.* U.S. Department of Health and Human Services, Public Health Service, Office of Disease Prevention and Health Promotion, in press.

U.S. DEPARTMENT OF HEALTH, EDUCATION, AND WELFARE. *The Health Consequences of Smoking. A Report of the Surgeon General: 1972.* U.S. Department of Health, Education, and Welfare, Public Health Service, Health Services and Mental Health Administration. DHEW Publication No. (HSM) 72-7516, 1972.

U.S. DEPARTMENT OF HEALTH, EDUCATION, AND WELFARE. *San Diego Smoking Research Project. Five Year Status.* U.S. Department of Health, Education, and Welfare, Center for Disease Control. DHEW Project No. 200-75-0516:1–7, 1976.

U.S. DEPARTMENT OF HEALTH, EDUCATION, AND WELFARE. *The Health Consequences of Smoking, 1977–1978.* U.S. Department of Health, Education, and Welfare, Public

Health Service, Officie of the Assistant Secretary for Health, Office on Smoking and Health. DHEW Publication No. (PHS) 79-50065, 1978.

U.S. DEPARTMENT OF HEALTH, EDUCATION, AND WELFARE. *Healthy People: The Surgeon General's Report on Health Promotion and Disease Prevention.* U.S. Department of Health, Education, and Welfare, Public Health Service, Office of the Assistant Secretary for Health and Surgeon General. DHEW Publication No. (PHS) 79-55071, 1979a.

U.S. DEPARTMENT OF HEALTH, EDUCATION, AND WELFARE. *Smoking and Health. A Report of the Surgeon General.* U.S. Department of Health, Education, and Welfare, Public Health Service, Office of the Assistant Secretary for Health, Office on Smoking and Health. DHEW Publication No. (PHS) 79-50066, 1979b.

U.S. DEPARTMENT OF HEALTH, EDUCATION, AND WELFARE. *Teenage Smoking. Immediate and Long-Term Patterns.* U.S. Department of Health, Education, and Welfare, National Institute of Education, November 1979c.

U.S. PREVENTIVE SERVICES TASK FORCE. Recommendations for smoking cessation counseling. *Journal of the American Medical Association* 259(19):2882, May 20, 1988.

U.S. PUBLIC HEALTH SERVICE. *Smoking and Health. Report of the Advisory Committee to the Surgeon General of the Public Health Service.* U.S. Department of Health, Education, and Welfare, Public Health Service, Center for Disease Control. PHS Publication No. 1103, 1964.

UNIVERSITY OF THE STATE OF NEW YORK. *Annotated Resource Guide for Alcohol, Tobacco and Other Drug Abuse/Misuse Prevention Education Programs. Secondary Level.* Albany, New York: University of the State of New York, State Education Department, Bureau of Drug Education, 1979.

WALTER, H.J., VAUGHAN, R.D., WYNDER, E.L. Primary prevention of cancer among children: Changes in cigarette smoking and diet after six years of intervention. *Journal of the National Cancer Institute*, in press.

WARNER, K.E. The effects of the anti-smoking campaign on cigarette consumption. *American Journal of Public Health* 67(7):645–650, July 1977.

WARNER, K.E. Possible increases in the underreporting of cigarette consumption. *Journal of the American Statistical Association* 73(362):314–318, June 1978.

WARNER, K.E. Cigarette smoking in the 1970's: The impact of the antismoking campaign. *Science* 211(4483):729–731, February 13, 1981.

WARNER, K.E. *Selling Smoke: Cigarette Advertising and Public Health.* Washington, D.C.: American Public Health Association, October 1986.

WARNER, K.E., ERNSTER, V.L., HOLBROOK, J.H., LEWIT, E.M., PERTSCHUK, M., STEINFELD, J.L., WHELAN, E.M. Public policy on smoking and health: Toward a smoke-free generation by the year 2000. A statement of a working group to the Subcommittee on Smoking of the American Heart Association. *Circulation* 73(2):381A–395A, February 1986.

WARNER, K.E., MURT, H.A. Impact of the antismoking campaign on smoking prevalence: A cohort analysis. *Journal of Public Health Policy* 3(4):374–390, December 1982.

WEISSMAN, W., GLASGOW, R., BIGLAN, A., LICHTENSTEIN, E. Development and preliminary evaluation of a cessation program for adolescent smokers. *Psychology of Addictive Behaviors* 1(2):84–91, 1987.

WHELAN, E.M. *A Smoking Gun: How the Tobacco Industry Gets Away With Murder.* Philadelphia: George F. Stickley, 1984.

WILBUR, C.S. The Johnson and Johnson Program. *Preventive Medicine* 12:672–681, 1983.

WILSON, D.M., TAYLOR, W., GILBERT, J.R., BEST, J.A., LINDSAY, E.A., WILLMS, D.G., SINGER, J. A randomized trial of a family physician intervention for smoking cessation. *Journal of the American Medical Association* 260(11):1570–1574, September 16, 1988.

WONG, W. Smoke-free rooms really will decide this California vote. Tobacco firms pour in money to fight proposal to ban indoor public puffing. *Wall Street Journal*, October 25, 1978, pp. 1, 23.

WORDEN, J.K., FLYNN, B.S., BRISSON, S.F., SECKER-WALKER, R.H., MCAULIFFE, T.L., JONES, R.P. An adult communication skills program to prevent adolescent smoking. *Journal of Drug Education* 17(1):1–9, 1987.

WORDEN, J.K., FLYNN, B.S., GELLER, B.A., CHEN, M., SHELTON, L.G., SECKER-WALKER, R.H., SOLOMON, D.S., SOLOMON, L.J., COUCHEY, S., CONSTANZA, M.C. Development of a smoking prevention mass media program using diagnostic and formative research. *Preventive Medicine*, in press.

YOUNG, S.R., CHEN, T.T.L., CERNADA, G.P. An evaluation of a biofeedback smoking education program. *International Quarterly of Community Health Education* 2(4):329–337, 1981–1982.

CHAPTER 7

SMOKING CONTROL POLICIES

CONTENTS

INTRODUCTION

This Chapter describes and evaluates policy measures that have affected, have been intended to affect, or might be expected to affect, smoking behavior. For current purposes, the term policy refers to a set of rules that guide the present and future behavior of individuals and organizations to achieve a specific goal. Smoking control policies encompass a diverse group of actions in both the public and private sectors. They share the common potential for reducing the burden of tobacco-induced illness by decreasing the prevalence and intensity of cigarette smoking in the United States.

The smoking control policies discussed here interact with and often complement nonpolicy activities, such as smoking cessation and prevention programs, described in Chapter 6. The distinction made here is that policies primarily involve the setting of rules, whereas nonpolicy activities are usually offered on a voluntary basis to smokers or potential smokers and attempt to influence directly the decision to smoke. The notion of policymaking is often associated primarily with government, but private sector organizations, such as schools, businesses, and health care facilities, have also set policies that influence smoking. Conversely, nonpolicy actions, such as voluntary smoking cessation programs, may be undertaken by Government units like Federal agencies or the Armed Forces, although most such activities are conducted by private organizations.

This Chapter covers tobacco control policies that have been adopted or seriously considered by Federal, State, and local governments and by the private sector, focusing on developments since the release of the first Surgeon General's Report in 1964. Each section reviews the history and rationale for adopting a particular policy, analyzes what is known about its impact on smoking behavior, and discusses related policies under serious consideration. While it would be ideal to determine the independent effect of each policy on public knowledge and smoking behavior, in many cases this is difficult to assess. Smoking control policies occur in a context of multiple social influences on smoking; individual policies overlap in time with each other and with the nonpolicy influences on smoking described in Chapter 6. Because relatively few studies adequately control for potentially confounding influences on smoking, it is often difficult to identify the effect of an individual policy on smoking behavior or knowledge. Chapter 8 considers the aggregate impact of antismoking activities and changing social norms over the past 25 years, including both policy and nonpolicy actions, on smoking.

The focus of the Chapter is necessarily on cigarettes; they are the predominant form of tobacco use, the cause of the overwhelming majority of tobacco-related diseases, and the subject of most policy efforts. Nonetheless, the Chapter also includes policies that target other forms of tobacco use. As with the rest of this Report, the Chapter's scope is limited to the United States; smoking control policies outside the United States have been reviewed by Roemer (1982, 1986). Furthermore, the Chapter does not cover tobacco trade policy, because it has limited relevance to smoking prevalence in the United States.

The targets of smoking-related policies are diverse; they include not only consumers (smokers) or potential consumers of tobacco products, but also suppliers, growers, manufacturers, distributors, and vendors. To summarize the array of tobacco control policies that have been considered or adopted, this review follows a classification proposed by Walsh and Gordon (1986): (1) educational and persuasive efforts, (2) economic incentives, and (3) direct restraints on tobacco use, manufacture, or sales (Table 1). Policies in the first category aim to inform the public about the health risks of smoking and persuade individuals to stop, or not to start, smoking. The second group of policies involves market mechanisms that increase the costs of smoking to the manufacturer, the vendor, or the consumer of tobacco products. The third category includes public policies that directly reduce opportunities to smoke by limiting the sale or use of tobacco products or that attempt to reduce the toxicity of tobacco products by regulating their contents. In many instances, policies that are educational for consumers have a regulatory nature for suppliers. An example is the Federal Government's requirement that all cigarette packages carry a Surgeon General's warning. In these cases, policies are categorized according to their influence on consumers or potential consumers.

Although broad in its coverage, the Chapter is limited to policies that have been adopted or seriously considered for adoption in the near future. Considerations of space and emphasis have forced the exclusion of a few policies that have been discussed in both the news media and the academic literature. Perhaps most conspicuously, this Chapter includes no discussion of tobacco farm policy. In particular, the tobacco price support and allotment system (better known as the tobacco "subsidy") is not considered. The impact of this policy on smoking and health is indirect (Warner 1988). Similarly, no attempt is made in this Report to examine the issue of how governments might facilitate tobacco farmers' transition to other crops or careers (Warner et al. 1986b).

Furthermore, this Chapter does not discuss other activities that might have a substantial impact on smoking but are not properly categorized as policies. A prominent example is tobacco product liability suits, which seek to establish the legal liability of tobacco manufacturers for the tobacco-related illnesses of smokers (Daynard 1988). The lawsuits themselves are private matters, not policy issues, and while there are policy issues relevant to the lawsuits, the lack of a significant body of literature on the issues of interest precludes coverage of them. Finally, the Chapter does not treat in detail the strongest potential policy: a total ban on tobacco sales and use. Given the addictiveness of tobacco, the unique history of tobacco use (which was widespread and culturally accepted long before the hazards were fully appreciated) and the Nation's experience with alcohol prohibition, a total ban on tobacco is at present neither widely discussed nor likely to be adopted.

TABLE 1.—Past, present, and proposed tobacco control policies

Information and education	Economic incentives	Direct restraints on tobacco use
1. Require health warnings A. Packages B. Advertising	1. Increase tobacco taxation (e.g., excise tax)	1. Restrict smoking in certain places (e.g., public places, workplaces, schools, hospitals)
2. Require disclosure of constituents of tobacco products or smoke A. Tar, nicotine, carbon monoxide B. Tobacco product additives	2. Mandate insurance incentives A. Premium price differentials (smoker–nonsmoker) B. Cover smoking cessation treatment costs	2. Restrict distribution (sales) A. By age (minors) B. Via certain outlets (e.g., vending machines)
3. Mandate educational programs A. Schools B. Mass media	3. Reduce or eliminate tobacco price supports[a]	3. Regulate product composition
4. Issue Government reports	4. Establish legal liability of producers[a]	4. Ban manufacture, sale, or use[a]
5. Fund smoking research and programs		
6. Restrict or ban advertising and promotion		

[a]Not discussed in this Report.

SOURCE: Modified from Walsh and Gordon (1986).

PART I. POLICIES PERTAINING TO INFORMATION AND EDUCATION

The majority of Government activity on smoking and health has consisted of providing information and education to the public (Walsh and Gordon 1986). This encompasses a broad range of policies whose primary aim is to warn the public about the health risks of smoking. This information might discourage individuals from starting or continuing to smoke, or at minimum permit them to be informed smokers. The informational message on smoking and health has broadened considerably since 1964, when the first Surgeon General's Report stimulated efforts to educate the public about the health effects of cigarette smoking. As further scientific knowledge accumulated on related topics, the content of information conveyed to the public expanded to include the health effects of using other tobacco products (US DHHS 1986c), the health consequences of involuntary tobacco smoke exposure (US DHHS 1986b), the addictive nature of smoking behavior (US DHHS 1988), and methods for quitting smoking (US DHEW 1979; US DHHS 1988).

Government efforts to warn the public about the dangers of tobacco use have included these activities: (1) requiring that some information about health risks be placed on packages of cigarettes and smokeless tobacco products and on advertisements; (2) requiring that schools teach curricula on smoking and health; (3) reducing the influence of prosmoking messages by regulating or restricting some types of cigarette advertising and promotion; (4) mandating the broadcast of antismoking messages on the electronic media in the late 1960s under the Federal Communication Commission's Fairness Doctrine; and (5) requiring the preparation of reports that summarize information on smoking and health and review public and private tobacco control activities. In addition,the Federal Government has encouraged and monitored the tobacco industry's testing and disclosure of the levels of certain tobacco smoke constituents.

In the private sector, information and education on smoking behavior and the health consequences of smoking have been provided by voluntary actions of health organizations, schools, health professionals, the mass media, and other groups and individuals. These efforts are described in Chapter 6.

This Section covers Federal, State, and local government actions whose goals are to inform and educate. It describes public policies of the past 25 years in the United States, summarizes available data on their effectiveness, and reviews the current status of policies under consideration. Finally, because funding levels have influenced the extent of Government's educational efforts, this Section also reviews the magnitude of Government expenditures on smoking and health.

Warning Labels on Tobacco Products

For the purpose of this Report, the term labeling is used to refer to the provision of health-related information on packages and in advertising. Warning labels could include either brief statements printed on tobacco packages or more detailed information placed on package inserts, similar to those required for pharmaceutical products.

History and Current Status

One of the earliest and best known mechanisms that the Federal Government used to inform the public about the health hazards of smoking was requiring that a warning label be placed on cigarette packages. Warning labels developed largely as a consequence of policy initiatives originated by the Federal Trade Commission (FTC) and subsequently modified by congressional action. This effort began shortly after January 11, 1964, when the Surgeon General released the Report of the Advisory Committee on Smoking and Health (US PHS 1964). Eleven days after the release of the Report, the FTC proposed three rules that would have required health warnings on cigarette packages and advertisements and imposed certain restrictions on cigarette advertising (FTC 1964a). The proposals were notable both for their comprehensiveness and for the speed with which they were published following the release of the Advisory Committee's Report. The FTC's proposed Rule 1 would have required that every cigarette advertisement and every pack, box, carton, and other container in which cigarettes were sold to the public carry one of the following warnings:

> CAUTION: CIGARETTE SMOKING IS A HEALTH HAZARD: The Surgeon General's Advisory Committee on Smoking and Health has found that "cigarette smoking contributes substantially to mortality from certain specific diseases and to the overall death rate."
>
> CAUTION: Cigarette smoking is dangerous to health. It may cause death from cancer and other diseases.

After a 6-month comment period and public hearings, the FTC issued its final rule on June 22, 1964; this was published in the *Federal Register* on July 2, 1964 (FTC 1964b). The final rule resembled Proposed Rule 1; it required that all cigarette advertising and every container in which cigarettes were sold to consumers disclose clearly and prominently that cigarette smoking is dangerous to health and may cause death from cancer and other diseases. However, the final rule did not specify the exact wording of the warning, which was left up to the tobacco companies to determine. January 1, 1965, was set as the effective date for the package warning, and July 1, 1965, for the warning on advertisements. The effective date for the package label was later delayed until July 1, 1965, in response to a congressional request (Fritschler 1969).

The FTC regulation was preempted before it took effect by the Federal Cigarette Labeling and Advertising Act of 1965 (Public Law 89-92), which was approved by Congress on July 1, 1965, and signed into law on July 27. This Act was the outcome of lengthy congressional debate in 1964 and 1965 about cigarette labeling requirements and advertising restrictions (Ernster 1988). The law, which became effective on January 1, 1966, was the first of a series of Federal statutes enacting labeling requirements for tobacco products (Table 2). Overall, the provisions of the law were less stringent than the FTC regulations they replaced. The law required that all cigarette packages contain the health warning "Caution: Cigarette Smoking May Be Hazardous to Your Health." However, it required no label on cigarette advertisements and temporarily (through June 1969) prohibited any government body, such as Federal regulatory agencies or States, from requiring a health warning in cigarette advertising. The Act also prohibited any health warning on cigarette packages other than the statement required by the Act itself. According to the Act's "Declaration of Policy," the warning was required so that "the public may be adequately informed that cigarette smoking may be hazardous to health." The day after the Act was signed into law, the FTC issued an order vacating its trade regulation rule (FTC 1965).

The Federal Cigarette Labeling and Advertising Act also required that the FTC transmit annually to Congress a report on the effectiveness of cigarette labeling, current cigarette advertising and promotion practices, and recommendations for legislation. In its first report to Congress, submitted in June 1967, the FTC recommended that the health warning be extended to cigarette advertisements and be strengthened to read: "Warning: Cigarette Smoking Is Dangerous to Health and May Cause Death from Cancer and Other Diseases" (FTC 1967). On May 20, 1969, just before expiration of the congressionally imposed moratorium on its action, the FTC announced a proposed rule that would have required all cigarette advertisements "to disclose, clearly and prominently, ... that cigarette smoking is dangerous to health and may cause death from cancer, coronary heart disease, chronic bronchitis, pulmonary emphysema, and other diseases" (FTC 1969a).

During this time, hearings were being held in Congress on cigarette labeling and advertising issues. On April 1, 1970, the Public Health Cigarette Smoking Act of 1969 (Public Law 91-222), which banned cigarette advertising on television and radio, was signed into law. The labeling provisions of this law, like its predecessor's, were less stringent than the FTC regulations they preempted. The Act (effective November 1, 1970) did strengthen the health warning on cigarette packages to read: "Warning: The Surgeon General Has Determined That Cigarette Smoking Is Dangerous to Your Health." However, it continued to prohibit any other health warning requirement for packages and to prohibit the FTC (through June 1971) from issuing regulations that would require a health warning in cigarette advertising.

In late 1971, after the second congressionally mandated moratorium on its actions had expired, the FTC announced its intention to file complaints against cigarette companies for failure to warn in their advertising that smoking is dangerous to health. Subsequent negotiations between the FTC and the cigarette industry resulted in consent orders on March 30, 1972, requiring that all cigarette advertising display "clearly and conspicuously" the same warning required by Congress on cigarette packages (FTC 1981b).

The 1972 consent order specified the type size of the warning in newspaper, magazine, and other periodical advertisements of various dimensions. For billboard advertisements, the size of the warnings was specified in inches (FTC 1972). In 1975, the U.S. Government filed a complaint in the U.S. District Court for the District of Columbia for alleged violations of the consent order, including failure to display the health warning in some advertising, billboard warnings in letters smaller than required, and improper placement of the warning in some advertisements (FTC 1982). This action ultimately led to judgments in 1981 by the U.S. District Court for the Southern District of New York against the six major cigarette companies (*U.S.A.* v. *Liggett et al.* 1981; *U.S.A.* v. *R.J. Reynolds* 1981). Among other things, these judgments required the cigarette companies to use larger lettering in billboard advertisements. Under this settlement, the format and size of the warning for advertisements of various dimensions

TABLE 2.—Major legislation related to information and education about tobacco and health in the United States

Law	Date	Major provisions and Federal agency affected			
		Labeling requirements	Advertising	Congressional reporting requirements	Other
Federal Cigarette Labeling and Advertising Act (PL 89-92)	1965	Health warning on cigarette packages		Annual report to Congress on health consequences of smoking (DHEW)	
		Preempted other package warnings		Annual report to Congress on cigarette labeling and advertising (FTC)	
		Temporarily preempted any health warning on cigarette advertisements (FTC)			
Public Health Cigarette Smoking Act (PL 91-222)	1969	Strengthened health warning on cigarette packages	Prohibited cigarette advertising on television and radio (DOJ)	Annual report to Congress on health consequences of smoking (DHEW)	
		Preempted other warnings on packages	Preempted any State or local requirement or prohibition based on smoking and health with respect to cigarette advertising or promotion	Annual report to Congress on cigarette labeling and advertising (FTC)	
		Temporarily preempted FTC requirement of health warning on cigarette advertisements[a] (FTC)			
Little Cigar Act (PL 93-109)	1973		Extended broadcast ban on cigarette advertising to "little cigars" (DOJ)		

TABLE 2.—Continued

Law	Date	Major provisions and Federal agency affected: Labeling requirements	Advertising	Congressional reporting requirements	Other
Comprehensive Smoking Education Act (PL 98-474)	1984	Replaced previous health warning on cigarette packages and advertisements[a] with system requiring rotation of four specific health warnings Preempted other package warnings		Biennial status report to Congress on smoking and health (DHHS)	Created the Federal Interagency Committee on Smoking and Health (DHHS) Cigarette industry must provide a confidential list of cigarette additives[c] (DHHS)
Comprehensive Smokeless Tobacco Health Education Act (PL 99-252)	1986	Rotation of three health warnings on smokeless tobacco packages and advertisements (in circle-and-arrow format on advertisements) Preempted any other health warning on smokeless tobacco packages or advertisements (except billboards)	Prohibited smokeless tobacco advertising on television and radio (DOJ)	Biennial status report to Congress on smokeless tobacco (DHHS) Biennial report to Congress on smokeless tobacco sales, advertising, and marketing practices (FTC)	Required public information campaign on health hazards of using smokeless tobacco (DHHS)[b] Smokeless tobacco companies must provide a confidential list of additives and a specification of nicotine content in smokeless tobacco products (DHHS)[c]

NOTE: DHEW, Department of Health, Education, and Welfare (now the Department of Health and Human Services (DHHS)); FTC, Federal Trade Commission; DOJ, Department of Justice.

[a]The requirement for a health warning on cigarette packages was extended to cigarette advertisements by an FTC consent order in 1972 (see text).

[b]No funds have been appropriated to carry out this campaign.

[c]List of additives does not identify company or cigarette brand. No public disclosure of additives on packages or advertisements required and no other public disclosure allowed.

were specified in acetate exhibits that are maintained on file at the FTC. The Comprehensive Smoking Education Act of 1984 (Public Law 98-474) again increased the size of the letters, but in the case of billboard ads, it did so only by requiring that all letters be uppercase. This Act was the first to codify into law the requirement for and the sizes of the warnings on ads.

In 1981, the FTC sent a staff report to Congress that concluded that the warning appearing on cigarette packages and in advertisements was no longer effective. The report noted that the warning did not communicate information on the significant, specific risks of smoking and concluded that the warning had become overexposed and "worn out" (FTC 1981b). The report recommended changing the shape of the warning to a circle-and-arrow format (for example, see Figure 1), increasing the size of the warning, and replacing the existing warning with a system of short rotational warnings.

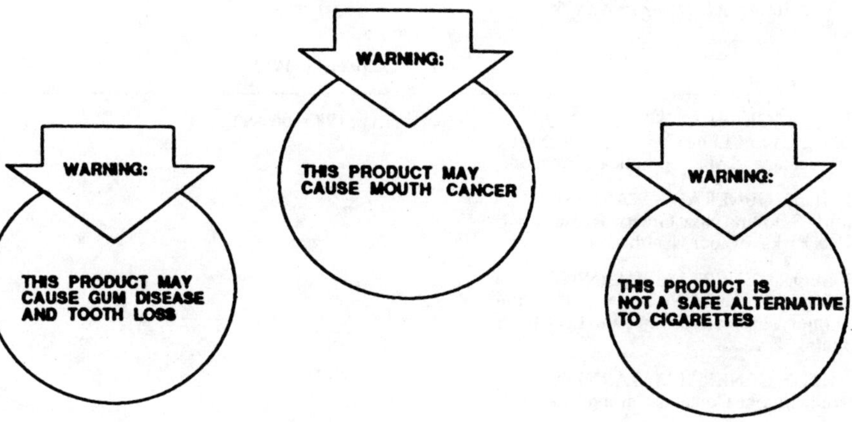

FIGURE 1.—Health warnings required for smokeless tobacco advertisements (except billboards)

Some of these recommendations were enacted by Congress as part of the Comprehensive Smoking Education Act (Public Law 98-474), which was signed into law on October 12, 1984. Effective October 12, 1985, it required cigarette companies to rotate four warnings on all cigarette packages and in advertisements (see Table 3). This was the first time that health warnings on cigarette advertisements were the result of legislative rather than regulatory action. The four warnings mandated for cigarette advertisements on outdoor billboards were slightly shorter versions of the messages required in other advertisements and on packages. The Act did not amend the existing prohibition of any other health warnings on cigarette packages and the preemption of State action, but it did not impose a similar preemption of other health warnings by Federal authorities in cigarette advertising.

The Comprehensive Smoking Education Act of 1984 required each cigarette manufacturer to obtain FTC approval for its plans to implement the rotational warning

TABLE 3.— Health warnings required on tobacco packages and advertisements in the United States.

CIGARETTES

Warning(s)	Effective dates	Applicability	
		Packages	Advertise-ments
CAUTION: Cigarette Smoking May Be Hazardous to Your Health.	January 1, 1966–October 31, 1970	X	
WARNING: The Surgeon General Has Determined That Cigarette Smoking Is Dangerous to Your Health.	November 1, 1970–October 11, 1985	X	
	1972–October 11, 1985		X[a]
SURGEON GENERAL'S WARNING: Smoking Causes Lung Cancer, Heart Disease, Emphysema, and May Complicate Pregnancy. SURGEON GENERAL'S WARNING: Quitting Smoking Now Greatly Reduces Serious Risks to Your Health. SURGEON GENERAL'S WARNING: Smoking by Pregnant Women May Result in Fetal Injury, Premature Birth, and Low Birth Weight. SURGEON GENERAL'S WARNING: Cigarette Smoke Contains Carbon Monoxide.	October 12, 1985–present	X	X[b]

SMOKELESS TOBACCO

Warnings	Effective dates	Applicability	
		Packages	Advertise-ments
WARNING: This product may cause mouth cancer. WARNING: This product may cause gum disease and tooth loss. WARNING: This product is not a safe alternative to cigarettes.	February 27, 1987–present	X	X[c]

[a]Required by Federal Trade Commission consent order. All other warnings required by Federal legislation.

[b]The four warnings mandated for cigarette advertisements on outdoor billboards are slightly shorter versions of the same messages.

[c]The warnings on advertisements must appear in a circle-and-arrow format (see Figure 1). No warnings are required on outdoor billboards.

system. Legislation was subsequently enacted that permitted certain smaller manufacturers and importers to display simultaneously all four warnings on packages instead of by quarterly rotation (Nurse Education Amendments of 1985, Section 11, amending section 4(c) of the Federal Cigarette Labeling and Advertising Act, 15 U.S.C. 1333(c)). This practice is now followed by 20 to 25 small manufacturers and importers.

More recently, Congress has extended requirements for warning labels to smokeless tobacco products. In early 1986, two national review groups, a National Institutes of Health Consensus Development Conference (US DHHS 1986a) and the Surgeon General's Advisory Committee on the Health Consequences of Using Smokeless Tobacco (US DHHS 1986c), issued reports concluding that smokeless tobacco can cause oral cancer and a number of noncancerous oral conditions. Between 1985 and 1986, the State of Massachusetts adopted legislation requiring warning labels on packages of snuff, and 25 other States considered similar legislation (Connolly et al. 1986).

The Massachusetts law was preempted before it took effect by the Federal Comprehensive Smokeless Tobacco Health Education Act of 1986 (Public Law 99-252), which was signed into law on February 27, 1986. The Act requires one of three warnings to be displayed on all smokeless tobacco packages and advertisements (except billboards) (Table 3). It requires that the three package warnings "be randomly displayed ... in each 12-month period in as equal a number of times as is possible on each brand of the product and be randomly distributed in all parts of the United States in which such product is marketed." On advertisements, the law requires rotation of each warning every 4 months for each brand. The warnings on advertisements are required to appear in the circle-and-arrow format recommended earlier by the FTC for cigarette warnings (FTC 1981b) (Figure 1). The Act prohibits Federal agencies or State or local jurisdictions from requiring any other health warnings on smokeless tobacco packages and advertisements (except billboards). No other Federal, State, or local actions were preempted by the Act. The FTC issued regulations implementing the law on November 4, 1986 (FTC 1986b).

Package inserts provide the opportunity to present more detailed information to the consumer than is possible with a warning label. They are a standard way of providing consumers with information about pharmaceutical products, but they have not been proposed for tobacco products in the United States. When used for prescription pharmaceuticals, patient package inserts have been generally effective in providing patients with information (US DHHS 1987d; Morris, Mazis, Gordon 1977) but have not been demonstrated to be effective in altering behavior (Dwyer 1978; Morris and Kanouse 1982). Information about smoking risks is included in the package insert for one class of pharmaceutical agents marketed in the United States. After several studies published between 1975 and 1977 reported that smoking increases the cardiovascular disease risks associated with oral contraceptive use (US DHEW 1978), the Food and Drug Administration (FDA) issued a regulation on January 31, 1978 requiring that as of April 3, 1978, packages of oral contraceptives contain a printed leaflet with the following boxed warning:

> Cigarette smoking increases the risk of serious adverse effects on the heart and blood vessels from oral contraceptive use. This risk increases with age and with heavy smoking (15

or more cigarettes per day) and is quite marked in women over 35 years of age. Women who use oral contraceptives should not smoke (FDA 1978).

The information provided to consumers of another nicotine-containing product contrasts with the information provided to consumers of tobacco products. The patient package insert for nicotine polacrilex gum, a nicotine-containing product approved by the FDA as an adjunct to smoking cessation programs, informs users of the addictiveness of nicotine and its potential effects on the fetus (US DHHS 1988). The product insert does not mention the risks of cigarette smoking, but it does state: "Warning to female patients: Nicorette contains nicotine which may cause fetal harm when administered to a pregnant woman. Do not take Nicorette if you are pregnant or nursing." The insert also warns that dependence on Nicorette "may occur when patients who are dependent on the nicotine in tobacco transfer that dependence to the nicotine in Nicorette gum."

Effectiveness of Cigarette Warning Labels

In May 1987, the Assistant Secretary for Health, Department of Health and Human Services, transmitted a report to Congress on the effects of health warning labels (US DHHS 1987d). Based on a review of the research literature, the report reached three major conclusions. First, health warning labels can have an impact on consumers if designed to take account of factors that influence consumer response to warning labels (e.g., a consumer's previous experience with the product, previous knowledge of the risks associated with product use, and education and reading levels). Second, health warning labels can have an impact upon the consumer if the labels are designed effectively (e.g., visible format and providing specific rather than general information). Third, studies that have examined the impact of health warning labels in "real world" situations have concluded that the labels did have an impact on consumer behavior. The report cautioned, however, that the results of these studies "cannot be regarded as conclusive evidence that health warning labels are necessarily effective in all situations." This Section reviews evidence related to the effectiveness of cigarette warning labels in the United States.

As noted above, the Federal Cigarette Labeling and Advertising Act of 1965 (Public Law 89-92), which required the first warning label on cigarette packages, stated that the health warning was required so that "the public may be adequately informed that cigarette smoking may be hazardous to health." More specific communications objectives were not set by legislation mandating warning labels. Generally, however, the goal of warning labels has been to increase public knowledge about the hazards of cigarette smoking. Such knowledge might deter individuals from starting or continuing to smoke.

Despite the fact that cigarette warning labels have been required since 1966, there are few data about their effectiveness in meeting any objective. As described below, empirical evidence is available about the cigarette warnings' visibility to consumers, and it is consistent with analyses based on communications theory. However, there are no controlled studies to permit a definitive assessment of the independent impact of cigarette warning labels on knowledge, beliefs, attitudes, or smoking behavior. In particular, there has been little evaluation of the impact of the rotating warning labels required since 1985.

If warning labels are to have any effect, they must actually appear on packaging and in advertising as required by law. Available evidence indicates that the tobacco industry has complied with disclosure obligations. For example, a study examining health warnings in magazine ads as an indicator of the industry's compliance with the 1984 labeling legislation found that the industry complied with the law (Davis, Lyman, Binkin 1988). The U.S. Department of Justice is empowered to enforce the disclosures required by the various labeling laws. According to the FTC (FTC 1967, 1969b, 1974, 1982, 1986a, 1988a,b) no actions have been brought by the Department of Justice for violations of labeling regulations, and the Commission has brought no action for failure to include the warnings in advertising (with the exception of the billboard and transit advertising enforcement proceedings discussed above). As of October 1988, no action had been sought against a cigarette manufacturer for a violation of the Comprehensive Smoking Education Act of 1984.

Despite the industry's compliance with the required warning labels, there is empirical evidence that the public did not pay much attention to the pre-1985 labels in advertisements; little information is available about the visibility of warning labels on packaging. In a Starch Message Report Service test of 24 different magazines in 1978, only 2.4 percent of the adults exposed to the cigarette ads read the pre-1985 Surgeon General's warning in those ads (FTC 1981b). Similarly, a study of seven Kool ads conducted in 1978 for the Brown and Williamson Tobacco Company found that only 2.4 percent of the respondents read the entire warning; the average time spent examining the warning was less than 0.3 seconds. In an advertising copy test conducted for the Liggett and Meyers Tobacco Company in 1976, no respondents read the entire warning (FTC 1981b). More recent studies of later cigarette and smokeless tobacco advertisements suggest that little attention is paid to the post-1984 health warnings. An eye-movement study examined the rotational cigarette warnings in magazine ads in a sample of 61 adolescents. Over 40 percent of the subjects did not view the warning at all; another 20 percent looked at the warning but did not read it (Fischer et al. 1989). Similarly low levels of warning recall were found for the recently introduced smokeless tobacco warnings (Popper and Murray 1988).

These findings are consistent with analyses of the visual imagery of tobacco advertising, which note that the structures of the ads draw consumers' attention away from the warnings contained in the ads (Richards and Zakia 1981; Zerner 1986). It has also been argued that the sheer volume of cigarette advertising, all applying the basic themes of product satisfaction, positive image associations, and risk minimization (Popper 1986b), overwhelm the in-advertisement warnings (Schwartz 1986).

In some advertising media, the cigarette warnings may not be readable. In a study of cigarette advertisements on 78 billboards and 100 taxicabs, Davis and Kendrick (1989) compared the readability of the Surgeon General's warning with recognition of the content of the cigarette advertisement. Under typical driving conditions, they found that a passing motorist could read the warning in about half of street billboard advertisements and in only 5 percent of highway billboard advertisements. The warning could not be read by a stationary observer in any of the taxicab advertisements. In contrast, the brand name could be read and notable imagery in the advertisements could be identified in almost all cases. Cullingford and coworkers (1988), using a model to assess the optical limits of the eye, showed that only about half of the health warnings on 37 billboard cigarette advertisements in Australia were legible to passing motorists; on the other hand, 98 percent of the brand names were legible.

Despite these findings, a national survey conducted by Lieberman Research, Inc. (1986) showed moderate recall of the post-1984 warnings 9 months after they began to appear on packages and advertisements. In this random survey of 1,025 Americans 18 years of age and older, 64 percent of all respondents and 77 percent of cigarette smokers said they recalled seeing one or more of the new warnings on cigarette packages. Lieberman concluded that this "represents a high level of penetration in a relatively short time period."

Respondents were also asked whether they recalled seeing each of the four warnings as well as the pre-1985 warning and a fictitious warning ("Smoking reduces life expectancy by an average of 6 years"). Recall of the true warnings ranged from 28 to 46 percent of all respondents (40 to 55 percent of smokers); recall of the carbon-monoxide warning was lowest among the four. Recall of the pre-1985 warning was substantially higher (85 percent of all respondents, 94 percent of smokers). Recall of the fictitious warning was 10 percent for the total sample as well as for smokers. Because the fictitious warning differed in style from the true warnings by presenting quantitative information, it is possible that stated recall of the fictitious warning was lower, at least in part, because of inferences made by respondents (as opposed to genuine differences in recall). The proportion who believed that a particular warning was "very" or "fairly" effective in convincing people that smoking is harmful ranged from 40 percent for the carbon-monoxide warning to 76 percent for the warning about lung cancer, heart disease, emphysema, and complications of pregnancy (the corresponding proportion for the pre-1985 warning was 56 percent).

Analyses of the wording and format of mandated health warnings have identified reasons why their impact may be limited even if they are noticed and read. Use of conditional words such as "can" or "may" anywhere in the warning can dramatically reduce the effect of the entire warning (Linthwaite 1985). Two of the current rotational warnings include the word "may." The other two warnings ("Quitting Smoking Now Greatly Reduces Serious Risks to Your Health" and "Cigarette Smoke Contains Carbon Monoxide") are not warnings but statements of fact; linguistically, consumers might be expected to minimize their impact (Dumas, in press). Furthermore, information in the current warnings is presented technically and abstractly rather than in a concrete and personal manner. A reader is more likely to read and learn information that is made personally relevant as opposed to that which is abstract and technical (Fishbein 1977). Researchers who have addressed the format of warnings have found that consumers' attention will be most effectively caught by novel formats (Cohen and Srull 1980). This line of study has suggested that the communications effectiveness of the post-1984 warnings may have been diminished because the same rectangular shape of the pre-1985 warnings was maintained (Bhalla and Lastovicka 1984).

The analysis of time trends in national survey data provides an opportunity to assess the effect of health warning labels on public knowledge of the health risks of smoking. As described in Chapter 4, public knowledge of these health effects has increased since 1966, when the first health warning label was required. Because warning labels were only one of a number of educational influences during this period, most researchers have concluded that it is impossible to isolate the effect of the warnings from other information sources (US DHHS 1987d; FTC 1974; Murphy 1980). Similarly, it is impossible to determine any independent effect of health warnings on aggregate cigarette sales (FTC 1967, 1969b). In sum, there are insufficient data to determine either the independent contribution of cigarette warning labels to changes in knowledge or smoking behavior or the precise role played by warning labels as part of a comprehensive antismoking effort.

Perhaps the most powerful indirect index of the effect of health warnings, along with other sources of information, is the number of smokers and consumers in general who remain unaware of the health risks of smoking. After a comprehensive review of studies on health risk awareness, including publicly generated studies and those conducted by the tobacco industry, the FTC concluded that significant numbers of consumers in general and even higher numbers of smokers were unaware of even the most rudimentary health risk information about smoking (FTC 1981b). It was this lack of consumer awareness that led the FTC to call for revised and expanded rotational warnings for cigarettes. More recent data reveal that a substantial minority of smokers still does not believe that smoking causes lung cancer, heart disease, emphysema, and other diseases, and the majority of smokers underestimate the degree of increased health risk posed by smoking. (See Chapter 4.)

Summary

As a result of policies described in this Section, a system of rotating health warning labels is currently required for all cigarette and smokeless tobacco packaging and advertisements in the United States. This system, established by congressional legislation in 1984 (for cigarettes) and 1986 (for smokeless tobacco products), achieves a portion of one of the Health Objectives for the Nation for 1990:

> By 1985, the present cigarette warning should be strengthened to increase its visibility and impact, and to give the consumer additional needed information on the specific multiple health risks of smoking. Special consideration should be given to rotational warnings and to identification of special vulnerable groups.

The 1984 Act provided the consumer with some of that "needed information," although the four mandated warnings provide less information than would have been provided by the 16 warnings described to the U.S. Congress in the 1981 FTC Report (FTC 1981b; Keenan and McLaughlin 1982). There is no legislated mechanism for monitoring the visibility or communications effectiveness of existing warning labels, and there are insufficient data to determine whether the visibility and impact of the warnings have increased as a result of the 1984 Act. Furthermore, current legislation does not provide a mechanism for updating the content of labels to reflect advances in knowledge about health effects and smoking behavior. One example of changing knowledge is the growing scientific awareness of the addictive nature of tobacco use, which was the subject of the 1988 Surgeon General's Report (US DHHS 1988). In that Report, the Secretary of Health and Human Services, the Assistant Secretary for Health, and the Surgeon General recommended that a new health warning label on the addictive nature of tobacco use be required on cigarette and smokeless tobacco packages and advertisements. On the day of the Report's release (May 16, 1988), legislation was introduced in the U.S. Senate that would require a warning to read: "Smoking is addictive. Once you start, you may not be able to stop" (S. 2402). Other bills that include provisions calling for a warning label on addiction have also been introduced in Congress. As of November 1988, this legislation was not enacted.

Currently, labels are not required on cigarettes made for export or on cigarettes manufactured abroad by U.S. tobacco companies. Federal law does not require warning labels on other tobacco products, such as cigars, pipe tobacco, and roll-your-own cigarette tobacco, despite the established health risks associated with cigar and pipe smoking (US DHEW 1979; US DHHS 1982a, 1984; Chapter 2). During the early 1970s, there was particular concern about the health risks for individuals who smoke "little cigars" (US DHEW 1973). In its 1974 report to Congress (FTC 1974), the FTC recommended that the following warning be required on little-cigar packages: "Warning: Smoking Little Cigars May be Dangerous to Your Health if Inhaled and Smoked in the Same Quantities as Cigarettes." The Little Cigar Act of 1973 (Public Law 93-109) extended the broadcast advertising ban for cigarettes to little cigars, but neither this Act nor subsequent legislation extended requirements for health warnings to little cigars (Table 2).

A warning label will appear on cigars and pipe tobacco sold in California, as a result of an agreement reached on October 18, 1988, between tobacco manufacturers and the State of California. Twenty-five tobacco manufacturers, along with eight retailers, had been sued by California's Attorney General for failing to comply with the State's Safe Drinking Water and Toxic Substances Enforcement Act, which requires warnings on all consumer products containing chemicals known to cause cancer or reproductive toxic effects (Wilson 1988a; Kizer et al. 1988). Because existing distribution systems for cigars do not easily permit the labeling of cigars destined only for California, the president of the Cigar Association of America indicated that most cigars sold in the United States would carry warning labels (Wilson 1988a). As of October 1988, the effect of the settlement on warning labels for pipe tobacco sold outside California was unknown.

Tobacco labeling requirements in other countries (Roemer 1982, 1986) provide comparisons for current labeling practices in the United States. Outside the United States, six countries (Finland, Iceland, Ireland, Norway, Sweden, and the United Kingdom) have enacted a rotational warning requirement. A Swedish law, adopted in 1976, requires the rotation of 16 warning statements on cigarette packages. Ireland requires the rotation of three brief, direct statements on cigarette packages and advertisements: "SMOKING CAUSES CANCER," "SMOKERS DIE YOUNG," and "SMOKING KILLS!" In the United Kingdom, one of six rotated warnings indicates smoking-attributable mortality: "More than 30,000 People Die Each Year in the UK from Lung

Cancer." Since 1985, Iceland has required the rotation of pictorial warnings (Figure 2). Several countries also require health warnings on packages of cigars and pipe tobacco. On packages of cigars, cigarillos, and pipe tobacco, for example, Ireland requires the warning: "SMOKING SERIOUSLY DAMAGES YOUR HEALTH." On June 29, 1988, Canada's House of Commons enacted a new labeling law as part of a comprehensive package of smoking restrictions, the Tobacco Products Control Act (House of Commons of Canada 1988). Canada's current cigarette warning labels will be replaced by a mandatory package insert that details all known health risks of smoking.

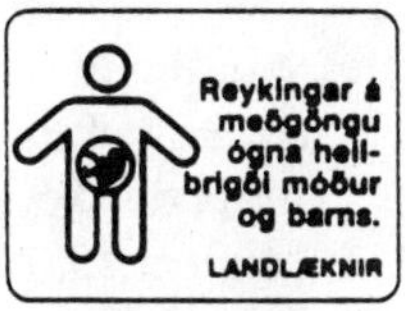

Reykingar á
meðgöngu
ógna heil-
brigði móður
og barns.
LANDLÆKNIR

1. Smoking during pregnancy endangers the health of mother and child.

DIRECTOR GENERAL OF PUBLIC HEALTH.

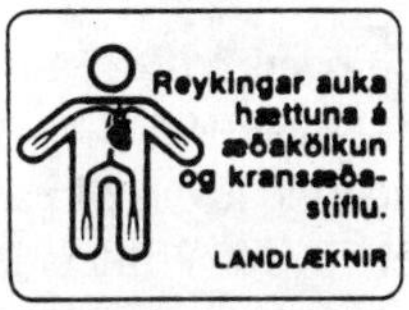

Reykingar auka
hættuna á
æðakölkun
og kransæða-
stíflu.
LANDLÆKNIR

2. Smoking may damage your arteries and cause heart attack.

DIRECTOR GENERAL OF PUBLIC HEALTH.

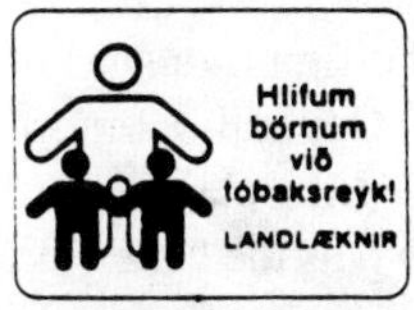

Hlífum
börnum
við
tóbaksreyk!
LANDLÆKNIR

3. Protect children from tobacco smoke.

DIRECTOR GENERAL OF PUBLIC HEALTH.

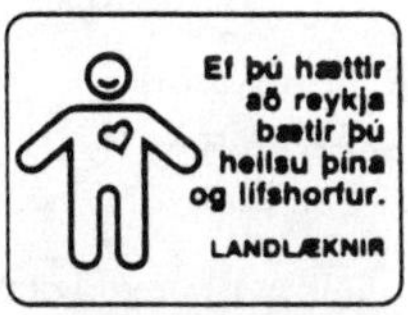

Ef þú hættir
að reykja
bætir þú
heilsu þína
og lífshorfur.
LANDLÆKNIR

4. If you stop smoking you improve your health and increase your life expectancy.

DIRECTOR GENERAL OF PUBLIC HEALTH.

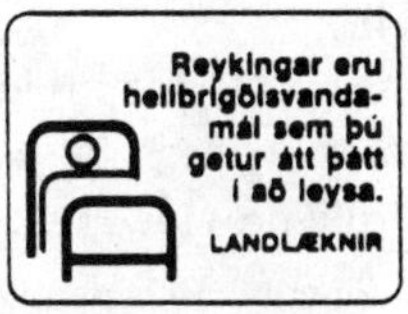

Reykingar eru
heilbrigðisvanda-
mál sem þú
getur átt þátt
í að leysa.
LANDLÆKNIR

5. Smoking is a health problem you can help to solve.

DIRECTOR GENERAL OF PUBLIC HEALTH.

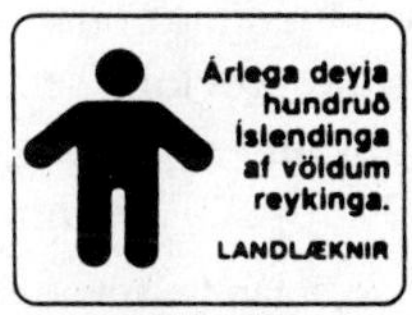

Árlega deyja
hundruð
Íslendinga
af völdum
reykinga.
LANDLÆKNIR

6. Hundreds of Icelanders die each year due to smoking.

DIRECTOR GENERAL OF PUBLIC HEALTH.

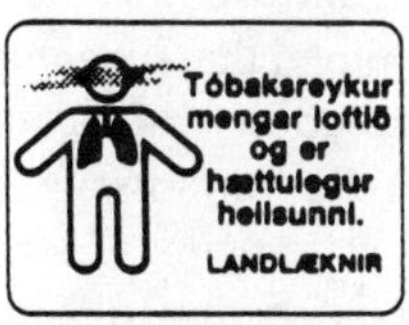

Tóbaksreykur
mengar loftið
og er
hættulegur
heilsunni.
LANDLÆKNIR

7. Tobacco smoke pollutes the air and is a health hazard.

DIRECTOR GENERAL OF PUBLIC HEALTH.

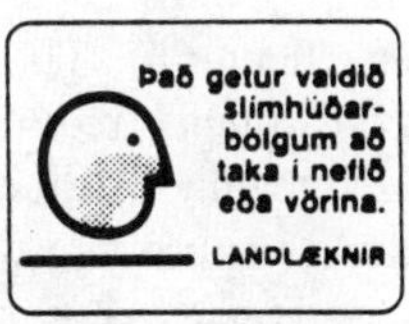

Það getur valdið
slímhúðar-
bólgum að
taka í nefið
eða vörina.
LANDLÆKNIR

8. Snuff and chewing-tobacco may damage the mucous membranes.

DIRECTOR GENERAL OF PUBLIC HEALTH.

Cigarettes, labels no. 1,2,3,4,5 and 6
Cigars and pipe tobacco, labels no. 3 and 7
Snuff and chewing tobacco, label no. 8

FIGURE 2.—Health warnings on tobacco packages in Iceland according to regulation no. 499/1984

SOURCE: Blondal and Magnusson (1985).

Disclosure of Tobacco Product Constituents

History and Current Status

The FTC has also been concerned with the disclosure, on packaging and in advertising, of information about the constituents of tobacco smoke (e.g., tar, nicotine, and carbon monoxide). More recently, there has also been growing interest in the identity and amounts of other ingredients added to tobacco products during the manufacturing process.

The first industrywide regulation occurred even before the release of the first Surgeon General's Report. In the mid- to late 1950s, many cigarette advertisements made conflicting claims for the tar and nicotine levels of various brands. This period became known as the "Tar Derby" (Wagner 1971a; Whiteside 1971). On September 15, 1955, after a year of conferences with the cigarette industry, the FTC promulgated cigarette advertising guidelines "for the use of its staff in the evaluation of cigarette advertising" (FTC 1964b). These guidelines, among other things, sought to prohibit cigarette advertising that made unsubstantiated claims about the level of nicotine, tars, or other substances in cigarette smoke. By 1960, the FTC obtained agreements from the leading cigarette manufacturers to eliminate from their advertising unsubstantiated claims of tar and nicotine content (FTC 1964b).

As the previous section noted, the FTC proposed three rules addressing cigarette labeling and advertising shortly after the release of the 1964 Surgeon General's Report (FTC 1964a). The third proposed rule provided that:

> No cigarette advertisement shall contain any statement as to the quantity of any cigarette-smoke ingredients (e.g., tars and nicotine) which has not been verified in accordance with a uniform and reliable testing procedure approved by the FTC.

This recommendation was not among the final regulations promulgated by the FTC nor in subsequent congressional legislation.

Shortly after passage of the Federal Cigarette Labeling and Advertising Act of 1965, the FTC identified a uniform testing system for measuring the tar and nicotine yield of cigarettes (Pillsbury et al. 1969; see Chapter 5). The FTC determined that meaningful disclosure of tobacco product constituents required the availability of accurate information obtained by standardized testing methods. In 1966, the Commission sent a letter to U.S. cigarette manufacturers approving their factual statements of tar and nicotine content in advertising, if based on tests conducted using the approved method. In 1967, the FTC activated its own laboratory to analyze the tar and nicotine content of cigarette smoke. At the request of the Chairman of the Senate Commerce Committee, the FTC began to test and report periodically to Congress the tar and nicotine content of various cigarette brands (FTC 1981a). In 1981, the FTC first published carbon monoxide yields, based on its own laboratory tests, along with data on tar and nicotine yields (FTC 1981a).

In 1983, the FTC determined that its testing procedures may have "significantly underestimated the level of tar, nicotine and carbon monoxide that smokers received from smoking" certain low-tar cigarettes and sought comments pursuant to modifying its testing procedures (FTC 1988a). One cigarette brand, Barclay, manufactured by the

Brown and Williamson Tobacco Company, was permanently enjoined from including in its advertising, packaging, or promotion the tar rating the brand received using the FTC test methods because of problems with the testing methodology and consumers' possible reliance on that information (*FTC* v. *Brown and Williamson* 1983).

On April 15, 1987, the FTC announced the closing of its in-house laboratory that tested cigarettes for tar, nicotine, and carbon monoxide levels. The FTC attributed its decision to the cost of running the laboratory and the fact that the information was available from the cigarette industry's laboratories, whose methodology was identical to that used by the FTC. The FTC stated that it would collect tar, nicotine, and carbon monoxide ratings from the industry for inclusion in its annual report to Congress pursuant to the Federal Cigarette Labeling and Advertising Act (FTC 1987; MacLeod 1987).

As a result of these actions, a mechanism has been in place whereby information about tar, nicotine, and carbon monoxide yields of cigarettes becomes part of the public record. However, this information is not as readily accessible to consumers as it would be if it were disclosed on all packages of tobacco products or in advertising. Recommendations for uniform disclosure of cigarette constituents have been made previously by the FTC and the Department of Health and Human Services, and a specific goal was set by the Public Health Service's 1990 Health Objectives for the Nation (US DHHS 1986d):

> By 1985, tar, nicotine, and carbon monoxide yields should be prominently displayed on each cigarette package and promotional material.

In 1981, the Department of Health and Human Services (DHHS) recommended that "manufacturers should list yields of 'tar', nicotine and other hazardous components on their packages and in their advertising with appropriate explanatory information on the health significance of these measurements" (US DHHS 1981a (transmittal letter)). As early as 1969, the FTC (FTC 1969b) recommended that disclosure of tar and nicotine yields be required on cigarette packages as well as in advertisements. The next year, the FTC proposed a regulation requiring cigarette companies to disclose the tar and nicotine content of cigarette brands in their advertisements, based on the most recent FTC test results (FTC 1970). The FTC suspended this proceeding to allow the major manufacturers to implement a voluntary plan for such disclosure. Since 1971, all manufacturers have complied with this plan and voluntarily disclose the tar and nicotine content of cigarette brands in advertisements (FTC 1981b).

There is no industrywide disclosure of tar and nicotine content on cigarette packages; such disclosure is often made voluntarily for cigarettes yielding 8 mg or less of tar but rarely for higher tar brands (unpublished data, Office on Smoking and Health 1988). Carbon monoxide yields are neither required nor voluntarily disclosed on packages or in advertising, despite a 1982 FTC recommendation that they be required on cigarette packages (Muris 1982). Currently, there are no government requirements for the disclosure of tobacco smoke constituents to consumers, although, as noted above, levels of some constituents are disclosed voluntarily in advertisements and on some packages by cigarette manufacturers.

In addition to tobacco, tobacco products contain other ingredients added in the process of manufacture. The identity of these additives is regarded as confidential information by manufacturers. The Comprehensive Smoking Education Act of 1984 and the Comprehensive Smokeless Tobacco Health Education Act of 1986 required, for the first time, that the manufacturers, packagers, and importers of cigarettes and smokeless tobacco products provide annually to the Secretary of Health and Human Services a list of additives used in the manufacture of these products. The Secretary is required to treat the lists as "trade secret or confidential information," but may report to Congress on research activities about the health risks of these additives and may call attention to "any ingredient which in the judgment of the Secretary poses a health risk to cigarette smokers" (Public Law 98-474, Public Law 99-252). However, the Secretary is granted no specific authority to regulate any such hazardous products. Regulations describing the procedures for protecting the confidentiality of this information have been published (US DHHS 1985a). Analysis of the information on cigarette additives is in progress.

Federal legislation on smokeless tobacco (Public Law 99-252) now requires that manufacturers provide to the Secretary of Health and Human Services a specification of the nicotine content of smokeless tobacco products, but it does not require that nicotine content be listed on packages or in advertisements. Currently, one brand of smokeless tobacco is marketed as "light" snuff, and the nicotine content is disclosed on its packaging and advertising.

Effects of Disclosure of Tobacco Product Constituents

Current Federal law neither requires the disclosure of tobacco product or tobacco smoke constituents on packages and advertising, nor provides for the monitoring of communications effects of voluntary disclosures. The principal public health rationale for requiring disclosure is to inform consumers about the amount of hazardous substances to which they are exposed, so that consumers will be better informed and so that those who do not abstain completely may be able to reduce their health risks by selecting a brand with a lower concentration of hazardous substances.

There is some information that this has occurred. As noted in Chapter 5, the rapid growth in the market share of cigarettes with reduced tar and nicotine yields during the 1970s indicates that consumers can and will make choices based on information about tobacco constituents (US DHHS 1981a). However, there is no clear evidence of substantial health benefits to consumers who switch to lower tar and nicotine cigarettes. The potential health benefit to smokers of making such discriminations is at best limited, because there is no known safe level of tobacco product consumption (US DHHS 1981a). As mentioned in Chapter 5, concerns about low-yield cigarettes center around: (1) compensatory smoking behavior among smokers who switch to low-nicotine brands, which might even increase total tobacco smoke intake in some smokers; (2) the increased use of additives with possible adverse health effects in low-yield cigarettes; and (3) the possibility that some smokers who believe these cigarettes to be safe or less hazardous will be less inclined to quit.

It is also possible that if smokers saw a more complete listing of the harmful constituents of tobacco on packages or in ads, some would stop smoking rather than merely choosing a different brand. Evidence to test this hypothesis has not been collected. The impact of informing smokers about the identity of tobacco product additives, about which consumers know little, is unknown. It is possible that this information might encourage smokers to stop smoking, or at least to reduce their daily cigarette consumption.

Mandated Education About Health Risks

Government activities to educate the public on smoking and health are not limited to product-oriented warnings to the tobacco consumer. Government policy has required schools to educate students and teachers about the health hazards of tobacco use. Educational messages in the broadcast media were also mandated by Federal policy from 1967 through 1970.

School Education

Current Status

Both public and private efforts to reduce the initiation of smoking by children have targeted schools. Education on tobacco and health may be provided voluntarily in school curricula or may be required by legislation or regulation. For the purposes of this review, such education is considered voluntary if it is based on a decision of the individual teacher or on an action taken by an individual school or school district. A "policy" refers to Federal or State legislation or regulation mandating instruction on tobacco and health. Voluntary initiatives on school education on smoking and health are considered in Chapter 6. Policies restricting smoking in schools by students and teachers are reviewed in Part III of this Chapter.

The Federal Government has taken no action to mandate education on tobacco in the Nation's schools. Federal legislation was introduced in the 100th Congress (Adolescent Tobacco Education and Prevention Act, H.R. 3658; Atkins 1987) that would require tobacco to be included in drug abuse and education programs established under Sections 4124-4125 of the Drug-Free Schools and Communities Act of 1986 (Public Law 99-750), but this legislation was not enacted. The Surgeon General, the Secretary of Health and Human Services, and the Assistant Secretary for Health have recommended that prevention of tobacco use be included, along with instruction on illicit drug use, in school health education curricula (US DHHS 1988).

A number of States have enacted laws mandating education about smoking and health in schools. The usual content of mandated instruction is the health effects of tobacco use, often included as a component of general health education or a drugs-and-alcohol curriculum. Few school-based educational programs provide education on cessation methods for students who have already started to smoke (Chapter 6). Policies may require the education of either students or teachers, the latter sometimes as a prerequisite to receiving a teaching certificate.

TABLE 4.—State requirements for school health education on drugs/alcohol/tobacco (1974–81) and on tobacco use prevention (1987)

State	State requirement for instruction in drugs/alcohol/tobacco[a]			State requirement for instruction in tobacco prevention
	1974	1977–1978	1981	1987
Alabama		M	M	M
Alaska				
Arizona	O	O	O	M
Arkansas	M	M	M	M
California	M	M	M	
Colorado	M	M	M	
Connecticut	M	M	M	
Delaware	M	M	M	M
District of Columbia	M	M	M	M
Florida	M	M	M	
Georgia	M	M	M	M
Hawaii	M	M	M	M
Idaho	M	M	M	
Illinois	M	M	M	M
Indiana	M	M	M	
Iowa	M	M	M	
Kansas				
Kentucky		M	M	
Louisiana	M-S	M-S	M	
Maine				M
Maryland	M	M	M	
Massachusetts				
Michigan	M	M	M	
Minnesota	M	M	M	
Mississippi			M	
Missouri	M	O	O	
Montana	M-S			
Nebraska			M	M
Nevada				M
New Hampshire	M	M	M	
New Jersey	M-S	M-S	M-S	
New Mexico	M	O	M	
New York	M	M	M	M

TABLE 4.—Continued

	State requirement for instruction in drugs/alcohol/tobacco[a]			State requirement for instruction in tobacco prevention
	1974	1977–1978	1981	1987
North Carolina	M	M	M	M
North Dakota	M	M	M	
Ohio	M	M	M	M
Oklahoma				
Oregon		M	M	
Pennsylvania	M	M	M	
Rhode Island		M	M	M
South Carolina	M	M	M	
South Dakota				
Tennessee	M	M	M	M
Texas	M	M	M	M
Utah	M	M	M	M
Vermont	M	M	M	
Virginia	M	M	M	M
Washington	M	M	M	
West Virginia				M
Wisconsin	M	O	M	
Wyoming				
TOTAL (mandatory)	35	35	39	20

NOTE: Thirty-four States required instruction in drugs/alcohol/tobacco in 1985. The individual States were not identified in the report (ASHA 1987).

[a]M, mandated; O, optional/permissive; S, secondary school level. Unless otherwise noted, policies refer to both elementary and secondary levels.

SOURCE: ASHA (1976, 1979, 1981); Lovato, Allenworth, Chan, in press.

Surveys of State requirements for school health education for the years 1974, 1977, 1978, 1981, 1985, and 1987 have been conducted by the American School Health Association (ASHA 1976, 1979, 1981, 1987; Lovato, Allensworth, Chan, in press). Questionnaires were sent to State school health consultants, when identifiable, or to State commissioners of education or health. Between 1974 and 1985, the number of States (including the District of Columbia) mandating school education in the category labeled "drugs/alcohol/tobacco" varied from 34 to 39, with no clear trend over time (Table 4; data not shown for 1985, for which only the total number of States—34—was provided). In fact, several States apparently weakened or repealed preexisting requirements. In most jurisdictions, the requirement pertained to both elementary and secondary school levels. The extent to which education in this broad category specifically required tobacco education is unknown. The results do not suggest that the number of States requiring instruction on the health effects of tobacco use is increasing. In the 1987 survey, mandated curriculum on tobacco use was reported separately from curricula on drug and alcohol use. The prevention of tobacco use is mandated curriculum in 20 States (Lovato, Allensworth, Chan, in press).

A separate survey of State legislation enacted as of December 1985 reported similar findings. It found that 18 of 21 States providing data required elementary and secondary schools to include instruction on the dangers of using tobacco as part of their health education programs (Table 5) (US DHHS 1986e).

Several States also require teacher training. Three States (Alabama, Connecticut, and Oklahoma) have directed their departments of education to establish and implement in-service training programs to educate teachers, school administrators, and other school personnel about the effects of nicotine or tobacco use. All educational institutions in Minnesota that provide teacher training must offer programs on the use of and dependence on tobacco. Connecticut law requires universities that train teachers to provide instruction on the effects of nicotine and tobacco use and on the best methods for instructing students on these topics. To receive a certificate to teach or supervise in any public school in Connecticut, a person must pass an examination on the effects of nicotine and tobacco use (US DHHS 1986e).

Compliance and Effects

Little is known about the level of compliance with these State regulations. A 1986 survey of a random sample of 2,000 school districts conducted by the National School Boards Association found that 61, 64, and 62 percent of school districts provide anti-smoking education in elementary school, middle or junior high school, and high school, respectively (NSBA 1987). The generalizability of the survey is limited by a low response rate (36 percent). It is unclear to what degree this instruction is voluntary or the result of a State requirement.

Even less is known about the content or quality of curricula developed to comply with government mandates. Evaluations of voluntary school-based smoking prevention programs (Chapter 6) suggest that they can be effective if done well. The extent to which government-mandated school education programs match these results is unknown. Consequently, it is impossible to determine the extent to which government-mandated school education has contributed to greater awareness by children of the health consequences of smoking or to reductions in the initiation of smoking.

TABLE 5.—States requiring school health education on tobacco use effects

State	School health education	In-service teacher training	Instruction required for teacher certification	Instructional material must be accurate	Other
Alabama	X	X			
Alaska	X				
Arizona	X				
California				X	
Connecticut	X	X	X		X[a]
Florida				X	X[b]
Georgia	X				
Idaho	X				
Illinois	X				
Indiana	X				
Iowa	X				
Massachusetts	X				
Michigan	X				
Minnesota			X		
Nebraska	X				
Ohio	X				
Oklahoma	X	X			
Oregon	X				
Utah	X				
Vermont	X				
Wisconsin	X				

[a]Connecticut law provides that no certificate to teach or supervise shall be granted to any person who has not passed a satisfactory examination on the effects of nicotine and tobacco. Conn. Gen. Stat. Ann., Section 10-145a (West Supp. 1964).

[b]Florida's Cancer Control and Research Act provides that proven causes of cancer, including smoking, should be publicized and should be the subject of educational programs for the prevention of cancer. Fla. Stat. Ann., Section 381.2712(2)(c) (West Supp. 1965).

SOURCE: US DHHS (1986e).

Broadcast Media

History

In 1949, the U.S. Federal Communications Commission (FCC) promulgated its Fairness Doctrine (FCC 1949). Under this doctrine, which the FCC repealed in August 1988, licensed broadcasters were obligated

> to encourage and implement the broadcast of all sides of controversial public issues over their facilities, over and beyond their obligation to make available on demand opportunities for the expression of opposing views (FCC 1987).

This meant that, as a condition of retaining the required license, broadcasters were required to air both sides of a controversial issue if one side was presented. Subsequent decisions by the FCC indicated that the Fairness Doctrine could require a station to grant free time, even when one viewpoint was presented under paid sponsorship. The FCC did not, however, require that a broadcaster provide equal time for opposing views; only a "reasonable opportunity" for the presentation of opposing views was required (Columbia Law Review 1967).

In January 1967, John Banzhaf, an attorney acting as a private citizen, petitioned the FCC to apply the Fairness Doctrine to cigarette advertising. On June 2, 1967, the Commission ruled that the doctrine applied to cigarette advertising on television and radio and required broadcasters who aired cigarette commercials to provide "a significant amount of time" to citizens who wished to point out that smoking "may be hazardous to the smoker's health" (FCC 1967). In a subsequent press interview, the FCC's chief counsel gave his informal opinion that a ratio of one antismoking message to three cigarette commercials seemed to him to constitute "a significant amount of time" (Whiteside 1971).

The ruling applying the Fairness Doctrine to cigarette advertising went into effect on July 1, 1967. Thereafter, broadcasters began to air an array of antismoking public service announcements (PSAs), developed primarily by voluntary health organizations and government health agencies (Whiteside 1971). The time "donated" for the antismoking spots amounted to approximately 75 million dollars (in 1970 dollars) per year from 1968 through 1970 (Lydon 1970). As discussed in the next section, subsequent Federal legislation, the Public Health Cigarette Smoking Act of 1969, banned cigarette advertising on television and radio, effective January 2, 1971. Once this occurred and cigarette ads were removed from radio and television, the Fairness Doctrine basis for requiring broadcasters to carry antismoking PSAs was eliminated. Antismoking messages then had to compete for public service advertising time donated by broadcasters. As a result, the frequency of the antismoking spots declined dramatically. According to Lewit, Coate, and Grossman (1981), the number of antismoking PSAs declined by almost 80 percent after 1970, relative to the number aired in 1969, and they were shown at times when youths in particular were not likely to be watching television.

Effectiveness

The antismoking messages mandated by the Fairness Doctrine might have been expected to increase public knowledge and change public attitudes about smoking. Indirectly, they might reduce smoking prevalence and tobacco consumption by stimulating cessation and retarding initiation. The degree to which the messages achieved these goals has been assessed by measuring trends in public beliefs concerning the health hazards of smoking, in smoking prevalence, and in cigarette sales before, during, and after the 1968–70 period. PSAs were only one of a number of societal influences on smoking during that period. Because of the broad reach of the mass media, it is impossible to control for these concurrent influences by examining a group that was not exposed to PSAs. Consequently, changes in these indices cannot be unequivocally attributed to the presence of PSAs. Nonetheless, they offer strong circumstantial evidence for an effect of the PSA campaign.

Survey data indicate that PSAs were in fact seen and recalled by large numbers of Americans. O'Keefe (1971) surveyed 621 students below 21 years of age and 300 adults in Central Florida. Ninety percent of the sample recalled seeing at least one antismoking PSA, and about half of them were able to recall a specific commercial. When asked about the effect of PSAs on their own smoking behavior, 32 percent of smokers reported that they had cut down, 37 percent said they thought more about the effects of smoking than before, and 11 percent said they stopped smoking temporarily as a result of the commercials. This study, based on the self-reported smoking behavior of a small sample, does not provide definitive evidence for an effect of PSAs on knowledge or cigarette consumption.

Analysis of trends in national survey data provides a stronger quality of evidence for the effects of PSAs on knowledge or behavior. National survey data collected before, during, and after the 1968–70 period show consistent but small increases in public knowledge of the health hazards of smoking (see Chapter 4). According to the Adult Use of Tobacco Surveys (AUTSs), the proportion of adults who believed that smoking is hazardous to health was already high before the airing of PSAs. It increased slightly during and after the period when PSAs were shown, from 85 to 87 to 90 percent in 1966, 1970, and 1975, respectively. Similar trends were seen for public beliefs concerning the causal relationship between smoking and specific diseases, including lung cancer, heart disease, and chronic obstructive lung disease (Chapter 4). One might expect that the personal and emotional messages in many of the PSAs (Whiteside 1971) would have a particularly salient effect on personalized acceptance of health risks from smoking (Chapter 4). AUTS data show a larger increase in this factor, coincident with the PSAs. The percentage of smokers who were concerned about the effects of smoking on their own health increased from 47 percent in 1966, before the Fairness Doctrine, to 69 and 68 percent in 1970 and 1975, respectively. One must be cautious in attributing these changes solely to the PSA campaign, because increases in public knowledge sometimes continued after the campaign ended and because other informational activities, such as cigarette warning labels, occurred concurrently in both the public and private sectors.

The effect of PSAs on smoking behavior has been assessed by analyzing trends in cigarette sales and smoking prevalence. Analyses of temporal trends in tobacco consumption, as measured by cigarette sales, provide evidence for an effect of PSAs in restraining smoking, at least temporarily. For the 3-year periods before (1965–67), during (1968–70), and after (1971–73) the Fairness Doctrine PSAs, per capita cigarette sales increased by 2.0 percent, decreased by 6.9 percent, and increased by 4.1 percent, respectively (Chapter 5). Warner (1977) compared actual sales figures for the Fairness Doctrine period to projected sales figures (for the same years) based on the trend in sales during the period 1947–67. He predicted that in the absence of PSAs and subsequent publicity, consumption would have been 19.5 percent higher than it actually was by 1975. In a regression analysis of the effects of both cigarette ads and the Fairness Doctrine PSAs, Hamilton (1972) found that the antismoking messages retarded per capita cigarette consumption by 530.7 cigarettes per year, while the cigarette ads boosted it by 95.0 per year. Schneider, Klein, and Murphy (1981) concluded that the PSAs reduced per capita tobacco consumption by 5 percent. Findings from these and related studies are reviewed in Chapter 8.

If PSAs had motivated large numbers of smokers to quit smoking, one would expect to have observed a decline in the prevalence of cigarette smoking, as well as in tobacco consumption, during the period when they were shown. Prevalence data have some limits compared with cigarette consumption data. Estimates of smoking prevalence are based on individuals' self-reported behavior in national surveys, which is a less objective measure than consumption estimates based on sales data. Furthermore, data on prevalence are collected less frequently than are sales data, making prevalence a less sensitive index of short-term effects. Data on the self-reported prevalence of cigarette smoking from 1965–85 show a highly consistent linear trend downward during the entire period (Chapter 5). These data do not provide evidence for an independent effect of the PSA campaign on overall smoking prevalence and contrast with the cigarette consumption data cited above. However, Lewit, Coate, and Grossman (1981), who analyzed the effect of PSAs on the smoking prevalence of teenagers, reported an effect in that age group. They found that the teenage smoking rate was 3.0 percentage points lower during the Fairness Doctrine period than during the 16-month period prior to the Doctrine; most of this effect occurred during the time when PSAs were shown.

Warner (1978) compared cigarette sales data to self-reported cigarette consumption for the years 1964–75. He found that the ratio of self-reported cigarette consumption to cigarette sales ("consumption ratio") decreased from a level of 72 and 73 percent in 1964 and 1966, to 66 percent in 1970, and to 64 percent in 1975. The decrease between 1966 and 1970, years spanning the Fairness Doctrine period, was statistically significant. Between 1966 and 1970, actual aggregate sales dropped 1 percent, while reported consumption dropped 9.5 percent. One explanation for this decline is a greater underreporting of current smoking because of growing awareness of the health hazards of smoking and the declining social acceptability of smoking (Chapter 5). Warner suggested that the Fairness Doctrine PSAs, by causing changes in knowledge and attitudes, may have been responsible for increased underreporting. More recent data from 1974–85 show that the consumption ratio has remained stable at approximately 72 percent, despite further reductions in the social acceptability of smoking (Chapter

5). As mentioned in Chapter 5, the decrease in the consumption ratio reported by Warner may be related to the fact that the self-reported data for 1970 and 1975 were collected by telephone surveys, while the 1964 and 1966 data were collected by in-person interviews; the latter technique generally provides slightly higher smoking prevalence estimates than do telephone surveys.

In summary, both per capita cigarette consumption changes and regression studies comparing actual cigarette sales to projected sales based on prior trends are consistent with the conclusion that the Fairness Doctrine PSAs affected smoking behavior, at least in the short term. Changes in public knowledge about the health effects of smoking as assessed in national surveys also occurred during the period PSAs were aired. Because of other social influences on smoking during this period, it is impossible to attribute changes in cigarette consumption or public knowledge solely to the airing of PSAs. However, as described further in Chapter 8, they were a prominent component of antismoking activities, which in the aggregate had marked effects on smoking prevalence and tobacco consumption in the 25 years since the release of the 1964 Surgeon General's Report. It is unclear whether and to what degree any short-term effects could have been sustained with an ongoing campaign. If PSAs had continued, it is possible that their short-term effects could have been sustained only with the types of message variation, pulsed media placement patterns, and ongoing communications measurement

TABLE 6.—Cigarette advertising and promotional expenditures, 1970–86 ($ millions)

Year	Advertising	Promotional	Total	Total in constant (1986) dollars	Advertising as percentage of total
1970	314.7	46.3	361.0	1019.4	87.2
1971	251.6	NA	NA	NA	NA
1972	257.6	NA	NA	NA	NA
1973	247.5	NA	NA	NA	NA
1974	306.8	NA	NA	NA	NA
1975	366.2	125.1	491.3	1000.9	74.5
1976	430.0	209.1	639.1	1231.0	67.3
1977	552.0	247.5	799.5	1446.6	69.0
1978	600.5	274.5	875.0	1470.6	68.6
1979	749.0	334.4	1083.4	1636.6	69.1
1980	829.9	412.4	1242.3	1653.0	66.8
1981	998.3	549.4	1547.7	1865.9	64.5
1982	1040.1	753.7	1793.8	2037.6	58.0
1983	1081.0	819.8	1900.8	2091.9	56.9
1984	1097.5	997.7	2095.2	2211.7	52.2
1985	1075.0	1401.4	2476.4	2524.1	43.4
1986	931.8	1450.6	2382.4	2382.4	39.1

NOTE: NA, not available.
SOURCE: Warner (1986b); Federal Trade Commission (1988b).

and tracking characteristics of ongoing national advertising campaigns (Aaker and Meyers 1987), including those of the cigarette companies themselves.

Restrictions on Tobacco Advertising and Promotion

Cigarettes are one of the most heavily marketed consumer products in the United States (FTC 1981b; Davis 1987). Cigarette advertising and promotional expenditures totaled 2.4 billion dollars in 1986 (FTC 1988b). In both actual and constant dollars, these expenditures increased consistently between 1975 and 1985 but fell slightly in 1986, the last year for which data are available (Table 6). A study reviewing 1985 data found that cigarettes were the most heavily advertised category of products in the outdoor media (e.g., billboards), the second most heavily advertised category in magazines (after passenger cars), and the third most heavily advertised subcategory in newspapers (after passenger cars and airlines) (Davis 1987). All six of the major cigarette manufacturers were included among the 100 companies with the highest advertising expenditures in 1985 (Davis 1987). According to FTC reports to Congress for the years 1982 and 1983, the major advertising themes associated cigarette smoking with high-style living, healthy activities, and economic, social, and professional success (FTC 1985).

Tobacco advertising includes both traditional advertising (in newspapers and magazines, on billboards, and in transit facilities) and promotional activities. Promotional activities are diverse and include the distribution of free product samples, coupons for price reductions, and offers for discounted products (often bearing the name of the cigarette brand). Promotional activities also encompass industry sponsorship of cultural, sporting, and entertainment events, and sponsorship of community or political organizations. Incentives paid to distributors or retailers are another form of tobacco promotion. Over the past decade, the balance of expenditures has shifted from traditional advertising to promotional activities (Davis 1987), so that by 1986, promotional expenditures accounted for 60 percent of the tobacco marketing dollar, compared with only 25 percent of the total in 1975 (FTC 1988b) (Table 6).

This Section reviews previous, current, and proposed government policies to regulate tobacco advertising and promotion. It considers the central public health issue—whether advertising and promotion increase tobacco consumption—and reviews available evidence on this question. The focus of this review is on cigarette advertising and promotion because cigarettes account for the vast majority of both tobacco use and advertising/promotional expenditures. The effects of advertising for other tobacco products have not often been studied. The discussion includes coverage of the smaller body of information about promotional activities beyond traditional advertising because of their growing importance in tobacco marketing.

Effects of Tobacco Advertising and Promotion

Public health concern about tobacco advertising and promotion is based on the premise that these activities encourage the initiation of smoking and stimulate tobacco consumption, especially by children, while retarding cessation efforts, particularly by adults. It has been suggested that ads promoting low-tar and -nicotine cigarettes may allay the anxiety of current smokers, shifting their attention away from the decision to stop smoking by presenting the option of switching to an ostensibly less hazardous brand (Davis 1987). It has also been suggested that tobacco advertising interferes with efforts to inform the public of the health hazards of smoking because media that accept tobacco advertising provide less coverage about the health hazards of tobacco use. Proponents of this view contend that restricting tobacco advertising would reduce both the number of prosmoking messages and their alleged restraining influence on the flow of antitobacco information from the media, thereby making antismoking efforts more visible and potentially more effective (Warner 1985).

By contrast, both tobacco products manufacturers and representatives of the major associations of advertisers have consistently denied that advertising and promotion encourage smoking and the use of other tobacco products. They claim that the purpose and effect of marketing are merely to provide information and to influence brand selection among current users of tobacco products (Waterson 1982; O'Toole 1986; Weil 1986). The statement might also be made that cigarette advertising has permitted tobacco companies to successfully market new brands with reduced tar and nicotine yields and will allow for the future promotion of new products with reduced tar and nicotine. However, because of considerable controversy about the health effects of low-tar and low-nicotine cigarettes (US DHHS 1981a, 1988), the public health benefit of switching to these products remains in doubt (See Chapters 2 and 5).

Mechanisms by Which Advertising and Promotion May Affect Consumption

From a marketing perspective, advertising and promotion have different roles (Popper 1986a; Davis and Jason 1988). Conceptually, both tobacco advertising and promotion could increase tobacco consumption through several direct and indirect mechanisms (Warner 1986b; Warner et al. 1986a). Direct mechanisms all relate to the immediate impact of marketing techniques on the consumer or potential consumer. Indirect mechanisms are those that influence some factor other than the consumer (e.g., the behavior of other institutions such as the news media), which in turn affects the use of tobacco products.

Four direct mechanisms by which tobacco advertising and promotion may increase tobacco consumption have been suggested.

1. Advertising and promotion could encourage children or young adults to experiment with tobacco products and initiate regular use. This is the central focus of the public health concern about advertising and promotion. Initiation could be encouraged when the images presented in cigarette advertising change children's and young adults' attitudes about cigarettes (in general and about specific brands) in a way that makes them more likely to start using tobacco products (McCarthy 1986). Promotion could directly lead to experimentation via the distribution of free samples and the creation of environments (cigarette-sponsored concerts and sporting events) where sample distribution is facilitated and cigarette trial is actively encouraged (Popper 1986b).
2. Advertising and promotion could increase tobacco users' daily consumption of tobacco products. Advertising could serve as a cue to tobacco use by creating

attitudes and images that reinforce the "desirability" of smoking and remind smokers of occasions that are associated with smoking (Glosser 1984; Warner 1986b; Davis 1987). Promotion could act as an economic incentive to increase tobacco users' daily consumption (Popper 1986b). Coupons (either for price reductions or free products) reduce the financial cost of smoking for the consumer, which can encourage increased consumption via the price elasticity of demand (see Part II).

3. Advertising and promotion could reduce current tobacco users' motivation to quit. Tobacco ads, with their attractive imagery and implicit alleviation of fears (Altman et al. 1987), could diminish users' cessation intentions. Advertising of low-tar and -nicotine cigarettes may, in particular, have this effect (Popper 1988; Davis 1987). Promotion could weaken current tobacco users' resolve to quit by reducing the financial cost of smoking (Popper 1986b).
4. Advertising and promotion could encourage former smokers to resume smoking. Quitters experience both physiological and psychological withdrawal (US DHHS 1988). Advertising presents smokers with images reminding them of the reasons and situations in which they smoked, thereby increasing the difficulties associated with withdrawal. Promotional events (sponsored sporting events or concerts) create environments where former smokers are encouraged to resume smoking. They provide cues to smoke in the social situations in which former smokers had been likely to smoke. This effect may be enhanced by the distribution of free cigarette samples that often occurs at tobacco-sponsored events (Popper 1986b; Davis and Jason 1988).

Three indirect mechanisms by which advertising and promotion might increase tobacco consumption have also been suggested.

1. Media dependence on advertising revenues from the tobacco companies may discourage full and open discussion of the hazards of tobacco use. Reduced media attention may reduce the extent of public understanding of the health hazards. This might reduce the public's understanding of the risks of tobacco use and thereby increase tobacco use relative to what it would be in an environment in which media coverage was more extensive and was influenced solely by the inherent interest and importance of the subject (Warner 1985).
2. A number of institutions have to some degree become financially dependent on the promotional, charitable, and public relations spending of the tobacco industry, including professional sports, cultural institutions, and minority organizations. This institutional dependence on tobacco spending may create political support for, or mute opposition to, the industry's marketing and policy objectives (Taylor 1984; Warner 1986b). In turn, this may reduce public knowledge about the risks of tobacco and indirectly, encourage initiation and maintenance of tobacco use.
3. Still more broadly, the ubiquity and familiarity of tobacco advertising and promotion may contribute to an environment in which tobacco use is perceived by users to be socially acceptable, or at least less socially objectionable and less hazardous than it is in fact. Smokers might interpret the legality of tobacco advertising and promotion as an implicit message that "Smoking can't really be

all that dangerous; otherwise the government would ban cigarette advertising." Presented with that statement in a British Government survey, 44 percent of smokers agreed (Chapman 1986). This environment may contribute to the initiation of tobacco use by children and the maintenance of use by adults.

Evidence

Evidence pertaining to the effects of tobacco advertising and promotion on the consumption of tobacco products is diverse in its nature and conclusions. The research includes formal empirical analysis, informal empirical observations, and logic. Although some evidence specifically addresses issues of direct or indirect impact, much of it applies generally to the overall effect of tobacco advertising on consumption. Promotion has received less attention in the research published to date. In the following sections, the evidence cited applies to the overall effect, except as indicated. Most of the existing evidence, both analytical and experiential, relates to cigarettes and advertising. Little work has examined the effects of other promotional techniques or addresses the advertising of tobacco products other than cigarettes.

Formal Empirical Analysis

Formal empirical analysis is primarily of two types: (1) statistical studies of the relationship between aggregate cigarette advertising expenditures and aggregate cigarette consumption, using the method of regression analysis, and (2) survey research and experimental studies of smokers' and potential smokers' reactions to and recall of cigarette ads.

Regression Analyses

More than a dozen studies using regression analysis have evaluated the statistical correlation between cigarette advertising expenditures and cigarette sales in at least four western countries. Several of these analyses have found no statistically significant correlation (Schmalensee 1972; Lambin 1976; Metra Consulting Group 1979; Schneider, Klein, Murphy 1981; Johnson 1985; Baltagi and Levin 1986). At least two studies have raised the possibility that advertising expenditures are a function of cigarette sales, rather than the reverse; that is, manufacturers devote a relatively fixed proportion of revenues to advertising, and ad expenditures rise or fall as company sales increase or decrease (Schmalensee 1972; Schneider, Klein, Murphy 1981). Other analyses have identified a statistically significant relationship and concluded that, in the aggregate, increased advertising expenditures do lead to increased sales, although typically the estimated effect of advertising expenditures on consumption is small (Peles 1971; McGuinness and Cowling 1975; Lewit, Coate, Grossman 1981; Reuijl 1982; Porter 1986; Radfar 1985; Roberts and Samuelson 1988; Chetwynd et al. 1988). Still other researchers have reported consistently finding a small positive effect, but one that is not generally statistically significant (Hamilton 1972).

Only one regression study has addressed the relationship between cigarette advertising and smoking by teenagers (Lewit, Coate, Grossman 1981), despite the fact that adolescence is the period in which the vast majority of smokers initiate cigarette use

(Chapter 5). As discussed above, Lewit and colleagues examined the issue in the context of the broadcast ad ban, estimating that teenagers' smoking prevalence fell by 0.6 percent from 1970 to 1974 as a result of the ban. Although not a quantitatively substantial effect in percentage terms, it was a statistically significant finding. Given the large population of teenage smokers, even a small percentage change in smoking translates into substantial absolute numbers.

The regression studies vary considerably in methods, sophistication, and quality. Most of the studies rely on time series analysis, introducing the inherent methodological risk of unstable parameter estimates due to correlations among variables over the time periods studied. Findings may also vary because of differences in the time period studied, differences among countries, and variability in functional form specification. The better studies attempt to control for other variables that might influence the movement of both advertising expenditures and consumption, but this is handled inconsistently. Some of the studies treat advertising as having an impact only in the year of expenditure, whereas others examine both current and later (residual) effects of advertising expenditures (Peles 1971). A few use a measure of cumulative advertising expenditures, rather than single-year expenditures, in constructing the principal independent variable (Schneider, Klein, Murphy 1981). A recent study found that quarterly data produced more meaningful results than annual data; the authors speculated that "the longer time period [i.e., annual data] may mask significant relationships" (Chetwynd et al. 1988). At least one study has adopted a nondollar measure of advertising (Lewit, Coate, Grossman 1981), recognizing that the assumption of homogeneity over time in the dollar measure may not hold (Calfee 1986).

None of the studies has properly distinguished between and incorporated both conventional advertising and other promotional expenditures. This omission is particularly germane to the late 1980s, the first period in which tobacco product promotional expenditures exceeded conventional advertising (FTC 1988b) (Table 6). Moreover, regression studies have not taken into account other means of interbrand competition besides advertising and promotion. The one exception is a recent study by Roberts and Samuelson (1988), who simultaneously analyzed the effects of advertising expenditures and numbers of brands sold on the market shares of rival manufacturers. In analyses of the low-tar and high-tar U.S. cigarette markets during 1971–82, they found that firms' advertising primarily affected the level of market demand, while individual firms' market shares depended upon the number of brands sold.

Methodological differences and problems such as these restrict the meaningful interpretation and comparison of findings. Furthermore, inherent limitations in the method of regression analysis diminish the ultimate value of these analyses in addressing the two fundamental questions of interest: How much, if at all, do advertising and promotion affect the level of tobacco consumption? Would restrictions or a ban on advertising and promotion affect the level of consumption? Regression analysis is designed to assess the statistical relationship between marginal changes in an independent variable and marginal changes in the dependent variable, controlling for other factors for which data are available. Regression results do not assess the effect of large (or complete) changes in the independent variable. Consequently, the findings of regression studies, pertaining to small changes in ad expenditures, may not relate at all to the change contemplated in a ban—the complete elimination of all advertising and promotion (Cox 1984).

There is a second theoretical reason why regression analysis might not be expected to find a sizable, significant relationship between advertising and consumption. If advertising both expands the overall market and helps firms capture existing market share from competitors, the rational level of advertising expenditure will exceed that which increases aggregate consumption alone. Thus, on the margin, the function of advertising dollars will be to compete for existing market share, not to expand the overall market. Hence, regression analyses, examining marginal effects, would not be expected to demonstrate a strong correlation between advertising expenditures and aggregate consumption (Warner et al. 1986a). In these circumstances, the fact that several of the regression studies have found statistically significant correlations has been interpreted as evidence that advertising does increase consumption (Tye, Warner, Glantz 1987).

Survey Research and Experimental Studies of Reactions to Advertisements

The second category of empirical analysis includes studies testing the hypothesis that advertising encourages children to try tobacco products and initiate related behaviors. Two types of studies fall in this category: surveys assessing recall of and reaction to cigarette ads and experimental analysis of subjects' responses to ads.

Among the surveys, the most direct approach to assessing the relationship between advertising and cigarette consumption has been to ask children or adults about the factors that influenced them to smoke. These studies typically find that advertising is ranked quite low on the list of relevant factors. Marketing experts have questioned the validity of this approach because conscious response to advertising is deemed to be a poor index of actual response (Bergler 1981; Chapman 1986). As such, studies with a similar method and opposite findings also offer little insight into the actual effects of advertising. An example is a study by Fisher and Magnus (1981), which found that most children believe that cigarette ads encourage children to smoke.

An alternative approach that employs both surveys and experiments is to assess reactions to ads and their imagery, often (then or later) correlated with subjects' reported smoking behavior. Analyses of this type range from studies asking subjects to recall cigarette brands and ad themes to experiments measuring subjects' eye contact with magazine ads (Fischer et al. 1989). Several studies have associated recognition and approval of cigarette ads with subsequent propensity to smoke (O'Connell et al. 1981; Chapman and Fitzgerald 1982; Alexander et al. 1983; McCarthy 1986; Goldstein et al. 1987). These studies are representative of the research methods used by the cigarette companies themselves to test the communications effects of their advertising (see advertising-related research presented in *Cippolone* v. *Liggett Group* 1988 and *FTC* v. *Brown and Williamson* 1983).

Collectively, these latter studies present data suggesting that cigarette ads are effective in getting children's attention and that they are recalled. In these studies, recall of prominent cigarette brand names and of ad themes is usually high. (By contrast, attention paid to the Surgeon General's health warnings and recall of them are much lower (Fischer et al., in press).) The studies find that strength of interest in the ads correlates with smoking behavior, either current or anticipated. However, the studies do not examine the causal links between this recall and smoking behavior. It is possible that smoking, or an interest in smoking, might affect awareness of ads, rather than ads encouraging smoking, a point acknowledged by the authors of some of these studies (e.g., Goldstein et al. 1987),but this possibility has not been examined with regard to cigarette advertising. The hypothesis is supported by the well-documented psychological phenomenon of perceptual vigilance (Spence and Engel 1970), whereby consumers are more aware of advertising for products they use. The opposite phenomenon, perceptual defense or selective perception (Spence 1967), helps explain why smokers avoid perceiving the warning labels and other risk-related information (FTC 1981b).

Additional Empirical Observations and Logical Arguments

The principal evidence for evaluating the role of tobacco advertising and promotion derives from the experience of advertising industry professionals and from logical analyses. Some of the latter are empirical, while others are not.

At the core of the argument that tobacco advertising affects only brand share among competitors and does not increase consumption is the contention that the market for tobacco products is a mature market, one in which market expansion cannot be achieved (O'Toole 1986). Advertising professionals who disagree have argued that market expansion is invariably a purpose of advertising. Furthermore, they have observed that it is principally in connection with two industries "under siege," tobacco and alcohol, that both producers and advertisers have made the brand-share-only argument (Foote 1981; Sharp 1986).

Proponents of the mature market argument have noted that adult per capita cigarette consumption has fallen annually since 1973; aggregate consumption has fallen each of the last 6 years (Tobacco Institute 1988); and per capita tobacco consumption is at an all-time low for this century (Grise 1984). The prevalence trends accounting for this change are particularly evident in cohort analyses that show younger birth cohorts taking up smoking in much smaller percentages than their predecessors (Chapter 5). Even in a mature market, however, the role of cigarette advertising could play a role in market maintenance, in addition to vying for brand share. In a mature or declining market, one standard strategy is to retain customers through defensive advertising and promotion (Kotler 1988). This strategy would be particularly important in the case of the cigarette market, in which an estimated 5 percent of its adult consumers are lost each year due to smoking cessation or death (from diseases related or unrelated to smoking) (Warner 1986b). It has been argued that such defensive strategies can be seen in the tobacco industry's advertising of low- and "ultra-low-tar" brands, where the goal of the campaign is not simply a shift between brands but a shift to a lower tar brand as opposed to total cessation (Popper 1988).

In opposition to the mature market argument, analysts have emphasized that although the market as a whole may be declining, segments of it appear to be actual or potential growth markets, including young women, children, blue-collar workers, and certain minority groups (Sharp 1986; Davis 1987). Industry advertising and promotion trends show increases in the relative shares of marketing budgets devoted to several of these subpopulations (Englander 1986; Albright et al. 1988).

Analysts have cited the past decade's growth in smokeless tobacco use as evidence that tobacco companies believe that advertising and promotion can be used to attract new consumers, at least for smokeless tobacco products (Connolly et al. 1986; Tye, Warner, Glantz 1987). Consequently, the mature market concept does not apply to smokeless tobacco products. Industry documents describing the marketing strategy for one smokeless tobacco product demonstrate that the company designed the low-nicotine product to serve as a "starter" product. Advertising for the product was concentrated in publications that have a high teenage male readership (Connolly 1986; Feigelson 1983). In other documents, the smokeless tobacco industry has referred to the "graduation" process from the low-nicotine starter products to more "full-flavored" products, that is, those higher in nicotine (Connolly 1986). In addition, advertisements for smokeless tobacco products have provided detailed instructions on how to use the products (Christen 1980), evidence that the marketing campaigns have been intended to attract new users.

Opponents of the position that tobacco advertising serves only to increase or maintain market share have also argued that this position is not financially consistent with the tobacco industry's marketing expenditures. A study of the economics of tobacco advertising concluded that advertising and promotion were unlikely to make financial sense if they served only brand-share function (Tye, Warner, Glantz 1987). Fewer than 10 percent of smokers change brands in any given year (Marketing and Media Decisions 1985). The current advertising and promotion expenditures of the domestic cigarette companies are greater than the sales revenues represented by those brand switchers (Popper 1986b). Furthermore, two companies, Phillip Morris and R.J. Reynolds, control more than two-thirds of the American cigarette market. Much of the limited brand switching that occurs is necessarily between brands of the same company. Based on such observations, it has been argued that the behavior of the tobacco industry itself supports the conclusion that the industry perceives a positive association between advertising and consumption (Warner 1986b).

Much of the empirically based evidence pertaining to the effects of advertising comes from international comparisons. Support for the view that cigarette advertising serves to expand the market comes from the observation that in several countries in which cigarettes are a state monopoly, the state enterprise advertises. If advertising served solely to redistribute smokers among brands, there would be no reason to advertise in such countries (Chapman and Vermeer 1985). Support for the view that advertising does not influence consumption levels has been sought in the experience of countries that have never permitted cigarette advertising, such as the Communist bloc countries, where cigarette consumption is high and has grown rapidly in the absence of advertising (Waterson 1982; Boddewyn 1986). The relevance of this observation has been challenged, however, on the ground that the issue is not whether advertising is the only, or even the most important, determinant of smoking trends. The relevant question, which these comparisons of countries do not and cannot address, is whether the rate of increase in tobacco consumption would have been affected by advertising (Warner et al. 1986a).

Indirect Mechanisms: Media Coverage of Smoking

The variety of potential indirect influences of tobacco advertising and promotion reflects the magnitude and diversity of expenditures (Taylor 1984; Warner 1986b; FTC 1988b). A substantial body of evidence exists only in one case: the relationship between cigarette advertising revenues and coverage of smoking and health in the media, especially in magazines. The public health relevance of this relationship is based on the assumption that discussion of the hazards of tobacco alters public knowledge of and opinions about tobacco use. Through a complex set of social and individual response mechanisms, knowledge and attitude changes evolve into reductions in smoking. Thus, if the media have restricted coverage of the hazards of tobacco for fear of losing advertising revenue, the public has been deprived of information that might have improved knowledge or changed social opinion more rapidly or extensively, thereby leading to reduced levels of smoking and the associated disease toll (Warner 1985).

Most of the evidence linking the level of cigarette advertising revenue to the degree

TABLE 7.—Cigarette advertising revenues and coverage of smoking and health, selected magazines

	Years surveyed	Percentage of health articles discussing smoking	Cigarette advertising revenue as percentage of total ad revenue
Reader's Digest	1965–81	34.4	0
Good Housekeeping	1965–81	22.1	0
Prevention	1967–78	15.4	0
Vogue	1965–81	11.7	5.1
U.S. News and World Report	1965–81	7.4	14.6
Ladies' Home Journal	1968–81	7.1	16.3
Time	1965–81	6.9	17.2
Harper's Bazaar	1968–81	4.5	7.1
McCall's	1969–80	4.5	15.1
Newsweek	1969–81	2.9	15.8
Cosmopolitan	1971–81	2.3	9.4
Mademoiselle	1966–81	1.9	7.3
Ms.	1972–81	0	14.8
Redbook	1970–81	0	16.1

NOTE: Magazines listed included a minimum of 60 health-related articles in the years surveyed.
SOURCE: Dale (1982).

of media coverage of smoking and health has been developed recently; some of it, however, dates back half a century (Seldes 1941). Formal analytical studies of the phenomenon that control for potential confounding influences are limited in number;

existing analyses are based primarily on correlations between magazines' cigarette advertising revenues and their coverage of smoking and health (Whelan et al. 1981; Dale 1982; Jacobson and Amos 1985; White and Whelan 1986; Warner and Goldenhar, in press).

One of these studies found that between 1967 and 1979, there were a total of 8 feature articles that seriously discussed quitting or the dangers of smoking in 10 prominent women's magazines that carry cigarette advertisements. Of the 10 magazines, 4 carried no antismoking articles in the entire 12-year period. By contrast, 2 prominent magazines that do not accept cigarette advertising, *Good Housekeeping* and *Seventeen*, ran 11 and 5 such articles, respectively. On average, the magazines that accepted cigarette advertisements published from 12 to 63 times as many articles on individual topics such as nutrition, contraception, stress, and mental health as they did on the antismoking theme. The ratio was much smaller for *Good Housekeeping* and *Seventeen* (Whelan et al. 1981). In another empirical study by the same organization, researchers examined coverage of smoking and health in prominent magazines recognized for their general interest in health matters. Publications selected for study published at least 60 articles on health topics between 1965 and 1981. The proportion of health articles devoted to smoking was compared with the proportion of advertising revenues derived from cigarette advertisements. Only four of the magazines had as many as 10 percent of their health-related articles devoted to smoking. Of these four, the top three did not accept cigarette advertising. The fourth had the lowest proportionate share of advertising income derived from cigarette ads of the remaining magazines. There was no substantial correlation between the volume of advertisements and smoking coverage within the remaining magazines (Dale 1982; Table 7).

A more recent study compared changes over time in coverage of smoking and health by 39 national magazines that published cigarette ads and 11 magazines that did not. The study also compared these changes with those found in coverage by *The New York Times* and *The Christian Science Monitor*, as well as with the collective cigarette advertising revenue of the first group of magazines. The two newspapers were selected as measures of the "inherent newsworthiness" of the subject. Comparing two 11-year periods, one preceding the broadcast media ban on cigarette advertising (1959–69) and the other following it (1973–83), the authors found that (1) the magazines that included cigarette ads experienced an increase in real cigarette ad revenues, controlling for inflation, of 727 percent (cigarette ads rose from 1.9 percent of total magazine ad revenues in the first period to 11.0 percent in the second); (2) these magazines decreased their coverage of smoking and health by 65 percent, while the magazines that did not carry cigarette ads decreased their coverage by 29 percent, a statistically significant difference; (3) the two newspapers' coverage fell by 21 percent (the *Times*, which accepts cigarette advertising) and 3 percent (the *Monitor*, which accepts no cigarette advertising). Both decreases were significantly smaller than that of the magazines that included cigarette ads, but not significantly different from that of the magazines not including cigarette ads (Warner and Goldenhar, in press).

In addition to these correlational studies, there is extensive anecdotal evidence about the influence of advertising revenues on magazine coverage of smoking and health. Writers, editors, and publishers have described numerous instances of purported censorship attributed directly to publications' fears of alienating cigarette advertisers (Smith 1978; Whelan et al. 1981; Bagdikian 1983; Warner 1985; Okie 1985; Magnus 1986). Although the anecdotal evidence pertains mainly to magazines, it includes other media, including newspapers (ABC News 1983; Gitlitz 1983) and the broadcast media prior to the removal of cigarette ads (Bagdikian 1983). Furthermore, there are allegations of advertising-induced censorship related to other tobacco products, such as smokeless tobacco (Connolly 1986).

Federal Advertising Restrictions

The Federal agency responsible for regulating the advertising of tobacco and other consumer products is the FTC. The Federal Trade Commission Act of 1914, amended in 1938, empowers the FTC "to prevent persons, partnerships, or corporations . . . from using unfair or deceptive acts or practices in commerce" (Wagner 1971b).

The FTC's efforts to regulate unsubstantiated claims in tobacco advertisements began well before 1964. From the 1930s through the 1950s, many cigarette advertisements made claims that smoking the advertised brand improved health or at least offered health benefits compared with smoking other brands (Neuberger 1963; Tye 1986). Between 1938 and 1968, the Commission invoked its adjudicatory (quasi-judicial) authority 25 times with respect to cigarette advertising (Fritschler 1969). Between 1945 and 1960, the Commission completed seven formal cease-and-desist order proceedings against cigarette manufacturers involving medical or health claims made in advertising (FTC 1964b). For example, according to Wagner (1971b):

> A 1945 complaint lodged against R.L. Swain Tobacco prohibited representations that respondent's cigarettes were endorsed or approved by the medical profession; that they would soothe the nose, throat, or mouth; that they contained no irritating properties; and that they produced little or no stain on fingers and teeth. In 1950, the FTC moved successfully to curb R.J. Reynolds Tobacco Company from claiming that Camels aided digestion; did not impair the wind or physical condition of athletes; would never harm or irritate the throat or leave an aftertaste; were soothing, restful, and comforting to the nerves; and contained less nicotine than any of the four other largest selling brands. A 1942 complaint against Brown and Williamson Tobacco Company prohibited claims that Kools would keep the head clear in winter and give extra protection against or cure colds.

Because the adjudicatory judgments obtained by the FTC applied only to the parties to the case, other cigarette companies engaging in the same or similar deceptive acts were not immediately affected. Fritschler (1969) concluded that "in the case of cigarette advertising, the Commission found itself putting out brush fires of deception while the inferno raged on." The FTC first promulgated industrywide cigarette advertising guidelines in September 1955. These guidelines were "for the use of its staff in the evaluation of cigarette advertising" (FTC 1964b), as opposed to formal trade regulation rules, which would have the force of law. The guidelines, among other things, sought to prohibit: (1) representations in cigarette advertising of medical approval of cigarette smoking in general or of smoking a particular brand; (2) advertising claims that referred either to the presence or absence of any physical effects relating to cigarette smoking in general or smoking a particular brand, or relating to filters or filtration; and (3) unsubstantiated advertising claims relating to tar and nicotine levels.

In June 1962, the FTC announced the adoption of general rule-making procedures, which it used on three occasions the following year to regulate various nontobacco products (Fritschler 1969). As noted in the section on warning labels, 11 days after the release of the 1964 Report of the Surgeon General's Advisory Committee on Smoking and Health, the FTC announced three proposed trade regulations on cigarette labeling and advertising (FTC 1964a). Rule 2 would have strictly regulated the imagery and copy of cigarette ads in order to prohibit explicit or implicit health claims. However, the proposed rule was vacated (FTC 1965) after the Federal Cigarette Labeling and Advertising Act of 1965 (Public Law 89-92) was signed into law. In the meantime, in April 1964, the major U.S. cigarette manufacturers had adopted their own Cigarette Advertising Code, intended to apply to broadcast advertising. It prohibited making health claims in advertisements and directing advertising to young people. Cigarette manufacturers agreed to avoid ads that represented "cigarette smoking as essential to social prominence, distinction, success, or sexual attraction" and to avoid showing smokers engaged in activities "requiring stamina or athletic conditioning beyond that of normal recreation" (Ernster 1988; Friedman 1975).

In its 1968 report to Congress, the FTC recommended a ban on cigarette advertising on television and radio (FTC 1968). In February 1969, the FCC announced a proposed trade regulation rule that would have banned cigarette commercials from television and radio (FCC 1969). On July 8, 1969, the National Association of Broadcasters announced a plan to phase out all cigarette advertising on the air over a 3-year period beginning January 1, 1970 (Whiteside 1971). At a Senate subcommittee hearing 2 weeks later, the cigarette industry offered voluntarily to end all cigarette advertising on television and radio by September 1970, provided that Congress would grant the companies immunity from antitrust laws to allow them to act in concert (Whiteside 1971). Ultimately, Congress approved the Public Health Cigarette Smoking Act of 1969, which was signed into law on April 1, 1970. The Act prohibited cigarette advertising in the broadcast media effective January 2, 1971.

Subsequent Federal legislation extended the ban on advertisements in the broadcast media to little cigars and to smokeless tobacco products. In September 1973, the Little Cigar Act of 1973 (Public Law 93-109) banned broadcast advertising of "little cigars," defined as "any roll of tobacco wrapped in leaf tobacco or any substance containing tobacco . . . as to which one thousand units weigh not more than three pounds." Over a decade later, smokeless tobacco advertising in the broadcast media was banned by the Comprehensive Smokeless Tobacco Health Education Act of 1986 (Public Law 99-252). The ban took effect on August 27, 1986.

In recent years, the FTC has again had its attention drawn to the content of print advertising. As discussed in a prior section, the FTC successfully obtained an injunction against one manufacturer for incorrectly stating the tar yield of one cigarette brand, Barclay, in packaging and advertising (*FTC* v. *Brown and Williamson* 1983). In addition, the Tobacco Institute (Tobacco Institute 1983) and R.J. Reynolds (RJR) have advertised in national print media with statements that challenged the link between smoking (active and involuntary) and disease.

During 1985, RJR published an advertisement (R.J. Reynolds 1985a) entitled "Of Cigarettes and Science," which discussed, among other things, the procedures that scientists use to test scientific hypotheses, and presented information about the Multiple Risk Factor Intervention Trial (MRFIT) (MRFIT Research Group 1982). In April 1985, the American Heart Association, the American Cancer Society, and the American Lung Association, acting through the Coalition on Smoking OR Health, petitioned the FTC with regard to this ad. On June 16, 1986, the FTC issued a complaint alleging that the advertisement falsely and misleadingly represented that the purpose of the MRFIT study was to determine whether heart disease is caused by smoking, that the MRFIT study provides credible scientific evidence that smoking is not as hazardous as the public has been led to believe, and that the MRFIT study tends to refute the theory that smoking causes coronary heart disease. The complaint also charged that in light of the representations made in the ad, the advertisement failed to disclose certain material facts about the study, specifically, that the men in the study who quit smoking had a significantly lower rate of coronary heart disease than men who continued to smoke and that the study results are consistent with previous studies showing that those who quit smoking experience a substantial decrease in coronary heart disease mortality.

On June 26, 1986, RJR moved to dismiss the complaint on the grounds that the advertisement was noncommercial speech that was fully protected by the first amendment, even if it was false and deceptive. An Administrative Law Judge agreed and dismissed the complaint on August 4, 1986. In an order and decision dated March 4, 1988, the FTC reversed the judge's order, holding that "the content of the Reynolds advertisement includes words and messages that are characteristic of commercial speech." RJR unsuccessfully appealed this decision to the U.S. Court of Appeals of the District of Columbia; trial before an FTC Administrative Law Judge on this matter is set for January 30, 1989. (Also see White 1987.) (As of October 1988, all documents related to this administrative matter were maintained in FTC Docket No. 9206.)

State and Local Advertising Restrictions

The preemption clause of the Public Health Cigarette Smoking Act of 1969 (Public Law 91-222) prevents States from regulating or prohibiting cigarette advertising or promotion for health-related reasons. The Act defines "State" to include "any political division of any State." This preemption was left intact by subsequent congressional legislation, including the 1984 Comprehensive Smoking Education Act (Public Law 98-474), which amended other sections of the original law, such as the requirement for warning labels. The stated purpose of the preemption was "to avoid the chaos created by a multiplicity of conflicting regulations" (U.S. Senate 1970). There is no preemption of State and local advertising restrictions for smokeless tobacco in the Comprehensive Smokeless Tobacco Health Education Act of 1986 (Public Law 99-252), although the Act does prevent States from requiring additional warning labels on smokeless tobacco products or advertisements.

States and localities may have some jurisdiction in regulating the location of advertising when the medium is not national in scope. For example, cities may be able to prohibit tobacco advertising on their transit systems. The extent of such jurisdiction is not clear from the preemption clause itself, and there is no body of case law. Several States and local jurisdictions have adopted statutes or regulations banning certain types of purely local cigarette advertising or promotion. The most common restrictions, described below, are bans on transit advertising and on the distribution of free cigarette samples. In some cases, these regulations apply to all tobacco products. None of these policies has been challenged in court.

The strongest State law has been adopted in Utah, where tobacco advertisements are banned on "any billboard, streetcar sign, streetcar, bus, placard, or on any other object or place of display" (Utah 1978). Bans on tobacco advertising in public transit systems have been adopted in several cities. In August 1984, the Board of Directors of the Regional Transportation District in the Denver, CO, area voted to prohibit transit advertising for tobacco products and alcoholic beverages on its buses and in its two downtown transit centers (Schmitz 1984). Similarly, the Massachusetts Bay Transportation Authority (MBTA) in the Boston metropolitan area adopted an administrative policy prohibiting tobacco advertisements on buses and trollies and in stations, effective October 1986 (Boston Herald 1986). The town of Amherst, MA, enacted a bylaw prohibiting tobacco advertising "on or in any bus, taxicab, or any other vehicle used for public transportation" within the town in 1987 (Amherst 1987). The Bay Area Rapid Transit (BART) District in the San Francisco Bay Area of California has eliminated the advertising of tobacco products and alcoholic beverages from its trains and stations. BART covers San Francisco, Alameda, and Contra Costa counties. Based on a vote of the BART Board of Directors, the policy was phased in between May 1987 and May 1988 to allow existing advertising contracts to expire (Collier 1987).

In Minnesota, the Metropolitan Sports Commission voted in January 1988 to end tobacco advertising in Minneapolis' professional sports stadium, the Hubert H. Humphrey Metrodome. The new policy will take effect after expiration of the existing 10-year cigarette advertising contract in 1992. Cigarette advertising revenue under this contract has been approximately 300,000 dollars per year (Marty 1987).

Cities and States have also acted to restrict or ban the distribution of free tobacco product samples, a major form of tobacco promotion. At least 14 cities have banned all distribution of free samples; these include Minneapolis, St. Paul, and Albert Lea, MN; Boston, Newton, Cambridge, Amherst, Somerville, and Worcester, MA; Honolulu, HI; Bowie, MD; Atlanta, GA (Davis and Jason 1988); Austin, TX (Austin 1988); and Cincinnati, OH (Smith 1988). The earliest of these ordinances were adopted by Minneapolis and St. Paul in 1979. Two States (Utah and Minnesota) have prohibited the distribution of free smokeless tobacco samples (Davis and Jason 1988). A larger number of States and cities have banned the distribution of free samples to minors, although the success in enforcing these selective sampling restrictions is uncertain. (See Part III, section on minors' access to tobacco.)

Effects of Government Actions to Restrict Tobacco Advertising

In general, there has been little formal evaluation of the impact of government actions concerning tobacco advertising and promotion.

The relationship between government policy and tobacco consumption has been studied only in the case of the Fairness Doctrine and the subsequent ban on cigarette advertising in the broadcast media. Evaluation of the effectiveness of the broadcast ad ban is complicated by three factors. First, the ban removed the obligation of stations to air the Fairness Doctrine PSAs. To the extent that the PSAs were effective in discouraging smoking, their disappearance serves to undermine any positive effect from the broadcast advertising ban. Second, the savings from reduced advertising in the short term may have allowed the cigarette companies to hold down the price of cigarettes temporarily, which in turn would have served to increase sales (Schneider, Klein, Murphy 1981). Third, after several years of reduced advertising expenditures following the broadcast advertising ban, the cigarette industry dramatically increased expenditures for print media advertising (especially billboards) and for promotional activities (Warner 1986b; Popper 1986a; Davis 1987). To the extent that cigarette advertising in these media and other promotional activities may increase total sales, this also may have served to decrease the net effectiveness of the broadcast ban.

As mentioned in the previous section on the broadcast media, per capita cigarette sales decreased by 6.9 percent during the 3-year period (1968–70) when PSAs were mandated by the Fairness Doctrine, but increased by 4.1 percent during the 3-year period (1971–73) following the end of Fairness Doctrine PSAs and the beginning of the broadcast advertising ban. This suggests that any beneficial effects of the broadcast ad ban may have been outweighed by disappearance of the PSAs, at least in the short run. In a regression analysis of the effects of both cigarette ads and the Fairness Doctrine PSAs, Hamilton (1972) found that the antismoking PSAs retarded per capita cigarette consumption far more than the cigarette ads boosted it. In an analysis taking into account cigarette price, advertising, and counteradvertising, Schneider, Klein, and Murphy (1981) concluded that the net effect of the broadcast advertising ban was to increase cigarette consumption. However, Hamilton (1972) and Warner (1979) both suggested that the net effect of the two policies may have been to increase cigarette consumption in the short term, although they cautioned that the net effect in the long term is difficult to gauge.

It is difficult to evaluate the effect on smoking behavior of FTC actions to regulate the content of advertising. FTC rulings did block misleading advertising, but as the MRFIT case demonstrates, the regulatory process is slow. Delays inherent in the regulatory process limit the impact of the ultimate decisions.

The effect on smoking behavior of State and local restrictions on cigarette advertising and promotion is not known because no evaluations have been conducted. No data are available regarding the effectiveness of sampling bans in reducing the availability of cigarettes. Even if such policies have no direct influence on smoking, however, these restrictions (and the publicity surrounding their enactment) may promote increased public awareness of the issue of smoking and health and may serve as important symbols of social disapproval of tobacco use.

More is known about the financial impact of local advertising bans on transit authorities, for whom the bans result in lost advertising revenue. Information from two of the four jurisdictions that have enacted transit tobacco advertising bans indicates that transit authorities have been able to recoup lost advertising revenue in a relatively short time. Cigarette advertisements accounted for approximately 800,000 dollars, or 36 percent, of MBTA's 2.2 million dollars in advertising revenue in 1985 (Boston Herald 1986; AdEast 1986). According to MBTA, it regained its previous (1985) level of advertising revenue in 1987 (Grealy 1988). Similarly, in San Francisco, BART officials reported only a minimal, temporary advertising revenue loss during the year of implementation (Healy 1988). The effect, if any, of transit and sampling bans on national advertising and promotional expenditures by tobacco companies is unknown.

Policies Under Consideration

Currently, as reviewed above, the Federal Government bans tobacco advertising in the broadcast media and regulates the content of tobacco advertising by FTC actions and by the requirement that warning labels appear on cigarette and smokeless tobacco advertisements. A number of proposals that would further restrict tobacco advertising and promotion are now under consideration by the public health community, State legislatures, and Congress. Some of the proposals are mutually exclusive and should be considered as alternatives, whereas others could coexist. Nationally prominent proposals are mentioned here. Their major strengths and weaknesses are considered in detail elsewhere (Warner et al. 1986a).

One group of proposals would have the Government more stringently regulate the imagery and content of advertising, either by developing and enforcing an advertising and promotion code or by severely restricting the permissible format of advertisements; the latter is so-called "tombstone advertising." With the former approach, a code defining permissible imagery in advertisements and a mechanism to ensure monitoring of and compliance with the code would have to be developed and implemented. For such a code to be effective, it would have to encompass both advertising and nonadvertising forms of promotion, the latter of which now represents over half of total cigarette advertising and promotional expenditures (FTC 1988b). The advantages and disadvantages of such a code have been discussed (Taylor 1984; FTC 1981b; Warner et al. 1986a). An alternative proposal would limit the imagery and graphics of tobacco advertisements to so-called "tombstone advertising," with no models, slogans, scenes, or colors permitted. The tombstone proposal does not address other forms of promotion. The merits of this proposal are considered elsewhere (e.g., FTC 1981b; Warner et al. 1986a).

A second set of proposals would restrict the availability of tobacco advertising and promotion. These range from a total ban on all advertising and promotion to more limited policies that would prohibit advertising in certain media; prohibit certain promotional techniques, such as the distribution of free tobacco product samples (Davis and Jason 1988); or ban advertising and promotion accessible to children. Currently, the most widely discussed proposal is to ban all forms of advertising and promotion for all tobacco products. The proposal's prominence reflects its advocacy by organizations such as the American Medical Association, American Cancer Society, American Heart Association, American Lung Association, and American Public Health Association, and the fact that it has been the basis of several bills before Congress (e.g., H.R. 1272, 100th Congress, 1st Session) and the subject of congressional hearings (Subcommittee on Health and the Environment 1986). A total ban on tobacco advertising and promotion was enacted in Canada in June 1988, scheduled to go into effect in stages beginning January 1, 1989 (Burns 1988; House of Commons of Canada 1988).

The ad ban proposal raises a wide range of complex issues whose full discussion is beyond the scope of this Report and has been covered elsewhere (Warner et al. 1986a). The most visible and fundamental is the question of commercial free speech: What is the right of the producers of a legal product to advertise and what is the right of consumers to have access through advertisements to information on legal products (White 1984; Miller 1985; Weil 1986; Neuborne 1986; Reimer 1986; Covington and Burling 1986; Blasi and Monaghan 1986, 1987)? Among the more pragmatic issues is concern that withdrawal of cigarette advertising and tobacco company sponsorship might jeopardize the existence of some publications, advertising agencies, and sports and arts institutions (Warner 1986b). From a public health perspective, the central issue is one of effectiveness: Would an advertising ban in fact achieve its desired end—reductions in smoking prevalence? If so, would a less restrictive policy achieve the same effect without raising first amendment concerns?

A third set of proposals seeks to neutralize the influence of advertising by mandating the publication or broadcast of antitobacco messages by the media. An example of this so-called "counteradvertising" was the FCC requirement for antismoking PSAs in the broadcast media under the Fairness Doctrine from 1967 through 1970; these were discussed in a previous section. The apparent effectiveness of these PSAs led to proposals for the Government to establish a source of substantial and continuous funding for an antitobacco advertising campaign (Warner 1986b,c). Several mechanisms have been proposed to raise the resources for a paid campaign. One would require tobacco advertisers to pay for an amount of counteradvertising space that is equivalent to or some fraction of what they devote to protobacco advertising. Another proposal would earmark a proportion of the Federal cigarette excise tax to fund a paid counteradvertising campaign (Warner 1986c).

A fourth approach seeks to create an economic disincentive for tobacco manufacturers to advertise by eliminating their ability to deduct tobacco advertising and promotional expenditures as business expenses for income tax purposes. This proposal has also been put into the form of congressional legislation (S. 446, 100th Congress, 1st Session, and H.R. 1563, 100th Congress, 1st Session) and its merits have been debated in congressional hearings (Weil 1986; Stark 1986; Bradley 1986).

The majority of proposals to restrict tobacco advertising and promotion are designed for action at the Federal level, because current Federal legislation preempts States from regulating cigarette advertising. Repeal of the Federal preemption clause has been proposed as a means of encouraging State and local regulatory actions (Bailey 1986; Warner et al. 1986a).

Summary

There is no scientifically rigorous study available to the public that provides a definitive answer to the basic question of whether advertising and promotion increase the level of tobacco consumption. Given the complexity of the issue, none is likely to be forthcoming in the foreseeable future. The most comprehensive review of both the direct and indirect mechanisms concluded that the collective empirical, experiential, and logical evidence makes it more likely than not that advertising and promotional activities do stimulate cigarette consumption. However, that analysis also concluded that the extent of influence of advertising and promotion on the level of consumption is unknown and possibly unknowable (Warner 1986b). This influence relative to other influences on tobacco use, such as peer pressure and role models, is uncertain. Although its effects are not wholly predictable, regulation of advertising and promotion is likely to be a prominent arena for tobacco policy debate in the 1990s. In part this reflects the high visibility of advertising and promotion; in part it reflects the perception that these activities constitute an influence on tobacco consumption that is amenable to government action.

Reporting Requirements

Current Federal legislation mandates that DHHS and the FTC issue reports to Congress on tobacco-related subjects at regular intervals. By virtue of the extensive media coverage and wide dissemination of many of these reports, they often provide information not only to Congress but also to the general public, journalists, other policymakers, health professionals, and researchers.

Surgeon General's Reports

As discussed in Chapter 1, the Federal Cigarette Labeling Act of 1965 and the Public Health Cigarette Smoking Act of 1969 require that the Secretary of Health, Education, and Welfare (now the Secretary of Health and Human Services) transmit an annual report to Congress on current information about the health consequences of smoking and such recommendations for legislation as he or she may deem appropriate. This Report is the 20th in the series of reports on the health consequences of smoking, generally referred to as Surgeon Generals' Reports, which began with the 1964 Report of the Surgeon General's Advisory Committee on Smoking and Health. The 1986 Report of the Advisory Committee to the Surgeon General, *The Health Consequences of Using Smokeless Tobacco* (US DHHS 1986c), was not produced in response to a specific legislative mandate.

Biennial Status Reports

The Comprehensive Smoking Education Act of 1984 requires the Secretary of Health and Human Services to transmit a report to Congress biennially containing the following information about smoking control efforts: (1) an assessment of Federal activities to inform the public; (2) a description of the extent of public knowledge about the health consequences of smoking; (3) a report of the activities of the Federal Interagency Committee on Smoking and Health, the research and educational activities of DHHS relating to smoking, and State and local laws relating to the use and consumption of cigarettes; (4) information on private actions taken to reduce the effects of smoking on health; and (5) recommendations for legislation and administrative action that the Secretary deems appropriate. The first such report, entitled *Smoking and Health: A National Status Report*, was released in November 1986 (US DHHS 1986e).

A similar reporting requirement exists for smokeless tobacco. The Comprehensive Smokeless Tobacco Health Education Act of 1986 requires that the Secretary of Health and Human Services transmit a report to Congress biennially on (1) the effects of health education efforts on the use of smokeless tobacco products, (2) the public's use of smokeless tobacco products, (3) the health effects of smokeless tobacco products and areas appropriate for further research, and (4) appropriate legislation and administrative action. The first report pursuant to this requirement was released in May 1987 (US DHHS 1987a).

Federal Trade Commission Reports

The Federal Cigarette Labeling and Advertising Act of 1965 and the Public Health Cigarette Smoking Act of 1969 require the FTC to transmit an annual report to Congress concerning (1) the effectiveness of cigarette labeling, (2) current practices and methods of cigarette advertising and promotion, and (3) such recommendations for legislation as it may deem appropriate. The first provision was eliminated by the Comprehensive Smoking Education Act of 1984. FTC Reports have been submitted annually to Congress since 1967. These reports generally include data on aggregate and per capita cigarette sales, domestic market share of filter and nonfilter cigarettes and menthol and nonmenthol cigarettes, domestic market share by cigarette length and tar and nicotine yields, and cigarette advertising and promotional expenditures broken down by type of advertising or promotion and type of cigarette (FTC 1988b). The tar, nicotine, and carbon monoxide yields of all cigarettes are to be provided in future reports.

The Comprehensive Smokeless Tobacco Health Education Act of 1986 requires that FTC report to Congress every other year on current sales, advertising and marketing practices, and recommendations for legislative or administrative action.

Effectiveness

One method for assessing the effectiveness of reporting requirements as a means of disseminating information is to evaluate the quantity and quality of information made available and the extent to which policymakers and the public are aware of the reports or their contents. The information in these reports may influence policy development, tobacco use, and public awareness of the health effects of smoking, but these relationships are difficult to measure. In fact, there has been little formal evaluation of reporting requirements or the reports themselves on any of these outcomes.

There is some empirical evidence that the Surgeon General's Reports, or at least the first Report in 1964, may have had a direct or indirect effect on cigarette consumption. Adult per capita consumption of manufactured cigarettes in the United States (total cigarettes consumed annually divided by the population 18 years of age and older) reached an all-time high of 4,345 in 1963. After the release of the 1964 Report of the

Surgeon General's Advisory Committee on Smoking and Health (US PHS 1964) and the attendant publicity, per capita consumption fell to 4,195 in 1964 before increasing to 4,259 in 1965 (Chapters 5 and 8). In an analysis comparing actual cigarette consumption to projections based on previous trends, Warner (1977, 1981, 1989) estimated that the Advisory Committee's Report and associated publicity induced a 5-percent decrease in cigarette consumption in 1964. Schneider, Klein, and Murphy (1981) estimated that the 1964 Report decreased per capita consumption of tobacco by 39 percent during the 1964–78 period. Similarly, British researchers (Russell 1973; Peto 1974) have credited the Royal College of Physicians' 1962 Report on Smoking and Health with decreasing cigarette consumption 4.6 to 9 percent that year. No published studies have evaluated the effects of other Surgeon General's Reports upon tobacco use. The impact of the 1964 Surgeon General's Advisory Committee Report may be unsurpassed, compared with that of subsequent reports, because of the widespread publicity surrounding the first Report and the "newness" of its findings.

Public knowledge of the health hazards of tobacco use has increased substantially since 1964 (Chapter 4). Because of the many factors that may have affected public knowledge and attitudes about smoking, it is difficult to estimate the degree to which the Surgeon General's Reports have by themselves influenced beliefs, attitudes, and opinions. Despite the lack of empirical data, it is widely acknowledged that the Surgeon General's Reports have become recognized as authoritative documents and summaries of the literature on the health consequences of smoking (Walsh and Gordon 1986). The quality of the reports can be attributed, at least in part, to the large number of expert contributors and an extensive peer review process (summarized in the acknowledgments of this and previous reports). Because of the large and expanding literature on tobacco and health, there is no doubt that the Surgeon General's Reports have served a useful purpose by providing detailed and current reviews of information on tobacco and health.

One of the principal intended audiences of the 1988 Surgeon General's Report on Nicotine Addiction (US DHHS 1988) was physicians. Two weeks after the release of the Report, Lakeside Pharmaceuticals sponsored a telephone survey of 159 randomly selected physicians from three primary care specialities. Ninety-one percent of physicians interviewed knew about the Report, and 70 percent thought that the conclusions of the Report would alter the way physicians treat patients for smoking (Ad Factors/Millward Brown 1988). These data suggest that the Report was effective in conveying information on smoking to health care providers.

The findings of the Surgeon General's Reports have often been cited as the scientific basis for public and private policies designed to reduce tobacco use. Similarly, the findings and legislative recommendations of FTC reports have been cited in support of strengthening existing cigarette warning labels. For example, in the legislative history of the Public Health Cigarette Smoking Act of 1969, the Senate Report (U.S. Senate 1970) recommended a stronger cigarette warning label by citing the findings of previous Surgeon General's Reports, the conclusion of the 1967 FTC Report that the original warning label was ineffective, and the legislative recommendation of the 1969 FTC Report for a stronger warning label. Thus, although empirical data are lacking, anecdotal reports suggest that the mandated Federal Government documents have played an important role in providing a knowledge base to support the development of smoking control policies.

Government Expenditures and State Smoking Control Plans

Government activities on smoking and health have, for the most part, been informational and educational. The extent of these activities is determined in part by the availability of funds to support them. Funding, in turn, reflects broad government priorities. Consequently, government decisions about expenditures on smoking and health can be considered as "policies" and will be reviewed in this Section.

Federal Expenditures

There are two sources of information about Federal expenditures on smoking and health. The Office on Smoking and Health (OSH), the successor of the National Clearinghouse for Smoking and Health (NCSH), is the only Federal office wholly devoted to smoking control. Its activities (Chapter 6) include providing information and education to health professionals, policymakers, and the general public and sponsoring national surveys of smoking behavior. Its budget is an index of categorical appropriations for activities related to smoking and health. In addition, since 1979, agencies within DHHS have reported their expenditures in 15 prevention priority areas, including smoking and health, to the Office of Disease Prevention and Health Promotion. This information has been published for fiscal years 1979 through 1981 and 1983 through 1986 (US DHHS 1981b, 1982b, 1985b, 1987b) and includes a list of projects funded by each reporting agency.

The budgets of OSH and NCSH are shown in Table 8 for fiscal years 1966 through 1988. Congressional appropriations designated for "smoking and health" have increased from 2.0 million dollars in 1966 to 3.5 million dollars in 1988. Expressed in constant 1966 dollars, the 1988 appropriation is 0.95 million dollars, 48.5 percent of the 1966 appropriation. For the past 5 years, the annual budget of OSH in current dollars has been approximately 3.5 million dollars.

Expenditures on smoking and health reported by agencies within DHHS for fiscal years 1979 through 1981 and 1983 through 1986 (US DHHS 1981b, 1982b, 1985b, 1987b) are shown in Table 9. Reported expenditures increased from approximately 21 million dollars in fiscal year 1979 to approximately 40 million dollars in fiscal year 1986. Increased expenditures by several agencies contributed to this change, but it is primarily attributable to sharply increased allocations by the National Cancer Institute (Chapter 6). Expenditures on smoking and health have accounted for a growing share of all DHHS prevention efforts, but remain a small proportion of the total prevention budget. In fiscal year 1986, smoking and health activities accounted for 1.0 percent of the DHHS prevention budget (4.1 billion dollars) and 1.2 percent of the Public Health Service's prevention budget (3.3 billion dollars) (US DHHS 1987b).

The data on expenditures reported by DHHS agencies should be interpreted with caution. These figures may vary slightly from figures contained in other documents because each agency applied its own criteria, within general guidelines, for identifying these expenditures. In addition, some prevention expenditures within certain block grants or certain programs (e.g., medicaid) are not accessible by current reporting systems and thus may not be included in these figures.

It should also be noted that these data do not include possible expenditures on smoking and health by other Federal departments or agencies. For example, the Department of Defense (DOD) has recently funded approximately 97,000 dollars in publications and 324,000 dollars in radio and television messages relating to smoking and health. Many of the radio and television spots are being used in the Armed Forces Radio and Television Network overseas (US DOD 1987). DOD has received assistance from voluntary health agencies in disseminating information and materials to military service members (US DOD 1987) (Chapter 6). These data also do not include Federal agency expenditures on tobacco where the goal is not smoking control. Examples of this are the Department of Agriculture's tobacco agriculture program (Warner 1988) and efforts by the Office of the U.S. Trade Representative to secure freer access to foreign markets for American cigarette manufacturers (Connolly 1987).

TABLE 8.—Appropriated funds and positions for the Office on Smoking and Health (OSH) (1978–87) and its predecessor, the National Clearinghouse for Smoking and Health (NCSH) (1966–77)

Fiscal year	Appropriated funds[a] (millions of dollars)[b]	Positions[c]
1966 (NCSH)	1.955	30
1967	2.144	37
1968	2.075	37
1969	2.100	35
1970	2.250	35
1971	2.156	29
1972	2.380	43
1973	1.600 (+ 0.306)[d]	43
1974	0.986 (+ 1.862)[d]	36
1975	1.028 (+ 0.813)[d]	35
1976	0.825 (+ 0.295)[d]	12
1977	1.200	12
1978	1.200	12
1979 (OSH)	2.500	12
1980	2.519[e]	25
1981	2.062[e]	25
1982	1.944	23
1983	2.098	21
1984	3.521	21
1985	3.538	17
1986	3.375[f]	17
1987	3.471	18
1988	3.466	18

[a]The difference between these figures and those in Table 9 reflect the fact that the figures in Table 9 may exclude salaries and other "overhead" expenditures (travel, postage, photocopying, etc.).

[b]Figures not adjusted for inflation.

[c]Beginning in 1980, the number of allocated "positions" was redefined as the number of allocated "full-time equivalents (FTEs)." FTEs allow the hiring of more than one person for a given FTE (e.g., two half-time employees for one FTE), which was not possible under the previous system.

[d]Additional funds transferred from other agencies.

[e]An additional 10 million dollars was appropriated to support a smoking and alcohol demonstration grant program for children and adolescents. This money was later transferred from the Office on Smoking and Health (which at that time was within the Office of the Assistant Secretary for Health) to the Centers for Disease Control.

[f]A total of 3.526 million dollars was originally appropriated, but 174,000 dollars were withheld ("sequestered") pursuant to Section 515 of Public Law 99-190.

SOURCE: Office on Smoking and Health (unpublished data).

TABLE 9.—Expenditures on smoking and health by DHHS, fiscal years 1979–81 and 1983–86

Agency	Fiscal year expenditures[a] (in thousands of dollars)						
	1979	1980	1981	1983	1984	1985	1986
ADAMHA	153		1,184	1,579	2,024	2,353	2,796
CDC[b]	213	4,400	445		50	380	755
HRSA[c]	377	457	386				
NIH[e]	18,550	16,150	12,931	13,810	21,520	26,850	33,112
NCI	12,845	13,235	10,182	9,476	16,721	21,131	27,099
NHLBI	2,550	2,900	2,637	2,210	2,700	3,375	3,360
OASH	1,853	2,074	1,555	2,024	3,273	2,503	2,862
OSH[b d]	1,706	1,961	1,555	1,895	3,148	2,495	2,857
TOTAL[e] (smoking and health)	21,146	23,081	16,501	17,413	26,867	32,086	39,525
TOTAL of all prevention activities	2,971,171	3,530,405	3,571,060	3,577,069	3,823,993	3,908,524	4,088,465
Smoking and health, as % of all prevention activities	0.7	0.7	0.5	0.5	0.7	0.8	1.0

NOTE: ADAMHA, Alcohol, Drug Abuse, and Mental Health Administration (includes National Institute on Drug Abuse); CDC, Centers for Disease Control; HRSA, Health Resources and Services Administration; NIH, National Institutes of Health; NCI, National Cancer Institute (part of NIH); NHLBI, National Heart, Lung, and Blood Institute (part of NIH); OASH, Office of the Assistant Secretary for Health; OSH, Office on Smoking and Health.

[a]Figures not adjusted for inflation.

[b]OSH was transferred administratively from OASH to CDC in September 1986.

[c]For fiscal years 1979–81, expenditures were reported separately for the Health Resources Administration and the Health Services Administration, but are combined in this table under HRSA, which now subsumes these two agencies.

[d]The difference between these expenditure figures for OSH and those in Table 8 reflect the fact that the figures in this table may exclude salaries and other "overhead" expenditures (e.g., travel, postage, photocopying).

[e]Figures differ slightly from published data because of revised NCI figures.

SOURCE: US DHHS (1981b, 1982b, 1985b, 1987b). The figures in this inventory may vary slightly from figures contained in other documents because each agency applied its own criteria, within general guidelines, for identifying these expenditures. Some prevention expenditures within certain block grants or certain programs (e.g., medicaid) are not available with current reporting systems and thus may not be included in the figures in this table. Figures for NCI budget year were provided by the Deputy Director, Division of Cancer Prevention and Control.

State Smoking and Health Plans

Data on expenditures relating to smoking and health by State and territorial health departments were not available for this Report. However, the existence of a State Smoking and Health Plan is an indicator of a well-developed State smoking control program.

State smoking control plans may be produced by a State health department acting alone or in conjunction with other public and private organizations in the State that are interested in smoking and health. They may also be produced by an advisory committee or "citizens' panel" on smoking and health appointed by the Governor or State health officer. Table 10 provides a list of selected State Reports on smoking and health. The most comprehensive reports provide State-specific information on tobacco use, smoking-attributable mortality and economic costs, current tobacco control activities, and recommendations for tobacco control programs and policies and for information collection. A similar report has also been produced by the City of New York (New York City Department of Health 1986).

The Minnesota Plan for Nonsmoking and Health (Minnesota Department of Health 1984, 1987b) is often cited as a particularly well-developed program. In 1983, the Minnesota Commissioner of Health established the Minnesota Center for Nonsmoking and Health. The three-member staff of the Center organized the Minnesota Technical Advisory Committee on Nonsmoking and Health, with representation from a variety of sectors: wholesale–retail sales; labor; medicine; nursing; hotels, resorts, and restaurants; law; large and small business; education; insurance; economics; advertising; State legislature; local government; and community action. In September 1984, the committee issued a 198-page document, *The Minnesota Plan for Nonsmoking and Health* (Minnesota Department of Health 1984), with 39 recommendations. During the same year, nearly 30 public and private organizations joined to form the Minnesota Coalition for a Smoke-Free Society by the Year 2000.

In June 1985, the Minnesota legislature ratified smoking control legislation, several provisions of which were based on recommendations of *The Minnesota Plan*. One of these provisions was a 5-cent increase in the State cigarette excise tax. One cent of the tax increase was earmarked for a public health fund, one-quarter of which was set aside for tobacco use prevention. The revenues have been used to fund special project grants for local smoking control projects, surveillance of adult and teenage use of tobacco in the State, a mass media educational campaign, and evaluation of the impact of these interventions.

Eight Western States (Arizona, Colorado, Montana, New Mexico, North Dakota, South Dakota, Utah, and Wyoming) are cooperating on the first regional tobacco-and-health "plan," the Rocky Mountain Tobacco-Free Challenge. The eight State health departments are coordinating a competition among these States to achieve specific goals by the year 2000. These goals include a 50-percent reduction in the prevalence of tobacco use by adults and youth, a 50-percent reduction in consumption of all tobacco products, and a 25-percent reduction in deaths related to tobacco use. The Governors of these eight States signed a declaration in early 1988 endorsing the competition and the year 2000 goals (Vilnius 1988).

TABLE 10.—Selected State and local reports on smoking and health

State	Year	Origin of report[a]	Information in report: Prevalence of smoking	Smoking-attributable mortality	Smoking-attributable costs	Recom-mendations
Colorado	1986	AC	X	X	X	X
Maine	1983	SHD	X	X	X	X
Massachusetts	1988	SHD	X	X	X	X
Michigan	1980	AC		X	X	X
	1984	SHD		X[b]		
Minnesota	1984	SHD	X	X	X	X
	1987	SHD	X	X	X	X
New Jersey	1988	AC	X	X	X	X
New York City	1986	AC	X	X	X	X
North Dakota	1986	SHD		X[c]		
Pennsylvania	1986	CC	X	X		X

[a]AC, Advisory Committee or Citizens' Panel; SHD, State Health Department; CC, Consensus Conference.
[b]By State Senate district.
[c]State- and county-specific data.
SOURCE: Colorado Department of Health (1986); Maine Department of Human Services (1983); Massachusetts Department of Public Health (1988); Michigan Department of Public Health (1980, 1984); Minnesota Department of Health (1984, 1987b); New Jersey Commission on Smoking or Health (1988); New York City Department of Health (1986); North Dakota State Department of Health (1986); Pennsylvania Plan for Tobacco or Health (1986).

PART II. ECONOMIC INCENTIVES

Economic as well as educational factors can influence tobacco consumption by increasing the costs of manufacturing, distributing, selling, or consuming cigarettes. Direct increases in consumer costs affect consumption patterns directly, but cost increases to suppliers ultimately affect consumers too, to the extent that supplier costs are passed on to consumers. This Section considers two economic instruments, taxation and insurance, and discusses how public and private policies have created economic disincentives for tobacco use.

The simplest economic disincentive to consumption is to raise the price of a product. Governments have done so by imposing a tax on tobacco, usually an excise tax, which offers the benefit of generating public revenue. Insurers' policies work more indirectly to discourage smoking. Premium differentials make insurance more expensive for smokers to purchase; this effectively increases the cost of being a smoker, although its impact is not felt directly at the point of cigarette purchase. Health insurers' decisions about the reimbursability of smoking cessation treatment costs also create economic incentives. For the smoker, reimbursement removes a financial impediment to cessation; for the provider, reimbursement presumably would stimulate the availability of cessation services. Unlike taxation, insurance mechanisms are largely private policies; however, they can be encouraged and supported by government actions. In addition, government acts as a health insurer through publicly funded programs, such as medicare, and theoretically could use insurance mechanisms to promote nonsmoking. It is important to note that taxation and insurance incentives may influence smoking behavior through more than purely economic mechanisms; they also remind smokers that smoking is a harmful and socially discouraged behavior.

Other policies that act via economic mechanisms are not discussed. Chief among these is the Federal policy of tobacco price supports and the allotment system. As an agricultural policy not oriented toward tobacco consumption (although it may have an indirect impact) (Warner 1988; Johnson 1984), it is not within the scope of this Chapter. Also not discussed in this Chapter is a current high-visibility antitobacco activity with potentially important economic effects relevant to consumption: the ongoing efforts to establish the legal liability of tobacco manufacturers for the diseases caused by their products (Daynard 1988). Although product liability suits themselves are not policies, policymaking pertaining to them could influence the number and ultimate impact of these suits. For example, recent legislative action in California attempts to limit the legal liability of tobacco manufacturers and vendors for claims brought in that State. California's Civil Liability Reform Act of 1987 (California Chapter 1498) includes a section specifically exempting manufacturers or sellers of tobacco products from product liability actions.

Economic incentives are not limited to public and private policies. Smoking cessation programs have used economic incentives to encourage participation or success, and employers have offered employees economic incentives not to smoke. These nonpolicy uses of incentives are identified in Chapter 6 and are discussed elsewhere (Warner and Murt 1984).

Tobacco Excise Taxation

Excise taxes are sales taxes on specific commodities such as tobacco products. Although accounting for only a small percentage of aggregate tax receipts in the United States today, excise taxes provide revenue for Federal, State, and local governments. The primary fiscal attraction of excise taxes is their low administrative cost relative to the revenue they can generate. In theory, to generate substantial revenue, excise taxes should be placed on commodities with a broad base of consumption that is not substantially reduced by the imposition of the tax. Hence, during the Middle Ages, the salt tax was an important source of revenue. In the United States, tobacco, alcohol, and gasoline have emerged as commodities subject to special excise taxes.

In addition to being an attractive source of revenue, excise taxes on tobacco have a history as measures designed to reflect public morality by taxing "sinful" behaviors. More recently, as attention has focused on the deleterious health effects of cigarette smoking, it has been recognized that excise taxes have the potential to enhance public health by reducing the consumption of tobacco. The capacity to simultaneously raise revenue and enhance public health has made the tobacco excise tax a particularly attractive public policy tool (Lewit 1985; Warner et al. 1986b).

This Section reviews the history and current status of cigarette excise taxation at the Federal, State, and local levels, focusing on the period since 1964. It examines the relationship between changes in taxes on cigarettes and changes in cigarette consumption, with particular attention to the consequences of the doubling of the Federal excise tax in 1983, and it identifies tax-related policies under serious consideration.

History and Current Status

Federal Excise Taxes

Tobacco was one of the first goods to be taxed in North America, first by the British and then by the newly independent Republic in the early 1790s (Tobacco Institute 1988). The early tax on snuff was eliminated in 1804 and revived briefly as a wartime measure in 1814. A number of Federal tobacco taxes, including a tax on cigarettes, were imposed in 1864 as part of a package of taxes to finance the Civil War. Federal excise taxes on tobacco in one form or another have remained a part of the Federal tax system since that time. The tax on tobacco was a particularly important source of revenue to the Federal Government prior to the enactment of the income tax in 1913.

Generally, the Federal tax on cigarettes over the 120-year period from 1864–1983 tended to fluctuate with the revenue requirements of the Government, corresponding to alternating periods of war and peace. The Federal tax on cigarettes, introduced during the Civil War, was raised briefly during the Spanish American War, and again during World Wars I and II. In November 1951, during the Korean War, the Federal excise tax was increased from 7 to 8 cents per pack. It remained at this level for over three decades, until March 1, 1983, when it was temporarily doubled to 16 cents per pack as part of the Tax Equity and Fiscal Responsibility Act of 1982. After several temporary extensions, Congress made the 16-cent rate permanent in 1986. A Federal excise tax on smokeless tobacco was levied by the Omnibus Budget Reconciliation Act of 1985, which imposed taxes of 24 cents per lb on snuff and 8 cents per lb on chewing tobacco. This is equivalent to a 1.8-cent tax on a 1.2-oz can of snuff and a 1.0-cent tax on a 2-oz pouch of chewing tobacco.

In the year ending June 30, 1987, Federal tobacco taxes grossed 4.8 billion dollars. Over 98 percent of Federal tobacco tax revenues were provided by the tax on cigarettes (Tobacco Institute 1988). Cigarette excise taxes have provided a declining share of total Federal revenue during the post-World War II period. Accounting for over 3 percent of Federal revenues in 1950, the share of total Federal revenues attributable to cigarette excise taxes fell from 1.76 percent in 1964 to 0.52 percent in 1987 (see Figure 3). This occurred despite a doubling of the tax in nominal terms in 1983 and an increase in total tax receipts of over 2.8 billion dollars between fiscal 1964 and fiscal 1987.

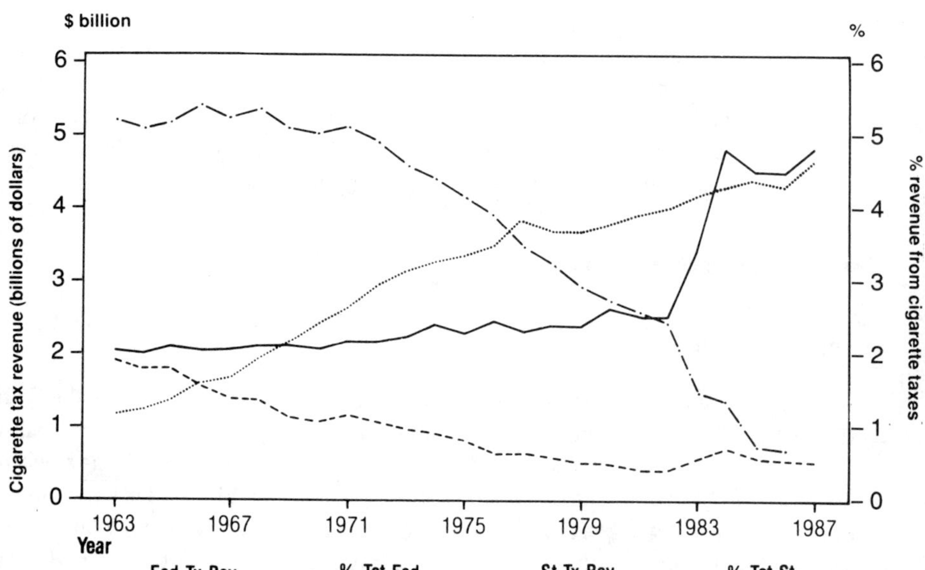

FIGURE 3.—Gross revenue and percentage of total revenue from cigarette tax, State and Federal Governments, 1963–87

NOTE: Figures in current dollars.

SOURCE: Tobacco Institute (1988b). Calculations by OSH.

The Federal excise tax has declined in real terms since 1964, despite the rising concern about the adverse effects of smoking on health that followed the release of the 1964 Surgeon General's Report and the adoption of specific Federal tobacco control policies. One reason for the decline was the lack of legislated increases in the tax rate. Only the prospect of huge Federal budget deficits that accompanied the 1981 tax cuts prompted renewed interest in the cigarette excise tax as a source of funds to help reduce the projected deficits (Toder 1985). Inflation also eroded the real excise tax rate because the excise taxes on cigarettes are unit rather than ad valorem taxes. A unit tax is a constant nominal rate per unit of a well-defined product, whereas the ad valorem tax is a constant fraction of either wholesale or retail price. Current Federal taxes on cigarettes, cigarette papers and tubes, smokeless and smoking tobacco, and small cigars, as well as most State and local taxes on cigarettes, are unit taxes. Federal taxes on large cigars and most State taxes on noncigarette tobacco products are ad valorem taxes.

Cigarette taxes fall relative to the price of cigarettes when cigarette taxes are not changed by at least as much as the rate of general inflation or the rate of increase in cigarette prices. The Federal tax has increased only once since 1951. Accordingly, the real tax (in 1987 value) fell from 30.4 to 9.8 cents per pack of 20 cigarettes between 1964 and 1982. The doubling of the nominal tax from 8 to 16 cents per pack in 1983 caused the tax to nearly double in real terms, to 19 cents (1987 value), between 1982 and 1983. However, inflation since 1983 has gradually eroded the tax to less than 16 cents (1987 value) today. During this same period, the Federal tax as a percentage of average retail price (including taxes) declined from 30.3 to 10.7 percent between 1964 and 1982, increased to 17.8 percent in 1983, and declined again to 13.7 percent in 1987 (Figure 4).

State and Local Excise Taxes

All States, the District of Columbia, and nearly 400 localities currently impose excise taxes on cigarettes in addition to the Federal tax. In 1921, Iowa became the first State to tax cigarettes. By 1964, 49 States had enacted cigarette taxes. The last State to enact an excise tax on cigarettes, North Carolina, did so in 1969. Since then, a number of States have modified their cigarette taxes, as described below. As of June 30, 1988, State excise tax rates ranged from a low of 2 cents per pack in North Carolina to a high of 38 cents in Minnesota. The average State tax was 18.2 cents per pack. In the year ending June 30, 1987, State tobacco taxes generated revenues of 4.8 billion dollars; almost 98 percent was provided by State cigarette taxes. In addition, 40 States and the District of Columbia imposed general sales taxes on cigarettes in 1987. In 35 States, the sales tax value base included the State excise tax. As a result, sales taxes added up to 10 cents per pack to the price of cigarettes in the highest tax States (Connecticut and Washington) in 1987. States have also increased their taxation of smokeless tobacco. In 1964, only 14 States taxed smokeless tobacco. By 1987, this number had nearly doubled to 27 (Tobacco Institute 1988).

During the local fiscal crises that resulted from the Depression of the 1930s, municipal governments also began to enact tobacco taxes. The spread of cigarette taxes has not been as rapid or extensive among municipal governments as it was among State

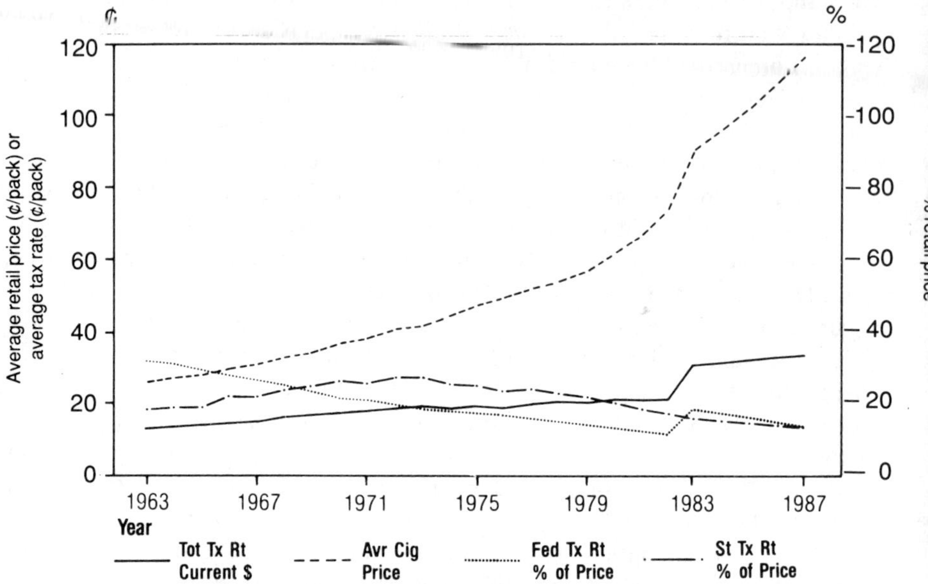

FIGURE 4.—Federal and State cigarette excise tax rates and retail cigarette prices, 1963–87

SOURCE: Tobacco Institute (1988b). Calculations by OSH.

governments. As of 1987, 369 cities and 20 counties in 6 States imposed local taxes on tobacco products. Taxes are levied by communities in Alabama, Illinois, Missouri, New York, Tennessee, and Virginia. In the year ending June 30, 1987, these taxes ranged from 1 to 15 cents per pack and yielded revenues of 197 million dollars. Over 70 percent of local cigarette tax revenues are collected in New York City and Chicago–Cook County, IL, where the local tax rates are 8 and 23 cents per pack, respectively.

During the period following the 1964 Surgeon General's Report, State cigarette excise tax receipts grew much more rapidly than Federal receipts (Figure 3), but their share of total State tax revenue declined. State tax receipts averaged a fairly constant 5 percent of total State revenues during the initial part of the period, but the proportion has declined steadily since 1972. Gross receipts from local taxes on cigarettes have grown from 58 million dollars in 1964 to 197 million dollars in 1987, less than the growth rate of State tax receipts but more rapid than Federal tax receipt change in the same period. The number of local jurisdictions taxing cigarettes has not increased appreciably (Tobacco Institute 1988).

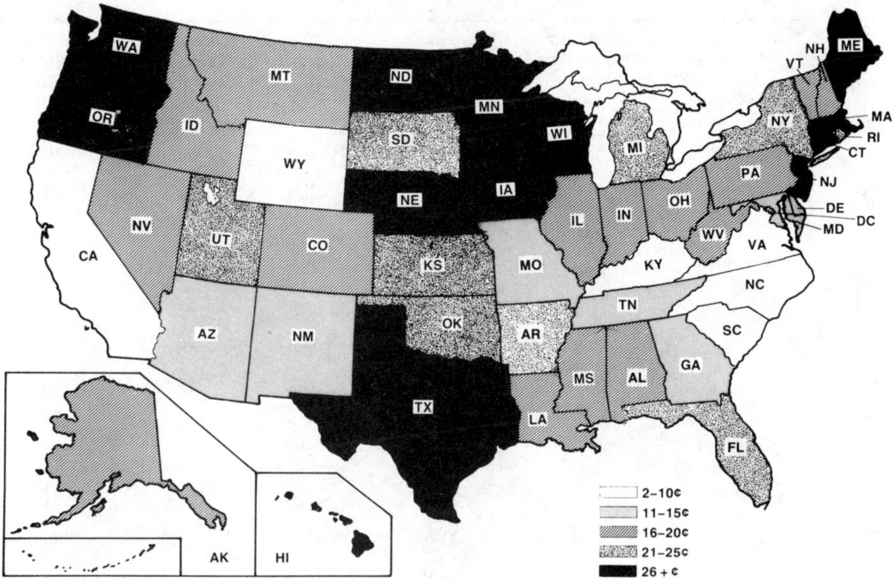

FIGURE 5.—State cigarette excise tax rates (as of June 30, 1988)

SOURCE: Tobacco Institute (1988a).

Between 1963 and 1987, the average State tax on cigarettes in current dollars increased almost annually, but because the rate of increase slowed relative to the rate of inflation after 1972, the real tax rate and the tax rate as a percentage of retail price have each declined by over 40 percent in the past 15 years. The rate of increase in State taxes accelerated after 1980, so that on average, it has kept pace with the general rate of inflation since that time (Figure 4).

Considerable differences in cigarette tax rates among States have persisted over the last 25 years (Figure 5). Not until 1969 did all States tax cigarettes. At that time, the maximum State tax rate was 16 cents, and the difference between the tax rate in the highest and lowest tax States was 14 cents (Table 11). The range of State cigarette taxes in constant dollars was greatest in 1971 and fell steadily through 1981. This decline occurred because the lowest tax State maintained a constant nominal tax rate and taxes in the high-tax States failed to keep pace with inflation. Since 1982, tax increases in high-tax States have tended to keep pace with the rate of inflation. The major tobacco-producing States of North Carolina, Kentucky, and Virginia have maintained low cigarette tax rates since 1964. The largest tax increases have occurred in Oregon, which did not even tax cigarettes in 1964, in Minnesota, and in California in November 1988.

Differences in cigarette tax rates among States and local jurisdictions can create problems with the enforcement of State and local tax laws and can result in lost revenues to some jurisdictions. In particular, large differences in cigarette tax rates among and within States provide an incentive for bootlegging; that is, purchasing of cigarettes in low-tax jurisdictions for consumption or resale in high-tax jurisdictions. A variety of tax evasion activities have been identified: casual smuggling (individuals buying

TABLE 11.—Dispersion in cigarette excise tax rates among States, 1963–87

Year	Number of taxing States[a]	Minimum tax, current dollars (cents/pack)	Maximum tax, current dollars (cents/pack)	Minimum tax, 1987 dollars (cents/pack)	Maximum tax, 1987 dollars (cents/pack)	Range, 1987 dollars (cents/pack)
1963	48	0.0	8.0	0.0	29.6	29.6
1964	49	0.0	8.0	0.0	29.3	29.3
1965	49	0.0	11.0	0.0	39.6	39.6
1966	50	0.0	11.0	0.0	38.5	38.5
1967	50	0.0	13.0	0.0	44.2	44.2
1968	51	0.0	15.0	0.0	49.0	49.0
1969	51	2.0	16.0	6.2	49.5	43.3
1970	51	2.0	18.0	5.8	52.6	46.8
1971	51	2.0	21.0	5.6	58.9	53.3
1972	51	2.0	21.0	5.5	56.9	51.5
1973	51	2.0	21.0	5.1	53.7	48.5
1974	51	2.0	21.0	4.6	48.3	43.7
1975	51	2.0	21.0	4.3	44.3	40.0
1976	51	2.0	21.0	3.9	41.9	37.9
1977	51	2.0	21.0	3.7	39.3	35.6
1978	51	2.0	21.0	3.5	36.5	33.0
1979	51	2.0	21.0	3.2	32.9	29.7
1980	51	2.0	21.0	2.7	28.9	26.2
1981	51	2.0	21.0	2.5	26.2	23.7
1982	51	2.0	25.0	2.4	29.4	27.0
1983	51	2.0	26.0	2.3	29.6	27.3
1984	51	2.0	26.0	2.2	28.4	26.2
1985	51	2.0	26.0	2.1	27.5	25.3
1986	51	2.0	31.0	2.1	32.1	30.0
1987	51	2.0	38.0	2.0	38.0	36.0

[a]Includes District of Columbia.
SOURCE: Tobacco Institute (1988).

cigarettes in neighboring lower tax jurisdictions for their own consumption), illegal organized or commercial smuggling for resale, tax-free mail order purchase of cigarettes (technically illegal since 1949), purchase of cigarettes through tax-free outlets (international ports of entry, military stores, and Indian reservations), and illegal diversion of cigarettes within the traditional distribution system (forged tax stamps and underreporting) (Advisory Commission on Intergovernmental Relations (ACIR) 1977, 1985).

As the differential in State tax rates increased during the late 1960s and early 1970s, the level of cigarette tax evasion increased substantially. Although casual smuggling between neighboring States (e.g., Massachusetts and New Hampshire, Washington and Oregon) had long been a problem, government officials reported a substantial increase in organized smuggling over long distances and in the illegal diversion of cigarettes from the legal distribution system (ACIR 1977). The problem was also reported in the media. In response, the Federal Cigarette Contraband Act was enacted. It prohibited the transportation, receipt, shipment, possession, distribution, or purchase of more than 60,000 cigarettes not bearing the indicia of the State in which the cigarettes were found. Enforcement of this Act was made the responsibility of the Bureau of Alcohol, Tobacco, and Firearms of the U.S. Treasury Department. A second study by the Advisory Commission on Intergovernmental Relations (1985) suggested that this act had been effective in reducing the level of organized smuggling. ACIR (1985) has suggested earmarking a portion of the revenue generated by increases in State cigarette excise taxes for antismoking law enforcement activities.

The law enforcement problems stemming from organized interstate cigarette bootlegging were also a factor in the deceleration of State tax increases in high-tax States (ACIR 1985). In real terms, the difference between the rate in the highest and lowest rate States (53 cents, 1987 value) peaked in 1971. The decline in the range of real prices means that interstate bootlegging has become less profitable since that time. This decline in profitability, combined with the increased Federal enforcement effort, probably accounted for the decline in bootlegging (Warner 1982). More recent increases in State taxes and the resultant widening of real differentials between high- and low-tax States have again increased the incentives for smuggling. In addition, many States and the FederalGovernment have reduced the level of resources allocated to enforcing State tax laws as the problem of bootlegging abated.

Cigarettes sold on military bases and Indian reservations are exempt from State and local tobacco excise taxes. Tax-exempt sales at these locations represent a revenue loss to the States, which would collect a tax on these sales if the tax-exempt options did not exist. These cigarette sales represent "the major sources of current revenue losses for most states" (ACIR 1985). In 1986, DOD discussed but did not adopt a proposal to remove the State and local tax exemption for cigarettes sold in the military, as part of an overall strategy to discourage smoking in the military (US DOD 1986c).

Effects of Excise Taxes on Smoking and Health

Price Elasticity of Demand for Cigarettes

One of the few nearly universal relationships in economics is the law of downward sloping demand; that is, demand for a commodity declines as its price increases. Numerous econometric studies have confirmed that this relationship holds for cigarettes. Because excise taxes increase the price of cigarettes, fluctuations in excise tax rates should influence the demand for cigarettes, and excise tax increases should reduce tobacco consumption.

The basis for estimating the consumption effects of a change in excise tax rates is an analysis of the price elasticity of demand for cigarettes. Elasticity, a measure of the degree of responsiveness of demand to changes in price, is defined as the percentage change in the quantity of cigarettes demanded divided by the percentage change in price. An elasticity of –0.5, for example, means that a 10-percent increase (decrease) in price would reduce (increase) by 5 percent the quantity of cigarettes demanded. Because cigarette taxes account for only a fraction of the total retail price of cigarettes, the price elasticity of demand would have to be multiplied by the percentage change in price that resulted from a tax change to determine the elasticity of demand with respect to the tax. Accordingly, the elasticity of demand with respect to a tax change will be less than the price elasticity of demand.

Numerous attempts have been made to measure the price elasticity of demand for cigarettes, with estimates ranging from –0.2 to –1.3. Miller (1982) suggested that –0.7 was the midpoint of recent studies and noted that the Tobacco Institute used that figure for its analyses of cigarette tax effects. Table 12 reports the results of studies published since 1980 on the price elasticity of demand for the United States. The substantial changes in the market for cigarettes and in the demographics of the smoking population that have occurred since 1964 suggest that earlier estimates may be inappropriate today.

The estimates reported in Table 12 derive from econometric studies that attempt to explain differences in cigarette consumption as functions of the price of cigarettes, income, and demographic variables. Some of the variability in results is a consequence of methodological differences among studies. The studies derive estimates of demand from different sources, including time series of per capita cigarette consumption (for the United States as a whole and for cross-sections of States) and cross-sectional survey data on the smoking behavior of individuals at a point in time and over time. Each of these methods has inherent limitations that can cloud the interpretation of results. In time series studies, the estimates of price and income elasticities are sensitive to the method of accounting for the effects of concurrent social influences on smoking, such as the growing public knowledge about its harmful effects and changing cigarette advertising policies. In addition, time series estimates are not stable because the independent variables tend to be highly correlated with each other. Moreover, price elasticities estimated with time series data may represent short-term responses to price fluctuations rather than the long-term responses that are typically of greater interest to policymakers.

On the other hand, estimates of cigarette price elasticities based on cross-sections of State tax-paid sales may be biased upward because some cigarettes sold in low-tax States are ultimately consumed by smokers in higher tax States. As a result, tax-paid sales may overstate actual consumption in low-tax States and understate consumption in high-tax States, and the estimated price elasticity of sales will exceed the price elasticity of actual consumption. Some studies have attempted to control for short-distance, casual smuggling (ACIR 1977, 1985; Becker, Grossman, Murphy 1987; Chaloupka and Saffer 1988) and long-distance, organized smuggling (Becker, Grossman, Murphy 1987; Chaloupka and Saffer 1988) by using a set of carefully constructed variables. While these are imperfect measures of the smuggling phenomena, the careful attempt to control for the problem should reduce the bias associated with the use of this type of data.

TABLE 12.—Recent estimates of the price elasticity of demand for cigarettes

Study	Estimated aggregate price elasticity	Method of estimation	Comments
Fujii (1980)	–0.45	Ridge regression	Time-series aggregate data, 1929–73
Schneider, Klein, Murphy (1981)	−1.23	Instrumental variables	Time-series aggregate data, 1930–78
Lewit, Coate, Grossman (1981) Teenage smoking	−1.44	Ordinary least-squares	U.S. Health Examination Survey, 12–17-year-olds, 1966–70
Lewit and Coate (1982) Adult smoking	–0.42	Ordinary least-squares	1976 Health Interview Survey, elasticities by age and sex, 20–74-year-olds
Young (1983)		Ridge regression	Fujii's model with asymmetrical responses
Price increase	–0.33		
Price decline	–0.61		
Bishop and Yoo (1985)	–0.45	Three-stage least-squares	Time-series aggregate data, U.S., 1954–80
ACIR (1985)	–0.45	Ordinary least-squares	Pooled-time series of State cross-sections, 1981–83
Mullahy (1985)	–0.47	Probit, instrumental variables	1979 Health Interview Survey, by sex
Baltagi and Levin (1986)	–0.14	Instrumental variables	Pooled-time series cross-section of 46 States, 1963–80
Porter (1986)	–0.27	Two-stage least-squares	Time-series aggregate data, 1947–82
Chaloupka (1988) Long run	–0.26– –0.40	Instrumental variables	HANES2 full sample; also by age, sex, race, or education
Becker, Grossman, Murphy (1987) Long run	–0.75	Instrumental variables	Pooled-time series of State cross-sections, 1956–85
Chaloupka and Saffer (1988)	–0.28	Two-step endogenous law model	Pooled-time series of State cross-sections, 1975–85

An additional limitation of most econometric studies is that they use aggregate or per capita cigarette consumption as their dependent variable. As a result, they provide estimates of the price elasticity of aggregate or per capita cigarette consumption but can provide no information on the effects of price changes on smoking rates, smoking cessation and initiation, or quantity and type of cigarette smoked by smokers. Also, they cannot identify differences by separate demographic groups in response to price changes. Accordingly, aggregate studies are useful for economic and fiscal planning but are of limited usefulness when considering the behavioral or health effects of changes in cigarette tax policy.

In contrast to studies focused on aggregate consumption effects, Lewit and colleagues (1981, 1982) used data on individuals from two national surveys to investigate the effects of price (tax) differences on smoking behavior. With data on a sample of 19,288 individuals aged 20 through 70 years from the 1976 NHIS, Lewit and Coate (1982) estimated an overall price elasticity of –0.42 for cigarettes. They corrected for bias in two ways: first, by using consumption reported by individuals rather than tax-paid sales as the unit of observation, and second, by removing from the sample those households within 20 miles of States with lower prices. The former eliminates some of the error in the measurement of consumption, and the latter partially corrects for errors in the price measure that result when households purchase cigarettes outside their own localities.

Lewit and Coate's study also gave a more detailed breakdown of the smoking response than in previous studies. They found that cigarette prices affected smoking primarily by reducing smoking prevalence (the "participation rate," or number of smokers). The estimated effects on the number of cigarettes per smoker were not statistically significant. There were also differences in the estimated price elasticities among groups; reported price elasticities were much higher for adult males than for adult females and much higher for people aged 20 to 25 years than for other age groups. Their estimates are summarized in Table 13.

In a methodologically similar study, Lewit, Coate, and Grossman (1981) analyzed teenage smoking by using data from Cycle III of the U.S. Health Examination Survey (HES), a national sample of 6,768 youths between the ages of 12 and 17 years who were surveyed between March 1966 and March 1970. They reported that price elasticities of demand for cigarettes among teenagers are larger in absolute value than price elasticities for adults. As in the adult study, smoking participation (or prevalence) is more responsive to price than is the quantity of cigarettes smoked. Their estimated smoking participation elasticity for teenagers was –1.20, and the quantity-smoked elasticity (conditional on smoking) was –0.25 (Table 13).

The estimated elasticities based on HES data for teenagers were generally confirmed in a related study by Grossman, Coate, and Lewit (1983) and summarized by Grossman (1983). The study used a similar methodology to estimate price elasticities for teenagers on the basis of the four U.S. National Surveys on Drug Abuse (NSDA) conducted in 1974, 1976, 1977, and 1979. Estimates based on these surveys must be interpreted with caution because they are based on much smaller samples than those from the previous studies. Adjusting for this fact, Grossman's summary estimate of NSDA

TABLE 13.—Estimates of the price elasticity of demand for cigarettes

	Elasticities		
Age group (years)	Total	Participation	Quantity per smoker
12–17	–1.40	–1.20	–0.25
20–25	–0.89	–0.74	–0.20
26–35	–0.47	–0.44	–0.04
36–74	–0.45	–0.15	–0.15
All adults (20–74)	–0.42	–0.26	–0.10
All ages (12–74)	–0.47	–0.31	–0.11

SOURCE: Lewit and Coate (1982); Lewit, Coate, Grossman (1981); Lewit (1985) and unpublished calculations by Lewit.

participation elasticity was –0.76, which is smaller in absolute value than the HES estimate but almost 3 times larger than the NHIS elasticity for adults.

Most economic studies of the demand for cigarettes, including those cited above, have not explicitly allowed for the addictive nature of cigarettes (US DHHS 1988). Part of the reason for this omission was that the consumption of addictive goods in general was not thought to conform to the rational, utility-maximizing model that is the paradigm of standard economic analysis. Recently, however, Becker and colleagues (Becker, Grossman, Murphy 1987; Becker and Murphy 1988), among others, have developed models of "rational addiction" that are conducive to economic analysis. In general, this work recognizes that the demand for cigarettes depends on the levels of both past and future consumption, permitting incorporation of the notions of tolerance, reinforcement, and withdrawal, which are generally used to distinguish addictive from nonaddictive substances.

The findings of preliminary empirical research are consistent with the characterization of smoking as an addiction and suggest that failure to consider addiction explicitly may lead to underestimation of the long-term response to changes in cigarette price (Becker, Grossman, Murphy 1987; Chaloupka 1988). The application of the rational addiction model to cigarette consumption is a recent development that will require further empirical investigation and theoretical refinement before its contribution to the understanding of smoking behavior can be fully evaluated. The range of estimates of the long-term price elasticity of demand for cigarettes derived under the assumptions of the model is not inconsistent with previously published estimates, however, which suggests that insights gained from analyses of recent tax increases are not likely to be invalidated by further refinement of the addiction model.

The principal message of this body of research on price elasticity of demand is that an increase in the price of cigarettes appears to curtail smoking, particularly the initiation of smoking by teenagers. Because adolescents are more responsive to changes in cigarette prices than are adults and because price changes appear to have stronger effects on smoking prevalence than on daily consumption by smokers, the studies suggest that excise tax increases may be useful tools to prevent or delay the onset of smoking by adolescents.

Because aggregate cigarette consumption and smoking prevalence are dominated by the behavior of adults, the short-term effects of an increase in cigarette excise taxes would likely be modest. The long-term impact of such an increase could, however, be considerably more substantial. If the current situation, in which very few individuals start smoking after age 20 (see Chapter 5) continued, it is possible that the cohort of young persons who do not begin to smoke as a result of a tax increase would never become smokers. If the tax increase were maintained in real terms, it could continue to discourage successive generations of youths from starting to smoke. Gradually, the smoking prevalence of adults might be reduced as these cohorts moved through the age spectrum. Over a period of several decades, aggregate smoking and its associated health effects might decline more substantially than would be evident in the years immediately following a tax increase.

In addition to its relevance for cigarette taxation, research demonstrating the inverse relationship between tobacco price and demand has implications for the armed forces. As described in Chapter 5, the prevalence of smoking among military personnel exceeds that of the general population. One factor probably contributing to the differential in smoking rates is the lower price paid by military personnel for tobacco products. The current pricing structure of the military resale system results in approximate 35-percent and 18-percent reductions in cigarette price in military commissaries and exchanges, respectively, when compared with commercial retail outlets (US DOD 1986c). Cigarettes sold in these military stores are exempt from State and local excise taxes and, if outside the United States, are also exempt from the Federal excise tax. Cigarette sales in the military resale system totaled 1,046 million packs in fiscal year 1985, though sales have been decreasing in the 1980s (US DOD 1986c, 1987). Price elasticity of demand data suggest that increasing the price of cigarettes could contribute to reducing tobacco use by military personnel. In 1986, DOD considered banning the sale of tobacco in commissaries or raising the price of tobacco products on military installations as part of a broad program to discourage tobacco use. Neither of these policies was adopted (US DOD 1987), although, as discussed in Part III and Chapter 6, DOD has instituted new smoking restrictions and has launched antismoking activities on a large scale.

Effects of an Excise Tax Increase

Research addressing the temporary doubling of the Federal excise tax in 1983 and its six temporary extensions prior to permanent adoption in 1986 generated several estimates of the effect of the tax increase on cigarette consumption and smoking prevalence. For example, Harris (1982) used the Lewit-Coate estimate of the adult-smoking participation price elasticity of –0.26 and the Lewit-Coate-Grossman estimate of the teenage-smoking participation price elasticity of –1.20 to forecast the impact of the doubling of the Federal excise tax rate in 1983. He predicted that the number of adult smokers would decline by 1.5 million and the number of teenage smokers by 0.7 million.

In an analysis performed in 1985, during the period of uncertainty as to whether the Federal tax increase would be extended permanently or allowed to lapse, Warner (1986a) used the Lewit-Coate and Lewit-Coate-Grossman age-specific elasticity estimates to project the changes in cigarette consumption that would have accompanied an 8-cent tax decrease or 8- and 16-cent tax increases (Table 14). Altogether he estimated that an 8-cent decrease in the tax would induce almost 2 million persons to smoke who would not do so if the tax were to remain unchanged at 16 cents per pack. In contrast, a doubling of the tax to 32 cents per pack would have encouraged almost 3.5 million Americans to forego smoking, a figure that included more than 800,000 teenagers and almost 2 million young adults aged 20 to 35 years.

TABLE 14.—Expected percentage changes in cigarette consumption resulting from changes in the Federal cigarette excise tax

	8-cent decrease		8-cent increase		16-cent increase	
Age group	Total consumption	Smoking prevalence	Total consumption	Smoking prevalence	Total consumption	Smoking prevalence
12–17	11.9	10.2	–11.1	–9.5	–21.1	–18.1
20–25	7.6	6.3	–7.0	–5.9	–13.4	–11.2
26–35	4.0	3.7	–3.7	–3.5	–7.1	–6.6
36–74	3.8	1.3	–3.6	–1.2	–6.8	–2.3
All adults (20–74)	3.6	2.2	–3.3	–2.1	–6.3	–3.9

SOURCE: Warner (1986a).

Lewit (1985) examined the actual decline in aggregate cigarette consumption following the 1983 tax increase. He noted that in anticipation of the January 1, 1983, tax increase, the tobacco companies increased the wholesale price of cigarettes four times between August 1982 and January 1983. Cigarette prices were increased twice again in 1983, and 16 States increased their cigarette excise taxes during 1982 and 1983. As a consequence, the average retail price of cigarettes increased by about 40 percent between November 1, 1981, and November 1, 1984, from approximately 70 cents per pack in 1981 to almost 98 cents in 1984 (Tobacco Institute 1988). During this same period, the price of cigarettes adjusted for inflation rose by 26 percent. Based on an overall price elasticity of –0.47 for adults and teenagers, per capita consumption should have declined by about 12 percent over this period. Department of Agriculture data indicate a decline of 11 to 12 percent. Although per capita cigarette consumption had been slowly declining at the rate of about 1 percent per annum since the mid-1970s, the very rapid acceleration in the rate of decline following the excise tax increase and associated price increases is consistent with the cross-sectional studies and serves as further evidence that excise taxes may be a potent tool to discourage smoking.

Harris (1987) conducted an extensive review of the 1983 Federal tax increase. On the whole, his findings for the period 1981–86 are consistent with those reported by Lewit (1985). Harris' discussion of the cigarette manufacturers' response to the tax increase is, however, of particular interest. It has been generally assumed that changes in tax rates would be fully passed on to consumers. Accordingly, Warner's analysis (1986a) and Harris' earlier analysis (1982) assumed that an 8-cent tax increase would raise the retail price of cigarettes by 8 cents. Harris (1987) reports evidence to suggest, however, that the preannounced 1983 Federal tax increase appeared to have served as a focal point for coordinating an oligopolistic price increase by tobacco producers that exceeded the amount of the tax. He concludes that "Quite contrary to the conventional view of the incidence of excise taxes, the federal excise tax may have actually had a multiplier effect upon price." He estimates that the 8-cent-per-pack tax increase induced a 16-cent-per-pack increase in the market price of cigarettes.

Health Consequences of Tax Changes

Given the deleterious health effects of cigarette smoking and the important changes in both cigarette consumption and smoking prevalence that would accompany a substantial tax change, it appears that a policy of aggressive increases in the tax on cigarettes would lead to large reductions in smoking-induced illness. To assess fully the effect of a cigarette tax change on the health of the population, information is needed on who actually cuts down on cigarettes, who quits, and who does not start smoking. Only a portion of such information is available.

However, both Warner (1986a) and Harris (1987) provide crude estimates of some of the health effects that may result from the 1983 Federal tax increase. Basing his estimates on the conservative assumption that one lifelong smoker out of every four dies of smoking-related illness (Mattson et al. 1987), Warner obtained upper bound estimates of the mortality impact of increases or decreases in the Federal excise tax. He estimated that an 8-cent tax increase, maintained in real value over time, would avert 450,000 premature deaths in the cohort of Americans 12 years of age and older in 1984 and that this number would rise to 860,000 following a 16-cent increase. An 8-cent tax decrease, however, would result in an increase of more than 480,000 premature smoking-induced deaths.

Focusing specifically on the post-1983 tax-induced price changes and their impact on consumption, Harris estimated that 100,000 additional persons will live to age 65 as a result of the tax increase. Of these 100,000, he estimated that 54,000 will result from having discouraged 600,000 teenagers from starting to smoke. Thus, the major effect of the tax increase on mortality will not be realized for decades. On the other hand, although no estimates of the impact of the tax increase on other health measures have been published, reductions in smoking-induced morbidity and disability should raise aggregate health levels long before the projected mortality reductions are fully realized.

Policies Under Consideration

Among the public policy tools with a potential to reduce tobacco use, the cigarette excise tax has received particular attention because its public health benefits are well documented, and it has the additional advantage of generating public revenues (Warner et al. 1986b). Currently discussed proposals to modify Federal, State, or local cigarette excise taxes fall into two categories: (1) proposals to increase the amount of the tax or the method of calculating the tax rate, and (2) proposals to channel the revenues generated from excise taxes for specific purposes. The first category includes proposals to increase the Federal excise tax rate, raise State and local excise tax rates (especially in States in which rates are currently below the national or regional average), and switch from a specific unit tax to an ad valorem tax, thereby tying the tax rate to a measure that changes with inflation. This last proposal often accompanies the others because it permits the real tax rate to keep pace with inflation. Proposals in the second category would dedicate (or earmark) some portion of tax receipts for purposes such as funding tobacco control programs or paying for the excess health care costs of smokers.

Tobacco Excise Tax Increases

Increasing the Federal excise tax beyond the 16-cent-per-pack level first set by Congress in 1983 and made permanent in 1986 is the most widely discussed and most broadly supported tax proposal. It has been endorsed by a wide range of voluntary health organizations and organized medical societies, including the American Medical Association, American Public Health Association, American Cancer Society, American Heart Association, and American Lung Association. Proponents of a Federal excise tax increase note that the real value of the tax has fallen since 1964 and that inflation since the last increase in 1983 has continued to erode the real value of the tax. Opponents of Federal excise tax increases have raised several issues, primarily based on tax equity considerations. Chief among them is that cigarette excise taxation is regressive, requiring the poor to pay a greater proportion of their income on the tax than the rich. More pragmatic concerns have been raised about the effect on State tax revenues. Because the consumption of cigarettes tends to decline as price rises, State cigarette tax receipts may fall after a Federal tax increase if State tax rates remain constant. In the aggregate, this did not happen after the 1983 Federal excise tax increase because State tax rates also increased.

Increases in State excise taxes have received less attention, although the effect of such a policy change on consumption and revenue would be expected to resemble that of a Federal tax change. The variability in State taxes adds an additional concern about interstate bootlegging of cigarettes, which could be avoided if excise tax rates were preferentially raised in States with relatively low tax rates. Beyond excise tax changes, cigarette taxes could also be increased in those States that now exempt cigarettes from the regular sales tax by removing that exemption. Massachusetts did so in June 1988, resulting in a 5-cent increase in the tax on cigarettes (Mohl 1988).

Switch to an Ad Valorem Tax

With the exception of the State excise tax in Hawaii, all Federal, State, and local cigarette taxes are specific unit taxes; that is, the tax rate is a constant nominal amount per unit. While a specific unit excise tax has the advantage of administrative simplicity, it has the disadvantage that the real revenue yield tends to decline with inflation. Unit excise taxes must be raised periodically if real revenues—and consequent impact on tobacco consumption—are to be maintained. Replacing unit taxes on cigarettes and other tobacco products with equivalent-yield ad valorem taxes would allow revenues to keep pace with inflation-induced increases in cigarette prices, and real cigarette prices would be more likely to be maintained over time. As mentioned above, Federal taxes on large cigars and most State taxes on noncigarette tobacco products are ad valorem taxes. An alternative to switching to an ad valorem tax on cigarettes is to index the unit tax to changes in either the general price level or to a price index for cigarettes (Toder 1985). This would maintain the administrative simplicity of per-unit taxes and eliminate the need to periodically reevaluate the unit tax rate to maintain real revenues.

Earmarking of Revenues

Tobacco taxes may also be earmarked (dedicated) for specific tobacco- or health-related purposes. Proposals have included using tax revenues to support the cost of health care for tobacco-related illnesses or to fund tobacco prevention and cessation programs delivered in schools or via the media (Warner 1986c). Earmarking a portion of the Federal cigarette excise tax to fund the medicare program has been proposed to Congress (Committee on Ways and Means 1986), and survey data show that a majority of the public would support an increase in the cigarette excise tax to fund medicare (Chapter 4).

Several States have used cigarette tax revenues to finance tobacco-related health programs. In Nebraska, revenue from a 1-cent-per-pack cigarette tax is used to fund the State's Cancer and Smoking Disease Research Program (CDC 1987). In Minnesota, the Omnibus Nonsmoking and Disease Prevention Act of 1985 increased the cigarette excise tax by 5 cents per pack and earmarked 1 cent of the additional revenues for a public health fund. As noted previously, one-quarter of this fund is dedicated to assist local school boards to implement tobacco use prevention programs. Funds are also provided for an active public tobacco control and prevention program overseen by the Commissioner of Health (Minnesota Department of Health 1987a,b). In Utah, a portion of revenues generated from an 11-cent increase in the State cigarette excise tax is dedicated for tobacco control programs (Utah 1987). A newer proposal would earmark a portion of the estimated excise tax revenue generated from sales of tobacco products to minors to support tobacco prevention and cessation programs for youth (Slade 1988a). In Indiana, a portion of the State tobacco excise tax is earmarked to support subsidized child care programs (Lewin 1988).

The most substantial earmarking of tobacco excise tax revenues is in California, the result of passage of a ballot initiative in November 1988 raising the State's cigarette excise tax by 25 cents per pack. With the exception of funds to cover the administrative and collection costs associated with the tax, three-quarters of all revenues are dedicated to health education, research, medical treatment, and environmental conservation programs. In its first full year of operation, the tax is expected to generate 650 million dollars for these purposes (Tobacco Tax and Health Protection Act of 1988; Wilson 1988b).

Insurance and the Treatment of Smokers

At the time of the 1964 Surgeon General's Report, whether a person smoked was not a consideration in the premiums paid for insurance. No major life, health, disability, homeowner, or auto insurer offered discounts to nonsmokers, and no major health insurer covered the expenses of smoking cessation programs. In fact, the consensus of a panel of the Society of Actuaries convened in 1963 was that consideration of smoking in calculating life insurance premiums seemed to be impractical (November et al. 1964).

Over the subsequent 25 years, this situation has changed considerably, but changes have come at different rates in the three major segments of the insurance industry—life, health and disability, and property and casualty. Currently, almost all life insurers, including two that are subsidiaries of major tobacco firms, offer premium discounts to individuals who do not smoke cigarettes (Trenk 1986). In contrast, only about 15 percent of companies writing health and disability insurance policies offer discounts to nonsmokers, and even fewer reimburse health care providers for smoking cessation treatment (National Association of Insurance Commissioners (NAIC) 1987c). Only 1 of the 10 leading writers of homeowner and personal passenger auto policies offers discounts to nonsmokers on both (Wasilewski 1987a,b). Although the underwriting practices and administrative exigencies vary considerably among these three types of insurance, sentiment has been building for insurers, primarily those in life and health, to offer premium differentials and cover the costs of smoking cessation treatment (Brailey 1980; Stokes 1983; Davis 1986; Engstrom 1986; Walsh and Gordon 1986; US DHHS 1988).

Premium differentials based on smoking behavior are generally referred to as nonsmoker discounts rather than as smoker surcharges. The terminology, which implies that smoking is the majority condition, is no longer correct, but it persists for historical and marketing reasons; the premium differentials were developed when smoking was a more common behavior, and a discount sounds like a positive incentive, while a surcharge has the negative connotation of a penalty. Smoker–nonsmoker premium differentials are the result of insurer business decisions, based primarily on differences between insured smokers and nonsmokers in mortality rates, health care costs, and auto and homeowner claims. For the policyholder, a premium differential may serve as an economic disincentive for smoking.

This Section will examine separately each of the three major industry segments to address the extent to which insurers in each category consider policyholder smoking status when calculating premiums or coverage, reasons the three segments handle the issue differently, and the potential effects of the insurance industry's premium structure and reimbursement policies on smoking behavior.

Life Insurance

Life insurance policies are sold on an individual, family, or group basis. Policies purchased on an individual or family basis are referred to as ordinary life insurance and are the most common type of life insurance. Sixty-two percent of households in the United States had ordinary life insurance policies in 1987 (American Council of Life Insurance (ACLI) 1987).

Life insurers price their products according to the mortality experience of the insured population. Higher premiums are set for classes of individuals with greater mortality rates. Smoker–nonsmoker premium differentials were adopted by the industry when actuarial studies confirmed that the excess mortality of smokers, previously observed in epidemiologic studies, was also present in the insured population (Cowell 1985). Some insurers offer an alternative to smoker–nonsmoker premium differentials. These policies are based on overall health behavior or health status and are typically available only to applicants who meet health standards with regard to weight, blood pressure, and exercise and who do not smoke.

History of Premium Differentials

Three months after the 1964 Surgeon General's Report was released, State Mutual Life Assurance Company became the first company to offer life insurance to nonsmokers at discounted rates. The company believed that its statistical evidence of "much higher death rates among persons who smoke was so overwhelming that the company could no longer ignore it in pricing insurance" (Cowell 1985; Cowell and Hirst 1980). This action was consistent with a position that nonsmokers should not subsidize the higher insurance costs resulting from smokers' excess death claims.

Between 1965 and 1975, more than 30 other companies introduced premium discounts for nonsmokers, based on their estimates of the effects of smoking on mortality in the insured population. Their estimates resulted at least partly from examination of mortality studies discussed in the early Surgeon General's Reports (Crowne and Shapiro 1980). However, most of the industry did not develop nonsmoker premium discounts at that time. Their reluctance derived primarily from a paucity of actuarial data. Furthermore, only half of the primary market of policyholders—adult males—stood to benefit from these discounts, because in 1965, 50 percent of adult males smoked (Chapter 5). Companies also had to address the uncertainties of marketing and administering a new product. These factors were sufficient to slow the adoption of smoker–nonsmoker premium differentials (Cowell 1985; Cowell and Hirst 1980).

In 1979, State Mutual analyzed the mortality differences between its insured smokers and nonsmokers. The analysis showed that the overall mortality of smoking policyholders was 2 to 2 1/2 times that of nonsmoking policyholders. The higher death rates of smokers were not confined to older ages but were apparent even at early ages. These findings were statistically significant and large enough to be used for insurance underwriting and pricing purposes (Cowell and Hirst 1980). This landmark report was a stimulus to rapid change in the industry. After State Mutual made public its experience, so did other life insurers, including those that had previously not issued their findings in the mistaken belief that the differences were too large to be true. Within 3 years, 400 companies offered discounted premiums to nonsmokers (Shaman 1982).

In 1983, at the request of NAIC, a Society of Actuaries' task force examined the smoking-related mortality data of insurance companies. The Task Force on Smoker/Nonsmoker Mortality determined the mortality differences between smoking and nonsmoking insured persons of ages 15 to 99 years and divided the mortality tables used to value the reserves on life insurance into those appropriate for pricing separate smoker and nonsmoker products. The group did not specifically address the nature of the association between smoking and increased mortality that it so clearly observed. For their purposes, it was sufficient only that premium rates reflected the actual mortality experience of groups of insured smokers and insured nonsmokers (Society of Actuaries 1983).

By addressing these issues, the task force facilitated greater acceptance of smoker–nonsmoker premium differentials by insurance companies and the State government officials who regulate them. NAIC used the Society of Actuaries' work to develop the "Model Rule (Regulation) Permitting Smoker/Nonsmoker Mortality Tables For Use In Determining Minimum Reserve Liabilities and Nonforfeiture Benefits" (NAIC 1985b). The rule permitted insurers to use standard underwriting and actuarial practices to set different premium rates for smokers and nonsmokers, as insurers would for any other accepted risk classification in their normal conduct of business. Proposed in January 1984 to Commissioners of Insurance in all States, the model rule or a similar variation had become law in 33 States as of July 1987 (NAIC 1987f).

Once the empirical basis for smoker–nonsmoker premium differentials was established, life insurers had to consider how to market and administer the new products. A central concern was the possibility that individuals would misrepresent their smoking status (Lipson 1988). Misrepresentation is not a new problem; insurance companies have had to deal with it since their beginning. One solution was to require biochemical validation of nonsmoking status. A growing number of insurers now require this validation before selling a policy (Lyons 1986). One reason nonsmoking discounts are less often offered on group policies is that persons within groups are rarely examined or have their smoking status verified (Brailey 1980).

A second approach has been to investigate claims made by nonsmokers. When confronted with a claim from an individual who has misrepresented his or her smoking status, insurance companies have usually done one of the following: (1) reduced the benefit to the amount that the premium actually paid would have purchased for a smoker, (2) paid the claim in full, (3) returned the premiums paid with interest, (4) deducted the premium differential from the benefits, or (5) rescinded the policy and refused to pay. How often insurers use each of these options is not known, but the last option, by far the most severe deterrent to misrepresentation, has recently garnered much industry support (Lyons 1986). It has also been upheld in the courts. In a January 4, 1988, decision in *Mutual Benefit Life Insurance Company* v. *JMR Electronics Corp.*, the U.S. District Court of the Southern District of New York absolved the insurer of liability for a policy where the insured had misrepresented his smoking status:

> To allow recovery would condone such fraudulent Statements, for applicants would have everything to gain and nothing to lose by gambling on getting full coverage and at worst

getting the coverage they are actually entitled to (Tobacco Products Litigation Reporter 1988).

In May 1988, the U.S. Court of Appeals upheld that opinion (Hagedorn 1988).

Current Status of Premium Differentials

In 1987, 89 percent of 215 companies responding to an industry survey reported that they offered health-behavior-related discounts on individual life insurance policies; 14 percent also offered them on group life insurance policies. Almost all of these health-behavior-related discounts included discounts to nonsmokers (Center for Corporate Public Involvement 1987).

Thirty percent of all individual life insurance policies purchased in the United States and 39 percent of the amount of coverage are so-called universal life policies, which offer the policyholder the option of varying the amount of coverage or the timing of premium payments (ACLI 1986). All of the top five life insurers, which as a group are responsible for 23.4 percent of life insurance premiums generated in the United States, offer nonsmoking discounts on universal policies, varying by the age of the insured by as much as 30 percent (A.M. Best 1987a). Nineteen of the top 25 companies, responsible for 46 percent of the total amount of life insurance premiums, offered universal policies in 1987 (A.M. Best 1987a). Of those 19 companies, 16 gave discounts to nonsmokers, some as high as 40 percent for both males and females. Discounts varied by the age and sex of the insured (Table 15). The discounts were smallest for younger persons, increased steadily to a peak at age 45 years, and dropped slightly for older individuals. At all ages, discounts were larger for men than for women. The average discounts for newly insured males and females in 1987 ranged from 12.5 to 22.5 percent.

TABLE 15.—Average premium discount (%) offered to nonsmokers purchasing universal life insurance policies, 1986–87

	Average age (years)			
	25	35	45	55
Male	14.5	18.1	22.5	20.4
Female	12.5	14.3	17.0	16.5

NOTE: Discounts based on the minimum amount of insurance that can be purchased.
SOURCE: A.M. Best (1987a).

The average dollar amount of discounts varied not only by sex and age but also by policy amount (Table 16). Savings for nonsmokers increased with the amount of the policy and the age of the insured, and they were larger for men than for women. The average size of an ordinary life insurance policy *in force* in 1986 was 25,538 dollars (ACLI 1987). On a 25,000 dollar policy written for males, the annual savings in premium cost ranged from 15 dollars at age 25 to 114 dollars at age 55. Savings on the same size policy written for females varied between 10 dollars at age 25 and 61 dollars

TABLE 16.—Average difference ($) between annual premiums paid by smokers and nonsmokers purchasing universal life insurance policies, 1986–87

	Age (years)			
Policy amount	25	35	45	55
$25,000 policy[a]				
Male	15	30	72	114
Female	10	18	39	61
$50,000 policy[b]				
Male	48	79	170	299
Female	34	55	109	192

NOTE: Figures are based on policies offered by the 25 largest life insurers.
[a]Average value of an ordinary (individual) life insurance policy in force in 1986 was 25,538 dollars (ACLI 1987). Not all companies offer this amount of coverage.
[b]Average value of an ordinary (individual) life insurance policy purchased in 1986 was 55,535 dollars (ACLI 1987).
SOURCE: A.M. Best (1987a).

at age 55 (A.M. Best 1987a). The average size of ordinary life insurance policies *purchased* in 1986 was 55,535 dollars (ACLI 1987). Annual savings on a 50,000 dollar policy averaged from 48 dollars at age 25 years to 299 dollars at age 55 in men, and from 34 dollars at age 25 years to 192 dollars at age 55 in women (A.M. Best 1987a).

Health Insurance

Approximately 85 percent of Americans are covered by health insurance, which is most frequently offered by commercial carriers, Blue Cross–Blue Shield (BC/BS) plans, and health maintenance organizations (HMOs). Unlike life insurance, which is largely sold to individuals and families, 80 percent of health insurance is purchased on a group basis, usually as an employment benefit (Health Insurance Association of America (HIAA) 1987). As a result, these policies are seldom tailored to individual health profiles or health risks to the degree common in individual life insurance underwriting, where a physical examination is typically required before a policy is written. In keeping with this situation, smoker–nonsmoker premium differentials are much less commonly offered by health than by life insurers, as described below.

Current Status of Premium Differentials

Individual health insurance policies are far less common than group plans. They account for only 20 percent of the health insurance market (HIAA 1987). The most complete study of premium differentials for individual health and disability policies was conducted in 1987 by NAIC (NAIC 1987a,b,c,d), which sent a survey to all 603 carriers offering individual health and disability insurance in Illinois and all BC/BS plans in the United States. Seventy-six percent of commercial carriers and 77 percent of

BC/BS plans responded. Fourteen percent of the commercial carrier respondents either offered discounts to nonsmokers or imposed surcharges on smokers for health (hospital–medical) or disability (loss of income) policies. Sixteen percent of BC/BS plans offered discounts to nonsmokers on hospital–medical policies. Average nonsmoker discounts on health insurance offered by commercial carriers ranged from 9 to 15 percent, with an industry average of 10 percent. Average discounts offered by the BC/BS plans ranged from 8 to 10 percent, with an industry average of 9 percent. For disability policies, the average nonsmoker discount ranged from 3 to 14 percent, with an industry average of 8 percent, whereas the average smoker surcharges ranged from 10 to 14 percent, with an industry average of 13 percent.

Health insurers are much less likely to offer nonsmoker discounts with their group health products, despite an NAIC resolution supporting premium differentials in group as well as in individual health policies (NAIC 1985a). In 1980, Provident Indemnity Life Insurance Company became the first to use smoking as a risk factor in establishing health insurance premiums for small groups (less than 25 employees) (Hellauer 1988). Few insurers have followed suit.

The use of smoking status in the calculation of premiums for HMOs has been slowed by Federal regulations. Federally qualified HMOs were required by the original HMO Act of 1973 (Public Law 93-222) to calculate their group premiums by community rating, reflecting the health cost experience of the overall community, not of special groups such as young, healthy employees. In the HMO Amendments of 1981 (Public Law 97-35), Congress modified that requirement and allowed HMOs to become more competitive by setting their community rates by class. Classes subsequently permitted by the Secretary of Health and Human Services include age, sex, family size, and industry of the insured. Because smoking status is not one of these, each HMO must individually petition the Federal Government to use smoking as one of its classification factors. As of March 1988, only one had applied for permission and received it. The Contra Costa Health Plan in 1987 became the first federally qualified HMO to use smoking as a factor in calculating its group health premiums. To do so, it received approval by the Office of Prepaid Health Care, Department of Health and Human Services. Contra Costa based its request, and the Federal office its approval, on a study (Brink 1987) that reported that nonsmokers incurred 18.5 percent lower health care costs than smokers (Contra Costa Health Plan 1987).

In summary, as of 1987, approximately one in seven commercial health carriers and BC/BS plans offered nonsmoking discounts on individual policies; these discounts ranged from 3 to 15 percent. A few carriers have introduced discounts of 2 to 3 percent on group policies where certain percentages of the groups are nonsmokers. Only one federally qualified HMO offers a nonsmoker discount; it is approximately 5 percent of premium cost.

Factors Influencing Decisions About Premium Differentials

Several factors have contributed to the slower development of smoker–nonsmoker premium differentials by health and disability insurers compared with life insurers. First, there are fewer actuarial data to document that nonsmokers incur fewer health care costs. Second, most health insurance is purchased on a group basis, which makes calculating discounts more difficult and makes validation of smoking status nearly impossible because no individual examination is undertaken. Third, as discussed above, current Federal regulations for HMOs preclude the use of smoking status in calculating premiums.

Health insurers have offered nonsmoker discounts with little supportive actuarial experience that nonsmokers incur fewer claims. Many insurers have not developed such data because they have not had the ability to separate the claims experience of smokers from nonsmokers. In addition, smaller companies may not have the statistical resources to collect or analyze such data. In one recent survey, only 32 percent of commercial carriers with premium differentials and 70 percent of BC/BS plans had the ability to develop the appropriate actuarial data (NAIC 1987c).

The first major compilation of claims data was made in 1987 by NAIC (1987c). It supported smoker–nonsmoker premium differentials in most cases. Analysis of the claims experience of eight commercial carriers justified a nonsmoking discount of 28 percent on hospital–medical policies, whereas a similar analysis of five BC/BS plans justified a 19-percent discount (Table 17). Claims data from all five BC/BS plans justified nonsmoking discounts that were more than or equal to that offered. The experience was not so clearcut for commercial carriers. The data from one company, with more than half of the total claims experience, supported a larger discount. However, claims experience justified nonsmoker discounts for only three of the seven smaller companies. This inconsistency may be explained by the misclassification of smokers in the "nonsmoker" policyholder category. This is suggested by the fact that only 20 percent of all adjusted earned premiums were held by policyholders classified as smokers, a much lower percentage than the prevalence of smoking in the general population. This discrepancy may result from smokers misrepresenting their status,

TABLE 17.—Summary of smoker–nonsmoker health and disability claims experience

	Adjusted earned premiums ($)		Loss ratio[a]	
	Nonsmoker	Smoker	Nonsmoker	Smoker
Hospital/medical insurance				
Commercial carrier	120,694,007	29,857,057	49.1	68.7
Blue Cross–Blue Shield	55,791,022	32,449,964	71.6	88.2
Disability insurance				
Commercial carrier				
Nonsmoker discount	11,445,976	3,931,357	30.4	25.1
Smoker surcharge	50,404,495	5,182,015	31.3	61.1
Blue Cross–Blue Shield	26,226,456	10,822,819	76.9	104.8

[a]Ratio of claims incurred to earned premiums, multiplied by 100. A loss ratio of 100 indicates that claims incurred equal earned premiums.
SOURCE: NAIC (1987c).

from excessively lenient eligibility standards for nonsmoker status, or from certain plans having an excess number of older former smokers who had quit smoking because of smoking-related illness.

For disability insurance policies, a nonsmoking discount of 25 percent was justified by the analysis of seven commercial carriers and one BC/BS plan (Table 17). However, as with hospital–medical policies, the claims experience of a single large insurer overwhelmed those of the others. Only one of the other carriers had experience that justified a discount. On the other hand, analysis of claims data from the five commercial carriers that charged smokers a premium surcharge rather than offering nonsmokers a discount supports these increased rates for smokers.

Another reason health insurers have been reluctant to offer nonsmoking discounts is that most insurance is purchased by groups. Premiums paid by groups are commonly "experience rated"; premiums paid in a given year are based largely on the overall costs of claims incurred by the group in the previous year or years. In theory, the experience rating mechanism should eventually result in lower premiums to groups with relatively more nonsmokers, if their health care costs are in fact lower than those of smokers. A group with fewer smokers should incur fewer health care costs, which should be reflected in their subsequent premiums. Adding a premium discount based on the proportion of nonsmokers in the group simply adds administrative problems with determining and validating the proportion of nonsmokers in the group. Finally, because the difference in health care costs between smokers and nonsmokers differs across various age groups, computation of discounts is complicated and must involve adjustment by the age mix of the employee group (Hellauer 1988).

Property and Casualty Insurance

There is a clear rationale for offering nonsmoker discounts on homeowner policies. Between 1981 and 1985, smoking materials caused 7.1 percent of all home fires, 8.0 percent of all home fire property damage, and 31.3 percent of all home fire civilian deaths (National Fire Protection Association 1987). In 1985 alone, smoking materials in the United States caused almost a quarter million home fires. Associated with those fires were 1,703 deaths, 3,997 injuries, and 422 million dollars in direct property damage (Hall 1987).

Smoker–nonsmoker premium differentials on auto insurance are based on studies demonstrating that nonsmokers have fewer motor vehicle accidents. Farmers' Insurance Group, the first property and casualty insurer to offer these discounts, instituted its nonsmoker discounts because of an early study reporting an association between smoking and vehicular accidents (Adams and Williams 1965, 1966). Farmers' own internal study of several thousand of its policyholders revealed that its nonsmokers had a lower accident rate and fewer claims than smokers. Subsequent claims experience has confirmed the original findings, as has nonindustry research (McGuire 1972; Grout et al. 1983; DiFranza et al. 1986).

The specific reason for the better safety record of nonsmokers is not clearly understood, and the relationship may not be causal. Several potential explanations for smokers' higher accident rate have been suggested: (1) smoking while driving may result in less attentive driving; (2) smokers may engage in more risk-taking behavior in operating their vehicles; (3) smokers use alcohol and illegal drugs more frequently than nonsmokers; and (4) nicotine or some other constituent of cigarette smoke may impair complex behaviors such as driving (DiFranza et al. 1986). In the industry's view, whether there is a causal link between smoking and motor vehicle accidents is irrelevant; the better safety record of nonsmokers has been shown repeatedly and is the basis for the discounts. Periodic reviews by Farmers' have been kept proprietary but support continuing discounts for nonsmokers (Clemans 1988). Similarly, Hanover Insurance Group's experience—that smokers have a 24-percent higher rate of claims than do nonsmokers—demonstrates that actuarial differences support premium differentials (DiFranza et al. 1986).

The first property and casualty insurer to offer premium discounts to nonsmokers, the Farmers' Insurance Group of Companies, includes the third largest private passenger auto insurer and the third largest homeowner insurer in the United States. Nonsmoking discounts were offered on auto policies beginning in 1971 and on homeowner policies in 1974 (Clemans 1988). This company remains the only 1 of the 10 leading writers of homeowner and private passenger auto insurance to offer discounts to nonsmokers on both types of policies (Wasilewski 1987a,b). Currently Farmers' offers nonsmokers and former smokers who have not smoked for at least 24 months discounts of 3 to 7 percent on homeowner policy base rates and discounts of 10 to 25 percent on auto policies, depending on State of residence.

Other insurers that offer nonsmoker discounts on auto policies include Preferred Risk Group and Hanover Insurance Company (NAIC 1987e). On the basis of its own claims experience, Hanover increased discounts from the original 5 percent, instituted between 1974 and 1978, to the current 10 percent. The company provides the discounts on both auto and homeowner policies nationwide, except in States where regulatory bodies prohibit them. Fifty-two percent of its policyholders have nonsmoker discounts (Weinman 1988).

Factors that have prevented the more widespread industry adoption of nonsmoker discounts on auto and homeowner policies include difficulties in the verification of smoking status and regulations in some States that prohibit nonsmoking discounts or prohibit rescission of benefits in cases of misrepresentation.

Effects of Insurance Premium Differentials on Smoking Behavior

Insurers' use of smoking behavior as a factor in setting premiums may have both economic and educational effects that discourage smoking. Premium differentials may serve as economic disincentives for smoking because they effectively, if indirectly, increase the cost of smoking cigarettes. This may reduce tobacco consumption and encourage cessation. In addition, payment of a higher premium may reinforce smokers' knowledge of the harm caused by smoking and serve as another social message to smokers about the disadvantages of smoking and desirability of cessation. It is less likely that insurance premium differentials will have a strong role in discouraging smoking initiation, because most individuals make decisions about smoking during adolescence, before many purchase insurance.

Empirical studies, reviewed in the previous section, have demonstrated that changes in cigarette prices affect tobacco consumption. Elasticities have been calculated for the effect on demand of changes in the price of cigarettes at the point of purchase, but not for economic policies that indirectly alter a smoker's costs. No empirical studies have examined the effect on smoking prevalence or cigarette consumption of higher insurance premiums for smokers or of reimbursement for the cost of smoking cessation programs. The potential educational effects of premium differentials on public knowledge or attitudes have not been studied; effects will be difficult to distinguish from other social influences discouraging smoking.

The expected effects of excise taxes and premium differentials are not identical, because of inherent differences between buying cigarettes and purchasing insurance. A smoker can respond to higher excise taxes by reducing consumption without giving up smoking, but a smoker can reduce insurance premiums only by stopping smoking altogether. Insurance premium differentials may be less powerful economic incentives than are changes in actual cigarette prices, because higher insurance premiums do not translate directly into an increase in the price of cigarettes at the point of sale. Furthermore, a smoker buys cigarettes far more often then he or she pays insurance premiums. On the other hand, the magnitude of an insurance premium differential is greater than a tax-induced change in the price of a pack of cigarettes.

Other factors may blunt the impact of insurance premium differentials based on smoking behavior. First, smokers may forget or not even know that they are being penalized if there is no reminder of that fact on their insurance bill or payroll receipt. Some life and health insurers may not inform smoking policyholders that they use controllable risk factors when setting premiums. The educational value of the premium differential is largely lost after the policy is issued if periodic reminders of the basis of premium are not sent with the insurance bill. Furthermore, part of the economic incentive is lost if no mechanism exists for smokers who quit smoking after the policy is issued to become eligible for a lower premium. Second, the individual may not pay the full cost of insurance premiums. Health and life insurance is often included in employee benefit packages, with the employee paying only a portion of the total premium. The employee's contributions to the insurance premiums may be small or nonexistent. Third, most health insurance policies are group policies that do not include smoker–nonsmoker differentials. Those that do set premiums based on the smoking prevalence of the group, so that a smoker's higher premium cost is partly borne by nonsmoking members of the group. Finally, because not all insurers offer nonsmoking discounts, even smokers purchasing individual insurance have the option of purchasing insurance from companies that do not tie premiums to smoking behavior.

Health Insurance Coverage for Smoking Cessation Treatment

Insurers who reimburse for the costs of attending a smoking cessation program or of purchasing a cessation aid effectively reduce the cost of quitting smoking, thereby removing a financial disincentive to quit. This reimbursement may also serve as an economic incentive to the provider of the treatment to offer more services, thereby increasing availability of cessation treatment.

Currently, few health insurance carriers cover the costs of smoking cessation programs. Only 11 percent of 263 health insurance carriers surveyed in 1985 included smoking cessation treatment as a covered benefit. Insurers that reimbursed for smoking cessation programs did so only to treat established smoking-related diseases, not to prevent these diseases (Gelb 1985). Among BC/BS plans, smoking cessation is usually not an approved benefit for groups unless it is included as part of a wellness package purchased by the employer (Moore 1988). A similar situation holds for the reimbursement of pharmacologic treatment to promote smoking cessation. Health insurers usually limit reimbursement of drug treatment to drugs that are approved by the Food and Drug Administration (FDA) and are prescribed for treatment of a diagnosed medical illness in a patient who has prescription drug coverage. Currently, nicotine polacrilex gum is the only drug approved by the FDA to aid in smoking cessation. Nevertheless, its prescription is usually not reimbursable for smokers who do not already carry a diagnosis of a smoking-related disease (Moore 1988).

Several barriers impede greater coverage of smoking cessation treatment by health insurers. Traditionally, health insurance has covered the cost of treating, not preventing, illness. A major reason for this was that insurers' were not convinced of the financial feasibility of covering preventive services, however socially desirable such a policy might be. Similarly, insurers have only gradually come to cover the costs of drug and alcohol treatment (American Hospital Association 1987). Smoking cessation programs might be classified as either preventive care or as treatment of substance abuse. Regardless of how it is classified, it appears that insurers are not convinced of the financial feasibility of covering smoking cessation treatment. In part, this stems from a lack of data with which to make appropriate calculations.

To be in the health insurers' economic interests, the cost of a treated smoker (the cost of cessation treatment in addition to other health claims) must be less than the claims paid to a smoker who does not attend a cessation program. This calculation requires the estimation of several factors that have not been well studied, including the difference in annual health care costs of current and former smokers, the costs and success rates of different smoking treatments, the likelihood that a smoker will quit without a program, the length of time that the smoker remains insured by the same insurer, and the discount rate at which future costs are evaluated. Furthermore, because health insurance is usually provided by employers, and employees change jobs, it is possible that the health insurer who pays for a policyholder's smoking cessation may not reap the benefits of any reduced health care costs that individual experiences.

Even if reimbursement for smoking cessation treatment were shown to be financially advantageous for insurers, practical problems would remain to slow the implementation of reimbursement. For example, insurers would have to define which programs, drugs, or other aids would be covered and which providers would be reimbursed.

Summary

The Public Health Service's 1990 Health Objectives for the Nation include two goals for smoking and insurance:

1. By 1985, the collection and publication by insurers of actuarial experience on differential life experience and hospital utilization by specific cause among smokers and nonsmokers, by sex;

2. By 1990, differential insurance premiums for smokers and nonsmokers by major life and health insurers (US DHHS 1981b, 1986d).

Progress has been made toward meeting both of these goals. The actuarial basis for life insurance premium differentials has been established, and data are beginning to be collected on hospitalization rates (US DHHS 1986d). However, more information on the total health care costs of smokers and nonsmokers, including ambulatory care, would help to establish a firmer rationale for offering premium discounts for health and disability insurance and for covering the costs of smoking cessation treatment. The second objective has been partially met. Although nearly all life insurers offer nonsmoker discounts, only a minority of health insurers do. This is partly because, unlike life insurance, most health insurance is sold to groups, which, as discussed above, presents greater operational obstacles to the development and implementation of nonsmoker discounts.

Much of the accomplishment to date is a result of the insurance industry's voluntary initiatives, which seem likely to continue (Walsh and Gordon 1986). Collection and publication of claims experience by industry groups such as the Society of Actuaries are steps that could be taken to increase the use of smoker–nonsmoker premium differentials in health and disability insurance. State and Federal governments have the opportunity to act as facilitators and educators to encourage insurers—especially health insurers—to offer premium discounts to nonsmokers and to reimburse for smoking cessation treatment. Government officials at both levels could act to remove those legal barriers that prevent insurers from adopting nonsmoker discounts and to disseminate research findings that support these discounts and coverage for smoking cessation. HMOs may be more likely to use smoking status as a factor in setting premiums if current Federal restrictions preventing it, except on a case-by-case basis, are removed.

Although the insurance industry is State regulated, regulation has generally been limited to ensuring the financial integrity of insurers. Some have suggested that a State-regulated industry could be subject to other controls in the public interest (Hiam 1987/88). Since the 1960s, all States have mandated certain types of coverage that insurers must provide as a condition of doing business in the State (Glantz 1985). State health insurance commissioners or legislatures could require smoker–nonsmoker premium differentials as a condition for writing policies within their States. In several States, bills have been filed that would mandate insurance premium differentials, although none have been enacted (CDC 1980, 1981). The few remaining life insurers without premium differentials might be encouraged to adopt them if the NAIC model rule regarding smoker–nonsmoker mortality tables were adopted by legislatures and insurance commissioners in the States that have not yet done so (NAIC 1985b).

Publicly funded health insurance such as medicare and medicaid is more directly amenable to government action. Measures have been introduced into Congress that would restructure medicare premiums to offer discounts to nonsmokers and to cover preventive care, including smoking cessation treatments (past bills include S. 357 and S. 358 in 1985). In the preface to the 1988 Surgeon General's Report (US DHHS 1988), the Surgeon General stated, "Treatment of tobacco addiction should be more widely available and should be considered at least as favorably by third-party payors as treatment of alcoholism and illicit drug addiction." Research to establish the cost-effectiveness of preventive care coverage by insurers, especially for smoking cessation, would be useful in reaching that goal.

PART III. DIRECT RESTRICTIONS ON SMOKING

The policies discussed so far discourage tobacco use indirectly, either by educating the public about the health hazards or by creating economic disincentives to smoke. A third category of public policies acts more directly; their aim is to reduce smoking by limiting either public access to tobacco products or the opportunity to use them. The most extreme potential policy in this category would be a total ban on the sale, possession, or use of tobacco products, analogous to current statutes on such other addictive drugs as heroin or cocaine. Short of that are policies that restrict or ban smoking in specific places, such as indoor public places and workplaces, prohibit the sale of tobacco products in particular places, or prohibit the use of tobacco by a particular group of individuals, namely minors.

Tobacco occupies a position unlike that of any other consumer product (or pharmaceutical agent) in the United States; it was widely used, socially accepted, and economically vital to strong agricultural and manufacturing interests long before its adverse health effects and addictive potential were appreciated. These facts have made the most stringent regulatory option—total ban on sale or use—impractical and undesirable. Such a policy did exist in some States in the early part of this century, when a moral crusade against cigarettes like that against alcohol led to the passage of laws in a dozen States banning the sale of tobacco products (Walsh and Gordon 1986). These laws proved difficult to enforce and were all repealed by 1927.

Although a total prohibition on tobacco is unlikely, there is a long tradition of restricting children's and adolescents' access to tobacco. According to established social convention, the rational use of certain products, like tobacco, alcohol, or the material sold in adult bookstores, requires an informed decision that minors are deemed to be too young to make. The growing awareness of the addictive nature of nicotine (US DHHS 1988) strengthens that convention in the case of tobacco products. Policies limiting smoking in public places or workplaces have a different rationale; they restrict the smoker's behavior for the sake of the nonsmoker. Although the primary aim of these policies is to protect the nonsmoker from the health consequences of involuntary tobacco smoke exposure, they may have the side effect of discouraging tobacco use by reducing opportunities to smoke and changing public attitudes about the social acceptability of smoking.

The direct restrictions discussed so far address the consumer (smoker or potential smoker). Policies directed at tobacco manufacturers include regulations on the contents of tobacco products to reduce their harmfulness. Such policies have the inherent difficulty of defining an acceptable level of tobacco or smoke exposure because, as documented in Chapter 2, there is no known safe level of tobacco use.

This Section considers three types of policies that put direct restrictions on smoking or tobacco products. First, it examines policies that restrict smoking in public places and workplaces, including both government actions and policies initiated in the private sector. Second, policies that would restrict minors' access to tobacco products are discussed. Finally, the Section considers the treatment of tobacco products by Federal regulatory agencies.

Government Actions to Restrict Smoking in Public Places and Workplaces

In 1986, the Surgeon General's Report documented "a wave of social action regulating tobacco smoking in public places" (US DHHS 1986b) that was then occurring. It reviewed public and private policies designed to protect individuals from environmental tobacco smoke (ETS) exposure by regulating the circumstances in which smoking is permitted. Since the 1986 Report, the pace of action appears to have increased in both the public and private sectors. Restrictions on smoking in public places are the result of government actions at the Federal, State, and local levels, particularly State and local legislation. The Federal Government has largely acted via regulatory mechanisms and has addressed smoking in Federal facilities and in public transportation. The major exception is recent congressional legislation restricting smoking on commercial airliners. Accompanying government actions are a wide range of private initiatives; these have become widespread in this decade. Smoking restrictions in the workplace are the most common private sector action, but hospitals, schools, hotels and motels, and other institutions are also adopting no-smoking policies. This trend reflects two forces: a growing scientific consensus about the health risks of involuntary smoking (US DHHS 1986b; NAS 1986b) and changing public attitudes about the social acceptability of smoking. As documented in Chapter 4, a growing majority of Americans now supports the right of nonsmokers to breathe smoke-free air and favors restricting smoking in public places and the workplace.

This Section addresses the scope and impact of government actions to restrict smoking in public places and workplaces. Private initiatives to regulate smoking are discussed in the subsequent section. Both sections summarize and update the findings of Chapter 6 of the 1986 Surgeon General's Report.

Smoking Restrictions in Public Places

A public place has usually been defined as any enclosed area to which the public is invited or in which the public is permitted (Americans for Nonsmokers' Rights (ANR) 1987a, b). This broad definition encompasses a diverse range of facilities that share the characteristic of being indoor enclosed spaces that permit the general public relatively free access. Beyond this general agreement, laws and regulations differ in their operational definition of public place. They even differ in the degree to which the concept is specified. Public place is commonly interpreted to include government buildings, banks, schools, health care facilities, public transportation vehicles and terminals, retail stores and service establishments, theaters, auditoriums, sports arenas, reception areas, and waiting rooms. Although they fit the definition, restaurants are usually treated separately in these laws. Private businesses are also separately addressed, and private homes specifically excluded.

As noted in the 1986 Surgeon General's Report, the degree to which smoking is restricted in public places also depends on history or tradition, the level of involuntary smoke exposure that is likely (determined by size, ventilation, and amount of smoking), the ease with which smokers and nonsmokers can be separated, and the degree of inconvenience that smoking restrictions pose to smokers. Public places may be owned by government or private interests. As a consequence of these factors and others, there is considerable variability in the methods by which new regulations have been proposed and the ease with which they have been adopted. Smoking restrictions have been most easily adopted in public facilities, especially facilities where smoking has traditionally been prohibited for safety reasons, where smoking is not associated with the activity taking place, and where the public spends limited time. Such considerations explain the relatively slower acceptance of smoking restrictions in restaurants, bars, and private businesses (US DHHS 1986b).

Federal Actions

Until recently, actions at the State and local Government level— primarily legislation—accounted for the bulk of smoking regulations in public places. Since 1986, the Federal Government has taken new steps, including the first congressional actions (covered below), to restrict smoking in two categories of public places: transportation facilities and Government worksites. The Federal Government has enacted no restrictions on smoking that apply to a broad range of nongovernmental public places.

State Legislation

Although the health hazards of smoking were not widely appreciated until the 1960s, the fire hazard was recognized much earlier, giving rise to the first State laws regulating smoking. For nearly a century cigarette smoking has been regulated by State law to prevent fires and prevent the contamination of food being prepared or packaged for public consumption. This was the extent of State law in 1964, when the first Surgeon General's Report was issued. At that time, 19 States prohibited smoking near explosives or fireworks, in or near mines, or near hazardous fire areas. Five States banned smoking in food processing factories or restaurant preparation areas (US DHHS 1986e; BNA 1987). These laws affected only a small proportion of the population and did not alter smoking in public places.

In addition, by 1964, 13 States had adopted some restrictions on smoking in specific public places. This legislation, also enacted to prevent fires, had some potential to reduce smoking in public places, even though that was not its primary intent. Six States permitted employers to ban smoking in mills and factories as long as signs were posted, and six States restricted smoking in public transportation vehicles or terminals or in auditoriums and theaters. The remaining laws sought to discourage smoking by children: three States prohibited smoking (at least by minors) on school grounds, buildings, or buses (US DHHS 1986b; BNA 1987). This remained the basic extent of smoking restrictions through the 1960s as the health hazards of smoking became widely known.

In the 1970s, a new form of smoking legislation emerged, differing in both intent and content. The specific rationale behind this legislation was the safety and comfort of nonsmokers, reflecting growing interest and, later, scientific evidence of the health hazards of passive smoke exposure (US DHHS 1986b; BNA 1987). These Clean Indoor Air Acts regulated smoking in a larger number of places and for the first time mandated smoking restrictions in private facilities. Over time, the language of the laws became more restrictive, first permitting, then requiring nonsmoking sections, then making nonsmoking the principal condition, with an option for smoking areas. The legislation was developed and promoted by the growing nonsmokers' rights movement, for the most part a grassroots movement consisting of Californians for Nonsmokers' Rights (later changed to Americans for Nonsmokers' Rights) and a number of other State and local groups, many using the name Group Against Smoking Pollution (GASP). These organizations focused their attention on achieving legislative goals at the State and local levels (see Chapter 6). In doing so, they sometimes worked in conjunction with the voluntary health organizations.

The prevalence and content of State legislation on smoking changed dramatically over the ensuing two decades (Figure 6). Current smoking restrictions in public places are largely the product of legislation enacted at the State level beginning in the early 1970s (Tables 18 and 19). Between 1970 and 1979, smoking restrictions were enacted by legislatures in 24 additional States; in 7 others, existing restrictions were extended. In 1975 alone, 13 States enacted laws, more than double the number that had done so in the previous decade (1964–74).

Not only the quantity but also the content of these laws was different. In 1973, Arizona became the first State to restrict smoking in a number of public places, and the first to do so explicitly because smoking was a public health hazard. Although not comprehensive by current standards, the law was regarded as comprehensive when passed. The first State law to include smoking restrictions in restaurants was passed in Connecticut in 1974. Coverage of worksite smoking also began at this time with the landmark Minnesota Clean Indoor Air Act. Passed in 1975, it extended smoking restrictions to many public places, restaurants, and both public and private worksites. It became the model for other comprehensive State legislation that began to be passed in the mid-1970s.

After a relative lull in the early 1980s, there was another notable increase in passage of State laws in the middle of the decade, probably reflecting greater scientific consensus about the health consequences of involuntary smoking. By the end of 1985, 41 States and the District of Columbia had passed laws regulating smoking in at least one public place (US DHHS 1986b). In 1987, the year after two national groups separately reviewed the evidence on passive smoking and reached similar conclusions about its health effects (US DHHS 1986b; NRC 1986b), 20 States passed legislation regulating smoking, more than ever before in a single year. Moreover, the legislation being passed grew more comprehensive in its coverage. From the start of 1985 to the end of the 1987 legislative sessions, there was a doubling in the number of States restricting smoking

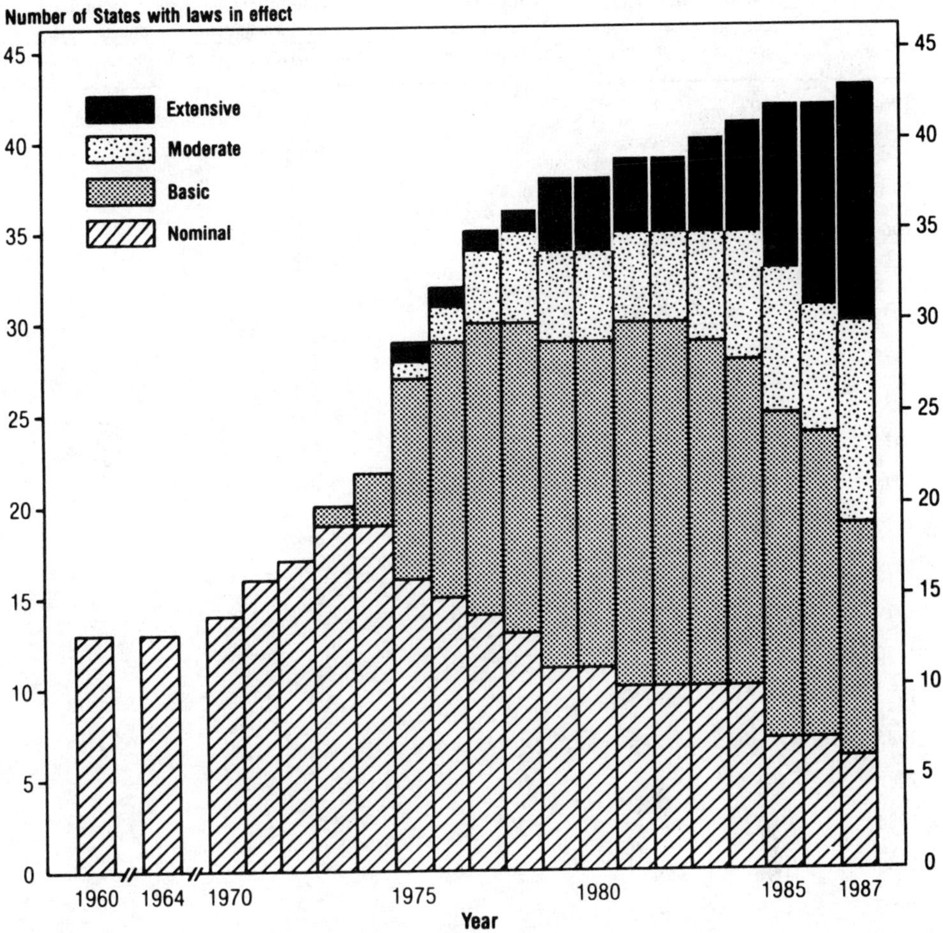

FIGURE 6.—Prevalence and restrictiveness of State laws regulating smoking in public places, 1960–1987

NOTE: Index of restrictiveness: 0 = none, no statewide restrictions; 0.25 = nominal, State regulates smoking in one to three public places, excluding restaurants and private worksites; 0.50 = basic, State regulates smoking in four or more public places, excluding restaurants and private worksites; 0.75 = moderate, State regulates smoking in restaurants but not private worksites; 1.00 = extensive, State regulates smoking in private worksites.

SOURCE: US DHHS (1986b); unpublished data, OSH.

TABLE 18.—State laws restricting smoking, 1964–87

Year	Number of States enacting laws	Cumulative number of States with laws	Number of States restricting smoking in restaurants Enacting/cumulative		Number of States restricting smoking in private worksites Enacting/cumulative		Number of States restricting smoking in public worksites Enacting/cumulative	
1964	0	13						
1965–66	0	13						
1967–68	2	14						
1969–70	0	14						
1971	2	16						
1972	1	17						
1973	3	20						
1974	3	22	1	1				
1975	13	29	2	3	1	1	4	4
1976	5	32	3	6	1	2	1	5
1977	6	35	2	7	0	2	3	8
1978	2	36	1	8	0	2	1	9
1979	6	38	2	10	2	4	2	11
1980	1	38	0	10	0	4	0	11
1981	7	39	1	11	0	4	3	13
1982	1	39	0	11	0	4	0	13
1983	4	40	1	12	1	5	2	15
1984	3	41	1	12	0	5	2	15
1985	9	42	4	16	4	9	5	20
1986	6	42	1	16	3	11	4	22
1987	20	43 (84%[a])	10	23 (45%)	4	13 (25%)	15	31 (61%)

NOTE: Includes the District of Columbia.
[a]Percentage of total States.
SOURCE: BNA (1987); US DHHS (1986b); individual State laws.

in private workplaces (from 4 to 13), public workplaces (15 to 31), and restaurants (10 to 23) (Table 18).

Recently adopted laws are more likely to include three provisions that strengthen the position of nonsmokers: (1) protection against discrimination for supporters of worksite smoking policies, (2) priority to the wishes of nonsmokers in any disagreement about the designation of an area as smoking or nonsmoking, and (3) permission for cities and counties to enact more stringent ordinances. In 1985, Maine was the first of five States to adopt a nondiscrimination provision, which makes it illegal for employers to discipline, discharge, or otherwise discriminate against employees who assist in the implementation of nonsmoking policies (BNA 1987). The second provision first appeared

TABLE 19.—State laws regulating smoking in public places and worksites, through October 1, 1988

	AL	AK	AZ	AR	CA	CO	CT
YEAR(S) LEGISLATION ENACTED		1975 1984	1973, 81 1986, 87	1977 1985, 87	1971, 76 1980, 81 1982, 87[a]	1977 1985[a]	1973, 74 1983, 87
PUBLIC PLACES WHERE SMOKING IS RESTRICTED							
Public transportation[b]		X	X	X	X[c]	X	X
Elevators		X[c]	X			X	X[c]
Indoor cultural or recreational facilities		X	X		X	X	
Retail stores[d]		X			X		X
Restaurants[e]		X			X	X	X
Schools		X	X	X	X	X	X
Hospitals		X	X	X	X	X	X
Nursing homes		X	X		X		X
Government buildings		X	X		X	X	X
Public meeting rooms		X			X		X
Libraries		X					
Other[f]		X	X	X			
WORKSITE SMOKING RESTRICTIONS[g h]							
Public worksites		D	B,D	B,D	B	C,D[a]	C
Private worksites		A					C
IMPLEMENTATION PROVISIONS							
Nonsmokers prevail in disputes			X				
No discrimination against nonsmokers			X				
ENFORCEMENT (PENALTIES)							
Against smokers[i]		X	X	X	X		X
For failure to post signs[j]		X					X
LOCAL ORDINANCES							
Specifically allowed					X	X	
Specifically preempted							
OVERALL RESTRICTIVENESS OF STATE LAW[k]	0	3	2	2	3	2	4

TABLE 19.—Continued

	DE	DC	FL	GA	HI	ID	IL
YEAR(S) LEGISLATION ENACTED	1960	1975, 79 1988	1974, 83 1985	1975	1976, 87	1975, 85	
PUBLIC PLACES WHERE SMOKING IS RESTRICTED							
Public transportation[b]	X	X	X[c]	X[c]		X	
Elevators		X	X[c]	X[c]	X	X	
Indoor cultural or recreational facilities			X		X	X	
Retail stores[d]		X	X		X	X	
Restaurants[e]		X	X		X	X	
Schools		X	X			X	
Hospitals		X	X		X	X	
Nursing homes		X	X		X	X	
Government buildings		X	X			X	
Public meeting rooms		X	X		X	X	
Libraries			X		X		
Other[f]			X				
WORKSITE SMOKING RESTRICTIONS[g h]							
Public worksites			B,D		B,D	D	
Private worksites			B,D				
IMPLEMENTATION PROVISIONS							
Nonsmokers prevail in disputes							
No discrimination against nonsmokers							
ENFORCEMENT (PENALTIES)							
Against smokers[i]	X	X	X	X	X	X	
For failure to post signs[j]		X	X		X		
LOCAL ORDINANCES							
Specifically allowed					X		
Specifically preempted			X				
OVERALL RESTRICTIVENESS OF STATE LAW[k]	1	3	4	1	3	3	0

TABLE 19.—Continued

	IN	IA	KS	KY	LA	ME	MD
YEAR(S) LEGISLATION ENACTED	1987	1978, 87	1975, 87 1988	1972		1954, 81 1983, 85 1987, 88	1957, 75 1987[a] 1988
PUBLIC PLACES WHERE SMOKING IS RESTRICTED							
Public transportation[b]		X	X[c]				X
Elevators		X	X[c]				X
Indoor cultural or recreational facilities		X	X			X	
Retail stores[d]		X	X			X	X
Restaurants[e]		X	X			X	
Schools	X	X	X	X		X	
Hospitals	X	X	X			X	X
Nursing homes	X	X	X			X	X
Government buildings	X	X	X			X	X[a]
Public meeting rooms	X	X	X			X	
Libraries	X	X	X				
Other[f]						X	
WORKSITE SMOKING RESTRICTIONS[g h]							
Public worksites	C,D	D	C,D			B,D	B[a]
Private worksites		D				B,D	
IMPLEMENTATION PROVISIONS							
Nonsmokers prevail in disputes							X
No discrimination against nonsmokers						X	
ENFORCEMENT (PENALTIES)							
Against smokers[i]	X	X	X	X		X	X
For failure to post signs[j]		X	X			X	
LOCAL ORDINANCES							
Specifically allowed	X		X				
Specifically preempted							
OVERALL RESTRICTIVENESS OF STATE LAW[k]	2	4	3	1	0	4	2

TABLE 19.—Continued

	MA	MI	MN	MS	MO	MT	NE
YEAR(S) LEGISLATION ENACTED	1947, 75 1987, 88	1967, 68 1978, 81 1986, 87 1988	1971, 75 1987	1942		1979	1979 1986
PUBLIC PLACES WHERE SMOKING IS RESTRICTED							
Public transportation[b]	X[c]	X	X	X		X	X
Elevators	X[c]	X	X			X[c]	X
Indoor cultural or recreational facilities	X	X	X			X	X
Retail stores[d]	X	X	X			X	X
Restaurants[e]	X	X	X			X	X
Schools	X	X	X			X	
Hospitals	X	X	X			X	X
Nursing homes	X	X	X			X	X
Government buildings	X	X	X			X	X
Public meeting rooms	X	X	X			X	X
Libraries	X		X				X
Other[f]	X	X	X				
WORKSITE SMOKING RESTRICTIONS[g h]							
Public worksites	C,D[a]	D	C,D			D	D
Private worksites			C,D			D	D
IMPLEMENTATION PROVISIONS							
Nonsmokers prevail in disputes			X				X
No discrimination against nonsmokers							
ENFORCEMENT (PENALTIES)							
Against smokers[i]	X	X	X	X			X
For failure to post signs[j]		X				X	
LOCAL ORDINANCES							
Specifically allowed							
Specifically preempted							
OVERALL RESTRICTIVENESS OF STATE LAW[k]	3	3	4	1	0	4	4

TABLE 19.—Continued

	NV	NH	NJ	NM	NY	NC	ND
YEAR(S) LEGISLATION ENACTED	1911, 75 1979 1987	1981 1986 1987	1953 1979 1985	1985	1921, 53 1975 1976		1977 1987
PUBLIC PLACES WHERE SMOKING IS RESTRICTED							
Public transportation[b]	X	X	X		X		X
Elevators	X	X	X	X			X
Indoor cultural or recreational facilities	X	X	X		X		X
Retail stores[d]	X	X	X				
Restaurants[e]	X	X	X				X
Schools	X	X	X				X
Hospitals	X	X	X				X
Nursing homes	X	X	X				X
Government buildings	X	X	X	X			X
Public meeting rooms	X	X	X	X			X
Libraries	X	X	X	X	X		X
Other[f]	X	X			X		
WORKSITE SMOKING RESTRICTIONS[g h]							
Public worksites		D	B,C	C,D			C,D
Private worksites	A	B	B,C		A		
IMPLEMENTATION PROVISIONS							
Nonsmokers prevail in disputes			X				
No discrimination against nonsmokers							
ENFORCEMENT (PENALTIES)							
Against smokers[i]	X	X	X	X	X		X
For failure to post signs[j]		X	X				X
LOCAL ORDINANCES							
Specifically allowed							
Specifically preempted			X				
OVERALL RESTRICTIVENESS OF STATE LAW[k]	3	4	4	2	2	0	3

TABLE 19.—Continued

	OH	OK	OR	PA	RI	SC	SD
YEAR(S) LEGISLATION ENACTED	1953, 81 1981, 84 1988	1975 1987	1973, 75 1977 1981	1927 1947 1977	1976 1977 1986	1937	1974 1987
PUBLIC PLACES WHERE SMOKING IS RESTRICTED							
Public transportation[b]	X	X	X[a]		X	X	X
Elevators	X	X	X		X		X
Indoor cultural or recreational facilities	X	X	X	X	X		X
Retail stores[d]			X	X	X		
Restaurants[e]		X	X		X		
Schools	X	X	X		X		X
Hospitals	X	X	X	X	X		X
Nursing homes	X	X	X	X	X		X
Government buildings	X	X	X		X		
Public meeting rooms	X	X	X				
Libraries		X			X		X
Other[f]	X		X		X		X
WORKSITE SMOKING RESTRICTIONS[g h]							
Public worksites	D	C,D	D		B		
Private worksites					B		
IMPLEMENTATION PROVISIONS							
Nonsmokers prevail in disputes		X			X		
No discrimination against nonsmokers					X		
ENFORCEMENT (PENALTIES)							
Against smokers[i]	X	X	X	X	X		X
For failure to post signs[j]			X		X		
LOCAL ORDINANCES							
Specifically allowed							
Specifically preempted		X					
OVERALL RESTRICTIVENESS OF STATE LAW[k]	2	3	3	2	4	1	2

TABLE 19.—Continued

	TN	TX	UT	VT	VA	WA	WV
YEAR(S) LEGISLATION ENACTED		1975 1987	1976 1979 1986	1892 1987		1984 1985	1913 1919 1985
PUBLIC PLACES WHERE SMOKING IS RESTRICTED							
Public transportation[b]		X	X			X[c]	X
Elevators		X	X	X[c]		X[c]	
Indoor cultural or recreational facilities		X	X			X[c]	
Retail stores[d]			X			X[c]	
Restaurants[e]			X			X	
Schools		X	X			X[c]	X
Hospitals		X	X			X	
Nursing homes		X	X	X		X	
Government buildings			X			X	
Public meeting rooms		X	X	X[c]		X[c]	
Libraries			X			X	
Other[f]				X			X
WORKSITE SMOKING RESTRICTIONS[g h]							
Public worksites			D	B,D		D	
Private worksites			D	B,D		D	A
IMPLEMENTATION PROVISIONS							
Nonsmokers prevail in disputes			X				
No discrimination against nonsmokers			X	X			
ENFORCEMENT (PENALTIES)							
Against smokers[i]		X	X	X		X	X
For failure to post signs[j]				X		X	
LOCAL ORDINANCES							
Specifically allowed			X				
Specifically preempted							
OVERALL RESTRICTIVENESS OF STATE LAW[k]	0	2	4	4	0	4	1

TABLE 19.—Continued

	WI	WY	TOTAL STATES N	TOTAL STATES %
YEAR(S) LEGISLATION ENACTED	1983			
PUBLIC PLACES WHERE SMOKING IS RESTRICTED				
Public transportation[b]	X		36	70.6
Elevators	X		32	62.7
Indoor cultural or recreational facilities	X		30	58.8
Retail stores[d]	X		25	49.0
Restaurants[e]	X		24	47.1
Schools	X		32	62.7
Hospitals	X		34	66.7
Nursing homes	X		32	62.7
Government buildings	X		31	60.8
Public meeting rooms			27	52.9
Libraries			21	41.1
Other[f]				
WORKSITE SMOKING RESTRICTIONS[g h]				
Public worksites	D		31	60.8
Private worksites			13	25.5
IMPLEMENTATION PROVISIONS				
Nonsmokers prevail in disputes			8	15.7
No discrimination against nonsmokers			5	9.8
ENFORCEMENT (PENALTIES)				
Against smokers[i]	X		40	78.4
For failure to post signs[j]			17	33.3
TOTAL			41	80.4
LOCAL ORDINANCES				
Specifically allowed	X		7	13.7
Specifically preempted			3	5.9
OVERALL RESTRICTIVENESS OF STATE LAW[k]	3	0		

TABLE 19.—Continued

NOTE: Laws cited do not include restrictions on smoking near explosives, fireworks, or hazardous areas; in or near mines; or in food preparation or handling areas of restaurants or food processing factories.

[a]Executive order.

[b]In school buses only in AR, FL, and SC. Smoking is prohibited on all forms of intrastate transportation in CA.

[c]Smoking is never permitted in this area.

[d]Proprietors of retail stores in CO are encouraged to establish no-smoking areas. Smoking is prohibited only in grocery stores in AK, CA, CT, MA, NV, and RI.

[e]Proprietors of restaurants in NJ and CO are encouraged to establish no-smoking areas. In AK, FL, HI, MI, NH, OK, RI, and WI, restaurants seating 50 or more persons must have a no-smoking section. In CA, restaurants in a publicly owned building seating 50 or more must have a no-smoking section. In CT and MA, restaurants seating 75 or more must have a no-smoking section.

[f]Smoking is restricted in jury rooms in AK, FL, ME, MA, MI, MN, OR, and SD; in day-care centers in AK, AZ, AR, MA, and MN; in mills, factories, barns, or stables in ME, MA, NV, RI, VT, and WV; in polling places in NH and NY; in prisons, at the prison officials' discretion, in FL and PA; and in the asbestos hazard abatement project in OH.

[g]A, employer must post a sign where smoking is prohibited; B, employer must have a written smoking policy; C, employer must have a policy that provides for a nonsmoking area; D, no smoking except in designated areas. Only B, C, and D count as having a worksite policy in calculation of totals.

[h]Employers must post signs designating smoking and no-smoking areas in AK, MI, MN, NE, NJ, and UT public worksites, and in MN, NE, NJ, and UT private worksites; in smoking areas only in FL, ND, and WI public worksites; and in no-smoking areas in NH and NM public worksites. Depending upon their policy, employers must post either smoking or no-smoking signs in MT public and private worksites. Smoking is not restricted in factories, warehouses, and similar worksites not usually frequented by the public in MN and NE. Smoking is prohibited in any mill or factory in which a no-smoking sign is posted in NV, NY, VT, and WV.

[i]Persons who smoke in a prohibited area are subject to the following maximum fines: $5, AK, KY, VT; $10, IA, OR, PA; $20–25, CT, DE, HI, KS, NM, WI; $50, ID, ME, NH; $100, AR, CA, DC, GA, NE, NV, NY, ND, OK, RI, WV; $100 per day, WA; $200, NJ; $300, MD; $500, FL, MI; $50 or up to 10 days jail or both, MA; minor misdemeanor, OH; petty misdemeanor, MN; misdemeanor, MS, TX; petty offense, AZ, SD; infraction, IN, UT.

[j]Persons who are required to and fail to post smoking and/or no-smoking signs are subject to the following maximum fines: $10, IA; $20–25, MT; $50, KS, NH; $100, ME, ND, OR, VT; $200, NJ; $300, AK, DC; $500, FL, MI; $500 per day, HI, RI; civil action, WA; infraction, CT.

[k]Restrictiveness key: 0, none (no statewide restrictions); 1, nominal (State regulates smoking in 1–3 public places, excluding restaurants and private worksites); 2, basic (State regulates smoking in 4 or more public places, excluding restaurants and private worksites); 3, moderate (State regulates smoking in restaurants but not private worksites); 4, extensive (State regulates smoking in private worksites).

SOURCE: BNA (1987); Tobacco-Free America Project 1987, 1988a, b; US DHHS (1986b); individual State laws.

in the Minnesota Clean Indoor Act (1975) and is incorporated into statutory language in six other States. Seven States include the third provision, which specifically permits local governments to enact ordinances more stringent than the State law (BNA 1987). Conversely, following intense legislative debate that included heavy lobbying by the tobacco industry, Florida (1985) enacted a State law that preempted more stringent local laws, as have Oklahoma (1987) and New Jersey (BNA 1987). Similar legislation has been proposed in other States.

By the end of 1987, smoking was restricted in at least 1 public place in 42 States and the District of Columbia. Table 19 summarizes the provisions of these laws, which most often restrict smoking in public transportation facilities (36 States), hospitals (34 States), schools (32 States), elevators (32 States), government buildings (31 States), and recreational facilities (30 States). As of January 1988, over 82 percent of the United States population resided in States that restricted smoking in at least one public place; this compares with a previous estimate of 8 percent in 1971 (US DHHS 1986b). Over

17 percent of Americans lived in States with laws requiring smoking restrictions at the worksite for nongovernment workers, whereas over half lived in States with such restrictions for State government employees. More than 40 percent of Americans live in States requiring no-smoking areas in restaurants, and two-thirds live in States that limit smoking in health care facilities.

The 1986 Surgeon General's Report documented geographical variation in State smoking laws. Southern States had fewer and less comprehensive laws. This remains true (Table 20). Excluding the major tobacco-producing States (North Carolina, Kentucky, South Carolina, Virginia, Tennessee, and Georgia), over 80 percent of States in each region, including the South, have enacted smoking restrictions. Of the major tobacco-growing States, only Georgia, which ranked sixth in production, had enacted restrictions on smoking in any public places other than school facilities or vehicles.

State laws also vary in their implementation and enforcement provisions. Health departments are responsible for policy implementation in most States (US DHHS 1986b). Nearly all States with laws (40 of 43) provide penalties for smokers who violate restrictions (Table 19). Seventeen States also have penalties for employers and proprietors who do not establish nonsmoking policies or post signs as required (BNA 1987). It is not known how often these penalties are actually imposed.

Local Legislation

As noted in the 1986 Report, efforts to pass Clean Indoor Air Laws spread from the State to the local level in the 1980s, spearheaded by actions in California (US DHHS 1986b). Local ordinances generally extend the scope of smoking restrictions beyond that provided for in corresponding State laws. Usually they include provisions to restrict or ban smoking in restaurants and public and private worksites, in addition to a broad range of public places. An accurate record of local ordinances nationwide is difficult to obtain because there is no single reference library for local legislation. Recently, two organizations have monitored local no-smoking ordinances on a nationwide basis. Their data indicate that local ordinances are being enacted at a rapid pace. As of August 1988, ANR (1988b) identified 321 local ordinances with provisions for significant nonsmoker protection. The Tobacco-Free America Project (1988c) reported in October 1988 that 380 local communities had passed laws restricting smoking in public places. These numbers represent a nearly fourfold increase in the estimate of 89 communities with smoking ordinances in 1986 (US DHHS 1986b).

The most complete information on the prevalence and content of local ordinances is available for California, where ANR has kept an ongoing compilation of laws (ANR 1988a). According to their records, the first local ordinances were passed in 1979. In 1982, San Diego became the first large California city to enact a workplace ordinance. Although not the first local action to include the private workplace, the passage of San Francisco's worksite smoking ordinance in 1983, in the face of heavily subsidized tobacco industry opposition, attracted widespread publicity and stimulated further action (US DHHS 1986b). The following year, Los Angeles passed a law requiring smoking policies in workplaces with five or more employees (ANR 1988a).

TABLE 20.—Regional variation in restrictiveness of State laws limiting smoking

Region[a]	Total States	Mean restrictiveness[b] in October 1988	States with laws[c] N	(%)	Mean restrictiveness[b] of laws in effect October 1988	States with different degrees of restrictiveness[b] 1.00	0.75	0.50	0.25	0.00
Northeast	9	.861	9	(100)	.861	6	1	2	0	0
Midwest	12	.625	10	(83)	.750	3	4	3	0	2
West	13	.692	12	(92)	.750	3	6	3	0	1
South	17	.324	12	(71)	.458	1	2	3	6	5
Major tobacco producer	6	.125	3	(50)	.250	0	0	0	3	3
Other	11	.432	9	(82)	.528	1	2	3	3	2
Total	51	.583	43	(84)	.692	13	13	11	6	8

[a]Regions are defined by the Bureau of the Census
Northeast: CT, MA, ME, NH, NJ, NY, PA, RI, VT
Midwest: IA, IL, IN, KS, MI, MN, MO, ND, NE,OH, SD, WI
West: AK, AZ, CA, CO, HI, ID, MT, NM, NV, OR, UT, WA, WY
South: AL, AR, DC, DE, FL, GA, KY, LA, MD, MS, NC, OK, SC, TN, TX, VA, WV
Major tobacco producers: GA, KY, NC, SC, TN, VA
[b]Index of restrictiveness (from US DHHS 1986b):
0.00 = None; no statewide restrictions.
0.25 = Nominal; State regulates smoking in one to three public places, excluding restaurants and private worksites.
0.50 = Basic; State regulates smoking in four or more public places, excluding restaurants and private worksites.
0.75 = Moderate; State regulates smoking in restaurants, but not private worksites.
1.00 = Extensive; State regulates smoking in private worksites.
[c]Difference in prevalence of laws, South versus all other: chi square (using Yates correction)=13.40, $p<0.005$.
SOURCE: BNA (1987), US DHHS (1986b), individual State laws.

As a result of this early action, California holds the distinction of having more cities, towns, and counties restricting smoking than any other State. As of April 1988, 125 California cities, towns, and counties had significant nonsmoker protection laws, including all California cities with populations greater than 250,000 and more than one-third of all other communities with populations greater than 25,000 (ANR 1988a). Smoking was restricted in private worksites in 117 California communities; these laws applied to nearly 15 million citizens, more than 55 percent of the State's population. Restaurant nonsmoking sections are required in 118 California communities.

A stringent restaurant law was passed in Beverly Hills in April 1987. It banned all smoking in restaurants except those in hotels or bars. Amid enforcement problems and restaurateurs' reports of losing business to neighboring communities with less stringent laws, the city subsequently amended the ordinance to permit smoking areas in restaurants with air filtration systems, as long as nonsmoking sections are at least 50 percent of seating capacity (ANR 1988a; Malnic 1988; New York Times 1987). This remains the only widely known example of a State or local ordinance that has been revised to become less stringent.

A total ban on smoking in restaurants has been adopted successfully by one city, Aspen, CO. In September 1985, Aspen passed a Clean Indoor Air Act that contained an even more stringent restaurant provision: a ban on smoking in all restaurants (Aspen 1985). Six months after the law passed, a survey of 30 restaurants revealed that 87 percent of managers favored the law; 77 percent reported no effect of the ordinance on their business, 10 percent said they lost business, and 13 percent were uncertain of the effect (Dunlop 1986).

Outside California, Massachusetts has the largest number of local smoking ordinances. As of June 1988, 56 cities and towns restricted smoking in restaurants and 9 communities restricted smoking in private workplaces. Since 1984, Massachusetts communities have been passing restaurant laws at the rate of over 10 per year, and there has been an increase in the minimum required size of nonsmoking sections (GASP 1988a,b).

Communities in more than 20 other States restrict smoking, including 6 of the 8 States without statewide restrictions. Two of the major tobacco-producing States, Virginia and South Carolina, each have several counties that restrict smoking. In Virginia, which has no statewide restrictions, Arlington, Fairfax, and Prince William Counties, as well as the city of Norfolk, restrict smoking in restaurants and other public places. In South Carolina, which has statewide limits only for school buses, smoking is restricted in government buildings in five counties. In 1987, the city of Greenville became the first in South Carolina to restrict smoking in private worksites and restaurants (Tobacco-Free Young America Project 1987).

Other States with several communities regulating smoking in public places or worksites are Texas, Colorado, Maryland, Ohio, Arizona, and New York. Among the major cities not already cited that restrict smoking in private worksites and various public places are New York, NY; Cleveland OH; Denver, CO; Kansas City, MO; Phoenix and Tucson, AZ; Pittsburgh, PA; Austin, Dallas, El Paso, and Houston, TX; and Seattle, WA (ANR 1988b).

The city ordinance affecting the largest number of people is the Clean Indoor Air Act that took effect in New York City on April 6, 1988. It applies to over 7 million people, almost 3 percent of the United States population, and bans or restricts smoking in a wide variety of public places. Restaurants seating more than 50 persons must designate at least half of their seating as nonsmoking, and employers with more than 15 employees must maintain a written smoking policy and provide, "to the extent reasonably practicable, smoke-free work areas for nonsmoking employees who sit in common work areas." Smoking is also prohibited in hallways, restrooms, and other shared areas at work (New York City Department of Health 1988).

Smoking Restrictions in Public Transportation Facilities

Buses and Trains

For interstate public transportation, prior Federal regulatory actions have been accompanied by more recent congressional legislation. In the 1970s, the Interstate Commerce Commission (ICC) and the Civil Aeronautics Board (CAB) issued smoking restrictions for buses and airliners, respectively. In 1971, the ICC issued regulations requiring that smoking on buses traveling interstate routes be confined to designated smoking sections. Upheld in a 1973 court case and amended in 1976, the current regulations require smoking sections to be at the rear of buses and to consist of no more than 30 percent of total seating capacity (49 CFR 1061, 1987). In 1971, the ICC also required that smoking on trains traveling on interstate routes be confined to designated areas (Public Law 91-518; 49 CFR 1124.1). The legislation mandating these regulations for trains was repealed in 1979.

More recently, congressional legislation passed in 1987 led indirectly to a ban on smoking on commuter rail lines serving New York City. The law would have withheld Federal funds to the New York Metropolitan Transportation Authority unless smoking was banned on the Long Island Railroad (LIRR) (101 Stat. 1329–382, 1987). In response, the Authority banned smoking, effective February 15, 1988, on all LIRR and Metro-North Commuter Railroad trains. The action affected 452,000 daily riders of these commuter lines, which connect New York City with Long Island and Westchester County, NY, and Connecticut. Railroad officials had previously favored a ban, but the Authority's board had rejected a total ban until the threatened loss of an estimated 539 million dollars in Federal funds (Schmitt 1988).

Commercial Airlines

Smoking on commercial airline flights has been the subject of longstanding Federal regulation and more recent congressional legislation. The CAB promulgated its first regulations in 1971 (14 CFR Part 252.2). These required that all commercial airline flights provide nonsmoking sections large enough to accommodate every passenger who desired to sit in them. In 1983, the CAB issued new regulations that banned smoking on flights of 2 hr or less; however, the CAB reversed its decision almost immediately, allegedly in response to outside pressure (Walsh and Gordon 1986).

Public pressure for a smoking ban on commercial airline flights continued to mount, however. In 1986, the National Academy of Sciences appointed a Committee on Airliner Cabin Air Quality to examine the issues. Their report recommended a ban on smoking on all commercial domestic airline flights, for several reasons: to increase the comfort of passengers and crew, to reduce potential health hazards of involuntary smoke exposure for the crew, to decrease the risk of fire caused by cigarettes, and to bring cabin air quality into line with established standards for indoor environments (NRC 1986a). That same year, the Adult Use of Tobacco Survey, which interviewed over 13,000 adults, found that nonsmoking sections were preferred by 82 percent of nonsmokers, 69 percent of former smokers, and even 14 percent of current smokers (CDC 1988).

In response to this evidence and growing pressure by the voluntary health organizations and nonsmokers' rights groups, Congress passed legislation in 1987 prohibiting smoking on all regularly scheduled commercial flights with scheduled flight times of 2 hr or less (Public Law 100-202). This includes approximately 80 percent of all domestic flights. The ban also prohibited tampering with aircraft smoke detection devices and authorized fines of up to 2,000 dollars for violations. The law, which became effective on April 23, 1988, will expire in 1990 in the absence of further congressional action (101 Stat. 1329–382, 1987).

Recent legislation in California and Canada has created more comprehensive smoking restrictions on a wider range of transportation vehicles. As of January 1, 1988, California banned smoking on all intrastate commercial airplane, train, and bus trips. Several carriers, including Amtrak, American Airlines, and Alaska Airlines, ignored the law on the grounds that their operations are regulated by Federal rather than State laws (Washington Post 1988). However, when both airlines complied with the Federal inflight smoking ban in April 1988, they effectively complied with the California law. In June 1988, the Canadian Parliament acted to ban smoking on flights less than 2 hr. The law also limits smoking on federally regulated ships, trains, and buses to designated areas separated from the main seating (Burns 1988).

Opinion surveys document support for greater restrictions on smoking in airliners (see Chapter 4). In a survey of more than 33,000 airline passengers in 39 States and 89 airports, conducted by the American Association for Respiratory Care prior to the passage of congressional legislation, 64 percent supported a total ban on smoking in flight, including 74 percent of nonsmokers and 30 percent of smokers (Milligan 1987). In another survey, California's smoking ban on intrastate flights was supported by 85 percent of 614 passengers and 94 percent of 63 airline flight crew surveyed at San Francisco's airport (Journal of the American Medical Association 1988b).

Less is known about smoking restrictions in airports. Preliminary data from a survey by the Airport Operators Council International (AOCI) of its 180 U.S. members showed that 50 of 59 respondents had smoking restrictions of some type (AOCI 1988; Yenckel 1988). However, after the institution of the congressionally mandated ban during flights of 2 hr or less, there were anecdotal reports of increased smoking in airports, as smokers appeared to compensate for on-board restrictions (Yenckel 1988).

Smoking Restrictions in the Workplace

Government Worksites

Federal, State, and local governments have used a combination of regulatory and legislative means to address the smoking in their own facilities. As a result of recent Federal regulations, most Federal workers are covered by policies that restrict but do not ban smoking in the workplace. In 1986, the General Services Administration (GSA), which is responsible for one-third of all Federal buildings and provides office space for 890,000 Federal employees, revised its 1973 smoking policy. The current regulations, which became effective on February 6, 1987, prohibit smoking except in designated areas, specify areas where smoking is to be banned and where it may be permitted, but do not require that all working areas be smoke free. The intent of these regulations was to provide a reasonably smoke-free environment for workers and visitors in GSA-controlled buildings. Smoking is prohibited in auditoriums, classrooms, conference rooms, elevators, medical care facilities, libraries, and hazardous areas. Smoking is banned in general office spaces unless they are designated for smoking and configured to protect nonsmokers from involuntary exposure to smoke. The regulations do not specify how to determine if nonsmokers are protected from exposure to ETS in cases where smoking areas are designated. Corridors, lobbies, restrooms, and stairways are also nonsmoking areas unless designated otherwise (41 CFR 101–20, 1987; GSA 1986).

In consultation with employees, agency heads have the authority to decide which areas are designated nonsmoking or smoking as well as to establish more stringent guidelines (GSA 1986). Response by the various executive departments has varied. DHHS has adopted the most stringent requirements: a complete ban in all Department buildings effective February 25, 1988. Previously, the Indian Health Service had banned smoking within its 45 hospitals (CDC 1987b). Other departments have permitted sections of food service facilities, restrooms, or corridors to become designated smoking areas (BNA 1987).

The second major Federal regulatory effort addressed smoking by Armed Forces personnel. DOD previously had a worksite smoking policy, dating from 1977, which prohibited smoking in auditoriums, conference rooms, and classrooms and required nonsmoking areas in all cafeterias. In March 1986, DOD established a new policy that was a component of the antismoking portion of the DOD comprehensive health promotion and education program (US DOD 1986a; Chapter 6). Its purpose was to create an environment that discouraged tobacco use. Although each of the military services has adopted branch-specific regulations, the departmentwide policy stipulates that smoking is prohibited in auditoriums, conference rooms, classrooms, elevators, buses, and vans. Smoking is not permitted in common work areas shared by smokers and nonsmokers unless adequate space is available for nonsmokers and ventilation is adequate to provide them with a healthy environment. Smoking is permitted only in designated sections of those common work areas, as in restricted sections of eating facilities, medical facilities, and schools (US DOD 1986a). The DOD policy covers nearly 2.2 million military and 1.2 million civilian personnel worldwide (US DOD 1986b).

Servicewide surveys taken in 1987 suggest that the DOD antismoking campaign is affecting smoking behavior. Between 1985 and 1987, the smoking prevalence in the Army dropped from 52 to 41 percent, in the Navy from 49 to 44 percent, and in the Air Force from 39 to 31 percent. The Marine Corps' last survey in 1985 indicated a smoking rate of 43 percent (Kimble 1987). It is impossible to determine how much of this drop is attributable specifically to the new smoking restrictions, because many other antismoking activities occurred during this time, both in the military and in the wider community. In the 6-month period ending April 30, 1987, monthly tobacco product sales in military commissaries decreased by approximately 18 percent. The rate of decreased sales does not necessarily directly reflect the rate of decreased consumption, because of possible purchases in the civilian market. Nevertheless, it is another suggestion of a decrease in tobacco consumption by military personnel (US DOD 1987).

In December 1988, the Veterans Administration (VA) announced its intent to establish smoke-free environments in acute-care sections within the 172 medical centers and more than 230 outpatient clinics that are part of the VA health care system (VA 1988).

In addition to Federal actions, smoking restrictions in State and local government offices have been imposed by legislation and regulation. Laws in 31 States now restrict smoking at public worksites, and additional States have restricted smoking by executive branch action.

Private Worksites

Governments have been slower to mandate smoking restrictions for private worksites than for their own employees. State laws in 13 States now require various levels of smoking restrictions at private sector worksites. Additionally, as discussed above, a growing number of city and county laws are also restricting smoking in private businesses. These actions have encouraged and supported ongoing initiatives by private businesses to restrict smoking, which are described in detail in the next section.

Judicial Actions

Decisions by both Federal and State courts have supported the authority of State and local governments to restrict or ban smoking in public places because of the health hazards, so long as the restrictions reasonably achieve desired results (Reynolds 1984). In a review of court opinions on workplace smoking restrictions, the Bureau of National Affairs found that challenges to the legality of governmental limitations have been rare (BNA 1987).

One widely publicized exception was the case of smoking regulations promulgated by the New York State Public Health Council in 1987. These broad restrictions on smoking in public places, restaurants, and workplaces were declared void by the highest level of State court on the grounds that the Public Health Council had usurped the legislature's prerogative to establish public policy (BNA 1987). Subsequently, the State legislature seriously considered several no-smoking bills, and New York City adopted a strong no-smoking ordinance (New York City Department of Health 1988).

Effects of Government Actions to Restrict Smoking

A summary of potential effects of smoking restrictions, methodological issues in their assessment, and the status of current evidence is included in Chapter 6 of the 1986 Surgeon General's Report (US DHHS 1986b). The following updates that discussion.

Implementation, Compliance, and Enforcement

No-smoking laws passed by State and local governments are generally implemented by health, rather than police, departments. Neither the adequacy of implementation nor the level of public compliance has been well studied. Their impact on smoking behavior and air quality has not been evaluated. These policies are often said to be "self-enforcing." This implies that the majority of smokers, being law abiding, obey smoking restrictions and that individuals assume responsibility for requesting compliance, thereby freeing the government from the need to actively monitor compliance or provide enforcement. Such a strategy requires substantial public awareness about the provisions of smoking laws or regulations, appropriate placement of signs, and the willingness, on the part of the public, to confront violators.

There has been little formal evaluation of the adequacy of implementation or level of compliance with smoking laws. Most available data are anecdotal. For example, newspaper accounts of the smoking ban on the LIRR reported the perception of railroad officials that cars were cleaner 2 weeks after the ban. After a well-publicized violation on the day that the ban went into effect, compliance appeared to be good (Schmitt 1988).

Prior to the implementation of New York City's no-smoking law in April 1988, a number of restaurant owners were interviewed. They anticipated great difficulty complying with the requirement that 50 percent of their seating capacity be nonsmoking. When these restaurateurs were reinterviewed 6 months after the law went into effect, they reported few problems with compliance. The city's Health Department reported receiving only a small number of complaints. Through August 24, 1988, only five hearings or complaints had been held, and only 700 dollars in fines were levied (Burns 1988).

One systematic study of implementation examined San Francisco's workplace smoking law. The city found that implementation required only a declining fraction of a single employee's time. Compliance was monitored passively; the city responded to complaints rather than doing active surveillance and equated the lack of complaints with good compliance (Martin 1988). This study's finding does not support the tobacco industry claim that smoking laws would be expensive to implement and enforce (Tobacco Institute 1983).

The implementation of a 1987 local ordinance restricting smoking in Cambridge, MA, was also studied systematically (Rigotti et al. 1988). To inform the public about the new law, the Health Commissioner relied on the news media; to inform city businesses about their new responsibilities, he mailed a brochure. The one employee in the Commissioner's office designated to handle communication about the ordinance kept a telephone log. Analysis of the log revealed a peak of calls in the first few weeks after the ordinance took effect, followed by a rapid decline. Most early calls were for information; later calls were to report complaints. Over the first 3 months, no individual or business was fined, and no judicial actions were taken.

Compliance was measured by direct observations of retail stores, which were required to ban smoking and to post signs. At 3-month followup, there was little smoking observed in stores but there were also very few signs. Only 22 percent of stores had no-smoking signs, and only 3 percent had signs worded as required by law. Compliance was also measured by a random survey of city residents. At 3 months, one-third of residents had recently noticed smoking where it was not permitted; the most common response to seeing a violation was to ignore it. The authors concluded that the reluctance of city residents to respond to violations of the law called into question the notion that the law was self-enforcing (Rigotti et al. 1988).

Public Opinion

As described in Chapter 4, a number of public opinion polls report that the majority of both smokers and nonsmokers favor restrictions on smoking in public places and workplaces. However, there have been relatively few surveys of residents of cities and States that have adopted a new policy. There is almost no information about what effect smoking laws have on knowledge of or attitudes about smoking.

The few existing surveys of public opinion after the implementation of a smoking law indicate that these policies are popular, especially with nonsmokers. Nearly three-quarters (73 percent) of a random sample of 676 New York City residents interviewed 3 months after the city's smoking law took effect were in favor of the law. This included 84 percent of nonsmokers and 43 percent of smokers (New York Times 1988). Similar results were found in Cambridge, MA: 77 percent of a random sample of 400 residents surveyed 3 months after the law became effective approved of the law. Although the policy was more popular among nonsmokers, 41 percent of smokers also approved of it. A separate survey of business managers in the city, also conducted 3 months after the law went into effect, found that the majority (64 percent) favored the law requiring the development of a smoking policy at the worksite (Rigotti et al. 1988). As noted above, the California State law banning smoking on intrastate airline flights was well accepted by both airline passengers and crew surveyed at the San Francisco airport (Journal of the American Medical Association 1988b).

Smoking Behavior

Smoking policies will be regarded as successful if they achieve their aim of reducing nonsmokers' exposure to smoke. They will assume added public health importance if, in so doing, they encourage cessation by smokers and discourage the initiation of smoking. Although there are suggestions that smoking restrictions may have these effects, evidence is lacking because the impact of these policies on attitudes or smoking behavior has not been systematically evaluated in controlled trials. In the previously mentioned study of the Cambridge smoking ordinance, there was no change over 3 months in smokers' self-reported actions or desire to quit and no change in smoking prevalence (Rigotti et al. 1988). Behavior change may require a longer time to occur. Furthermore, because of the relatively greater time that smokers spend at work compared with public places, worksite smoking restrictions may have a greater potential to change the behavior of smokers (US DHHS 1986b).

As noted previously, surveys of Armed Forces personnel indicate a drop in smoking prevalence in all services between 1985 and 1987, coincident with the adoption of a militarywide nonsmoking policy and an aggressive antismoking intervention program (Kimble 1987). The precise contribution of the policy to the overall decline is not possible to determine.

Lewit (1988) reported a relationship between smoking behavior and residence in a community having a State or local law restricting smoking. Using NHIS data, he compared the smoking prevalence and cigarette consumption of individuals living in communities with smoking laws to the smoking behavior of individuals living in areas without these laws. He reported that residence in a town with a highly restrictive ordinance (restricting smoking in restaurants and the worksite) was associated with a rate of smoking cessation that was up to 10 percentage points above the rate expected on the basis of personal characteristics alone. This applied to teenagers and young adults, as well as to the general adult population. Lewit found less of a relationship between the laws and daily cigarette consumption by continuing smokers. This is the first evidence of an association between smoking laws and smoking behavior and requires confirmation. Furthermore, as Lewit observed, the direction of causality between the existence of laws and reduced smoking, if any, is uncertain.

This assessment has been reinforced by new work by Chaloupka (1988) and Chaloupka and Saffer (1988) that concludes that, while smoking and the existence of laws are inversely related, the association reflects the higher probability of laws being passed in States with relatively low levels of smoking. Once this relationship was controlled, the authors found no significant effect of passage of the laws on smoking rates. They observed, however, that this did not mean enactment of laws would not decrease smoking, but rather that, thus far, laws have been passed primarily by States with low levels of smoking.

Summary

The Public Health Service's 1990 Health Objectives for the Nation included this goal:

> By 1990, laws should exist in all 50 States and all jurisdictions prohibiting smoking in enclosed public places, and establishing separate smoking areas at work and in dining establishments (US DHHS 1980).

As this Section has documented, there has been a rapid increase in the number of State and local government actions to restrict smoking in public places and worksites. Since 1980, 5 of 13 States without public place smoking laws have enacted them; similarly, 13 of 40 States without restaurant laws in 1980 have adopted them; and 9 of 46 States without worksite restrictions have passed such laws. However, gaps in statewide legislation remain. Eight States currently have no smoking restrictions at all, 27 States do not include provisions for restaurants, and 37 States do not have laws restricting smoking at private worksites. Although both the number and comprehensiveness of Statewide laws have grown rapidly since 1980, it is unlikely that this 1990 Health Objective will be fully achieved by the target date.

Some of the present gaps in State legislation are now being filled by community ordinances. A recent analysis estimated that, as of August 1988, there were 321 local smoking ordinances nationwide, covering a total population of over 45 million (ANR 1988b). Another compilation counted 380 local laws (Tobacco-Free America Project 1988c). Local ordinances restricting smoking at the worksite now cover over half of California's population (ANR 1988a). If this trend occurs in other States, the level of protection for nonsmokers will increase and in certain States supplant the need for stronger State legislation. However, because of the potential for differing regulations, a patchwork of local legislation may be less desirable than broader State or Federal action. In the U.S., Federal actions have restricted smoking in transportation facilities and Federal offices. The first congressional action, the 1988 ban on smoking on short commercial airline flights, will expire in 1990 without congressional action to extend it. Actions by the General Services Administration (GSA) and DOD have restricted smoking in the majority of Federal offices.

It appears that the trend toward increasingly comprehensive State and local smoking restrictions, identified in the 1986 Surgeon General's Report, is continuing. Additional legislation is being adopted, and with one exception (Beverly Hills, CA), none has been rescinded or substantially weakened. If present trends continue, smoking restrictions in cities and States can be expected to be the norm by the end of the century. A potential obstacle to the growth of local legislation is the inclusion in State legislation of a provision prohibiting cities and towns from taking stronger actions than has the State. This has occurred in at least three States (Florida, New Jersey, and Oklahoma).

Currently, little is known about the effects of no-smoking laws on attitudes toward smoking or smoking behavior. As smoking laws become more common, public health interest may shift from enactment to implementation of these laws and address issues of compliance and impact on smoking behavior.

Smoking Restrictions in the Private Sector

In 1986, the Surgeon General's Report noted the new development of policies regulating smoking in the private sector, particularly policies restricting smoking in the workplace (US DHHS 1986b). Evidence accumulated since then indicates that this trend, which began in the early 1980s, is continuing and possibly accelerating. A growing number of businesses, schools, health care facilities, and other institutions have adopted smoking policies to protect the health of employees, students, teachers, and patients. Not only are more private institutions adopting smoking policies, but also the policies they are adopting are further limiting the areas in which smoking is permitted. Survey data summarized in Chapter 4 demonstrate that this trend is strongly supported by public opinion.

The previous section summarized smoking restrictions that have been adopted as a result of government actions at the Federal, State, and local levels. This Section addresses smoking restrictions adopted voluntarily, that is, by private initiative. However, surveys on smoking restrictions in the private sector often do not distinguish between restrictions adopted voluntarily and those adopted to comply with legislation. This Section focuses on activities of businesses, schools, and health care facilities, because trends in these areas are the best recorded. Similar efforts are also being made for public transportation, restaurants, hotels and motels, and other sites; these are covered in the previous Report (US DHHS 1986b).

Workplace Smoking Restrictions

Walsh and Gordon (1986) cite a number of reasons for labeling the worksite as a "lightning rod" for those concerned about the health consequences of involuntary smoking. Along with growing evidence about the adverse health effects of involuntary tobacco smoke exposure (Eriksen, LeMaistre, Newell 1988; US DHHS 1986b), there is appreciation that the workplace is a major source of involuntary smoke exposure for all employed adults and is the most important source of exposure for adults who live in nonsmoking households (CDC 1987a). Furthermore, employees have less choice about their place of work, and hence their ETS exposure at work, than they do about where they spend time outside work. From the employer's standpoint, there are medical, legal, legislative, and economic reasons to consider workplace smoking control initiatives (Eriksen 1986). Nonsmokers' right to clean air at work has been supported by common law precedent (US DHHS 1985c; Walsh and Gordon 1986). Smoking policies have also attracted the interest of behavioral scientists interested in the potential of the worksite as a base for activities that alter worksite norms about smoking, restrict opportunities to smoke, and increase motivation to quit (US DHHS 1985d).

A broad range of smoking policies has been developed by businesses. A taxonomy of these policies is presented and discussed in the 1986 Surgeon General's Report (US DHHS 1986b). Briefly, the options can be categorized as follows: (1) no explicit policy, (2) environmental alterations, (3) restricting smoking to designated areas, (4) banning smoking at work, and (5) preferential hiring of nonsmokers. In addition to these actions to control workplace smoking, private businesses have also developed worksite-based smoking cessation programs (Chapter 6).

History and Prevalence

There is a long tradition of smoking restrictions in the workplace to protect the safety of the worker, workplace, and product from hazards such as fires, explosions, or contamination. Such policies were supported by State legislation as far back as 1892. Although there are very few systematic data about prevalence or nature of workplace policies prior to the late 1970s, available data indicate that at the time of the 1964 Surgeon General's Report, there were essentially no restrictions on smoking in the workplace except where restrictions were needed because of fire or explosion hazards or sensitive equipment (US DHHS 1986b).

During the 1970s, workplace smoking regulations for the sake of employee health and comfort were included in clean indoor air legislation proposed at the State level and adopted by private businesses. By the late 1970s, private consulting firms, universities, and public health agencies began to assess the prevalence and characteristics of these policies. Most surveys have included large businesses only; consequently, less is known about the prevalence of smoking restrictions in smaller businesses.

The Dartnell Corporation (1977), a private organization that conducts survey research for businesses, made one of the first attempts to estimate the prevalence of workplace smoking policies. In its 1977 survey of U.S. and Canadian office administrators, the organization reported that 30 percent of U.S. and 25 percent of Canadian offices had smoking policies. Since then, a number of State and national surveys have been conducted. The prevalence of policies reported by surveys done in the 1970s ranged from a low of 8 percent in California (Fielding and Breslow 1979) to a high of 64 percent in Massachusetts (Bennett and Levy 1980). During the 1980s, the estimates of workplace smoking policies have ranged from a low of 32 percent (Human Resources Policy Corporation 1985) to a high of 54 percent (BNA 1987).

Attempts to compare the results of different surveys are complicated by differences in survey design, types of companies studied, definitions of "policy," measurement instruments, and analytical techniques. Furthermore, the low response rate of some surveys limits their generalizability. Particularly in the earlier surveys, the variability in results may have been attributable as much to differences in research methodology as it was to differences in the actual prevalence of policies. The 1986 Surgeon General's Report includes a comprehensive review of the results and methodological limitations of the surveys measuring the prevalence of workplace smoking policies (US DHHS 1986b). It concluded that the prevalence of worksite smoking policies was increasing. Recently, Walsh and McDougall (1988) reviewed the trends in workplace smoking policies, noted the methodological limitations, and tentatively concluded that about 30 percent of employers have some type of smoking policy.

The conclusion that worksite smoking policies are becoming more common is supported by the results of two surveys conducted by the Bureau of National Affairs (BNA). These were two national surveys, in 1986 and 1987, of random samples of members of the American Society of Personnel Administration (BNA 1986, 1987). Although the generalizability of the results is limited by low response rates (34 percent in 1986 and 29 percent in 1987), the similarity of the two surveys' methodologies permits limited comparisons between years and provides an indication of general trends. In 1986, BNA reported a 36-percent prevalence of workplace smoking policies; in 1987, the estimate was 54 percent. Taken together, these results indicate a 50-percent increase in the proportion of companies with policies between 1986 and 1987. This conclusion was supported by the finding that 85 percent of companies with a smoking policy in 1987 reported that it had been adopted in the past 3 years (1985 to 1987). In addition to the companies that had a policy in 1987, 4 percent of companies were planning to establish a policy by the end of 1988, and 21 percent were considering workplace smoking restrictions at the time of the survey. Thus, only 22 percent of responding companies did not have either a smoking policy in place or one under consideration.

These results are consistent with those from a large random sample survey of U.S. businesses participating in the 1985 National Survey of Worksite Health Promotion Activities. Of the 35 percent of companies that had smoking control activities, over three-quarters (76.5 percent) reported having a formal smoking policy in place (US DHHS 1987c). Formal smoking policies were the most common component of workplace smoking control programs. The one discrepant result was obtained by a survey restricted to New York City businesses (CDC 1987a). Done in August 1986, it reported that only 4 percent of 573 companies responding to the survey had written smoking policies. It is notable that this is the only one of these surveys to include a large number of smaller businesses. Half of the sample consisted of businesses with fewer than 10 employees, and they were less likely than larger companies to have a smoking policy. Another possible explanation for the discrepancy is that businesses were asked about having a written smoking policy. Some small businesses may have unwritten policies in place.

A separate line of evidence supports these estimates of worksite smoking policy prevalence. The 1986 Adult Use of Tobacco Survey provides an estimate of the extent of worksite smoking policies from the employee's, not the employer's, perspective (CDC 1988). The results are based on a national probability sample of over 13,000 adults. Of employed adults, 45 percent reported having some smoking restrictions at their place of work; smoking was restricted for 42 percent and banned for 3 percent. Of the 55 percent working in places without smoking restrictions, two-thirds reported at least some exposure to ETS (CDC 1988).

Most surveys of workplace smoking policies have assessed their prevalence in private businesses. Recently, however, there have been some attempts to assess the prevalence of smoking policies at public worksites. The 1987 BNA survey reported that organizations classified as "non-business" tended to establish their smoking policy before their business counterparts did; however, the opposite was reported in a systematic random-sample survey of private businesses and public agencies in Texas (Gottlieb, Hedl, Eriksen et al., in press). In that survey, over 50 percent of both private and public employers reported having a restrictive smoking policy, with only minor differences between them. These Texas surveys were conducted at the same time as the national BNA survey (1987), and each reported the prevalence of restrictive smoking policies to be over 50 percent. In another study of public agencies, Timmins (1987) surveyed a random sample of public agency personnel managers and reported that 38 percent had either formal or informal personnel policies dealing with smoking at work. This percentage is consistent with the prevalence of workplace smoking policies reported for private corporations in 1986 (BNA 1986). Although there are some small differences in rationale and timing, there appear to be more similarities than differences between public and private workplaces regarding the establishment of restrictive smoking policies. Overall, smoking restrictions currently exist in approximately one-half of large American businesses.

Level of Restrictiveness

Not only the prevalence but also the restrictiveness of worksite smoking policies is increasing. According to the BNA surveys (1987), the proportion of company smoking policies that stipulated a total ban on smoking in all company buildings doubled from 1986 to 1987, from 6 to 12 percent. The proportion of company policies that prohibit smoking in all open work areas also increased, from 41 percent in 1986 to 51 percent in 1987. In addition to open work areas, smoking was more likely to be prohibited in 1987 than in 1986 in each of six specific areas addressed in the surveys, including hallways, conference rooms, and private offices. When workplace smoking policies are revised, the revisions are typically more restrictive, sometimes becoming total smoking bans. In the 1987 BNA survey, 13 percent of companies had revised their policies since first being adopted and another 17 percent were anticipating changes before 1989, with the "vast majority" becoming more restrictive than the original ones (BNA 1987). The most restrictive smoking policy, the preferential or exclusive hiring of nonsmokers, is uncommon. According to the BNA survey (BNA 1987), only 12 percent of companies give a hiring preference to nonsmokers and only 1 percent restrict hiring to nonsmokers. There was no indication that this trend is increasing over time.

Reasons for Adopting Smoking Policies

In their review of current smoking policies, Walsh and McDougall (1988) identify reasons businesses have adopted restrictive smoking policies: (1) to protect equipment; (2) to impress customers; (3) to protect the health of smoking employees; (4) to reduce the health risks of involuntary smoke exposure for nonsmoking employees; (5) to respond to employees' complaints; (6) to comply with regulations; and (7) to avert insurance and productivity losses.

As noted above, the first workplace smoking policies were implemented primarily for safety and productivity reasons (Bennett and Levy 1980), whereas the majority of the recent policies have been implemented to protect employee health (Walsh and McDougall 1988). According to the National Survey of Worksite Health Promotion Activities (US DHHS 1987c), the major reasons companies established restrictive smoking policies were to protect the health of nonsmoking employees (40.4 percent) and to comply with regulations (39.5 percent). Of secondary importance was the need to protect equipment (12.7 percent). In the 1987 BNA survey, the leading reason reported for adopting a smoking policy was a concern for the comfort and health of employees. The second most common reason was in response to employee complaints, followed by the need to comply with State or local law. Both surveys illustrate the impact of the nonsmokers' rights movement and the flurry of local and State legislation on the adoption of workplace smoking policies.

The most common barrier to adopting a restrictive smoking policy is perceived lack of employee demand. In the 1987 BNA survey, two-thirds of the companies without policies cited insufficient employee demand as the reason for not adopting a policy, twice the proportion citing anticipated enforcement problems and lack of support from top management, the next most common reasons given. In addition, some employers fear a negative reaction from smoking employees, conflict between smokers and nonsmokers, and the possibility of legal action and grievances by smokers demanding the right to smoke at work (Thompson, Sexton, Sinsheimer 1987; US DHHS 1987c). Also, sometimes unions have not supported smoking policies, a fact that may have discouraged management in some companies from adopting smoking restrictions (BNA 1986). However, in a recent survey, 82 percent of union members favored smoking restrictions (Brown et al. 1988).

Another reason employers may be reluctant to implement a restrictive smoking policy is concern about its impact on workplace norms. Until recently, smoking was sanctioned at work and many aspects of the work environment actually reinforced smoking. Smoking breaks were times for employee socialization and were often included in collective bargaining agreements. Concern for smokers' needs to satisfy their addiction to nicotine and the fear of productivity losses resulting from frequent smoking breaks outside the immediate work area may also deter some employers from implementing a restrictive smoking policy (Schilling, Gilchrist, Schinke 1985). On the other hand, there is some indication that societal norms about smoking are changing rapidly in the work environment. For example, a 1987 *Wall Street Journal* article (Freedman 1987) cited anecdotal evidence to support the notion that cigarette smoking could serve as a barrier to the career development of white-collar workers.

Correlates of Worksite Smoking Policies

Worksite smoking policies are more common in larger businesses. In a survey of personnel managers (BNA 1987), 63 percent of those with 1,000 or more employees reported having a smoking policy, compared with 52 percent of companies with fewer employees. In the same survey, smaller companies were half as likely as larger ones to have a policy under consideration (12 vs. 24 percent). Similar findings were reported by the National Survey of Worksite Health Promotion Activities, in which larger worksites were more likely than smaller ones to report smoking control activities (US DHHS 1987c). As noted above, in a survey of private New York City businesses, only 4 percent (21/539) of companies with fewer than 100 employees had a written smoking policy (CDC 1987a).

The prevalence of smoking policies also varies by type of industry. In general, companies with the greatest potential for respiratory hazards (manufacturing and processing) and the highest prevalence of smoking employees (US DHHS 1985c) are also the ones least likely to have smoking policies (Administrative Management Society 1986; BNA 1986, 1987). One study has shown a relationship between the smoking status of the top administrator and the likelihood of having a smoking policy. A business whose manager was a current smoker was less likely to have a written smoking policy (CDC 1987a).

Health Care Facilities

Like the worksites described above, health care facilities, especially hospitals, have become focal points of private efforts to restrict smoking. There are compelling reasons for these facilities to adopt strong smoking restrictions (US DHHS 1986b). Many patients treated in health care facilities have smoking-related illnesses; nonsmoking is part of their treatment. Permitting smoking in hospitals may undermine the advice given by physicians to patients to stop smoking. Other patients have illnesses whose symptoms can be worsened by exposure to tobacco smoke. The majority of hospital fires are caused by smoking in bed. Furthermore, hospitals are also workplaces; like any other worksite, employees have numerous reasons for having smoking restrictions. Smoking restrictions in health care facilities are supported by surveys of patients (Kottke et al. 1985) and have been endorsed by numerous medical organizations (US DHHS 1986b).

Despite the strong rationale and favorable public attitudes, smoking restrictions in health care facilities have lagged behind those in private businesses. This has occurred despite the fact that, much more often than businesses, health care facilities have been required by State and local laws to have smoking restrictions. As noted in the previous Section, two-thirds of States now require hospitals to restrict smoking to designated areas. These legislative efforts have not led to strong protection of patients in many cases because the laws do not specify the nature or size of smoke-free areas. Most smoking restriction has been the result of private initiative, often beginning with the medical staff (US DHHS 1986b).

Two recent surveys indicate that almost all hospitals have adopted some smoking restrictions. A survey of 774 hospital administrators by the American College of Healthcare Executives (ACHE) (1988) reported that 90 percent of hospitals currently restrict smoking and another 6 percent are currently developing a smoking policy. Similar results were obtained in a study of hospitals accredited by the Joint Commission on Accreditation of Healthcare Organizations (JCAHO): 93 percent of the 2,165 responding hospitals reported having a formal written smoking policy (Holland 1988).

Although these national surveys of hospital administrators indicate that nearly all hospitals restrict smoking in at least some areas, they do not indicate the extent of these smoking restrictions. Other surveys suggest that patient care areas are not uniformly free of smoke. For example, over 90 percent of Indiana hospitals allow inpatients, outpatients, and visitors to smoke, at least in designated areas (Torabi, Seffrin, Brashear 1987). In Texas, where 78 percent of hospitals have written smoking policies, only two-thirds of hospitals provide smoke-free rooms, and even then, smoke-free rooms are often available only on a "when available" basis, and patient requests are often denied (Zamrazil 1984).

A number of hospitals are beginning to ban smoking entirely. In the ACHE survey, 7 percent (28/394) of the responding hospitals with current smoking restrictions reported that smoking was entirely prohibited, although some of these hospitals allowed smoking by patients under the written order of a physician. Although the survey of JCAHO-accredited hospitals did not ask if the facility was smoke free, by analyzing the response to questions regarding smoking in specific areas, the authors estimate that approximately 5 percent of surveyed hospitals are smoke free. In Minnesota, 26 percent of hospitals have already banned smoking in preparation for compliance with a recently enacted State law that will require all hospitals to become smoke free by 1990 (Kirn 1988). All 20 of the nation's comprehensive cancer centers are or will soon become mostly or totally smoke free (Neville 1988). The requirement that a doctor's order be written before a patient is allowed to smoke appears to be becoming a common component of hospital smoking policies. These are intended for use in unusual situations, for example, in the case of terminal patients. It is not clear how often this option is used when available. For example, at Saint Cloud Hospital in Minnesota, only 10 doctors' smoking orders were written in the 18 months following the effective date of the smoking ban (ACHE 1988).

Health care facilities report somewhat different reasons for adopting smoking restrictions than do other worksites. The national survey of ACHE members indicated that the most often cited rationale for smoking restrictions was that they were a moral obligation of health care providers. Other reasons included improvement of employee health and air quality.

Hospital policies other than smoking restrictions also discourage smoking. In one recent survey, 3 percent of hospitals reported that they do not hire smokers (ACHE 1988). Most hospitals prohibit the sale of cigarettes. In 1976, a survey of hospital administrators found that 58 percent of Indiana hospitals sold cigarettes. When a similar survey was repeated in 1986, the proportion of hospitals selling cigarettes had dropped to 13 percent (Torabi, Seffrin, Brashear 1987). In Texas, 26 percent of surveyed hospitals never sold cigarettes; as of 1984, 28 percent of hospitals continue to sell them (Zamrazil 1984). Voluntary (nonpolicy) efforts by health care professionals to discourage smoking are discussed in Chapter 6.

There is virtually no information about the prevalence of smoking restrictions in physician offices. One small study of primary care physician offices reported that ashtrays were found in 9 of 51 waiting rooms and that "no smoking" signs were posted in only 20 of 51 offices (Radovsky and Barry 1988). Medical organizations are themselves also beginning to restrict smoking in their facilities. In an informal telephone survey conducted by the American Medical Association (AMA), 45 of the 65 medical organizations represented in the AMA House of Delegates had some type of smoking policy (Journal of the American Medical Association 1988a; Goldsmith 1988).

Many pharmacies sell tobacco products, in addition to dispensing medications for the treatment of smoking-related illnesses. Only 11 of 100 San Francisco pharmacies surveyed in 1978 did not sell tobacco products (Schroeder and Showstack 1978). The extent to which this situation may have changed in the subsequent decade is unknown. During that time, pharmacists have been exhorted to stop selling tobacco products (Richards and Blum 1985), and at least one advocacy group compiles an ongoing list of pharmacists who have made this decision (New Jersey GASP 1988). The American Pharmaceutical Association has endorsed the position that pharmacists should not sell tobacco products (Taylor, Richards, Fischer 1987). A survey of 136 pharmacists in Georgia in 1986 revealed that 74 percent sold cigarettes (Taylor, Richards, Fischer 1987).

Schools

Secondary schools have traditionally regulated smoking by students, but for reasons other than concern about involuntary smoke exposure (US DHHS 1986b). School smoking restrictions are part of broader societal efforts to prevent children and adolescents from starting to smoke by educating them about the hazards of tobacco use and by restricting their access to tobacco products. Because most smokers start smoking before age 20 (Chapter 5), efforts to reduce the initiation of smoking have focused on schools. As noted in Part I, school education about the health consequences of smoking is mandated by law in 20 States (Lovato, Allensworth, Chan, in press) and has also been the result of voluntary efforts by individual schools (Chapter 6).

Smoking by secondary school students is also restricted by State laws and regulations. Currently, 32 States restrict or ban smoking in schools (Table 19). Smoking by students is banned in schools in 15 States and restricted to designated areas in an additional 17 States (Tobacco-Free America Project 1988a). Furthermore, as discussed in the next section, laws in 43 States and the District of Columbia prohibit the sale of cigarettes to minors below a designated age; in most cases this is age 18 years or higher. In 16 States, not only the sale but also the use or possession of tobacco products is banned with respect to minors. Consequently, secondary schools have banned student smoking for at least two major reasons: to comply with State law and to discourage the initiation of smoking by students.

Recognition of the health effects of involuntary smoke exposure provides an additional reason for school smoking restrictions and a reason to expand attention from students to teachers. Smoking by teachers has traditionally been permitted only in areas away from students, partly out of concern that teachers' smoking could serve as role model behavior for students. Available evidence indicates that there are far fewer restrictions on smoking by teachers and other school staff than on smoking by students. Nearly as many States restrict faculty smoking as restrict student smoking; however, whereas 15 State laws totally ban smoking by students, only 1 State, Kansas, bans smoking by teachers. A history and description of school smoking policy restrictions can be found in the 1986 Surgeon General's Report (US DHHS 1986b). There is little information about smoking restrictions in colleges and universities. In 1988, the American College Health Association adopted a statement endorsing stringent smoking restrictions and a prohibition of tobacco sales and advertising on college and university campuses (ACHA 1988).

The most comprehensive and recent information about the prevalence of school smoking policies was reported by the National School Boards Association (NSBA), which surveyed a stratified random sample of 2,000 school districts nationwide in 1986 (NSBA 1986, 1987). The 36-percent response rate, although relatively low, was consistent with response rates reported for other workplace surveys (Walsh and McDougall 1988). Eighty-seven percent of the responding school districts reported having written policies or regulations on smoking in schools. Nearly half of the districts (47 percent) had a comprehensive policy that prohibited student smoking in school buildings, on school grounds, and at school-sponsored functions. There were fewer restrictions on smoking by faculty and staff. Although 91 percent of school districts prohibited student smoking in school buildings, these restrictions applied to teachers in only 10 percent of the districts. Most school districts (81 percent) provided designated smoking areas in school buildings for faculty and staff. Overall, only 2 percent of the school districts prohibited school-related tobacco use for students, faculty, and administration. The NSBA survey addressed school smoking policies only; it did not assess rules about smokeless tobacco usage.

School smoking policies, like those in other worksites, are becoming more restrictive. According to the NSBA survey (1986, 1987), 37 percent of school districts have revised their policies since 1981, with 80 percent instituting stricter rules for students and 56 percent strengthening restrictions for faculty and staff. The major reason given by school districts for implementing smoking policies was concern about health, followed by problems associated with smoking behavior (42 percent) and State or local legislation (35 percent). The reason for adopting smoking policies differed by location; rural districts tended to be influenced more by the belief that adult role models change student smoking behavior, whereas urban districts were influenced by municipal or State antismoking legislation.

Public Transportation

As noted in a preceding section, as of April 1988, smoking was banned by Federal legislation on all domestic U.S. airline flights scheduled for 2 hr or less. Shortly before that ban took effect, one airline, Northwest Airlines, the Nation's fifth largest carrier, adopted a policy stricter than the law required; it banned smoking on all its domestic flights, regardless of flight time, excluding those between Hawaii and the mainland (Northwest Airlines 1988). According to company information, the action was at least partially a marketing decision to capitalize on changing social norms related to smoker and nonsmoker rights (Northwest Airlines 1988). Little is known about private initiatives to ban smoking on trains or buses. In 1987, Air Canada, that nation's largest carrier, voluntarily banned smoking on a trial basis on selected flights within Canada and to the United States. This action preceded parliamentary action in June 1988 to ban smoking on all flights of 2 hr or less. Subsequently, in July 1988, Air Canada announced a ban on smoking on all its North American flights (Boston Globe 1988b).

Effects of Smoking Restrictions

Policies restricting smoking at the worksite have a number of possible direct and indirect effects that are outlined here (US DHHS 1986b). An adequately implemented smoking policy has the direct effect of limiting the circumstances in which smoking is permitted, thereby altering the behavior of smokers and eliminating or reducing the concentration of ETS in areas in which smoking is banned. Successful policy implementation requires that employees and managers be aware of the policy, comply with its provisions, and enforce it against violations. For smokers, the result is fewer opportunities to smoke during working hours, which should reduce cigarette consumption at work, may reduce overall consumption, and may trigger attempts at cessation. For nonsmokers, worksite restrictions have the potential to reduce an important source of involuntary smoke exposure, because adults spend more time at work than at any other place outside the home.

Beyond these direct effects, worksite smoking policies may have broader, indirect effects on public attitudes about tobacco use and smoking behavior outside work. Policies that restrict or ban smoking at work convey strong messages about the social acceptability of cigarettes and reinforce perceptions that nonsmoking is the norm. The combination of altered social norms and reduced opportunities to smoke has the potential to make a strong impact on smoking behavior at many points in its natural history. For worksite policies, hypothesized effects include reducing overall cigarette consumption and increasing the number and success of cessation attempts. The effects on behavior may be enhanced by a coexistent smoking cessation program. Worksite smoking restrictions may have other impacts, such as economic benefits, that are of interest to employers (US DHHS 1986b).

Smoking policies in schools may alter attitudes about the desirability of smoking and reduce social pressures to smoke, thereby discouraging smoking initiation. As in business, the impact may be enhanced by concurrent health education programs. In health care settings, smoking restrictions have the potential to influence smoking by patients, in addition to any impact on employees. Patients who develop acute illness, particularly cardiovascular disease manifestations, are more likely to quit smoking (Rigotti and Tesar 1985). Smoking restrictions in hospitals may enhance the effect of illness on smoking cessation and increase the effectiveness of health professionals' advice to stop smoking (US DHHS 1986b).

Although smoking policies have been increasingly adopted at worksites, especially in recent years, few have been subject to evaluation. Some businesses have conducted baseline surveys of employees to assess attitudes and behavior prior to policy implementation, but few have followed these with postimplementation surveys to assess their effects. Methodological issues in evaluation are reviewed in detail in the 1986 Surgeon General's Report and elsewhere (US DHHS 1986b; Rigotti 1989). The ideal study would assess variables before and after a policy is adopted and include a comparison group for whom no change occurs. This would permit controlling for concurrent outside influences on smoking behavior and attitudes, such as populationwide trends that are now occurring (Chapter 4), which may confound results. Such controlled evaluations are rare. Most available information is drawn from uncontrolled studies, often done retrospectively. The first evaluations of worksite smoking policies were done in a health care setting (Rigotti et al. 1986; Biener et al. 1989; Andrews 1983; Rosenstock, Stergachis, Heaney 1986). Evaluations of policies at other workplaces have begun to appear recently. The following section, which updates a review in the 1986 Surgeon General's Report, will describe the current state of knowledge about the impacts of smoking restrictions at worksites, schools, and health care facilities.

Implementation and Compliance

There has been little systematic evaluation of the degree of worksite smoking policy compliance by managers and employees, although descriptions of policy adoption by individual companies have not reported major problems (US DHHS 1986b; BNA 1986). On the other hand, data from the 1986 Adult Use of Tobacco Survey indicate that the presence of a policy does not guarantee smoke-free air (CDC 1988). A policy that is poorly implemented or enforced will result in little restriction of smoking and can be expected to have slight effect on air quality or smoking behavior. Model smoking policies for worksites and health care facilities and guidelines for implementation have been developed by several groups (BNA 1986, 1987; US DHHS 1985c; Kottke et al. 1986; American Hospital Association 1988).

Attitudes and Norms

Available studies indicate that smoking restrictions are well received by most employees. They are uniformly more popular with nonsmokers than with smokers. Four months after a stringent smoking policy was adopted at the Group Health Cooperative, a large health maintenance organization in the Pacific Northwest, 85 percent of surveyed employees approved of the decision to prohibit smoking, including nearly all nonsmokers and 36 percent of smokers. The level of approval of both smokers and nonsmokers was higher after implementation than it was when the policy was first announced, suggesting that policy implementation is better received than the initial policy announcement (Rosenstock, Stergachis, Heaney 1986). Rigotti and colleagues (1986) reported similar results among pediatric nurses after a smoking ban.

In another study of hospital employees by Biener and coworkers (1989), over 90 percent of the nonsmokers and two-thirds of the smokers approved of a smoking policy at both 6 and 12 months following its implementation. In another hospital, Andrews (1983) reported that 93 percent of the nonsmokers and 83 percent of the smokers, surveyed 20 months after the adoption of a strict smoking policy, approved of it. Outside the health care setting, similar results have been reported. Petersen and colleagues (1988) found that 67 percent of nonsmokers and 19 percent of smokers in an insurance company felt that a restrictive smoking policy had an overall positive impact on the work environment. At Ranier Bank (1986), headquartered in Seattle, the majority of all employees felt the company's smoking policy was effective and fairly implemented.

The attitude of smokers toward smoking policies depends on the restrictiveness of the policy and characteristics of the individual smoker. As would be expected, a policy is less popular with smokers when smoking is prohibited in work areas, as at the Connecticut insurance company (Petersen et al. 1988) and Group Health Cooperative (Rosenstock, Stergachis, Heaney 1986), than when the policy calls for designated smoking areas, as in the first phase of the Ranier Bank policy (1986) and the Rhode Island hospitals study (Biener et al. 1989). Thompson, Sexton, and Sinsheimer (1987) surveyed all employees in a Pacific Northwest high technology company that had recently implemented a restrictive smoking policy. Among smokers, those most likely to oppose the policy were females and heavy long-term smokers with fewer positive health practices. In addition, on discriminant analysis, a low desire to quit and a low probability of quitting were also significantly associated with opposition to the policy. These findings agree with another study associating support for smoking policies with greater interest in quitting, more concern for smoking health risks, and greater social support for nonsmoking (Sorensen and Pechacek 1989).

Although most studies have found the majority of smokers and nonsmokers to favor restrictive policies, both prior to and following policy implementation, there is little information available about the effect of policies on attitudes about smoking in general. In one case, Biener and associates (1989) found little change in nonsmokers' attitudes toward secondhand smoke or their assertiveness in confronting smokers after a restrictive smoking policy was adopted.

Smoking Behavior

Currently available studies indicate that worksite smoking restrictions reduce cigarette consumption at work, but there is little evidence about effects on overall smoking. All studies are limited by reliance on self-reports of smoking behavior. They tend to validate the hypothesis that implementation of a restrictive smoking policy has a positive effect on overall smoking behavior. Early studies monitored smokers' compliance with no-smoking signs (Dawley and Baldwin 1983; Dawley and Burton 1985) and oral reminders not to smoke in designated nonsmoking areas (Jason and Liotta 1982) and found these techniques to be effective.

Expanding upon these observational studies, researchers began to use survey methodology to investigate the impact of restrictive smoking policies on representative samples of an entire work force. Some of the earliest evidence of the impact of smoking policy on smoking behavior came from Group Health Cooperative of Puget Sound following the prohibition of smoking in its 35 facilities (Rosenstock, Stergachis, Heaney 1986). Four months after policy implementation, 29 percent of the surveyed current smokers reported they were smoking less and attributed the reduction to the policy. The average reduction, 2 cigarettes a day, was small but of statistical significance. However, prepolicy tobacco consumption was assessed after the policy took effect. Such retrospective assessment is subject to possible respondent bias that might overestimate the actual change. Four percent of the surveyed smokers reported that they quit smoking in association with the implementation of the policy; however, because it was only 4 months following the program, it is difficult to evaluate the long-term impact on cessation.

For these health maintenance organization employees, a smoking ban had relatively little impact on cessation rates, but contributed to reductions in the amount smoked. This relationship has also been reported among insurance company and hospital employees. Three months after a work area smoking ban was adopted by an insurance company in Connecticut, employees reported no increase in cessation rates, but an average reduction of 32 percent in the amount smoked. The average daily cigarette consumption fell from 0.95 pack per day to 0.67 pack per day, with 44 percent of smokers reporting a decrease in consumption (Petersen et al. 1988). The proportion of smokers reducing the amount smoked is similar to the decreases projected for employees in studies by Eriksen (1985) and Millar (1986).

Furthermore, there was a direct correlation between the amount smoked and the likelihood of reporting a consumption decrease in the Petersen study (1988). The heaviest smokers were the ones most likely to report a reduction in the amount smoked, with 93 percent of those who smoked at least 2 packs a day reporting a reduction following the policy. However, the conclusions of the study are limited by major weaknesses in design. First, employees reported their current and previous smoking behavior at the same time and on the same questionnaire. The retrospective assessment of prepolicy smoking behavior introduced the possibility of recall bias. Second, the survey instrument was administered to employees as they entered the company cafeteria. Using this technique, researchers reached 56.6 percent of all employees; however, because the respondents were not randomly selected, they are not necessarily representative of the entire work force and the findings cannot be generalized beyond the respondents. In fact, compared with the average company employee, the survey respondents were more likely to be white (87 vs. 82 percent), be college educated (69 vs. 59 percent), and have professional or technical jobs (63 vs. 52 percent).

The study with the strongest research design, that of Biener and colleagues (1989), used random, cross-sectional samples of employees to examine the impact of a restrictive smoking policy on hospital employee smoking behavior. Telephone interviews were conducted at baseline and 6 and 12 months in experimental and comparison hospitals. They found no difference in quit rates between the two hospitals, but a reduction in the number of cigarettes smoked during work in the experimental group. Because there was no apparent change in the number of cigarettes smoked outside of work, the authors conclude that there was a net reduction in the daily amount smoked. In their study of hospital nurses, Rigotti and coworkers (1986) also reported a significant reduction in the number of cigarettes smoked at work, but no change in the overall daily amount smoked.

In another hospital-based study, Andrews (1983) surveyed 36 percent of the hospital staff 20 months after the implementation of a restrictive smoking policy and reported a major impact on both cessation and reduction of smoking: 26 percent of those surveyed had stopped smoking and 33 percent smoked less since the policy went into effect. However, methodological problems prevent an unequivocal conclusion that change was attributable to the policy.

In summary, the current data about the impact of worksite smoking policies on smoking behavior are equivocal, and firm conclusions await studies with stronger designs. The conclusion of one study reporting an effect on cessation was weakened by methodological problems (Andrews 1983). Three studies reported no impact on cessation, but reductions in the amount smoked (Petersen et al. 1988; Rosenstock, Stergachis, Heaney 1986; Biener et al. 1989), and one study showed no effect on overall smoking behavior (Rigotti et al. 1986). The conclusion of the 1986 Surgeon General's Report still holds: "There is as yet no conclusive evidence that worksite smoking policies are associated with increases in smoking cessation attempts or reductions in smoking prevalence" (US DHHS 1986b).

Even less information is available about the effect of school smoking policies on smoking behavior. One study (Porter 1982) has linked smoking policies with reduced smoking initiation. Another study (Murray, Kiryluk, Swan 1984) found student smoking behavior to be associated with teacher smoking, along with other organizational variables. As with worksites and health care facilities, there are few studies that have attempted to determine the relationship between smoking policy and associated behavior.

Participation in Cessation Programs

Smoking control efforts are the most prevalent worksite health promotion activity, according to the National Survey of Worksite Health Promotion Activities (US DHHS 1987c). In 1987, over half (54 percent) of companies responding to the 1987 BNA survey were planning future activities to encourage employee smoking cessation, a doubling of the 1986 rate (27 percent). However, data on the level of program participation are mixed, and data on outcomes are virtually nonexistent.

Companies with smoking policies are much more likely (64 vs. 38 percent) to have attempted to help their employees to quit smoking than are companies without policies (BNA 1987). It has been hypothesized that the adoption of a smoking policy will increase participation in company-sponsored smoking cessation programs, reflecting the potential of smoking policies to increase smokers' motivation to quit smoking. However, the data on the influence of a workplace smoking policy on participation in a worksite smoking cessation program are mixed. In the Group Health Cooperative study, only 2 percent of surveyed smokers participated in a smoking cessation class offered during the implementation period (Rosenstock, Stergachis, Heaney 1986). In the Rhode Island hospital study (Biener et al. 1989), implementation of a restrictive policy did not lead to an increase in enrollment in a self-help smoking cessation program when compared with employee enrollment in a comparison hospital (13 vs. 14 percent). In the Connecticut insurance company study (Petersen et al. 1988), only 20 smoking employees (about 4 percent of the eligible smokers) enrolled in a company-subsidized smoking cessation program, and no smokers requested support through a volunteer buddy system. On the other hand, over 25 percent of the smoking employees at Pacific Northwest Bell participated in a company-sponsored smoking cessation program that was offered in conjunction with a ban on workplace smoking (Martin 1988; Walsh and McDougall 1988).

Air Quality

The primary goal of worksite smoking policies is to reduce individuals' involuntary tobacco smoke exposure, but the degree to which policies achieve this goal has been measured infrequently and only indirectly. Air quality has been assessed only by subjective measures, which ask employees to rate the concentration of smoke in the air. These studies have found improvements in perceived air quality after policy adoption in most cases. After establishing designated smoking areas as the first phase in an eventual prohibition of smoking, Ranier Bank (1986) surveyed over 3,300 employees regarding their reaction to the policy. Nearly two-thirds of all employees, smokers and nonsmokers alike, felt that the amount of smoke in common areas decreased following implementation of the policy. In the Rhode Island hospital study (Biener et al. 1989), employees in the hospital with a restrictive policy were less likely to report being bothered by smoke at work than were employees in the comparison hospital. This was true for offices and staff lounges, but not for lavatories, suggesting that this was an area of noncompliance in the policy hospital. Rigotti and colleagues (1986) reported a significant improvement in air quality for nurses 1 year following a smoking ban.

Data from the 1986 Adult Use of Tobacco Survey (CDC 1988) suggest that a substantial proportion of employees at worksites with smoking restrictions or bans are still exposed to tobacco smoke. Among employees working where smoking was restricted, 53 percent reported at least some exposure to ETS, compared with 65 percent of respondents from worksites without restrictions and 21 percent from worksites with complete smoking bans.

Other Effects

There is little empirical evidence about the economic impact of worksite smoking policies because systematic analyses have not been done. Employee absenteeism, productivity, turnover, or health care costs have rarely been assessed. Biener and colleagues (1989) investigated the effect of a restrictive smoking policy on work performance. Although the majority of smokers and nonsmokers felt the policy had no impact, 21 percent of the nonsmokers felt that their work had improved, whereas 19 percent of the smokers felt their performance had deteriorated. However, there is little evidence of negative impact from even the most restrictive policies. For example, there have been no lawsuits, grievances, or dismissals associated with a total ban on smoking at Pacific Northwest Bell (Martin 1988).

Summary

Available survey data on smoking policies in businesses, hospitals, and schools strongly suggest that the previously identified trend toward greater prevalence and increasing restrictiveness (US DHHS 1986b) is continuing, and may have accelerated since 1986. According to the BNA survey, 85 percent of the worksite smoking policies in place in 1987 were adopted within the last 3 years. Furthermore, there is no sign of reversal; policies that have been revised nearly always become more restrictive than the original ones (BNA 1987). The same situation holds for smoking restrictions in schools. Half of the school districts enacted their current smoking policies within the last 6 years, and virtually all policy revisions are becoming more restrictive and are expanding to include smoking by teachers and staff (NSBA 1986).

The growing number of State laws and community ordinances mandating smoking restrictions in the private sector worksite has contributed to this trend. For example, in the city of Cambridge, MA, 31 percent of businesses with a smoking policy had adopted it in the 6 months after the city passed a no-smoking ordinance requiring employers to have a smoking policy (Rigotti et al. 1988). Laws requiring smoking policies have also helped to overcome fears about loss of business for companies in service industries. For example, some hospitals have been reluctant to ban smoking for fear that some smokers might choose to be admitted to hospitals that will allow them to smoke. To eliminate this problem, the State of Minnesota passed a law prohibiting smoking in health care facilities, effective January 1, 1990 (Kirn 1988). By requiring every hospital to prohibit smoking (except for chemical dependency and mental health patients or under a physician's written order), this legislation avoids potential economic reasons for not restricting smoking.

Observers have noted that the tobacco industry is downplaying the existence and importance of the trend toward smoking restrictions in the hope that this may slow the momentum toward restrictive policies (Walsh and McDougall 1988). However, there is no evidence to support the industry's assertion of retrenchment and there is every indication to refute it (BNA 1987; US OTA 1986). If present trends in the prevalence of smoking restrictions continue, it can be expected that smoking will be permitted in fewer and fewer areas at work, in health care facilities, and in schools.

The impact of these restrictions on air quality and the behavior of smokers is less certain and probably will depend on the restrictiveness of the policy and the degree to which the policy is implemented as written. Current evidence permits no definitive conclusion about the actual impact of restrictive smoking policies on smoking behavior. The limited data available suggest that policies contribute to reductions in cigarette consumption by smokers, but not to cessation. However, comprehensive programs that include smoking restrictions along with other environmental changes and other health promotion activities may have a major impact on smoking prevalence, especially among high-risk employees (Shipley et al. 1988). Similarly, the same type of comprehensive program that aims to influence environmental factors may contribute to positive health outcomes in schools, including the prevention of smoking (Simons-Morton, Parcel, O'Hara 1988).

If worksite smoking policies, by themselves or in conjunction with health promotion programs, are shown to reduce tobacco consumption or smoking prevalence, they will need to reach high-risk groups and populations with high smoking rates to have a major impact upon public health. Blue-collar employees are an example of such a group. Data indicate that these employees are more likely to be occupationally exposed to respiratory hazards and are more likely to smoke (US DHHS 1985d). These employees are also less likely to work in the type of industry in which restrictive smoking policies are currently in force (Administrative Management Society 1986; BNA 1986, 1987).

Restrictions on Children's Access to Tobacco

Because only a very small percentage of smokers begin smoking as adults (Chapter 5), efforts at prevention must focus on children. Individuals who start smoking early have more difficulty quitting, are more likely to become heavy smokers, and are at higher risk for developing a smoking-related disease (US DHHS 1986e).

As reviewed in Chapter 4, surveys of adolescents indicate that many of those who start to smoke do not understand the nature of tobacco addiction and are unaware of or underestimate important health consequences of smoking. Their decision to smoke is, therefore, not a fully informed choice (Leventhal, Glynn, Fleming 1987). The difficulty that teenagers report in quitting smoking demonstrates that nicotine addiction can quickly become established in children (US DHHS 1988). Among 15-year-olds surveyed in Britain, 51 percent of those smoking 5 or more cigarettes per day had failed in their efforts to stop smoking, and 27 percent thought they would not be able to stop no matter how hard they tried (Revill and Drury 1980). A survey of American high school seniors found that 47 percent of those who were smoking daily would like to quit; however, only 17 percent of teenagers who smoked regularly quit by the time they were high school seniors (Johnston, O'Malley, Bachman 1987). The tenacity of smoking behavior appears to have changed little since the mid-1960s, when 80 percent of the teenagers who smoked regularly continued to smoke as adults (McKennell and Thomas 1967).

Given both the addictive nature of tobacco use and its health consequences, it is important to protect children and adolescents from using tobacco until they are capable of making a mature and informed decision. Policies to do this seek to reduce children's and adolescents' opportunities to experiment with tobacco products, and thereby develop a regular pattern of use, by making these products less available. Efforts to eliminate the availability of tobacco to children are supported by numerous medical and public health groups (WHO 1975, 1979, 1985; Hardes 1983; ACP 1986; AAP 1987; AMA 1987; DiFranza et al. 1987; Stanwick et al. 1987). It has been suggested, though not proved, that strict observance of prohibitions against the sale of tobacco to children might be the most powerful means for reducing the initiation of smoking by children (Reid 1985).

Restricting children's access to tobacco is only one approach to prevent the initiation of smoking. Other policies that specifically target children include prohibiting smoking in schools, mandating school curricula on the health effects of tobacco, and banning the promotional distribution of cigarettes to children. Additionally, policies such as increased excise taxation or proposed restrictions on advertising affect both adults and children, but may have a disproportionate impact on children and on the decision to smoke. Finally, restrictions on smoking in public places apply to children as well as to adults. These policies are discussed in other sections of this Chapter. They work synergistically with voluntary efforts (Chapter 6) to prevent the initiation of smoking. The remainder of this Section will focus on laws intended to prevent children from obtaining and using tobacco.

How Do Children Obtain Tobacco Products?

Recently, researchers have surveyed children and adolescents who smoke in order to determine how they obtain tobacco products. Although the published evidence is limited, these studies suggest that retailers, not parents or friends, are the primary sources of tobacco used by children. According to one Minnesota survey, the most common sources of cigarettes for 10th graders were gas stations, convenience stores, and vending machines, followed by friends, grocery stores, and drug stores. Only 19 percent of respondents reported that they commonly obtained cigarettes from home (Forster, Klepp, Jeffery, in press). In a survey cited by Slade (1988a), 90 percent of 472 adolescents between 12 and 18 years of age reported that they bought their own cigarettes. In another survey, 92 percent of 172 suburban New Jersey high school students who smoked reported that they had purchased their last pack of cigarettes in a retail store; 5 percent had used a vending machine; and 3 percent had obtained their last pack from a friend (Slade et al., unpublished manuscript). A Canadian survey revealed that although older children tended to purchase their own cigarettes, children from 8 to 15 years of age were more likely to rely on other children as a source of cigarettes. The youngest children were the most likely to use vending machines, presumably because of greater difficulty in purchasing cigarettes from a store clerk (Stanwick et al. 1987).

Thus, purchases from retailers or vending machines, either by the child or the child's friends or siblings, appear to represent the main source of cigarettes for children. This conclusion is consistent with studies, discussed below, in which the majority of retail stores were observed to sell cigarettes illegally to minors who requested them (DiFranza et al. 1987; Altman et al. 1989 ; Slade et al., unpublished manuscript).

Children also obtain cigarettes and other tobacco products as free samples distributed for promotional purposes. Although the tobacco industry's voluntary codes prohibit the distribution of cigarette samples to individuals under 21 years of age (Tobacco Institute 1981) and the distribution of smokeless tobacco to children under 18 (Smokeless Tobacco, Inc. 1986), there is evidence of widespread violation of this code (Davis and Jason 1988). Even in a State where the free distribution of tobacco to minors is illegal, 4 percent of elementary school children and 20 percent of high school students reported having received free samples (Davis and Jason 1988). In another survey of suburban New Jersey high school students, one-third of over 500 current and former smokers had received free cigarette samples before age 16 (Slade et al., unpublished manuscript).

Consistent with these apparent trends, policies intended to reduce the availability of tobacco products to children include those that (1) restrict the sale and free distribution of these products to minors, (2) ban the use or possession of tobacco by minors, and (3) ban or limit the location of vending machines.

History of Tobacco Access Laws

The Federal Government has taken no action to regulate the access of minors to tobacco. Almost all restrictions are the result of legislation by States. Every State in the Union has at one time restricted the sale of tobacco to children. The right of States to do so was established at the turn of the century by the U.S. Supreme Court, which ruled that it is within a State's authority to ban the sale of tobacco (*Austin* v. *Tennessee* 1900). Several decades later the authority of local officials to ban the sale of cigarettes from vending machines was upheld by the Federal Court of Appeals, which ruled that such sales could be prohibited to prevent "the evil . . . of the purchase of cigarettes by immature minors" (*Illinois Cigarette Service Co.* v. *City of Chicago* 1937).

In 1964, when the first Surgeon General's Report on smoking was released, 48 States and the District of Columbia had active laws prohibiting the sale or gift of tobacco to children (Hawkins 1964). Two States, Louisiana and Wisconsin, had repealed their tobacco access laws before 1964 on the grounds that the laws were neither enforced nor enforceable. Louisiana did so in 1942, when the State legislature concluded that enforcement was impossible (Jacobs 1974). Wisconsin followed suit in 1955; the rationale was that because the law was not being enforced, it invited a disrespect for authority (Hawkins 1964). In the 48 State laws in effect in 1964, the minimum age for the purchase of tobacco ranged from 15 to 21. Eighteen States differentiated among various forms of tobacco, reflecting the belief that cigarettes were more dangerous than other tobacco products; 14 States restricted the sale of cigarettes but not that of cigars, pipe tobacco, or snuff, and 4 other States set the minimum age for the purchase of cigarettes higher than that for other forms of tobacco.

Since 1964, tobacco access laws have been rescinded in several other States and subsequently reinstated in only a few. More States have lowered the minimum age for sales of tobacco to children than have raised it. In addition, enforcement of laws in effect declined during the 1970s, when many high schools established student smoking areas (Jacobs 1974). In some cases this occurred in States where children were not legally permitted to purchase or possess tobacco.

There are fewer restrictions on child tobacco use now than at any time in many decades, despite what has been learned since 1964 about the dangers of tobacco use, its addictive nature, and the early age of its initiation. This situation is in sharp contrast to virtually all other tobacco-related public policy measures, which have been strengthened since the release of the 1964 Surgeon General's Report.

Current Tobacco Access Laws

As of January 1, 1988, 43 States and the District of Columbia had some legal restriction on the sale of cigarettes to children, while 7 States allowed children of any age to purchase tobacco in any form (Table 21). Since that time, Wisconsin enacted a law scheduled to take effect in 1989, and several other States have strengthened existing restrictions. The most common provision of State laws is to ban the sale of cigarettes to minors below a specified age. All State access laws have this provision, except South Dakota, whose law applies only to smokeless tobacco. In 11 States, the vendor must post signs wherever cigarettes are sold stating that it is illegal to sell tobacco to minors. In 36 States, the ban on sales extends beyond cigarettes to apply to all tobacco products (cigarettes, cigars, pipe tobacco, chewing tobacco, and snuff). Laws in 21 States also restrict the distribution of some types of smoking paraphernalia, such as cigarette papers or pipes. All of these laws address tobacco *sales*. Sixteen States have a broader ban,

TABLE 21.—State laws restricting minors' access to tobacco products (as of January 1, 1988)

	AL	AK	AZ	AR	CA	CO	CT	DE	DC	FL	GA	HI	ID	IL	IN	IA	KS
Minimum age for sale or possession	19[a]	16	18	18	18		16	17	16	18	17	15	18	18	18	18	18[a]
Prohibits use or possession of tobacco by minors			X										X	X	X		X[a]
Prohibits the sale of all tobacco products to minors			X	X	X		X	X	X	X	X	X	X	X	X	X	
Prohibits the sale of cigarettes to minors	X	X	X	X	X		X	X	X	X	X	X	X	X	X	X	X
Prohibits the free distribution of tobacco to minors	X	X	X	X	X		X	X	X	X	X	X	X	X	X	X	X
Prohibits all free distribution of tobacco																	
Prohibits cigarette vending machines accessible to minors													X				
Requires signs posted at point of sale					X									X	X		
Requires a license to sell tobacco	X	X	X	X	X	X	X	X	X	X	X	X	X	X	X	X	X
Provides for license revocation												X					
Penalties[b]	B	B	F	B	B		F	B	B	B		F	B	B	F	B	B
Enforcement provisions										X[c]						X[c]	

TABLE 21.—Continued

	KY	LA	ME	MD	MA	MI	MN	MS	MO	MT	NE	NV	NH	NJ	NM	NY	NC
Minimum age for sale or possession			18	16	18	18[d]	18	18			18	18	18	16		18	17
Prohibits use or possession of tobacco by minors						X	X				X		X				
Prohibits the sale of all tobacco products to minors			X		X	X	X				X	X	X	X		X	X
Prohibits the sale of cigarettes to minors			X	X	X	X	X	X			X	X	X	X		X	X
Prohibits the free distribution of tobacco to minors			X	X	X	X	X	X			X	X	X	X			X
Prohibits all free distribution of tobacco							X										
Prohibits cigarette vending machines accessible to minors																	
Requires signs posted at point of sale					X		X						X			X	
Requires a license to sell tobacco	X	X	X	X	X	X	X	X	X	X	X	X	X	X	X	X	X
Provides for license revocation											X	X					
Penalties			F	B	F	B	B	B			B	F	F	F		B	B
Enforcement provisions											X[c]						

TABLE 21.—Continued

	ND	OH	OK	OR	PA	RI	SC	SD	TN	TX	UT	VT	VA	WA	WV	WI	WY	TOTAL
Minimum age for sale or possession	18	18	18	18	16	16[a]	18	18	18	16	19	17	16	18	18			
Prohibits use or possession of tobacco by minors	X					X		X	X		X		X		X			16
Prohibits the sale of all tobacco products to minors	X	X		X			X	X		X	X	X	X	X	X			34
Prohibits the sale of cigarettes to minors	X	X	X	X	X	X	X	X	X	X	X	X	X	X	X			43
Prohibits the free distribution of tobacco to minors	X	X	X	X	X	X	X	X	X	X	X	X		X	X			41
Prohibits all free distribution of tobacco																		1
Prohibits cigarette vending machines accessible to minors											X							2
Requires signs posted at point of sale		X							X		X	X						11
Requires a license to sell tobacco	X	X	X	X	X	X	X	X	X	X	X	X	X	X		X	X	50
Provides for license revocation									X									4
Penalties	B	B	B	B	B	F	B	U	B	F	B	F	F	B	F			
Enforcement provisions			X[c e]				X[e]		X[f]						X[c]			7

TABLE 21.—Continued

NOTE: Since January 1, 1988, the following States have new age restrictions on the sale of tobacco products: CO, 18 years; CT, 18 years; GA, 17 years; HI, 18 years; NJ, 18 years; WI (effective 1989), 18 years.

[a]Applies only to cigarettes.

[b]F, fine; B, both jail or fine; U, unspecified.

[c]Provisions to encourage minors to divulge source of tobacco.

[d]For cigarettes only; minimum age for smokeless tobacco sale is 17 years.

[e]Provides a bounty to informers.

[f]Provides that it is not entrapment to send a minor into a store.

SOURCE: DiFranza et al. (1987); US DHHS (1986e).

covering not only tobacco sales, but also the use or possession of some form of tobacco by minors (DiFranza et al. 1987).

The minimum age for the legal purchase of tobacco ranges from 15 to 19 years. Two-thirds of the laws require the purchaser to be 18 years or older. However, 7 States that prohibit the sale of tobacco to minors allow children of any age to purchase tobacco if they have a note from their parent or guardian. An age limit of 19 years or higher has the theoretical advantage of ensuring that most high school students cannot legally use tobacco products. This would automatically ban student smoking on school grounds, make it easier for schools to eliminate tobacco and support other school-based antismoking efforts (Chapter 6).

The enforcement of tobacco access laws is left to local law enforcement officials in most States. The exceptions are New Hampshire, where the Commissioner of Revenue Administration sets enforcement rules, and Massachusetts, where the Department of Public Health enforces the law requiring that signs be posted at point of sale. Violation of tobacco access laws is a misdemeanor or petty offense, punishable by fine, imprisonment, or both. Minors found guilty of possession of tobacco face a fine under most laws and either fine or imprisonment in 3 States.

A few States have special provisions to facilitate enforcement. In Oklahoma and South Carolina, a portion of any fine levied against a merchant found guilty of selling tobacco to a minor goes to the witness who informed authorities of the violation (DiFranza et al. 1987). Tennessee law specifies that it is not entrapment for law enforcement authorities to have minors purchase tobacco for the purpose of monitoring retailer compliance with the law. Five States (Florida, Iowa, Nebraska, Oklahoma, and West Virginia) require minors caught in possession of tobacco to identify the person or business that provided the tobacco. In Nebraska and West Virginia, a juvenile who furnishes the identity of the person who provided the tobacco will be free from further prosecution (US DHHS 1986e).

With the exception of Virginia, the 43 States prohibiting tobacco sales to children also ban the distribution of free cigarette samples to minors. Communities that have banned all free cigarette distribution have also effectively banned distribution to children; these are discussed in the advertising section (Part I). A ban on all free distribution of tobacco products has been endorsed by the Surgeon General, the American Medical Association, the American Academy of Family Physicians, the Department of Health and Human Services, and others. In addition, opinion polls demonstrate that such an action is supported by a majority of the public (Davis and Jason 1988; Chapter 4).

By their design and intent, vending machines do not require supervision and allow easy access to minors (DiFranza et al. 1987). Despite survey data cited above suggesting that vending machines are an important source of cigarettes for children, as of October 1988, laws in only five States restrict minors' access to vending machines (Tobacco-Free America Project 1988b). Utah, Idaho, Alaska, and New Hampshire specify that vending machines must be inaccessible to minors, whereas Maine requires that vending machines be supervised by an adult (Tobacco-Free America Project 1988b). Nine States require the owners, operators, or supervisors of tobacco vending machines to post signs stating that minors are prohibited from purchasing cigarettes from that machine (Tobacco-Free America Project 1988b). At least one locality has enacted a law requiring supervision of cigarette vending machines. King County, WA, will ban unsupervised vending machines in unincorporated areas as of February 1, 1989 (Coughlin 1988).

The World Health Organization, American Medical Association, American Cancer Society, American Heart Association, American Lung Association, and others have called for a ban on cigarette vending machines, citing them as a major obstacle to the enforcement of tobacco access laws (WHO 1975, 1976, 1985; Bennett 1985; AMA 1987; DiFranza et al. 1987). The analogy between alcohol and tobacco has been made: it is illegal to sell alcohol from vending machines, and the same standard could apply to tobacco (US DHHS 1988, Preface). According to Census Bureau data, in 1982, vending machine sales of cigarettes represented only 6.2 percent of all cigarette sales (US DHHS 1987e), suggesting that the absence of vending machines would result in little inconvenience to adult smokers.

In addition to laws restricting tobacco sales to minors, every State except West Virginia requires that an individual obtain a license before distributing, retailing, wholesaling, or manufacturing cigarettes and other tobacco products. This licensing requirement appears to be for the purpose of facilitating the collection of State excise taxes rather than for enforcing compliance with laws on tobacco sales. Only four States (Hawaii, Nebraska, Nevada, and Tennessee) permit a vendor's license to be revoked for selling cigarettes to minors (DiFranza et al. 1987).

Few community ordinances have addressed the sale of tobacco to minors, but in the past decade at least 14 local communities have banned the free distribution of tobacco products, generally for the purpose of limiting minors' access to tobacco (Davis and Jason 1988; Tobacco-Free America Project 1988b).

Compliance With Tobacco Access Laws

For a law to reduce or eliminate the commercial availability of tobacco products to minors, tobacco vendors must be aware of and comply with the law, and appropriate public officials must enforce it. Compliance with tobacco access laws has been evaluated by determining the degree of difficulty a minor has in obtaining tobacco products. Two methods have been used. The first is to ask children how difficult it is for them to obtain tobacco. In 1987, nearly 90 percent of a sample of Minnesota 10th grade students who smoked regularly reported that it would be very easy for them to obtain cigarettes, despite a State law banning cigarette sales to children under 18 years of age (Forster, Klepp, Jeffery, in press). A survey in New Jersey found that 90 percent of 508 current and former high school student smokers were always or nearly always able to buy tobacco products before age 16 (Slade et al., unpublished manuscript).

A second, more reliable method of assessing compliance is to observe directly the degree of compliance by individual merchants in an experimental situation. In a recent study, an 11-year-old girl was successful in 75 of 100 attempts to purchase cigarettes in Massachusetts, a State that prohibits the sale of cigarettes to children under 18 years of age (DiFranza et al. 1987). Compliance with the law was six times greater in stores where signs were posted compared with stores without signs. Similar data collected by two nonprofit organizations, STAT (Stop Teen-age Addiction to Tobacco) and DOC (Doctors Ought to Care), and other investigators suggest that compliance with access laws is low throughout the United States (Kirn 1987; Altman et al. 1989; Slade et al., unpublished manuscript). Using the same method of sending a child into a business establishment to test compliance with the law, they found that an average of 80 percent of the retailers in five States were violating the law (Kirn 1987).

Two reasons have been identified for thc failure of these laws to reduce children's access to tobacco: vendors are unaware of the laws, and State and local authorities fail to enforce the laws (DiFranza et al. 1987). Current laws provide no mechanism to inform tobacco vendors of their responsibility to prevent children from purchasing tobacco. As a result, many vendors are unaware that it is illegal to sell tobacco to minors. For example, in Massachusetts, one-third of tobacco vendors were unaware of the law (DiFranza et al. 1987), and in New York, 40 percent were uninformed (Cummings and Marshall 1988).

Knowledge of the law by tobacco vendors is necessary but not sufficient for the law to succeed; knowledgeable vendors must also comply with the law. In Massachusetts, 73 percent of vendors who knew that it was illegal to sell tobacco to minors sold cigarettes to an 11-year-old girl (DiFranza et al. 1987). This suggests that vendors either have little fear that noncompliance will be detected or are not deterred by the potential punishment. Retailers have a strong financial incentive to sell cigarettes to children. Although the size of the market is not known, one rough estimate is that cigarette sales to children under 18 years of age are worth nearly 500 million dollars per year, and smokeless tobacco sales to this age group are worth an additional 130 million dollars (Slade 1988a). As noted above, it appears that children purchase most of their cigarettes themselves. Compliance will be achieved only if retailers are not only aware of tobacco access laws but also deterred from violating them by adequate penalties and effective enforcement. It has been estimated that there are hundreds of millions of such violations annually, yet law enforcement officials throughout the country have difficulty recalling instances in which a vendor was charged with violating the law (Kirn 1987). Under these circumstances, tobacco vendors may have little fear of prosecution, and therefore, little incentive to comply with the law. They may also not appreciate the magnitude of harm caused by tobacco or the importance of their sales in the initiation of smoking.

There are several reasons why these laws are not enforced. The provisions of some laws make enforcement difficult. In Washington, DC, for example, an arrest cannot be made without a warrant, and the arresting officer must personally witness the crime. Indiana law provides that a vendor may use as a defense that he or she "reasonably believed that the buyer or taker was at least eighteen years of age." This places the burden on the prosecutor to prove not only that a child under 18 was sold tobacco, but also that the child would appear under age to a reasonable person.

A 1987 survey of law enforcement officials in 25 States identified attitudinal barriers to the enforcement of tobacco access laws (Uzych, unpublished manuscript). Overall, the officials felt that the laws could not, should not, or need not be vigorously enforced. The most commonly held belief was that the laws were unenforceable. There was substantial evidence that little or no effort was being made to enforce tobacco access laws.

The most common policy cited by survey respondents was to enforce the law "only if specific complaints have been received," or "only if violations are conspicuous." Some respondents felt the law was self-enforcing for retailers, while others felt enforcement of tobacco access laws was not the business of law enforcement officials, because tobacco sales to minors is a "health issue rather than a public safety issue"; "tobacco, a legal substance, does not have as a side effect anti-social behavior"; or "possession of tobacco by a minor is not . . . considered a grave offense" (Uzych, unpublished manuscript). These data suggest that widespread and substantial changes in the attitudes and priorities of law enforcement officials would be needed if conventional enforcement were to become effective. These changes include a shift in attitudes about the importance of smoking by children, the importance of enforcement, and the ability of law enforcement officers to enforce the law.

An alternative approach to enforcement that has been suggested is to transfer the responsibility from law enforcement agencies to public health departments (DiFranza, 1988). Public health departments traditionally have had both enforcement and licensing responsibilities. Public health inspectors routinely make unannounced visits to restaurants and food stores to monitor compliance with health and safety statutes. They are given the authority to issue citations or to revoke a vendor's license. Public health inspectors could also be assigned to ensure that tobacco vendors comply with tobacco access laws. It has been suggested that revenues from fines and the licensing of vendors might cover the cost of enforcement and even potentially be a source of State revenues (DiFranza 1988). It has also been suggested that some of the estimated excise tax revenues derived from the sale of tobacco to children be dedicated to enforcement. For New Jersey alone, this was recently estimated at 3 million dollars per year (Slade 1988a).

As an alternative to increasing enforcement, efforts could be made to increase tobacco vendors' knowledge of and compliance with existing laws. Educational efforts that target tobacco vendors have recently been developed in several States. They have shown promise in preliminary studies (Altman et al. 1989; Slade et al., unpublished manuscript). One study in Santa Clara County, CA, documented a significant reduction in illegal tobacco sales to minors after a 6-month campaign using mass media, direct merchant education, contact with management of chain stores and franchises, and community organization (Altman et al. 1989).

Legal tactics to increase compliance have also been pursued, so far without success. In *Parker* v. *City School Superintendent*, action was brought against school officials for providing students with a smoking lounge in a State that prohibited smoking by children under 18 (Jacobs 1974). The Supreme Court of Missouri ruled that smoking of cigarettes by minors was a misdemeanor and did not give rise to a civil cause of action. In another case, the Group Against Smoking Pollution (GASP) of Massachusetts filed a lawsuit on behalf of a 16-year-old girl who began smoking at the age of 14 and was illegally sold cigarettes for 2 years by a local convenience store. The suit charged the convenience store chain and the cigarette manufacturer with the "negligent entrustment of a dangerous instrumentality to minors" in violation of a State law prohibiting the sale of tobacco to minors. The case is pending (GASP 1987).

Effects of Current Access Laws

There has been little systematic evaluation of the impact of tobacco access restrictions. As described above, considerable evidence indicates that compliance is low and enforcement is poor, with the result that tobacco products are relatively easy for children to obtain. Under these circumstances, it is impossible to test hypotheses about the impact of tobacco access restrictions on smoking behavior.

It would be surprising if laws as currently implemented had much effect on the initiation of tobacco use by children. If tobacco access laws were adequately implemented, it would be possible to test the effect of a program of merchant education or strong enforcement on tobacco availability and, ultimately, on smoking behavior. However, comparisons of adolescent smoking rates in States with and without tobacco access laws or strong enforcement might be confounded by other cultural, economic, and demographic factors that can affect the prevalence of smoking among children.

Summary

Despite existing legislation in 43 States and the District of Columbia restricting the sale of cigarettes to minors, tobacco products are relatively easy for children to obtain. Tobacco vendors are often unaware of tobacco access laws, and law enforcement agencies do not enforce them. Furthermore, there are gaps in legislation. Seven States currently have no law prohibiting the sale or distribution of cigarettes to minors, and laws in many other States are not comprehensive. For example, some laws do not include all tobacco products, and a dozen permit children under 18 years of age to be sold tobacco. Only a few prohibit the use or possession of tobacco by children.

This situation could be ameliorated by improving the compliance with and enforcement of laws currently in effect, by amending current legislation, and by enacting new legislation. Because even new legislation would require adequate implementation to achieve its goals, efforts to ensure compliance with and enforcement of tobacco access laws are essential to achieve meaningful reductions in the availability of cigarettes to children. Moreover, interest in the enactment of new laws might be limited by the poor compliance record of past legislation, suggesting the importance of improving the implementation of existing laws.

The adoption of a uniform comprehensive tobacco access law throughout the United States has been proposed by several groups as one means to eliminate some of the loopholes through which children now legally obtain and use tobacco (AMA 1987; DiFranza et al. 1987; Stanwick et al. 1987; Cummings and Marshall 1988). The sale of tobacco to minors has been banned on a national level in Great Britain and Canada (Walker 1980; Stanwick et al. 1987). Model tobacco access laws, designed to protect children from tobacco, have been developed by the American Medical Association (AMA) and others (AMA 1987; DiFranza et al. 1987; Stanwick et al. 1987; Cummings and Marshall 1988). The provisions of these laws are similar. A number of provisions are borrowed from alcohol control efforts; these include banning all sales to minors, limiting sales to a small number of licensed vendors (which would eliminate vending machine sales), and requiring purchasers to show positive proof of age. Legislation was introduced in the 100th Congress (H.R. 3658) that would prohibit the sale of cigarettes and other tobacco products to anyone under the age of 18, limit sales to over-the-counter sales (that is, prohibit vending machine sales), and require every retail establishment selling tobacco products to post conspicuously a sign stating, "The Sale of Cigarettes to Minors is Strictly Prohibited" (Atkins 1987). Proponents of comprehensive access laws draw an analogy between alcohol and tobacco and express the view that the sale of tobacco should be considered as seriously as the sale of alcohol and other addictive drugs (US DHHS 1988, Preface; Stanwick et al. 1987).

Federal Regulation of Tobacco Products

Because the use of tobacco products is hazardous to the health and safety of consumers, the regulation of tobacco products would be consistent with the established tradition of health and safety regulation for other consumer products. However, with few exceptions (e.g., see Part I regarding labeling and advertising regulations), none of the Federal agencies charged with health and safety regulation has taken regulatory action against tobacco products, due in part to specific statutory restrictions. There are a number of possible reasons for the lack of regulation, including the fact that millions of Americans became addicted to tobacco before its hazards were understood (Walsh and Gordon 1986).

In contrast to its approach to tobacco, Congress has passed a number of laws over the last two decades that strictly regulate other hazardous consumer, environmental, and occupational exposures. The primary aim of these laws is to reduce the risk of cancer, reproductive hazards, and injuries. An analysis by Morrall (1986) of the impact of 26 final rules promulgated under these acts suggested that the estimated number of lives they saved collectively each year was far smaller than the annual number of lives lost because of cigarette smoking. Doll and Peto (1981) have estimated that the proportions of cancers attributable to occupational and environmental exposures are 4 and 2 percent, respectively, in contrast to the estimated 30 percent of cancer deaths that are caused by smoking (Chapter 3).

This Section examines the history of tobacco product regulation for health and safety purposes. The focus is on actions of the Federal Government, although relevant State actions are also mentioned.

Regulation of Tobacco Products Prior to 1964

In 1892, during a period in which several States were considering bans on cigarette sales, the U.S. Senate's Committee on Epidemic Diseases studied the cigarette issue and decided it was properly a State matter (Dillow 1981). By 1908, 11 States had banned the sale of cigarettes, primarily on the basis of aesthetic and moral objections and on the basis of health concerns that were poorly documented at that time. The laws proved unenforceable and were gradually repealed (Dillow 1981; Whelan 1984).

The Food and Drugs Act of 1906, the first Federal food and drug law, contained no express reference to tobacco products. It defined a drug as including medicines and preparations recognized in the United States Pharmacopeia (USP) or the National Formulary. Tobacco was listed in the 1890 edition of the USP, but it was deleted in the next edition, which was released in 1905. Neuberger (1963) stated that this deletion was rumored to have been made in exchange for support from tobacco-State Congressmen for passage of the law.

The 1906 Act also defined a drug as including substances intended to be used for the cure, mitigation, or prevention of disease in man or other animals. In 1914, the chief of the Bureau of Chemistry in the U.S. Department of Agriculture, the predecessor to the Food and Drug Administration (FDA), interpreted the 1906 Act by advising:

> [T]obacco and its preparations, when labeled in such a manner as to indicate their use for the cure, mitigation, or prevention of disease, are drugs within the meaning of the act, and, as such, are subject to the provisions thereof.
>
> On the other hand, tobacco and its preparations which are not so labeled and are used for smoking or chewing or as snuff and not for medicinal purposes are not subject to the provisions of the act (USDA 1914).

The 1906 Act was superseded in 1938 by the Federal Food, Drug, and Cosmetic Act (FFDCA), which gives FDA jurisdiction with respect to food, drugs, medical devices, and cosmetics. The definition of drug was expanded to include articles recognized in the Homeopathic Pharmacopeia. The current Homeopathic Pharmacopeia contains a monograph (i.e., a listing) for tobacco in the form of a tincture for application as a drug. Conventional cigarettes made from tobacco leaves are not recognized as drugs in any of the official compendia referred to in the "drug" definition of the FFDCA.

As further revised, the definition of "drug" in the FFDCA also includes "articles intended for use in the diagnosis, cure, mitigation, treatment, or prevention of disease in man or other animals" and "articles (other than food) intended to affect the structure or any function of the body of man or other animals" (FFDCA).

The FFDCA has not referred specifically to tobacco products as articles either within or outside the scope of jurisdiction under the Act. Tobacco products, as they have been customarily marketed, have not been considered by the FDA to fall within any of the categories over which the agency has jurisdiction (Young 1988). However, the agency has taken jurisdiction over tobacco products on the grounds that they are "drugs" when the manufacturer or vendor has made medical claims for the product (Young 1988). The FDA used this authority to assert jurisdiction over cigarettes in two cases during the 1950s, in which the FDA's jurisdiction was upheld in court. The first action involved Fairfax Cigarettes, which the manufacturer claimed to prevent respiratory and other diseases (*United States* v. *46 Cartons . . . Fairfax Cigarettes* 1953). The second action involved Trim Reducing-Aid Cigarettes, which contained the additive tartaric acid, which was claimed to aid the smoker in weight reduction (*United States* v. *354 Bulk Cartons . . . Trim Reducing-Aid Cigarettes* 1959).

In a 1952 court case that involved the Federal Trade Commission (FTC), the FTC contended that the manufacturer deceptively advertised Chesterfield cigarettes and that the cigarettes were a drug by a definition virtually identical to that in the FFDCA (*Federal Trade Commission* v. *Liggett and Myers Tobacco Company* 1952). The court ruled that Chesterfield cigarettes did not meet the definition of a drug at issue in the case. The FTC argument that the cigarettes were a drug was based in part on two types of representations by the manufacturer. The first type was that the cigarettes did not cause irritation of the throat and nose. The court ruled that this was not an affirmative claim of a beneficial effect or therapeutic purpose, but was merely a representation that the cigarettes had a nonadverse effect, and that such a representation was insufficient to find the product to be a drug. The second type of representation, which the FTC relied upon in asserting that the cigarettes were intended by the manufacturer to affect the functions of the body, was that the cigarettes had a "soothing effect." This was considered by the court to be not the type of bodily effect contemplated by the statute.

The FDA received new authority to regulate consumer products in 1960, with passage of the first Federal Hazardous Substances Labeling Act (FHSA), under which the definition of hazardous substance comprised six categories including toxic, corrosive, irritant, strong sensitizer, flammable, or pressure-generating substance, which may cause substantial personal injury or illness during or as a result of customary or reasonable use. Tobacco products were not specifically excluded. However, the FDA did not regulate tobacco products under that law.

In 1963, FDA expressed its interpretation that tobacco did not qualify as a hazardous substance under the FHSA. It noted that tobacco did not appear to fit within any of the FHSA's six classifications, and that at no time during the congressional consideration of the FHSA was there any indication that it was intended to cover tobacco (FDA 1963). In the same document, FDA also noted that the Surgeon General of the Public Health Service had recently appointed an Advisory Committee on Smoking and Health, and FDA stated its preference to withhold making any recommendations on Federal action regarding tobacco until the committee's report was issued (FDA 1963).

Regulation of Tobacco Products After 1964

Following the 1964 Surgeon General's Report, Congress considered a number of bills to regulate tobacco. From 1965 through 1978, over 75 bills were introduced into Congress on a wide variety of issues designed to address the smoking problem (Klebe 1979). The first U.S. House of Representatives bill dealing with smoking (H.R. 2248, 89th Congress) proposed amending the FFDCA to place cigarettes under the authority of the FDA. Because there was no known safe level for tar, nicotine, or other tobacco constituents, regulation would have likely resulted in prohibition of a product that was widely used. Instead, following considerable debate, the House Committee on Interstate and Foreign Commerce reported out H.R. 3014 (89th Congress), which called for warning labels on packages. This bill, along with its Senate counterpart, led to the first Federal cigarette labeling act (see Part I).

Other bills to regulate tobacco products indirectly by encouraging or requiring lower tar or nicotine levels were introduced. Of the bills filed during the next 6 sessions, 13 contained provisions for taxing cigarettes according to tar and nicotine content or cigarette length. Three other bills would have established maximum levels for tar and nicotine content or cigarette length. None of these bills became law.

Consumer health and safety laws enacted after 1964 might have led to the regulation of tobacco products. However, tobacco was specifically excluded in virtually all major bills passed after 1964. In 1970, Congress passed the Controlled Substances Act to prevent the abuse of drugs, narcotics, and other addictive substances. In view of the scientific knowledge of nicotine's effects subsequently reported in the 1988 Surgeon General's Report (US DHHS 1988), nicotine would seem to be the type of substance the statute was intended to regulate. However, the law specifically excluded tobacco from the definition of a "controlled substance" in 21 U.S.C. 802(6).

In 1972, Congress passed the Consumer Product Safety Act (CPSA) and established the Consumer Product Safety Commission (CPSC), an independent regulatory agency, to administer the law. The Act excluded tobacco and tobacco products from the definition of "consumer product" (15 U.S.C. 2052 (a)(1)(B)). The Act also transferred authority for FHSA from the FDA to CPSC. Tobacco had not been exempted from FHSA when it was first passed in 1960. The American Public Health Association and others petitioned CPSC to set a maximum level of 21 mg of tar in cigarettes, under the authority of FHSA. In 1974, CPSC voted 3 to 2 that it lacked the authority to do so. The decision was appealed, and in April 1975, the U.S. District Court for the District of Columbia ruled that CPSC had jurisdiction and ordered it to consider the petition (*American Public Health Association* v. *Consumer Product Safety Commission* 1975). On May 11, 1976, Congress amended FHSA to exclude tobacco or tobacco products from the definition of hazardous substances. After this action, the court's decision was moot (Klebe 1979). The Senate report on the action stated that the change was made to clarify Congress' original intent and "should not be interpreted as reflecting any new judgment on smoking and health" (Senate Report No. 94-251 (June 24, 1975) for Public Law 94-284).

In 1976, Congress passed the Toxic Substances Control Act. One purpose of the Act was to "regulate chemical substances and mixtures which present an unreasonable risk of injury to health or the environment . . . " (15 U.S.C. 2601 (b)). Evidence reported in the Surgeon General's reports indicates that tobacco and tobacco products could have otherwise met the definition of "chemical substance" under the Act. However, the Act excluded tobacco and tobacco products from that definition (15 U.S.C. 2602(2)(B)(iii)).

In 1977, the FDA was petitioned by Action on Smoking and Health (ASH) and others to assert jurisdiction over cigarettes as a "drug" or a "medical device" under the definitions of the FFDCA and to restrict the sale of cigarettes to pharmacies. FDA denied those requests (FDA 1977, FDA 1980), finding that the administrative records relating to the requests did not contain the requisite evidence of intended use to bring cigarettes within the drug or device definitions. ASH appealed the 1977 denial of its request that FDA assert jurisdiction over cigarettes as a drug. The U.S. Court of Appeals for the District of Columbia Circuit upheld the FDA's interpretation of the scope of its jurisdiction over cigarettes (*Action on Smoking and Health* v. *Harris* 1980). ASH did not appeal FDA's denial (FDA 1980) of the request by ASH that FDA assert jurisdiction over cigarettes as medical devices.

In 1988, the Coalition on Smoking OR Health petitioned the FDA to declare low-tar and low-nicotine cigarettes to be a drug, asserting that manufacturers market them with the intent of creating a consumer perception that they will mitigate or prevent disease (Coalition on Smoking OR Health 1988a). The petitioners introduced evidence obtained through the discovery process in a 1988 New Jersey tobacco product liability lawsuit that, in their view, documents manufacturer intent. In that suit, the jury found that the tobacco manufacturer had made express warranties to the consumer about the health aspects of its cigarettes (*Cipollone* v. *Liggett Group Inc. et al.* 1988). The petition was pending as of November 1988.

The issue of whether tobacco could be classified as a hazardous substance under FHSA was addressed again in 1984 in a tobacco product liability suit (*Palmer* v. *Liggett Group Inc.* 1984). The plaintiffs claimed that the tobacco manufacturer violated FHSA by failing to place warning labels on cigarette packages from 1960, when the first FHSA became law, until 1965, when the Federal Cigarette Labeling and Advertising Act preempted cigarette labeling except as required under the Cigarette Act. The U.S. District Court dismissed this claim, citing the legislative history of FHSA as evidence that the intent of the legislators was not to cover tobacco, but to protect against accidental poisonings by household chemicals.

In 1985, the Massachusetts Department of Public Health, acting under the authority of the State hazardous substance law, which was modeled after the Federal law, declared oral snuff to be a hazardous substance and required protective labeling on packages as of July 1985. The State law, unlike the Federal statute, was never amended to exclude tobacco. The Massachusetts action was followed by a wave of labeling bills in other States and, the following year, by Congress' passage of the Comprehensive Smokeless Tobacco Health Education Act of 1986 (Public Law 99-252). That Federal law preempted the Massachusetts labeling requirement. However, oral snuff is still classified as a hazardous substance in Massachusetts (Connolly et al. 1986).

Tobacco products have also been classified as hazardous substances in another State. In 1986, California adopted the Safe Drinking Water and Toxic Substances Enforcement Act, which requires warnings for and regulation of chemicals known to cause cancer and reproductive toxic effects (Kizer, Warriner, Book 1988). Tobacco has been identified as a carcinogen and reproductive toxicant under the law. In August 1988, four environmental groups announced plans to file a lawsuit that would require that a warning label about cancer and reproductive risks be placed on store shelves containing tobacco products that do not carry the Surgeon General's warning. These products include cigars, pipe tobacco, and roll-your-own cigarette tobacco (Matthews 1988). In a settlement reached on October 18, 1988, 25 tobacco manufacturers agreed to place a warning label on cigars and pipe tobacco sold in California (Wilson 1988a). Canada has also defined tobacco as a hazardous product in Federal legislation passed in 1988 (House of Commons of Canada 1988; C-204, 1988).

Currently, most Federal regulation of tobacco products is administered by the Bureau of Alcohol, Tobacco, and Firearms (BATF) of the Department of the Treasury, and by the Federal Trade Commission (FTC). Regulation by BATF involves tobacco taxation with no intended impact on public health concerns, while the FTC actions involve advertising of tobacco products and the disclosure of health risks, as described in detail in Part I of this Chapter.

Environmental Tobacco Smoke Exposure

The Occupational Safety and Health Act, passed in 1970, empowers the Labor Department's Occupational Safety and Health Administration (OSHA) to ensure that:

> Each employer shall furnish to each of his employees employment and a place of employment which are free from recognized hazards that are causing or are likely to cause death or serious physical harm to his employees.

OSHA has set standards limiting occupational exposure to 24 airborne materials that are present in tobacco smoke, including carbon monoxide and acrolein. Even though environmental tobacco smoke (ETS) is not excluded from OSHA's review, the agency has not sought to regulate it. A 1986 petition (Horne et al. 1986) requested OSHA to classify ETS as a category I potential occupational carcinogen. The petition was denied. In 1987, ASH, joined by the American Public Health Association and the Public Citizens Health Research Group, requested an emergency temporary standard to prohibit smoking in indoor workplaces under the authority of the OSHA law. As of November 1988, these petitions were pending (Public Citizen 1987).

The Clean Air Act of 1963 (Clean Air Act 1963) requires the Environmental Protection Agency (EPA) to regulate airborne pollutants. EPA has set standards for maximum acceptable exposures to pollutants that are also constituents of ETS, including carbon monoxide and nitrogen dioxide. However, EPA has interpreted the statute to apply to outdoor air pollutants only and has not moved to regulate exposure to ETS.

Tobacco Product Additives

Exclusion of tobacco and tobacco products from Federal health and safety laws also resulted in the exemption of tobacco product additives from regulatory review. The 1981 Surgeon General's Report, *The Changing Cigarette*, noted that additives may be in greater use in the low-tar brands to compensate for a loss in "flavor" brought about by tar reduction (US DHHS 1981a). The Report noted that it was impossible to assess the risks of the additives because manufacturers were not required to disclose the additives. The issue of additives was raised again in the 1984 Surgeon General's Report, citing the presence of powdered cocoa, which had been shown to enhance the carcinogenicity of tar. The Report observed:

> A characterization of the chemical composition and adverse biological potential of these additives is urgently needed, but is currently impossible because cigarette companies are not required to reveal what additives they employ in the manufacture of cigarettes (US DHHS 1984).

A 1978 amendment to the Public Health Service Act (Public Law 95-626) contained a number of tobacco-specific provisions. One called for a Department of Health and Human Services (DHHS) study of the health risks of cigarette additives. Attempts by DHHS to obtain complete, updated lists of additives from tobacco manufacturers were unsuccessful (Cummins 1983). As discussed in Part I of this Chapter, the Comprehensive Smoking Education Act of 1984 (Public Law 98-474) required manufacturers to provide the Secretary of DHHS with a list of all ingredients. However, the Secretary's authorities were limited to conducting research on the additives and reporting back to Congress with findings on their potential health effects. No authority was granted to restrict or eliminate ingredients found to be harmful.

In 1988, CA. Blockers, Inc., announced development of a cigarette additive that allegedly blocks the action of nitrosamines and its carcinogenic metabolites contained in tobacco smoke. The company intended to introduce the product into the market without FDA approval, stating that the company would make no health claims (CA. Blockers, Inc. 1988). However, the company's prospectus describes the action of the additive as blocking receptors in the lungs and states that its goal is "to eliminate a health risk associated with cigarette smoking" (CA. Blockers, Inc. 1987). The FDA has initiated an investigation of this matter, which was under review as of November 1988.

Fire Safety of Cigarettes

Over 1,500 deaths each year are caused by fires ignited by burning cigarettes (Hall 1987). Even though this number is low in comparison with the estimate of 390,000 deaths caused by smoking-related diseases (Chapter 3), public concern is high because many victims are nonsmoking infants and children or disabled persons (Botkin 1988). Congressional legislation calling for "fire-safe" (e.g., self-extinguishing) cigarettes was first introduced in 1974 and reintroduced in 1979. In 1983, eight States considered similar legislation but none was enacted (McGuire 1983; Garner 1985). In 1984, Congress passed the Cigarette Safety Act (Public Law 98-567). The purpose of the law was to

> determine the technical and commercial feasibility of developing cigarettes and little cigars that would be less likely to ignite upholstered furniture and mattresses (CPSC 1987).

The Act established an Interagency Committee (IAC) for Cigarette and Little Cigar Fire Safety that included representatives from CPSC, DHHS, and the U.S. Fire Administrator's Office. The IAC was advised by a Technical Study Group (TSG), which was charged with undertaking "such studies and other activities as considered necessary and appropriate to determine the technical and commercial feasibility" of developing a fire-safe cigarette. Following 2 years of work, TSG concluded that it is technically feasible and may be commercially feasible to develop a cigarette with a significantly reduced potential for igniting fires. After reviewing these findings, IAC concluded that issues concerning the economic feasibility, consumer acceptance, and health implications were unresolved. IAC recommended the formation and funding of a new advisory committee that, within 2 years of its formation, would develop and test a prototype of a less ignition-prone cigarette. Two months before IAC made its report to Congress, a major cigarette manufacturer announced the development of a new product, commonly referred to in the press as a "smokeless cigarette" that, when lying flat, is purportedly unlikely to ignite most materials with which it comes into contact (R.J. Reynolds Tobacco Co. 1987) (see below). Legislation was introduced in the 100th Congress to fund work of the new advisory committee and also to require the FDA to set fire safety standards (H.R. 3440, S. 1763).

Smokeless Tobacco Products

When the 1964 Surgeon General's Report was issued, the use of snuff and chewing tobacco was on the decline and there was little interest in Congress or the public health community in dealing with smokeless tobacco. In 1965, the Federal excise tax on smokeless tobacco products was repealed. Smokeless tobacco products, particularly moist snuff, were more aggressively marketed in the late 1970s by tobacco manufacturers and promoted as an alternative to the cigarette (Connolly et al. 1986).

In the absence of restrictions on advertising, moist snuff was marketed without warning labels on television and in other media. From 1978 through 1985, sales for moist snuff rose by 55 percent. By 1985, there were an estimated 13 million users nationally, of whom 3 million were below 21 years of age (US DHHS 1986c). Tobacco manufacturers developed low-nicotine snuff products that may be used as a "starter" to snuff use. A graduation strategy was employed in which the new users were encouraged to switch to higher nicotine brands over time (Connolly 1986; Connolly et al. 1986; Feigelson 1983).

As described in Part I, legislation to require health warning labels on smokeless tobacco packages was pending in 26 States when manufacturers, faced with the possibility of multiple different State labeling requirements, sought a uniform national law that preempted State action (Connolly et al. 1986). One State (Utah) considered but did not pass legislation to ban smokeless tobacco use (Utah House of Representatives 1986). Existing policies for cigarettes (excise taxes, prohibition on sales to minors, ban on television advertising, and warning labels on packages and print ads) were extended to apply to smokeless tobacco at the Federal and State levels.

Alternative Nicotine-Containing Products

Beginning in 1985, tobacco manufacturers introduced a variety of new products that delivered nicotine to the user and produced little or no smoke. The public health impact of the marketing of these new products is unknown because limited information is available about the products or their appeal. The 1988 Surgeon General's Report on nicotine addiction compared the use of the alternative nicotine delivery systems, in combination with regular cigarettes, with the "nonmedically approved use of methadone by opioid-dependent individuals when their drug of choice (e.g., heroin) is not available, and they are not involved in treatment for opioid dependence" (US DHHS 1988). The public health community has expressed concern that the alternative nicotine delivery systems will encourage experimentation among non-tobacco-using adolescents, will be used as an alternative to cessation by current smokers, may encourage relapse among former smokers, and may be used where smoking is prohibited (Slade 1988b; AMA 1988; Coalition on Smoking OR Health 1988b). The 1988 Surgeon General's Report called for an evaluation of the potential toxic and addictive effects of new nicotine-containing products (US DHHS 1988).

Whether these alternative nicotine delivery products are "drugs" or "devices" as defined by the FFDCA (and therefore subject to FDA jurisdiction) is being addressed on a case-by-case basis. The Commissioner of the FDA took the following position in testimony before Congress:

> [T]he Agency must attempt to differentiate between the traditional tobacco product marketed without medical claims, and therefore not regulated by FDA, and the newer innovations designed to deliver nicotine to satisfy a nicotine dependence or otherwise to affect the structure or function of the body. FDA must decide, on a case-by-case basis, which product is subject to the FDC Act (Young 1988).

The FDA has reviewed or is reviewing four nicotine-containing products described below. In three cases, the FDA exerted jurisdiction over the product; two of these were removed from the market and one was approved for sale as a new drug. A decision in the fourth case has not been reached, as of November 1988.

A device called the Favor Smokeless Cigarette was introduced in 1985. This cigarette-sized white plastic tube had a fibrous plug impregnated with nicotine at one end. Users sucked air through the other end, drawing a nicotine aerosol into the oral cavity. The product contained nicotine purportedly derived from tobacco but did not contain tobacco leaf. In February 1987, the FDA determined that Favor was "a nicotine delivery system intended to satisfy a nicotine dependence and to affect the structure and one or more functions of the body" (FDA 1987a; Young 1988; FDA letter to Congressman Waxman 1987b). As such, it met the FDA definition of a drug. The FDA also determined that Favor was a "new drug" within the meaning of the FFDCA because its composition was not generally recognized as safe and effective under the prescribed or recommended conditions of use (Young 1988). The FDA went on to state in the regulatory letter (FDA 1987a):

> The medical literature clearly recognizes that nicotine is well absorbed from the lungs; that it has potent pharmacologic effects, including effects on the nervous system; and that nicotine is a drug of dependence. . . . [I]t is our position that Favor is a nicotine delivery system intended to satisfy a nicotine dependence and to affect the structure and one or more functions of the body. Because of its intended uses, Favor is a drug as defined within section 201(g) of the Federal Food, Drug, and Cosmetic Act.

In 1987, the Pinkerton Tobacco Company introduced Masterpiece Tobacs, a tobacco chewing gum containing approximately 1 mg of nicotine. By the appearance and function of the product, the FDA determined that it was a food and because it contained tobacco, which is generally not considered safe for use in foods, it was an adulterated food. Both products, Favor Smokeless Cigarettes and Masterpiece Tobacs, have been removed from the marketplace (FDA letter to Congressman Waxman 1987b). A tobacco toothpaste containing ground snuff was introduced for sale in Indian food stores in the United States in 1987. Possible regulation was under review by the FDA as of November 1988.

The FDA has approved and allowed for sale nicotine polacrilex chewing gum, intended and labeled as a smoking cessation product and available only with a physician's prescription. The manufacturer subjected the gum to new drug safety and efficacy testing as a smoking cessation aid, and a New Drug Application for the product was approved in January 1984 (FDA letter to Congressman Waxman 1987b; Chapter 6).

In the fall of 1987, R.J. Reynolds Tobacco Company (RJR) announced the development of a new product whose exterior resembles a cigarette but whose composition is based on a technology not previously associated with conventional cigarettes. The device contains an insulated carbon fuel element at one end that is ignited and emits heat that is drawn across a bead-filled aluminum chamber, around which tobacco is wrapped. The chamber contains nicotine from a tobacco extract, flavorings, and a humectant. These are nebulized to form a smoke-like aerosol containing nicotine, carbon monoxide, carbon dioxide, and other ingredients. The company claims that less sidestream smoke is released into the environment. RJR also claims that the new product results in a substantial reduction in the number and concentration of compounds delivered to the user (RJR 1985b, 1987, 1988). However, many of the toxic and carcinogenic constituents typically present in the "tar" component of tobacco smoke (e.g., benzo(*a*)pyrene) are still present in the aerosol (RJR 1988). In addition, concern has been expressed that the product can be manipulated easily to allow it to be used to deliver "crack" cocaine (Cone and Henningfield 1989).

In October 1988, R.J. Reynolds began test marketing this product under the name Premier. The FDA has been petitioned by the American Medical Association and the Coalition on Smoking OR Health to exert jurisdiction over the new product on the grounds that it is a drug or medical device and that health claims are being made (AMA 1988, Coalition on Smoking OR Health 1988b). As of November 1988, the FDA had both petitions under review. (See Chapter 5.)

Summary

Since the first Surgeon General's Report in 1964, a number of proposals have been made for FDA or other agencies to regulate tobacco products or their ingredients because of their effects on health and safety. These efforts have been unsuccessful except in a few cases when manufacturers made health claims or when FDA deemed the product to be a food. Since there are no known safe levels for tar, nicotine, or other tobacco ingredients, in the absence of legislation, FDA regulation would probably have resulted in a ban of tobacco products, even those that might have been made less hazardous than conventional cigarettes. Instead of allowing regulation by Federal agencies, Congress in most cases reserved to itself jurisdiction over tobacco products, banned tobacco advertising in broadcast media, and required a disclosure of risks on packages and print ads (See Part I of this Chapter). This approach, however, allowed tobacco manufacturers to modify products and introduce new ones without subjecting them to the scrutiny of Federal agencies concerned with health and product safety.

During the early 1970s, low-yield cigarettes were introduced and implicitly promoted as being less hazardous than conventional products (Davis 1987; US DHHS 1981a; Chapter 5). Beginning in the late 1970s smokeless tobacco was more aggressively marketed as an alternative to smoked tobacco. Sheppard (1985) has described this as the "controlled" tobacco product cycle in which cigarette manufacturers manage existing demand and create new demand by varying the form of the tobacco product as public awareness about the dangers of traditional cigarettes increases.

Several approaches have been proposed to increase the regulation of tobacco products without resulting in a total ban. The first proposal would regulate new products or new product modifications while exempting existing products from regulatory review. An international example of this approach to product regulation concerns the introduction of smokeless tobacco products into countries with no established smokeless tobacco users. In 1987, the World Health Organization Study Group on Smokeless Tobacco recommended that such countries prohibit smokeless tobacco products before their use became common (WHO, in press). Based on this recommendation, four nations whose residents have no history of using oral snuff (Australia, New Zealand, Hong Kong, and Saudi Arabia) banned the manufacture, sale, or importation of oral snuff; Ireland banned the sale of snuff, and Great Britain had legislation pending as of November 1988. A second approach to tobacco product regulation would continue to recognize the special status of tobacco products but regulate their marketing and sales in line with the marketing of other drugs and alcohol. A third approach is to use legislation to bring tobacco products under the jurisdiction of Federal regulatory agencies without banning them by explicitly limiting the power of the Federal agency. Legislation introduced in Congress in 1987 included provisions that would bring tobacco products under regulatory control of the FDA and the CPSC (H.R. 2376 and H.R. 3294), but these bills were not enacted.

CONCLUSIONS

Part I. Policies Pertaining to Information and Education

1. The Federal Government's efforts to reduce the health consequences of cigarette smoking have consisted primarily of providing the public with information and education about the hazards of tobacco use. Two of the most well-known mechanisms are the publication of Surgeon General's Reports and the requirement of warning labels on cigarette packages. A system of rotating health warning labels is now required for all cigarette and smokeless tobacco packaging and advertisements.
2. Current laws do not require health warning labels on all tobacco products and do not require monitoring of the communications effectiveness of the warnings. Furthermore, existing laws do not provide administrative mechanisms to update the contents of labels to prevent the overexposure of current messages or to reflect advances in scientific knowledge, such as new information about the addictive nature of tobacco use.
3. There is insufficient evidence to determine the independent effect of cigarette warning labels, particularly the rotating warning labels required since 1985, on public knowledge about the health effects of smoking or on smoking behavior.
4. Information about tar and nicotine yields appears on all cigarette advertisements but not on all cigarette packages. Levels of other hazardous constituents of tobacco smoke, such as carbon monoxide, hydrogen cyanide, and ammonia, are not disclosed on packages or advertisements. Little information is available to the public about the identity or health consequences of the additives in tobacco products.

5. Declines in adult per capita cigarette consumption have occurred in years of major dissemination of information on the health hazards of smoking. These include 1964, the year of the first Surgeon General's Report on smoking and health, and 1967–70, when antismoking public service announcements were widely broadcast on radio and television, as mandated by the Federal Communications Commission's Fairness Doctrine.
6. In 1985, when cigarette advertising and promotion totaled 2.5 billion dollars, cigarettes were the most heavily advertised product category in the outdoor media (e.g., billboards), second in magazines, and third in newspapers. Over the past decade, the majority of cigarette marketing expenditures has shifted from traditional print advertising to promotional activities (e.g., free samples, coupons, sponsorship of sporting events).
7. An estimated 1 percent of the budget allocated to disease prevention by the U.S. Department of Health and Human Services is devoted specifically to tobacco control. These expenditures totaled 39.5 million dollars in 1986.

Part II. Economic Incentives

1. Cigarette excise taxes are imposed by the Federal Government (16 cents per pack), all State governments, and nearly 400 cities and counties. On average, Federal and State excise taxes add 34 cents per pack to the price of cigarettes. Cigarette excise tax rates have fallen since 1964 in real terms because the rate and magnitude of periodic tax increases have not kept pace with inflation.
2. Studies demonstrate that increases in the price of cigarettes decrease smoking, particularly by adolescents. It has been estimated that an additional 100,000 or more persons will live to age 65 as a result of the price increases induced by the 1983 doubling of the Federal excise tax on cigarettes.
3. In 1964, smoking status was not considered in the determination of insurance premiums. Currently, nearly all life insurers but only a few health, disability, and property and casualty insurers offer premium discounts for nonsmokers. Few health insurers reimburse for the costs of smoking cessation programs or treatment.

Part III. Direct Restrictions on Smoking

1. Restrictions on smoking in public places and at work are growing in number and comprehensiveness, as a result of both Government actions and private initiatives. Forty-two States and more than 320 communities have passed laws restricting smoking in public, and an estimated one-half of large businesses have a smoking policy for their employees.
2. The goal of these smoking restrictions is to protect individuals from the consequences of involuntary tobacco smoke exposure, but they may also contribute to reductions in smoking prevalence by changing the attitudes and behavior of current and potential smokers. Insufficient research has been undertaken to determine the extent, if any, of these effects.

3. There are fewer legal restrictions on children's access to tobacco products now than in 1964, despite what has been learned since then about the dangers of tobacco use, its addictive nature, and the early age of initiation of smoking.
4. As of January 1, 1988, laws in 43 States and the District of Columbia restricted the sale of cigarettes to minors. Nevertheless, tobacco products are relatively easy for children to obtain through vending machines and over-the-counter purchases because of low levels of compliance with and enforcement of current laws.
5. Tobacco products have been exempted by law or administrative decision from the jurisdiction of Federal regulatory agencies under whose authority they might otherwise fall.

References

22 MRSA c.265-B. Vending Machine Sales of Cigarettes. 1987.

41 Code of Federal Regulations. Part 101-20, 1987.

49 Code of Federal Regulations. Ch. X, Part 1061, 1987.

101 Stat. 1329-382, P.L. 100-202, 1987.

A.M. BEST COMPANY. *Best's Flitcraft Compend, 1987*. Oldwick, New Jersey: A.M. Best Company, April 1987a.

A.M. BEST COMPANY. The 500 leading life companies in total premium income. *Best's Review (Life/Health)* 88(4):99–103, August 1987b.

ABC NEWS. Growing up in smoke. *20/20*, transcript of Show No. 338, October 20, 1983.

AAKER, D.A., MEYERS, J.G. *Advertising Management*, Third Edition. Englewood Cliffs, New Jersey: Prentice-Hall, 1987.

ACTION ON SMOKING AND HEALTH V. HARRIS, 655 F.2d 236 (D.C. Cir. 1980).

AD FACTORS/MILLWARD BROWN. *A Study of the Attitudes Physicians Hold Toward the Surgeon General's Report on Nicotine Addiction*. Ad Factors/Millward Brown (Racine, Wisconsin), for Lakeside Pharmaceuticals, June 1988.

ADAMS, J.R., WILLIAMS, E.B. *The Association Between Smoking and Accidents: Overdependency as an Influencing Variable*. New York: Columbia University, Teachers' College, 1965.

ADAMS, J.R., WILLIAMS, E.B. The association between smoking and accidents: Overdependency as an influencing variable. *Traffic Quarterly* 20(4):583–588, October 1966.

ADEAST. MBTA wants to quit smoking (ads). *AdEast*, June 1986, p. 3.

ADMINISTRATIVE MANAGEMENT SOCIETY. *Executive Summary: Workplace Smoking Policies Survey*. Washington, D.C.: Administrative Management Society, 1986.

ADVISORY COMMISSION ON INTERGOVERNMENTAL RELATIONS. *Cigarette Bootlegging: A State AND Federal Responsibility*. Washington, D.C.: Advisory Commission on Intergovernmental Relations, May 1977.

ADVISORY COMMISSION ON INTERGOVERNMENTAL RELATIONS. *Cigarette Tax Evasion: A Second Look*. Washington, D.C.: Advisory Commission on Intergovernmental Relations, March 1985.

AIRPORT OPERATORS COUNCIL INTERNATIONAL. *Synopses of Airport Smoking Restrictions*. Washington, D.C.: Airport Operators Council International, June 1988.

ALBRIGHT, C.L., ALTMAN, D.G., SLATER, M.D., MACCOBY, N. Cigarette advertisements in magazines: Evidence for a differential focus on women's and youth magazines. *Health Education Quarterly* 15(2):225–233, Summer 1988.

ALEXANDER, H.M., CALCOTT, R., DOBSON, A.J., HARDES, G.R., LLOYD, D.M., O'CONNELL, D.L., LEEDER, S.R. Cigarette smoking and drug use in schoolchildren: IV—Factors associated with changes in smoking behaviour. *International Journal of Epidemiology* 12(1):59–66, 1983.

ALTMAN, D.G., FOSTER, V., RASENICK-DOUSS, L., TYE, J.B. Reducing the illegal sale of cigarettes to minors. *Journal of the American Medical Association* 261(1):80–83, January 6, 1989.

ALTMAN, D.G., SLATER, M.D., ALBRIGHT, C.L., MACCOBY, N. How an unhealthy product is sold: Cigarette advertising in magazines, 1960–1985. *Journal of Communications* 37(4):95–106, Autumn 1987.

AMERICAN ACADEMY OF PEDIATRICS. Tobacco use by children and adolescents. *Pediatrics* 79(3):479–481, March 1987.

AMERICAN COLLEGE HEALTH ASSOCIATION. Statement on tobacco use on college and university campuses. *Journal of American College Health* 37(1):45, July 1988.

AMERICAN COLLEGE OF HEALTHCARE EXECUTIVES. *Public Policy Opinion Poll: How Do Executives' Behavior and Views Match the Colleges' Public Statement.* Chicago: American College of Healthcare Executives, Division of Research and Public Policy, February 1988.

AMERICAN COLLEGE OF PHYSICIANS. *Cigarette Abuse Epidemic.* Philadelphia: American College of Physicians, April 9, 1986.

AMERICAN COUNCIL OF LIFE INSURANCE. *1986 Life Insurance Factbook.* Washington, D.C.: American Council of Life Insurance, 1986.

AMERICAN COUNCIL OF LIFE INSURANCE. *1987 Life Insurance Factbook Update.* Washington, D.C.: American Council of Life Insurance, 1987.

AMERICAN HOSPITAL ASSOCIATION. *Digest of National Health Care and Expense Indicators.* American Hospital Association, Office of Health Coalitions and Private Sector Initiatives, November 1987.

AMERICAN HOSPITAL ASSOCIATION. *Smoking and Hospitals Are a Bad Match! Policy Development and Implementation Strategies for a Smoke-Free Environment.* Division of Public Relations with assistance from Division of Ambulatory Care, Health Promotion, and Women's and Children's Health, American Hospital Association, 1988.

AMERICAN MEDICAL ASSOCIATION. Model legislation on the enforcement of laws to restrict children's access to tobacco. *AMA Proceedings, No. 193.* American Medical Association, 1987.

AMERICAN MEDICAL ASSOCIATION. Citizen petition to the Food and Drug Administration (Docket No. 88P-0155). Chicago: American Medical Association, April 25, 1988.

AMERICAN PUBLIC HEALTH ASSOCIATION V. CONSUMER PRODUCT SAFETY COMMISSION C.A. No. 74-1222 (D.D.C. April 23, 1975).

AMERICAN SCHOOL HEALTH ASSOCIATION. *School Health in America. A Survey of State School Health Programs.* Kent, Ohio: American School Health Association, 1976.

AMERICAN SCHOOL HEALTH ASSOCIATION. *School Health in America. A Survey of State School Health Programs*, Second Edition. Kent, Ohio: American School Health Association, August 1979.

AMERICAN SCHOOL HEALTH ASSOCIATION. *School Health in America. A Survey of State School Health Programs*, Third Edition. Kent, Ohio: American School Health Association, December 1981.

AMERICAN SCHOOL HEALTH ASSOCIATION. *School Health in America. An Assessment of State Policies to Protect and Improve the Health of Students*, Fourth Edition. Kent, Ohio: American School Health Association, 1987.

AMERICANS FOR NONSMOKERS' RIGHTS. *Model Smoking Pollution Control Ordinance.* Berkeley, California: Americans for Nonsmokers' Rights, 1987a.

AMERICANS FOR NONSMOKERS' RIGHTS. *Model Clean Indoor Air Act.* Berkeley, California: Americans for Nonsmokers' Rights, 1987b.

AMERICANS FOR NONSMOKERS' RIGHTS. *California City and County Smoking Ordinances.* Berkeley, California: Americans for Nonsmokers' Rights, April 29, 1988a.

AMERICANS FOR NONSMOKERS' RIGHTS. *Matrix of Local Smoking Ordinances.* Berkeley, California: Americans for Nonsmokers' Rights, August 1988b.

AMHERST. Article 53, Town By-Laws, Amherst, Massachusetts, May 18, 1987.

ANDREWS, J.L. JR. Reducing smoking in the hospital: An effective model program. *Chest* 84(2):206–209, August 1983.

ASPEN. Municipal Code of the City of Aspen, Colorado. Ordinance 35, Series of 1985, September 12, 1985.

ATKINS, C.G. The Adolescent Tobacco Education and Prevention Act. *Congressional Record*, E4552–E4553, November 19, 1987.

AUSTIN. Ordinance No. 880218-F. Austin, Texas, February 18, 1988.

AUSTIN V. TENNESSEE, 21 S.Ct. 132, 179 U.S. 343 (1900).

BAGDIKIAN, B.H. *The Media Monopoly*. Boston: Beacon Press, 1983.

BAILEY, W.J. A.L.A. calls for ban on cigarette ads in doctors' waiting rooms and asks for removal of Federal preemption clause. *Smoking and Health Reporter* 3(4):1, 4, July 1986.

BALTAGI, B.H., LEVIN, D. Estimating dynamic demand for cigarettes using panel data: The effects of bootlegging, taxation and advertising reconsidered. *Review of Economics and Statistics* 68:148–155, 1986.

BECKER, G., GROSSMAN, M., MURPHY, K.M. An empirical analysis of cigarette addiction. Working paper. National Bureau of Economic Research, 1987.

BECKER, G.S., MURPHY, K.M. A theory of rational addiction. *Journal of Political Economy* 96(4):657–700, August 1988.

BENNETT, D., LEVY, B.S. Smoking policies and smoking cessation programs of large employers in Massachusetts. *American Journal of Public Health* 70:629–631, 1980.

BENNETT, W. Cigarettes: Prevention or cure? *Harvard Medical School Health Letter* 10(5): 3–5, March 1985.

BERGLER, R. *Advertising and Cigarette Smoking*. Bern, Switzerland: Hans Huber Publishers, 1981.

BHALLA, G., LASTOVICKA, J.L. The impact of changing cigarette warning message content and format. In: Kinnear, T.C. (ed.) *Advances in Consumer Research*, Volume 6. Association for Consumer Research, 1984, pp. 303–310.

BIENER, L., ABRAMS, D.B., FOLLICK, M.J., DEAN, L. A comparative evaluation of a restrictive smoking policy in a general hospital. *American Journal of Public Health* 79(2): 192–195, February 1988.

BISHOP, J.A., YOO, J.H. "Health scare," excise taxes and advertising ban in the cigarette demand and supply. *Southern Economic Journal* 52(2):402–411, October 1985.

BLASI, V., MONAGHAN, H.P. The first amendment and cigarette advertising. *Journal of the American Medical Association* 256(4):502–509, July 25, 1986.

BLASI, V., MONAGHAN, H.P. Posadas and the prohibition of cigarette advertising. Legal memorandum. Columbia University Law School, February 3, 1987.

BLONDAL, T., MAGNUSSON, G. Innovation in Iceland: Graphic health warnings on tobacco products. *New York State Journal of Medicine* 85(7):405–406, July 1985.

BODDEWYN, J.J. (ed.) *Tobacco Advertising Bans and Consumption in 16 Countries*. New York: International Advertising Association, 1986.

BOSTON GLOBE. Canada antismoking laws are called models for U.S. *Boston Globe*, June 30, 1988a, p. 3.

BOSTON GLOBE. Air Canada broadens smoking ban on airplanes. *Boston Globe*, July 21, 1988b.

BOSTON HERALD. Breaking the habit. *Boston Herald*, February 25, 1986, p. 18.

BOTKIN, J.R. The fire-safe cigarette. *Journal of the American Medical Association* 260(2):226–229, July 8, 1988.

BRADLEY, B. Testimony at the Hearings on Advertising of Tobacco Products before the Subcommittee on Health and the Environment of the Committee on Energy and Commerce, House of Representatives, 99th Congress, 2d Session, Serial No. 99-167, July 18, August 1, 1986, pp. 10–12.

BRAILEY, A.G. JR. The promotion of health through health insurance. *New England Journal of Medicine* 302(1):51–52, January 3, 1980.

BRINK, S.D. *Health Risks and Behavior: The Impact on Medical Costs*. San Francisco: Milliman and Robertson, 1987.

BROWN, E.R., MCCARTHY, W.J., MARCUS, A., BAKER, D., FROINES, J.R., DELLENBAUGH, C., MCQUISTON, T. Workplace smoking policies: Attitudes of union members in a high-risk industry. *Journal of Occupational Medicine* 30(4):312–320, 1988.

BUREAU OF NATIONAL AFFAIRS. *Where There's Smoke: Problems and Policies Concerning Smoking in the Workplace.* Washington, D.C.: Bureau of National Affairs, 1986.

BUREAU OF NATIONAL AFFAIRS. *Where There's Smoke: Problems and Policies Concerning Smoking in the Workplace*, Second Edition. Washington, D.C.: Bureau of National Affairs, 1987.

BURNS, J.F. Canada passes law to ban tobacco ads and curb smoking. *New York Times*, June 30, 1988, pp. A1, A13.

BURROS, M. The smoking law revisited: Room enough for everyone. *New York Times*, October 12, 1988.

CA. BLOCKERS. *Prospectus.* Louisville, Kentucky: CA. Blockers, October 7, 1987.

CA. BLOCKERS. *Project Bloctin.* Louisville, Kentucky: CA. Blockers, 1988.

CALFEE, J.E. *Cigarette Advertising, Health Information and Regulation.* Federal Trade Commission, May 20, 1986.

CALIFORNIA CHAPTER 1498. Tort Reform—Attorney's Fees, Product Liability, and Punitive Damages. Senate Bill No. 241, Chapter 1498, Statutes of 1987.

CENTER FOR CORPORATE PUBLIC INVOLVEMENT. *1987 Social Report for the Life and Health Insurance Business.* Washington, D.C.: Center for Corporate Public Involvement, American Council of Life Insurance, Health Insurance Association of America, 1987.

CENTERS FOR DISEASE CONTROL. *State Legislation on Smoking and Health, 1979.* U.S. Department of Health and Human Services, Public Health Service, Centers for Disease Control, Bureau of Health Education. DHHS Publication No. (CDC) 80-8386, June 1980.

CENTERS FOR DISEASE CONTROL. *State Legislation on Smoking and Health 1980.* U.S. Department of Health and Human Services, Public Health Service, Centers for Disease Control, Center for Health Promotion and Education, April 1981.

CENTERS FOR DISEASE CONTROL. Survey of worksite smoking policies—New York City. *Morbidity and Mortality Weekly Report* 36(12):177–179, April 3, 1987a.

CENTERS FOR DISEASE CONTROL. Indian Health Service facilities become smoke-free. *Morbidity and Mortality Weekly Report* 36(22):348–350, June 12, 1987b.

CENTERS FOR DISEASE CONTROL. Passive smoking: Beliefs, attitudes, and exposures—United States, 1986. *Morbidity and Mortality Weekly Report* 37(15):239–241, April 22, 1988.

CHALOUPKA, F., SAFFER, H. The demand for cigarettes and restrictions on smoking in the workplace. Working paper. New York: National Bureau of Economic Research, July 1988.

CHALOUPKA, F.J. IV. *An Economic Analysis of Addictive Behavior: The Case of Cigarette Smoking.* Doctoral Dissertation. City University of New York, 1988.

CHAPMAN, S. Cigarette advertising and smoking: A review of the evidence. In: *Smoking Out the Barons: The Campaign Against the Tobacco Industry.* Chichester, England: John Wiley and Sons, 1986, pp. 79–97.

CHAPMAN, S., FITZGERALD, B. Brand preference and advertising recall in adolescent smokers: Some implications for health promotion. *American Journal of Public Health* 72(5):491–494, May 1982.

CHAPMAN, S., VERMEER, R. Tobacco marketing monopolies that advertise. (Letter.) *Lancet* 1(8431):758, March 30, 1985.

CHETWYND, J., COOPE, P., BRODIE, R.J., WELLS, E. Impact of cigarette advertising on aggregate demand for cigarettes in New Zealand. *British Journal of Addiction* 83:409–414, 1988.

CHRISTEN, A.G. The case against smokeless tobacco: Five facts for the health professional to consider. *Journal of the American Dental Association* 101(3):464–469, September 1980.

CIPPOLONE V. LIGGETT GROUP INC. ET AL. C.A. 83-8846 (D.N.J. June 7, 1988).

CLEAN AIR ACT OF 1963, 42 U.S.C.S., 1857-1857(L).

CLEMANS, J.G. Director, Media Relations, Farmer's Insurance Group of Companies. Personal communication to Chris Pashos, Institute for the Study of Smoking Behavior and Policy, John F. Kennedy School of Government, Harvard University, April 1988.

COALITION ON SMOKING OR HEALTH. Petition requesting classification of low tar and low nicotine cigarettes as drugs under the Food Drug and Cosmetic Act, (Food and Drug Administration Docket No. 88P-0155), 1988a.

COALITION ON SMOKING OR HEALTH. Petition to classify R.J. Reynolds new alternative nicotine delivery product to be subject to the jurisdiction of the Food and Drug Administration as a drug (Food and Drug Administration Docket No. 88P-0155), 1988b.

COHEN, J., SRULL, T. *Information Processing Issues Involved in the Communication and Retrieval of Cigarette Warning Information.* Report to the Federal Trade Commission, November 1980.

COLLIER, M. BART bans cigarette, liquor ads. *Oakland Tribune*, May 1, 1987, p. 1.

COLORADO DEPARTMENT OF HEALTH. *Report of the Technical Advisory Committee on Tobacco and Health for Colorado.* Colorado Department of Health, July 1986.

COLUMBIA LAW REVIEW. Fairness, freedom and cigarette advertising: A defense of the Federal Communications Commission. *Columbia Law Review* 67:1470–1489, 1967.

COMMITTEE ON WAYS AND MEANS. *Hearings on User Fees, Revenue Proposals Contained in President Reagan's 1986 Budget, and Other Revenue Measures.* Committee on Ways and Means, 1986.

CONE, E.J., HENNINGFIELD, J.E. Premier 'smokeless cigarettes' can be used to deliver crack. (Letter.) *Journal of the American Medical Association* 261(1):41, January 6, 1989.

CONNOLLY, G.N. Tobacco, politics and United States trade policy. *ACSH News and Views* 8(4):1–2, September–October 1987. (American Council on Science and Health, NY.)

CONNOLLY, G.N. Testimony at the Hearings on Advertising of Tobacco Products before the Subcommittee on Health and the Environment of the Committee on Energy and Commerce, House of Representatives, 99th Congress, 2d Session, Serial No. 99-167, July 18, August 1, 1986.

CONNOLLY, G.N., WINN, D.M., HECHT, S.S., HENNINGFIELD, J.E., WALKER, B. JR., HOFFMANN, D. The reemergence of smokeless tobacco. *New England Journal of Medicine* 314(16):1020–1027, April 17, 1986.

CONSUMER PRODUCT SAFETY COMMISSION. *Recommendations of the Interagency Committee on Cigarette and Little Cigar Fire Safety.* Consumer Product Safety Commission, December 1987.

CONTRA COSTA HEALTH PLAN. Contra Costa Health Plan is first in the Nation to use smoking in premium setting. Press release. Martinez, California: Contra Costa Health Plan, 1987.

COUGHLIN, D. County curbs cigarette machines. *Seattle Post-Intelligence*, September 20, 1988.

COVINGTON AND BURLING. Legal Memorandum: A Constitutional Analysis of Proposals to Ban or Restrict Tobacco Product Advertising. Washington, D.C.: Covington and Burling, July 18, 1986.

COWELL, M.J. An insurance company perspective on smoking. *New York State Journal of Medicine* 85(7):307–309, July 1985.

COWELL, M.J., HIRST, B.L. Mortality differences between smokers and non-smokers. *Transactions of the Society of Actuaries* 32:185–261, 1980.

COX, H.T. Smoking, tobacco promotion, and the voluntary agreements. *British Medical Journal* 288:303–305, January 28, 1984.

CROWNE, J.E., SHAPIRO, R.D. The nonsmoker as a preferred risk. *National Underwriter* 84:13, 16–17, August 23, 1980.

CULLINGFORD, R., DA CRUZ, L., WEBB, S., SHEAN, R., JAMROZIK, K. Legibility of health warnings on billboards that advertise cigarettes. *Medical Journal of Australia* 148:336–338, April 4, 1988.

CUMMINGS, K.M., MARSHALL, D.R. Awareness of the New York State law banning the sale of tobacco to minors. *New York State Journal of Medicine* 88:418–419, August 1988.

CUMMINS, K. Cigarette makers slow to give list of all additives. *Florida Times Union*, January 17, 1983, p. A2.

DALE, K.C. ACSH survey: Which magazines report the hazards of smoking? *ACSH News and Views* 3(3):1, 8–10, May–June1982.

DARTNELL CORPORATION. Smoking in the office—Is it a problem? *Dartnell Corporation Target Survey*, September 1977.

DAVIS, R.M. Legislative action at the State and local level to reduce tobacco consumption. *State Health Legislation Report* 14(1):1–15, February 1986, Chicago: AMA.

DAVIS, R.M. Current trends in cigarette advertising and marketing. *New England Journal of Medicine* 316:725–732, March 19, 1987.

DAVIS, R.M. Uniting physicians against smoking: The need for a coordinated national strategy. *Journal of the American Medical Association* 259(19):2900–2901, May 20, 1988.

DAVIS, R.M., JASON, L.A. The distribution of free cigarette samples to minors. *American Journal of Preventive Medicine* 4(1):21–26, January–February 1988.

DAVIS, R.M., KENDRICK, J.S. The Surgeon General's warnings in outdoor cigarette advertising: Are they readable? *Journal of the American Medical Association* 261(1):90–94, January 6, 1989.

DAVIS, R.M., LYMAN, A., BINKIN, N.J. The rotation of health warnings in cigarette advertisements. Compliance with the Comprehensive Smoking Education Act of 1984. *Journal of Public Health Policy* 9(3):403–410, Autumn 1988.

DAWLEY, H.H., BURTON, M.C. Smoking control in a hospital setting. *Addictive Behaviors* 10:351–355, 1985.

DAWLEY, H.H. JR., BALDWIN, J. The control of smoking: Smoking rate in designated smoking and no-smoking areas. *International Journal of the Addictions* 18(7):1033–1038, 1983.

DAYNARD, R.A. Tobacco liability litigation as a cancer control strategy. *Journal of the National Cancer Institute* 80(1):9–13, May 2, 1988.

DIFRANZA, J.R. Regulatory initiatives to prevent and treat nicotine addiction in children. In: *The Massachusetts Plan for Nonsmoking and Health.* Massachusetts Department of Public Health, Office for Nonsmoking and Health, September 1988.

DIFRANZA, J.R., NORWOOD, B.D., GARNER, D.W., TYE, J.B. Legislative efforts to protect children from tobacco. *Journal of the American Medical Association* 257(24):3387–3389, June 26, 1987.

DIFRANZA, J.R., WINTERS, T.H., GOLDBERG, R.J., CIRILLO, L., BILIOURIS, T. The relationship of smoking to motor vehicle accidents and traffic violations. *New York State Journal of Medicine* 86:464–467, September 1986.

DILLOW, G.L. *The Hundred-Year War Against the Cigarette.* Washington, D.C.: Tobacco Institute, 1981.

DOLL, R., PETO, R. The causes of cancer: Quantitative estimates of avoidable risks of cancer in the United States today. *Journal of the National Cancer Institute* 66(6):1191–1308, June 1981.

DUMAS, B.K. The adequacy of federally mandated cigarette package warnings. In: Levi, J., Walker, A.G. (eds.) *Language in the Judicial Process.* New York: Plenum Press, in press.

DUNLOP, T.S. *Memorandum. Report to City Council on Effectiveness of Ordinance 35.* Aspen, Colorado: Aspen–Pitkin Environmental Health Department, March 27, 1986.

DWYER, F.R. Consumer processing and use of supplemental drug label information. In: *Advances in Consumer Research*, Volume 10. Association for Consumer Research, 1978, pp. 220–226.

ENGLANDER, T.J. Cigarette makers shift ad strategies. *United States Tobacco and Candy Journal* 213(21):1, 46, April 3–23, 1986.

ENGSTROM, P.F. Cancer control objectives for the year 2000. *Progress in Clinical and Biological Research* 216:1–10, 1986.

ERIKSEN, M. Smoking policies at Pacific Bell. *Corporate Commentary* 1(4):24–34, June 1985.

ERIKSEN, M.P. Workplace smoking control: Rationale and approaches. *Advances in Health Education and Promotion* 1(A):65–103, 1986.

ERIKSEN, M.P., LEMAISTRE, C.A., NEWELL, G.R. The health hazards of passive smoking. *Annual Review of Public Health* 9:47–70, 1988.

ERNSTER, V.L. Trends in smoking, cancer risk, and cigarette promotion: Current priorities for reducing tobacco exposure. *Cancer* 62:1702–1712, 1988.

FEDERAL COMMUNICATIONS COMMISSION. Editorializing by broadcast licensees. Docket no. 8516. *Federal Communications Commission Reports* 13:1246–1270, 1949.

FEDERAL COMMUNICATIONS COMMISSION. *WCBS-TV, Pike and Fisher Radio Reg.*, 2d Series, Volume 9, pp. 1423–1425, 1967; affirmed on reconsideration, *Pike and Fisher Radio Reg.*, 2d Series, Volume 11, pp. 1901–1908, 1967.

FEDERAL COMMUNICATIONS COMMISSION. Advertisement of cigarettes. Notice of proposed rule making. *Federal Register* 34:1959–1962, February 11, 1969.

FEDERAL COMMUNICATIONS COMMISSION. Inquiry into Section 73.1910 of the Commission's rules and regulations concerning alternatives to the general Fairness Doctrine obligations of broadcast licensees. *Federal Communications Commission Record* 2:5272, August 17–28, 1987.

FEDERAL FOOD, DRUG, AND COSMETIC ACT. 52 Stat. 1040, 75th Congress, 3d Session, June 25, 1938, 21 U.S.C. 301 *et seq.*

FEDERAL TRADE COMMISSION. Advertising and labeling of cigarettes. Notice of rulemaking proceeding for establishment of trade regulation rules. *Federal Register* 29:530–532, January 22, 1964a.

FEDERAL TRADE COMMISSION. Unfair or deceptive advertising and labeling of cigarettes in relation to the health hazards of smoking. *Federal Register* 29:8324–8375, July 2, 1964b.

FEDERAL TRADE COMMISSION. Vacation of warning requirements in trade regulation rule concerning advertising and labeling of cigarettes. *Federal Register* 30:9484, July 28, 1965.

FEDERAL TRADE COMMISSION. *Report to Congress Pursuant to the Federal Cigarette Labeling and Advertising Act.* Federal Trade Commission, June 30, 1967.

FEDERAL TRADE COMMISSION. *Report to Congress Pursuant to the Federal Cigarette Labeling and Advertising Act.* Federal Trade Commission, June 30, 1968.

FEDERAL TRADE COMMISSION. Cigarettes in relation to the health hazards of smoking: Unfair or deceptive advertising and labeling. *Federal Register* 34:7917–7918, May 20, 1969a.

FEDERAL TRADE COMMISSION. *Report to Congress Pursuant to the Federal Cigarette Labeling and Advertising Act.* Federal Trade Commission, June 30, 1969b.

FEDERAL TRADE COMMISSION. Advertising of cigarettes. Notice of public hearing and opportunity to submit data, views, or arguments regarding proposed trade regulation rule. *Federal Register* 35(154):12671, August 8, 1970.

FEDERAL TRADE COMMISSION. Complaint in the matter of Lorillard, Philip Morris Inc., American Brands, Inc., Brown and Williamson Tobacco Corporation, R.J. Reynolds Tobacco Company, Liggett and Myers Incorporated, consent orders, etc., in regard to the alleged violation of the Federal Trade Commission Act, Complaints, March 30, 1972–Decisions, March 30, 1972. *Federal Trade Commission Decisions* 80:455–465, 1972.

FEDERAL TRADE COMMISSION. *Report to Congress Pursuant to the Public Health Cigarette Smoking Act.* Federal Trade Commission, December 31, 1974.

FEDERAL TRADE COMMISSION. *Report of "Tar," Nicotine and Carbon Monoxide of the Smoke of 187 Varieties of Cigarettes.* Federal Trade Commission, March 1981a.

FEDERAL TRADE COMMISSION. *Federal Trade Commission Staff Report on the Cigarette Advertising Investigation.* Federal Trade Commission, May 1981b.

FEDERAL TRADE COMMISSION. *Report to Congress Pursuant to the Federal Cigarette Labeling and Advertising Act for the Year 1980.* Federal Trade Commission, November 15, 1982.

FEDERAL TRADE COMMISSION. *Report to Congress Pursuant to the Federal Cigarette Labeling and Advertising Act for the Years 1982–1983.* Federal Trade Commission, June 1985.

FEDERAL TRADE COMMISSION. *Report to Congress Pursuant to the Federal Cigarette Labeling and Advertising Act, 1984.* Federal Trade Commission, 1986a.

FEDERAL TRADE COMMISSION. Regulations under the Comprehensive Smokeless Tobacco Health Education Act of 1986. *Federal Register* 51(213):40005–40023, November 4, 1986b.

FEDERAL TRADE COMMISSION. Press release. Federal Trade Commission, Office of Public Affairs, April 15, 1987.

FEDERAL TRADE COMMISSION. *Report to Congress Pursuant to the Federal Cigarette Labeling and Advertising Act, 1985.* Federal Trade Commission, February 1988a.

FEDERAL TRADE COMMISSION. *Report to Congress Pursuant to the Federal Cigarette Labeling and Advertising Act, 1986.* Federal Trade Commission, May 1988b.

FEDERAL TRADE COMMISSION V. BROWN AND WILLIAMSON. U.S. District Court for D.C. D# 83-1940, 1983.

FEDERAL TRADE COMMISSION V. LIGGETT AND MYERS TOBACCO CO., 108 F. Supp. 573 (S.D.N.Y. 1952), affirmed, 203 F.2d 955 (2nd Cir. 1953).

FEIGELSON, J. Skoal Bandits blitz kicks off N.Y. entry. *Advertising Age*, August 8, 1983.

FIELDING, J.E., BRESLOW, L. Healthy promotion programs sponsored by California employers. *American Journal of Public Health* 73(5):538–542, May 1983.

FISCHER, P.M., RICHARDS, J.W. JR., BERMAN, E.J., KRUGMAN, D.M. Recall and eye tracking study of adolescents viewing tobacco advertisements. *Journal of the American Medical Association* 261(1):84–89, January 6, 1989.

FISHBEIN, M. *Consumer beliefs and behavior with respect to cigarette smoking: A critical analysis of the public literature.* In: Federal Trade Commission Report to Congress Pursuant to the Public Health Cigarette Smoking Act for the Year 1976. Federal Trade Commission, 1977.

FISHER, D.A., MAGNUS, P. "Out of the mouths of babes . . ." The opinions of 10 and 11 year old children regarding the advertising of cigarettes. *Community Health Studies* 5(1):22–26, 1981.

FOOD AND DRUG ADMINISTRATION. Bureau of Enforcement Guideline, May 24, 1963. Reprinted in Hearings on Public Health Cigarette Amendments of 1971, U.S. Senate, 92d Congress, 2d Session, Serial No. 92-82, 1972, at 240.

FOOD AND DRUG ADMINISTRATION. Letter from Donald Kennedy, Commissioner of Food and Drugs, to John F. Banzhaf III, Action on Smoking and Health, December 5, 1977 (Docket No. 77P-0185).

FOOD AND DRUG ADMINISTRATION. New drugs requirement for labeling directed to the patient. *Federal Register* 43(21):4214–4234, January 31, 1978.

FOOD AND DRUG ADMINISTRATION. Letter from Mark Novitch for Jere E. Glyan, Commissioner of Food and Drugs, to John F. Banzhaf III and Peter N. Georgiades, Action on Smoking and Health, November 25, 1980 (Docket Nos. 77P-0185 and 78P-0338/CP).

FOOD AND DRUG ADMINISTRATION. Letter from Daniel L. Michels, Director, Office of Compliance, Center for Drugs and Biologics, to J. Philip Ray, Advanced Tobacco Products, Inc. (San Antonio, TX), February 9, 1987a.

FOOD AND DRUG ADMINISTRATION. Letter from Frank E. Young, Commissioner of Food and Drugs, to Congressman Henry A. Waxman, September 29, 1987b.

FOOTE, E. Advertising and tobacco. *Journal of the American Medical Association* 245(16): 1667–1668, April 24, 1981.

FORSTER, J., KLEPP, K.-I., JEFFERY, R.W. Sources of cigarettes for tenth graders in two Minnesota cities. *Health Education Research*, in press.

FREEDMAN, A.M. Cigarette smoking is growing hazardous to careers in business. *Wall Street Journal*, April 23, 1987, p. 29.

FRIEDMAN, K.M. *Public Policy and the Smoking–Health Controversy. A Comparative Study*. Lexington, Massachusetts: D.C. Heath, 1975.

FRITSCHLER, A.L. *Smoking and Politics: Policymaking and the Federal Bureaucracy*. New York: Appleton-Century-Crofts, 1969.

FUJII, E.T. The demand for cigarettes: Further empirical evidence and its implications for public policy. *Applied Economics* 12:479–489, 1980.

GARNER, D.W. Product liability in cigarette-caused fires. *New York State Journal of Medicine* 85(7):322–323, July 1985.

GELB, B.D. Preventive medicine and employee productivity. *Harvard Business Review* 63(2):12–13, March–April 1985.

GENERAL SERVICES ADMINISTRATION. *GSA Issues Smoking Rules for Federal Buildings*. GSA News Release No. 8687. General Services Administration, December 5, 1986.

GITLITZ, G. Cigarette advertising and The New York Times: An ethical issue that's unfit to print? *New York State Journal of Medicine* 83(13):1284–1291, December 1983.

GLANTZ, L.H. Mandating health insurance benefits in the private sector: A decision for State legislatures. *American Journal of Public Health* 75(11):1344–1346, November 1985.

GLOSSER, D.S. *Conditioned Craving in a Sample of Cigarette Smokers*. Doctoral Dessertation. Boston University. Ann Arbor, University Microfilms International, Thesis No. 84-13168, 1984.

GOLDSMITH, M. Medical organization policies about tobacco use. *Journal of the American Medical Association* 260(1):14, July 1, 1988.

GOLDSTEIN, A.O., FISCHER, P.M., RICHARDS, J.W., CRETEN, D. Relationship between high school student smoking and recognition of cigarette advertisements. *Journal of Pediatrics* 110(3):488–491, March 1987.

GOTTLIEB, N.H., HEDL, J.J. JR., ERIKSEN, M.P., CHAN, F. Smoking policies among private employers and public agencies in Texas: A statewide analysis. *Journal of the National Cancer Institute* 81(3):200–204, February 1, 1989.

GREALY, M., Massachusetts Bay Transportation Authority. Personal communication to the Director, Office on Smoking and Health, June 14, 1988.

GRISE, V.N. Tobacco: Background for 1985 Farm Legislation. U.S. Department of Agriculture, Economic Research Service, Agriculture Information Bulletin No. 468, September 1984.

GROSSMAN, M. Taxation and Cigarette Smoking in the United States. In: Forbes, W.F., Frecker, R.C., Nostbakken, D. (eds.) *Proceedings of the Fifth World Conference on Smok-*

ing and Health, Volume 1. Ottawa, Canada: Canadian Council on Smoking and Health, 1983, pp. 483–487.

GROSSMAN, M., COATE, D., LEWIT, E., SHAKOTKO, R.A. *Economics and Other Factors in Youth Smoking* New York: National Bureau of Economic Research, December 1983.

GROUP AGAINST SMOKING POLLUTION. Girl sues over illegal tobacco sales to children. *GASP of Massachusetts Newsletter*, Second Quarter 1987, pp. 1, 7.

GROUP AGAINST SMOKING POLLUTION OF MASSACHUSETTS. *Local Laws Regulating Smoking in the Workplace in Massachusetts.* Boston: GASP of Massachusetts, June 1, 1988a.

GROUP AGAINST SMOKING POLLUTION OF MASSACHUSETTS. *Local Laws in Massachusetts to Restrict Smoking in Restaurants.* Boston: Group Against Smoking Pollution of Massachusetts, June 8, 1988b.

GROUT, P., CLIFF, K.S., HARMAN, M.L., MACHIN, D. Cigarette smoking, road traffic accidents and seat belt usage. *Public Health* (London) 97:95–101, 1983.

HAGEDORN, A. Smoking lie voids insurance contract, appeals court rules. Electronics company loses benefit on late president with half-a-pack habit. *Wall Street Journal*, May 31, 1988.

HALL, J.R. *The U.S. Smoking-Material Fire Problem Through 1985.* Quincy, Massachusetts: National Fire Protection Association, December 1987.

HAMILTON, J.L. The demand for cigarettes: Advertising, the health scare, and the cigarette advertising ban. *Review of Economics and Statistics* 54:401–411, November 1972.

HARDES, G.R. The Hunter Region Childhood Smoking Prevention Program. In: Forbes, W.F., Frecker, R.C., Nostbakken, D. (eds.) *Proceedings of the Fifth World Conference on Smoking and Health, Winnipeg, Canada, 1983*, Volume 2. Ottawa, Canada: Canadian Council on Smoking and Health, 1983, pp. 209–213.

HARRIS, J.E. Increasing the Federal excise tax on cigarettes. *Journal of Health Economics* 1: 117–120, 1982.

HARRIS, J.E. The 1983 increase in the Federal Cigarette Excise Tax. In: Summers, L.H. (ed.) *Tax Policy and the Economy*, Volume 1. Cambridge, Massachusetts: Massachusetts Institute of Technology Press, 1987, pp. 87–111.

HAWKINS, C.H. Legal restrictions on minors' smoking. *American Journal of Public Health* 54(10):1741–1744, October 1964.

HEALTH INSURANCE ASSOCIATION OF AMERICA. *1986–1987 Source Book of Health Insurance Data.* Washington, D.C.: Health Insurance Association of America, 1987.

HEALY, M., Bay Area Rapid Transit District, Oakland, California. Personal communication to the Director, Office on Smoking and Health, June 14, 1988.

HELLAUER, J.C., President and Chief Executive Officer, Provident Indemnity Life Insurance Company. Personal communication to Chris Pashos, Institute for the Study of Smoking Behavior and Policy, John F. Kennedy School of Government, Harvard University, Cambridge, Massachusetts, April 1988.

HIAM, P. Insurers, consumers, and testing: The AIDS experience. *Law, Medicine and Health Care* 15(4):212–222, Winter 1987–88.

HOLLAND, R.P. *National Hospital Tobacco Smoking Policy Survey.* Lancaster County: American Lung Association of Lancaster County and the Pennsylvania Academy of Family Physicians, 1988.

HORNE, D.H., HORNE, R.H., HORNE, J.H., CHAMBERLAIN, C.R. Citizens petition: Classification of tobacco smoke as a potential occupational carcinogen. To Honorable William Brock, Secretary of Labor, August 21, 1985, pp. 1–17.

HOUSE OF COMMONS OF CANADA. Bill C-51. The Tobacco Products Control Act. House of Commons of Canada. Second Session, Thirty-Third Parliament, May 31, 1988.

HUMAN RESOURCES POLICY CORPORATION. *Smoking Policies in Large Corporations.* Los Angeles: Human Resources Policy Corporation, 1985.

ILLINOIS CIGARETTE SERVICE CO. V. CITY OF CHICAGO, 89 F 2d 610 (1937).

JACOBS, C. *Effects of State Tobacco Laws on High School Student Smoking Throughout the United States: Suggestions From High School Principals Concerning Student Smoking Problems.* Doctoral Dissertation. University of Utah. Ann Arbor, University Microfilms International, Thesis No. 74-29, 553, 1974.

JACOBSON, B., AMOS, A. *When Smoke Gets in Your Eyes: Cigarette Advertising Policy and Coverage of Smoking and Health in Women's Magazines.* London: British Medical Association Professional Division, May 1985.

JASON, L.A., LIOTTA, R.F. Reduction of cigarette smoking in a university cafeteria. *Journal of Applied Behavior Analysis* 15(4):573–577, Winter 1982.

JOHNSON, L.W. Advertising expenditures and aggregate demand for cigarettes in Australia. Research paper no. 302. Macquarie University, School of Economics and Financial Studies, June 1985.

JOHNSON, P.R. *The Economics of the Tobacco Industry.* New York: Praeger Publishers, 1984.

JOHNSTON, L.D., O'MALLEY, P.M., BACHMAN, J.G. *National Trends in Drug Use and Related Factors Among American High School Students and Young Adults, 1975–1986.* U.S. Department of Health and Human Services, Public Health Service, Alcohol, Drug Abuse, and Mental Health Administration, National Institute on Drug Abuse. DHHS Publication No. (ADM) 87-1535, 1987.

JOURNAL OF THE AMERICAN MEDICAL ASSOCIATION. Increasing number of medical organizations adopting policies relating to tobacco use. *Journal of the American Medical Association* 259(19):2812–2814, May 20, 1988a.

JOURNAL OF THE AMERICAN MEDICAL ASSOCIATION. New rules extinguish 'smoking lamp' in growing number of public places. *Journal of the American Medical Association* 259(19):2809–2810, 1988b.

KEENAN AND MCLAUGHLIN. *Cigarette Warning Project.* Comprehensive Smoking Prevention Act, Hearings before the Subcommittee on Health and the Environment, U.S. House of Representatives, Committee on Energy and Commerce, 1982.

KIMBLE, V. Smokers dwindling in military, survey finds. *Army Times*, November 23, 1987, p. 45.

KIRN, T.F. Laws ban minors' tobacco purchases, but enforcement is another matter. *Journal of the American Medical Association* 257(24):3323–3324, June 26, 1987.

KIRN, T.F. More "No Smoking" signs seen in hospitals. *Journal of the American Medical Association* 259(19):2814, May 20, 1988.

KIZER, K.W., WARRINER, T.E., BOOK, S.A. Sound science in the implementation of public policy. A case report on California's Proposition 65. *Journal of the American Medical Association* 260(7):951–955, August 19, 1988.

KLEBE, E.R. Actions of the Congress and the Federal Government on smoking and health. Congressional Research Service Report No. 79-219, September 26, 1979.

KNAPP J., SILVIS G., SORENSEN G., KOTTKE, T.E. *Clean Air Health Care. A Guide to Establish Smoke-Free Health Care Facilities.* Minneapolis: University of Minnesota, 1986.

KOTLER, P. *Marketing Management. Analysis, Planning, Implementation and Control,* Sixth Edition. Englewood Cliffs, New Jersey: Prentice-Hall, 1988.

KOTTKE, T.E., HILL, C., HEITZIG, C., BREKKE, M., BLAKE, S., ARNESON, S., CASPERSEN, C. Smoke-free hospitals. Attitudes of patients, employees, and faculty. *Minnesota Medicine* 68(1):53–55, January 1985.

LAMBIN, J.J. *Advertising, Competition and Market Conduct in Oligopoly Over Time.* Amsterdam: North-Holland Publishing, 1976.

LEVENTHAL, H., GLYNN, K., FLEMING, R. Is the smoking decision an "informed choice"? Effect of smoking risk factors on smoking beliefs. *Journal of the American Medical Association* 257(24):3373–3376, June 26, 1987.

LEWIN, T. Letting smokers pay for child care. *New York Times*, October 24, 1988.

LEWIT, E.M. Regulatory and legislative initiatives. In: *Proceedings of the Pennsylvania Consensus Conference on Tobacco and Health Priorities.* Pennsylvania Cancer Plan, Pennsylvania Department of Health, Pennsylvania Interagency Council on Tobacco and Health, Statewide Health Coordinating Council, October 1985, pp. 113–121.

LEWIT, E.M. *Clean Indoor Air Laws and Male/Female Smoking Differences. Final Report of Program Activities.* Grant No. DAO3641-02. Newark, New Jersey: University of Medicine and Dentistry of New Jersey, 1988.

LEWIT, E.M., COATE, D. The potential for using excise taxes to reduce smoking. *Journal of Health Economics* 1(2):121–145, 1982.

LEWIT, E.M., COATE, D., GROSSMAN, M. The effects of government regulation on teenage smoking. *Journal of Law and Economics* 24:545–569, December 1981.

LIEBERMAN RESEARCH. *A Study of Public Attitudes Toward Cigarette Advertising and Promotion Programs—Conducted for American Cancer Society, American Heart Association, American Lung Association.* Lieberman Research, October 1986.

LINTHWAITE, P. Health warnings. *Health Education Journal* 44(4):218–219, 1985.

LIPSON, B. Smokers who lie can expect rough treatment by insurers. *Boston Globe*, June 9, 1988, p. 48.

LOVATO, C.Y., ALLENSWORTH, D.D., CHAN, F.A. *School Health in America: An Assessment of State Policies to Protect and Improve the Health of Students.* American School Health Association, in press.

LYDON, C. Ban on TV cigarette ads could halt free spots against smoking. *New York Times*, August 16, 1970, p. 63.

LYONS, W.J. *Cologne Life Reinsurance Company Newsletter* 19(1):1–3, March 1986.

MACLEOD, W. Testimony before the Subcommittee on Transportation, Tourism and Hazardous Materials, Committee on Energy and Commerce, U.S. House of Representatives, May 7, 1987.

MAGNUS, P. Aspects of the tobacco-media story and cigarette advertising. Testimony presented to the Federal Interagency Committee on Smoking and Health, February 12, 1986.

MAINE DEPARTMENT OF HUMAN SERVICES. *Smoking in Maine. A Report on the Health and Economic Consequences of Cigarette Smoking in Maine.* Maine Department of Human Services, Bureau of Health, Division of Health Education, February 1983.

MALNIC, E. Postscript. *Los Angeles Times*, November 22, 1988.

MARKETING AND MEDIA DECISIONS. Cigarettes: At match point. *Marketing and Media Decisions*, 104–118, October 1985.

MARTIN, M.J. Smoking control—Policy and legal methods. (Letter.) *Western Journal of Medicine* 148(2):199, February 1988.

MARTY, J. Commentary. Dome ads help inflate a statistic: Cancer deaths. *Minneapolis Star-Tribune*, October 27, 1987, p. 1.

MASSACHUSETTS DEPARTMENT OF PUBLIC HEALTH. *The Massachusetts Plan for Nonsmoking and Health.* Massachusetts Department of Public Health, Office for Nonsmoking and Health, September 1988.

MATTHEWS, J. Groups take steps to put teeth in California's antitoxics law. *Washington Post*, August 3, 1988.

MATTSON, M.E., POLLACK, E.S., CULLEN, J.W. What are the odds that smoking will kill you? *American Journal of Public Health* 77(4):425–431, April 1987.

MCCARTHY, W.J. Testimony at the Hearings on Advertising of Tobacco Products before the Subcommittee on Health and the Environment of the Committee on Energy and Commerce, House of Representatives, 99th Congress, 2d Session, Serial No. 99-167, July 18, August 1, 1986.

MCGUINNESS, T., COWLING, K. Advertising and the aggregate demand for cigarettes. *European Economic Review* 6:311–328, 1975.

MCGUIRE, A. Cigarettes and fire deaths. *New York State Journal of Medicine* 83(13):1296–1298, December 1983.

MCGUIRE, F.L. Smoking, driver education, and other correlates of accidents among young males. *Journal of Safety Research* 4(1):5–11, March 1972.

MCKENNELL, A., THOMAS, R. *Adults' and Adolescents' Smoking Habits and Attitudes. Government Social Survey Report, SS353B*. London: Her Majesty's Stationery Office, 1967.

METRA CONSULTING GROUP. *The Relationship Between Total Cigarette Advertising and Total Cigarette Consumption in the UK*. Metra Consulting Group, 1979.

MICHIGAN DEPARTMENT OF PUBLIC HEALTH. *1980 Report of the Governor's Citizens' Panel on Smoking and Health*. Michigan Department of Public Health, 1980.

MICHIGAN DEPARTMENT OF PUBLIC HEALTH. *Smoking is Killing Your Constituents. Deaths Due to Smoking by Michigan State Senate Districts*. Michigan Department of Public Health, Division of Health Education, November 1984.

MILLAR, W.J. *Smoke in the Workplace: A Survey of Health and Welfare Employee Opinion*. Canadian Health and Welfare, Health Services and Promotion Branch, 1986.

MILLER, M. The first amendment and legislative bans of liquor and cigarette advertisements. *Columbia Law Review* 85(3):632–655, April 1985.

MILLER, R. Cigarettes: Consumption, situation and outlook. In: *Proceedings of the Fifty-Sixth Annual Meeting*, National Tobacco Tax Association, 1982.

MILLIGAN, S. AARC Airline Smoking Survey: Airline passengers prefer smoke-free environment. *AARC Times* 11(11):20–25, November 1987.

MINNESOTA DEPARTMENT OF HEALTH. *The Minnesota Plan for Nonsmoking and Health. Report and Recommendations of the Technical Advisory Committee on Nonsmoking and Health*. Minnesota Department of Health, September 1984.

MINNESOTA DEPARTMENT OF HEALTH. *The Minnesota Nonsmoking Initiative, June, 1985–December, 1986. A Report to the 1987 Legislature*. Minnesota Department of Health, Center for Nonsmoking and Health, 1987a.

MINNESOTA DEPARTMENT OF HEALTH. *The Path to Nonsmoking. Summary of the Minnesota Plan for Nonsmoking and Health*. Minnesota: Center for Nonsmoking and Health, 1987b.

MOHL, B. Dukakis signs 5 percent cigarette tax. *Boston Globe*, June 24, 1988, p. 1.

MOORE, E., Information Analyst, Communications Division, Blue Cross/Blue Shield Association. Personal communication to Chris Pashos, Institute for the Study of Smoking Behavior and Policy, John F. Kennedy School of Government, Harvard University, Cambridge, Massachusetts, June 1988.

MORRALL, J.F. A review of the record. *Regulation* 10(2):25–34, November–December 1986.

MORRIS, L.A., KANOUSE, D.E. Informing patients about drug side effects. *Journal of Behavioral Medicine* 5(3):363–373, 1982.

MORRIS, L.A., MAZIS, M., GORDON, E. A survey of the effects of oral contraceptive patient information. *Journal of the American Medical Association* 238(23):2504–2508, 1977.

MULLAHY, J. *Cigarette Smoking: Habits, Health Concerns, and Heterogeneous Unobservables in a Microeconomic Analysis of Consumer Demand*. Doctoral Dissertation. University of Virginia. Ann Arbor, University Microfilms International, Thesis No. 86-15599, 1985.

MULTIPLE RISK FACTOR INTERVENTION TRIAL RESEARCH GROUP. Multiple Risk Factor Intervention Trial: Risk factor changes and mortality results. *Journal of the American Medical Association* 248(12):1465–1477, September 24, 1982.

MURIS, T.J. Letter from Timothy J. Muris, Director, Bureau of Consumer Protection, Federal Trade Commission, to the Honorable John D. Dingell, U.S. House of Representatives, September 1, 1982.

MURPHY, R.D. Consumer responses to cigarette health warnings. In: Morris, L.A., Mazis, M.B., Barofsky, I. (eds.) *Product Labeling and Health Risks. Banbury Report No. 6.* Cold Springs Harbor, New York: Cold Springs Harbor Laboratory, 1980, pp. 13–18.

MURRAY, M., KIRYLUK, S., SWAN, A.V. School characteristics and adolescent smoking. Results from the MRC/Derbyshire Smoking Study of 1974–8 and from a follow up in 1981. *Journal of Epidemiology and Community Health* 38:167–172, 1984.

NATIONAL ASSOCIATION OF INSURANCE COMMISSIONERS. Resolution on financial incentives. December 1984. *NAIC Proceedings 1985* 1:638, 1985a.

NATIONAL ASSOCIATION OF INSURANCE COMMISSIONERS. NAIC Model rule (regulation) permitting smoker/nonsmoker mortality tables for use in determining minimum reserve liabilities and nonforfeiture benefits. *Model Regulation Service* 812.1–812.3, January 1985b.

NATIONAL ASSOCIATION OF INSURANCE COMMISSIONERS. Health Promotion and Chemical Abuse (B) Task Force. June 23, 1987 report. *NAIC Proceedings 1987* 2:648–650, 1987a.

NATIONAL ASSOCIATION OF INSURANCE COMMISSIONERS. ASH special report. Charging smokers more for health insurance is fair and legal. *NAIC Proceedings 1987* 2:653–659, 1987b.

NATIONAL ASSOCIATION OF INSURANCE COMMISSIONERS. Life and Health Actuarial (Ex5) Task Force results of field test of the Smoker/Nonsmoker Experience Exhibit. *NAIC Proceedings 1987* 2:687–705, 1987c.

NATIONAL ASSOCIATION OF INSURANCE COMMISSIONERS. NAIC Life and Health Actuarial Task Force results of field test of the Smoker/Nonsmoker Experience Exhibit. *NAIC Proceedings 1987* 2:717–722, 1987d.

NATIONAL ASSOCIATION OF INSURANCE COMMISSIONERS. Personal Lines—Property and Casualty (C) Committee. June 25, 1987 report. *NAIC Proceedings 1987* 2:769–771, 1987e.

NATIONAL ASSOCIATION OF INSURANCE COMMISSIONERS. NAIC model rule (regulation) permitting smoker/nonsmoker mortality tables for use in determining minimum reserve liabilities and nonforfeiture benefits. *Model Regulation Service* 812.4–812.7, January 1987f.

NATIONAL FIRE PROTECTION ASSOCIATION. *Major Causes of 1981–85 Home Fires.* Quincy, Massachusetts: National Fire Protection Association, 1987.

NATIONAL RESEARCH COUNCIL. *The Airliner Cabin Environment. Air Quality and Safety.* Washington, D.C.: National Academy Press, 1986a.

NATIONAL RESEARCH COUNCIL. *Environmental Tobacco Smoke. Measuring Exposures and Assessing Health Effects.* Washington, D.C.: National Academy Press, 1986b.

NATIONAL SCHOOL BOARDS ASSOCIATION. *Study on Nonsmoking Policies in the Nation's School Districts.* Washington, D.C.: National School Boards Association, 1986.

NATIONAL SCHOOL BOARDS ASSOCIATION. *No Smoking: A Board Member's Guide to Nonsmoking Policies for the Schools.* Alexandria, Virginia: National School Boards Association, June 1987.

NEUBERGER, M.B. *Smoke Screen: Tobacco and the Public Welfare.* Englewood Cliffs, New Jersey: Prentice-Hall, 1963.

NEUBORNE, B. Testimony at the Hearings on Advertising of Tobacco Products before the Subcommittee on Health and the Environment of the Committee on Energy and Commerce, House of Representatives, 99th Congress, 2d Session, Serial No. 99-167, July 18, August 1, 1986.

NEVILLE, H.R. Smoking banned in leading cancer centers. *Journal of the National Cancer Institute* 80(11):798–799, August 3, 1988.

NEW JERSEY COMMISSION ON SMOKING OR HEALTH. Preventing tobacco dependence. *New Jersey Medicine* 85(2):151–155, February 1988.

NEW JERSEY GROUP AGAINST SMOKING POLLUTION. New Jersey GASP salutes New Jersey's tobacco-free pharmacies. *New Jersey Medicine* 85(2):107, February 1988.

NEW YORK CITY DEPARTMENT OF HEALTH. *Report of the Mayor's Committee on Smoking and Health* (and Appendixes). New York City Department of Health, July 1, 1986.

NEW YORK CITY DEPARTMENT OF HEALTH. *The Clean Indoor Air Act: Smoking Regulations for New York City.* New York City Department of Health, 1988.

NEW YORK TIMES. Beverly Hills eases its ban on smoking in restaurants. *New York Times*, July 23, 1987.

NEW YORK TIMES. Support for smoking bans. *New York Times*, July 5, 1988, p. B2.

NORTH DAKOTA STATE DEPARTMENT OF HEALTH. *Smoking in North Dakota: Mortality and Low Birth Weight.* North Dakota State Department of Health, Preventive Health Section, December 1986.

NORTHWEST AIRLINES. Northwest Airlines to have only smoke free flights throughout North America system. Press release. New York: Northwest Airlines, March 23, 1988.

NOVEMBER, W.J., HAMMOND, E.C., HOCKETT, R.C., LERICHE, W.H. Mortality of smokers and nonsmokers. *Transactions of the Society of Actuaries* 16:D118–D145, April–May 1964.

O'CONNELL, D.L., ALEXANDER, H.M., DOBSON, A.J., LLOYD, D.M., HARDES, G.R., SPRINGTHORPE, H.J., LEEDER, S.R. Cigarette smoking and drug use in schoolchildren: II. Factors associated with smoking. *International Journal of Epidemiology* 10(3):223–231, 1981.

O'KEEFE, M.T. The anti-smoking commercials: A study of television's impact on behavior. *Public Opinion Quarterly* 35(2):242–248, 1971.

O'TOOLE, J. Testimony at the Hearings on Advertising of Tobacco Products before the Subcommittee on Health and the Environment of the Committee on Energy and Commerce, House of Representatives, 99th Congress, 2d Session, Serial No. 99-167, July 18, August 1, 1986.

OCCUPATIONAL SAFETY AND HEALTH ACT OF 1970, 29 U.S.C. 2655(G) and (C).

OCCUPATIONAL SAFETY AND HEALTH ADMINISTRATION. Letter to David Horne. Document No. 02026, 1987.

OKIE, S. Ad dollars seen inhibiting antismoking news: AMA seeks cigarette-promotion ban as publications defend record. *Washington Post*, December 11, 1985, pp. A1, A18.

PALMER V. LIGGETT GROUP, INC., C.A. 83-2445-MA (D. Mass. Feb 1, 1984).

PELES, Y. Rate of amortization of advertising expenditures. *Journal of Political Economy* 79:1032–1058, 1971.

PENNSYLVANIA PLAN FOR TOBACCO OR HEALTH. *Pennsylvania Consensus Conference on Tobacco and Health Priorities.* Pennsylvania Cancer Plan, Pennsylvania Department of Health, Pennsylvania Interagency Council on Tobacco and Health, Statewide Health Coordinating Council, 1986.

PETERSEN, L.R., HELGERSON, S.D., GIBBONS, C.M., CALHOUN, C.R., CIACCO, K.H., PITCHFORD, K.C. Employee smoking behavior changes and attitudes following a restrictive policy on worksite smoking in a large company. *Public Health Reports* 103(2):115–120, 1988.

PETO, J. Price and consumption of cigarettes: A case for intervention? *British Journal of Preventive and Social Medicine* 28:241–245, 1974.

PILLSBURY, H.C., BRIGHT, C.C., O'CONNOR, K.J., IRISH, F.W. Tar and nicotine in cigarette smoke. *Journal of Official Analytical Chemists* 52(3):458–462, 1969.

POPPER, E.T. *Sampling and Couponing Promotional Activity in the Domestic Cigarette Market. A Report to the Office on Smoking and Health.* Presented to Federal Interagency Committee on Smoking and Health, May 15, 1986a.

POPPER, E.T. Testimony at the Hearings on Advertising of Tobacco Products before the Subcommittee on Health and the Environment of the Committee on Energy and Commerce, House of Representatives, 99th Congress, 2d Session, Serial No. 99-167, August 1, 1986b, pp. 119–156.

POPPER, E.T. Statement in Support of Petition for FDA Jurisdiction Over Low Tar Cigarettes. Unpublished, April 1988.

POPPER, E.T., MURRAY, K.B. Format effects on in-ad disclosure. In: Srull, T. (ed.) *Advances in Consumer Research*, Volume 15. Association for Consumer Research, 1988.

PORTER, A. Disciplinary attitudes and cigarette smoking: A comparison of two schools. *British Medical Journal* 285:1725–1726, December 11, 1982.

PORTER, R.H. The impact of Government policy on the U.S. cigarette industry. In: Ippolito, P.M., Scheffman, D.T. (eds.) *Empirical Approaches to Consumer Protection Economics.* Federal Trade Commission, Bureau of Economics Conference, March 1986, pp. 447–484.

PUBLIC CITIZEN. Petition requesting an emergency temporary standard to prohibit smoking in indoor workplaces under the authority of the Occupational Safety and Health Act, May 6, 1987.

R.J. REYNOLDS TOBACCO COMPANY. Of cigarettes and science. *Time*, March 25, 1985a, p. 38.

R.J. REYNOLDS TOBACCO COMPANY. Smoking article. European Patent Application No. 0174645, filed Sept. 11, 1985b.

R.J. REYNOLDS TOBACCO COMPANY. R.J. Reynolds Tobacco Co. developing new cigarette. Press release. Winston-Salem, North Carolina: R.J. Reynolds Tobacco Company, September 14, 1987.

R.J. REYNOLDS TOBACCO COMPANY. *Chemical and Biological Studies on New Cigarette Prototypes That Heat Instead of Burn Tobacco.* Winston-Salem, North Carolina: R.J. Reynolds Tobacco Company, 1988.

RADFAR, M. The effect of advertising on total consumption of cigarettes in the U.K. *European Economic Review* 29(2):225–231, November 1985.

RADOVSKY, L., BARRY, P.P. Tobacco advertisements in physicians' offices: A pilot study of physician attitudes. *American Journal of Public Health* 78(2):174–175, February 1988.

RANIER BANCORPORATION. Survey response: Smoking policy improves work environment. *Venture*, August–September 1986, p. 10.

REID, D. Prevention of smoking among school children: Recommendations for policy development. *Health Education Journal* 44(1):3–12, 1985.

REIMER, R.A. *The Proposed Prohibition on Advertising Tobacco Products: A Constitutional Analysis.* Congressional Research Service, The Library of Congress, 1986.

REUIJL, J.C. *On the Determination of Advertising Effectiveness. An Empirical Study of the German Cigarette Market.* The Netherlands: Kluwer-Nijhoff Publishing, 1982.

REVILL, J., DRURY, C.G. An assessment of the incidence of cigarette smoking in fourth year school children and factors leading to its establishment. *Public Health* (London) 94:243–260, 1980.

REYNOLDS, O.M. JR. Extinguishing brushfires: Legal limits on the smoking of tobacco. *University of Cincinnati Law Review* 53(2):435–467, 1984.

RICHARDS, J.I., ZAKIA, R.D. Pictures: An advertiser's expressway through FTC regulation. *Georgia Law Review* (16):77–134, 1981.

RICHARDS, J.W. JR., BLUM, A. Pharmacists who dispense cigarettes. With reference to drug store chains and pharmaceutical companies. *New York State Journal of Medicine* 85(7):350–353, July 1985.

RIGOTTI, N.A. Trends in the adoption of smoking restrictions in public places and worksites. *New York State Journal of Medicine* 89(1):19–26, January 1989.

RIGOTTI, N.A., HILL PIKL, B., CLEARY, P., SINGER, D.E., MULLEY, A.G. The impact of banning smoking on a hospital ward: Acceptance, compliance, air quality and smoking behavior. (Abstract.) *Clinical Research* 34(2):833A, 1986.

RIGOTTI, N.A., STOTO, M.A., KLEIMAN, M., SCHELLING, T.C. Implementation and impact of a city's regulation of smoking in public places and the workplace: The experience of Cambridge, Massachusetts. In: *Smoking Behavior and Policy Discussion Paper Series.* Institute for the Study of Smoking Behavior and Policy, John F. Kennedy School of Government, Harvard University, January 1988.

RIGOTTI, N.A., TESAR, G.E. Smoking cessation in the prevention of cardiovascular disease. *Cardiology Clinics* 3(2):245–257, May 1985.

ROBERTS, M.J., SAMUELSON, L. An empirical analysis of dynamic, nonprice competition in an oligopolistic industry. *Rand Journal of Economics* 19(2):200–220, Summer 1988.

ROEMER, R. *Legislative Action to Combat the World Smoking Epidemic.* Geneva, Switzerland: World Health Organization, 1982.

ROEMER, R. *Recent Developments in Legislation to Combat the World Smoking Epidemic.* Geneva, Switzerland: World Health Organization, 1986.

ROSENSTOCK, I.M., STERGACHIS, A., HEANEY, C. Evaluation of smoking prohibition policy in a health maintenance organization. *American Journal of Public Health* 76(8):1014–1015, August 1986.

RUSSELL, M.A.H. Changes in cigarette price and consumption by men in Britain, 1946–71: A preliminary analysis. *British Journal of Preventive and Social Medicine* 27(1):1–7, February 1973.

SCHELLING, T.C. Economics and cigarettes. *Preventive Medicine* 15(5):549–560, September 1986.

SCHILLING, R.F. II., GILCHRIST, L.D., SCHINKE, S.P. Smoking in the workplace: Review of critical issues. *Public Health Reports* 100(5):473–479, September–October 1985.

SCHMALENSEE, R. *The Economics of Advertising.* Amsterdam, Holland: North-Holland Publishing, 1972.

SCHMITT, E. Smoke clears and trains are cleaner. *New York Times*, March 2, 1988, p. B1, B5.

SCHMITZ, G. Cigarette, liquor ads banned from RTD buses. *Denver Post*, August 1, 1984.

SCHNEIDER, L., KLEIN, B., MURPHY, K.M. Governmental regulation of cigarette health information. *Journal of Law and Economics* 24:575–612, December 1981.

SCHROEDER, S.A., SHOWSTACK, J.A. Merchandising cigarettes in pharmacies: A San Francisco survey. *American Journal of Public Health* 68(5):494–495, May 1978.

SCHWARTZ, T.M. The relevance of overpromotion in tobacco products litigation. *Tobacco Products Liability Reporter* 4:4.41–4.44, 1986.

SELDES, G. *Lords of The Press.* New York: Blue Ribbon Books, 1941.

SHAMAN, D. Nonsmokers make good risks, say insurance companies. *American Lung Association Bulletin* 68(7):2–6, September–October 1982.

SHARP, C. Testimony at the Hearings on Advertising of Tobacco Products before the Subcommittee on Health and the Environment of the Committee on Energy and Commerce, House of Representatives, 99th Congress, 2d Session, Serial No. 99-167, July 18, August 1, 1986.

SHEPPARD, P.L. Transnational corporations and the international cigarette industry. In: Newfarmer, R.S. (ed.) *Profits, Progress and Poverty*. South Bend, Indiana: University of Notre Dame Press, 1985, pp. 63–112.

SHIPLEY, R.H., ORLEANS, C.T., WILBUR, C.S., PISERCHIA, P.V., MCFADDEN, D.W. Effect of the Johnson and Johnson LIVE FOR LIFE Program on employee smoking. *Preventive Medicine* 17(1):25–34, January 1988.

SIMONS-MORTON, B.G., PARCEL, G.S., O'HARA, N.M. Implementing organizational changes to promote healthful diet and physical activity at school. *Health Education Quarterly* 15(1):115–130, Spring 1988.

SLADE, J. Learning to fight nicotiana tabacum. *New Jersey Medicine* 85(2):102–106, February 1988a.

SLADE, J. Testimony at the Hearings on the Health Consequences of Smoking: Nicotine Addiction, before the Subcommittee on Health and the Environment, Committee on Energy and Commerce, U.S. House of Representatives, 100th Congress, 2d Session, Serial No. 100-168, July 29, 1988b, pp. 163–277.

SLADE, J., APOSTOLOV, G., CONNOLLY, P., ZANETTI, C. Preventing cigarette acquisition by the young. Unpublished manuscript, 1988.

SMITH, J.F. Sample cigarettes outlawed. City council prohibits tobacco giveaways on streets. *Cincinnati Enquirer*, November 3, 1988, p. D1.

SMITH, R.C. The magazines' smoking habit. *Columbia Journalism Review* 16:29–31, January–February 1978.

SMOKELESS TOBACCO COUNCIL. *Advertising and Sampling Code for Smokeless Tobacco Products*. Washington, D.C.: Smokeless Tobacco Council, 1986.

SOCIETY OF ACTUARIES. *Task Force on Smoker/Non-Smoker Mortality*. Itaska, Illinois: Society of Actuaries, October 3, 1983.

SORENSEN, G., PECHACEK, T.F. Implementing nonsmoking policies in the private sector and assessing their effects. *New York State Journal of Medicine* 89(1):11–15, January 1989.

SPENCE, D.P. Subliminal perception and perceptual defense: Two sides to a single problem. *Behavioral Science* 12:183–193, 1967.

SPENCE, H.E., ENGEL, J.F. The impact of brand preference on the perception of brand names: A laboratory analysis. In: McDonald, P.R. (ed.) *Marketing Involvement in Society*. Chicago: American Marketing Association, 1970, pp. 267–271.

STANWICK, R.S., FISH, D.G., MANFREDA, J., GELSKEY, D., SKUBA, A. Where Manitoba children obtain their cigarettes. *Canadian Medical Association Journal* 137:405–408, September 1, 1987.

STARK, F.H. Testimony at the Hearings on Advertising of Tobacco Products before the Subcommittee on Health and the Environment of the Committee on Energy and Commerce, House of Representatives, 99th Congress, 2d Session, Serial No. 99-167, August 1, 1986.

STOKES, J. III. Why not rate health and life insurance premiums by risks? *New England Journal of Medicine* 308(7):393–395, February 17, 1983.

SUBCOMMITTEE ON HEALTH AND THE ENVIRONMENT. Hearings on Advertising of Tobacco Products. Committee on Energy and Commerce of the House of Representatives, 99th Congress, 2d Session, Serial No. 99-167, July 18, August 1, 1986.

TAYLOR, A.T., RICHARDS, J.W., FISCHER, P.M. The sale of tobacco in Georgia pharmacies. Unpublished manuscript, 1987.

TAYLOR, P. *The Smoke Ring: Tobacco, Money, and Multinational Politics*. New York: Pantheon Books, 1984.

THOMPSON, B., SEXTON, M., SINSHEIMER, J. Smoking policy at the worksite: Employee reactions to policy changes. In: *Advances in Cancer Control: The War on Cancer—15 Years of Progress*. Alan R. Liss, 1987, pp. 101–108.

TIMMINS, W.M. Smoking versus nonsmoking at work: A survey of public agency policy and practice. *Public Personnel Management* 16(3):221–234, Fall 1987.

TOBACCO-FREE AMERICA PROJECT. *State Regulations Limiting Smoking on School Property*. Washington, D.C.: Tobacco-Free America Project, June 1988a.

TOBACCO-FREE AMERICA PROJECT. *State Legislated Actions on Tobacco Issues*. Washington, D.C.: Tobacco-Free America Project, October 1988b.

TOBACCO-FREE AMERICA PROJECT. *State Legislated Actions: Limitations on Smoking in Public Places*. Washington, D.C.: Tobacco-Free America Project, October 1988c.

TOBACCO-FREE YOUNG AMERICA PROJECT. *State Legislated Actions on Clean Indoor Air, Cigarette Excise Taxes, and Sale of Cigarettes to Minors*. Washington, D.C.: Tobacco-Free Young America Project, October 1987.

TOBACCO INSTITUTE. *Code of Cigarette Sampling Practices*. Washington, D.C.: Tobacco Institute, 1981.

TOBACCO INSTITUTE. *Answers to the Most Asked Questions About Cigarettes*.Washington, D.C.: Tobacco Institute, 1983.

TOBACCO INSTITUTE. Monthly State cigarette tax report. *Cigarette Tax Data*, June 1988a.

TOBACCO INSTITUTE. *The Tax Burden on Tobacco. Historical Compilation*, Volume 22, 1987. Washington, D.C.: Tobacco Institute, 1988b.

TOBACCO PRODUCTS LITIGATION REPORTER. Mutual Benefit Life Insurance Company, Plaintiff, v. JMR Electronics Corp., Defendant. 61979 87 Civ. 1822 (RWS). *Tobacco Products Litigation Reporter* 3(3):2.64–2.65, March 1988.

TOBACCO TAX AND HEALTH PROTECTION ACT OF 1988. Proposition 99, California, 1988.

TODER, E.J. The effect of the Federal cigarette tax increase on State tax revenues. In: *Proceedings of the Fifty-Sixth Annual Meeting*. National Tobacco Association, 1982.

TODER, E.J. Issues in the taxation of cigarettes. In: *The Cigarette Excise Tax*. Cambridge, Massachusetts: Institute for the Study of Smoking Behavior and Policy, John F. Kennedy School of Government, Harvard University, April 17, 1985, pp. 65–87.

TORABI, M.R., SEFFRIN, J.R., BRASHEAR, R.E. A statewide survey of hospital policy and practice concerning cigarette sales: A follow-up study. *Indiana Medicine* 80(8):756–758, August 1987.

TRENK, B.S. Health insurers slow to accept non-smoker discounts. *American Medical News*, October 10, 1986, pp. 43–44.

TYE, J.B. Cigarette ads reveal a history of deceit. *Wall Street Journal*, August 5, 1986, p. 30.

TYE, J.B., WARNER, K.E., GLANTZ, S.A. Tobacco advertising and consumption: Evidence of a causal relationship. *Journal of Public Health Policy* 8(4):492–508, Winter 1987.

U.S. BUREAU OF THE CENSUS. *Statistical Abstract of the United States 1988*. U.S. Bureau of the Census, U.S. Department of Commerce, 1988.

U.S. DEPARTMENT OF AGRICULTURE, BUREAU OF CHEMISTRY. Service and Regulatory Announcements, No. 13 (1914).

U.S. DEPARTMENT OF DEFENSE. *Directive 1010.10: Health Promotion*. U.S. Department of Defense, March 11, 1986a.

U.S. DEPARTMENT OF DEFENSE. *Defense 86 Almanac*. U.S. Department of Defense, September–October 1986b.

U.S. DEPARTMENT OF DEFENSE. *Report on Smoking and Health in the Military*. U.S. Department of Defense, Office of the Assistant Secretary of Defense (Health Affairs), Office of the Assistant Secretary of Defense (Force Management and Personnel), March 1986c.

U.S. DEPARTMENT OF DEFENSE. *Updated Report on Smoking and Health in the Military*. U.S. Department of Defense, Office of the Assistant Secretary of Defense (Health Affairs), Office of the Assistant Secretary of Defense (Force Management and Personnel), June 1987.

U.S. DEPARTMENT OF HEALTH AND HUMAN SERVICES. *Promoting Health/Preventing Disease: Objectives for the Nation.* U.S. Department of Health and Human Services, Public Health Service, 1980.

U.S. DEPARTMENT OF HEALTH AND HUMAN SERVICES. *The Health Consequences of Smoking. The Changing Cigarette: A Report of the Surgeon General.* U.S. Department of Health and Human Services, Public Health Service, Office of the Assistant Secretary for Health, Office on Smoking and Health. DHEW Publication No. (PHS) 81-50156, 1981a.

U.S. DEPARTMENT OF HEALTH AND HUMAN SERVICES. *Prevention '80.* U.S. Department of Health and Human Services, Public Health Service, Office of Disease Prevention and Health Promotion. DHHS Publication No. (PHS) 81-50157, 1981b.

U.S. DEPARTMENT OF HEALTH AND HUMAN SERVICES. *The Health Consequences of Smoking: Cancer. A Report of the Surgeon General.* U.S. Department of Health and Human Services, Public Health Service, Office on Smoking and Health. DHHS Publication No. (PHS) 82-50179, 1982a.

U.S. DEPARTMENT OF HEALTH AND HUMAN SERVICES. *Prevention '82.* U.S. Department of Health and Human Services, Public Health Service, Office of Disease Prevention and Health Promotion. DHHS Publication No. (PHS) 82-50157, 1982b.

U.S. DEPARTMENT OF HEALTH AND HUMAN SERVICES. *The Health Consequences of Smoking: Chronic Obstructive Lung Disease. A Report of the Surgeon General.* U.S. Department of Health and Human Services, Public Health Service, Office on Smoking and Health. DHHS Publication No. (PHS) 84-50205, 1984.

U.S. DEPARTMENT OF HEALTH AND HUMAN SERVICES. Notice regarding requirements for submission of list of ingredients added to tobacco in cigarettes. *Federal Register* 50(232):49617–49619, December 3, 1985a.

U.S. DEPARTMENT OF HEALTH AND HUMAN SERVICES. *Prevention '84/'85.* U.S. Department of Health and Human Services, Public Health Service, Office of Disease Prevention and Health Promotion, 1985b.

U.S. DEPARTMENT OF HEALTH AND HUMAN SERVICES. *A Decision Maker's Guide to Reducing Smoking at the Worksite.* U. S. Department of Health and Human Services, Public Health Service, Office on Smoking and Health, Office of Disease Prevention and Health Promotion, 1985c.

U.S. DEPARTMENT OF HEALTH AND HUMAN SERVICES. *The Health Consequences of Smoking: Cancer and Chronic Lung Disease in the Workplace. A Report of the Surgeon General.* U.S. Department of Health and Human Services, Public Health Service, Office on Smoking and Health. DHHS Publication No. 85-50207, 1985d.

U.S. DEPARTMENT OF HEALTH AND HUMAN SERVICES, NATIONAL INSTITUTES OF HEALTH. Health applications of smokeless tobacco use. *Journal of the American Medical Association* 255(8):1045–1048, February 28, 1986a.

U.S. DEPARTMENT OF HEALTH AND HUMAN SERVICES. *The Health Consequences of Involuntary Smoking. A Report of the Surgeon General.* U.S. Department of Health and Human Services, Public Health Service, Centers for Disease Control. DHHS Publication No. (CDC) 87-8398, 1986b.

U.S. DEPARTMENT OF HEALTH AND HUMAN SERVICES. *The Health Consequences of Using Smokeless Tobacco. A Report of the Advisory Committee to the Surgeon General, 1986.* U.S. Department of Health and Human Services, Public Health Service. NIH Publication No. 86-2874, April 1986c.

U.S. DEPARTMENT OF HEALTH AND HUMAN SERVICES. *The 1990 Health Objectives for the Nation: A Midcourse Review.* U.S. Department of Health and Human Services, Public Health Service, Office of Disease Prevention and Health Promotion, November 1986d.

U.S. DEPARTMENT OF HEALTH AND HUMAN SERVICES. *Smoking and Health. A National Status Report. A Report to Congress.* U.S. Department of Health and Human Services, Public Health Service, Centers for Disease Control, Center for Health Promotion and Education, Office on Smoking and Health. DHHS Publication No. (CDC) 87-8396, 1986e.

U.S. DEPARTMENT OF HEALTH AND HUMAN SERVICES. *Report to Congress. Comprehensive Smokeless Tobacco Health Education Act of 1986, Public Law 99-252.* U.S. Department of Health and Human Services, Public Health Service, Centers for Disease Control, Center for Prevention Services, Dental Disease Prevention Activity, 1987a.

U.S. DEPARTMENT OF HEALTH AND HUMAN SERVICES. *Prevention '86/'87. Federal Programs and Progress.* U.S. Department of Health and Human Services, Public Health Service, Office of Disease Prevention and Health Promotion, 1987b.

U.S. DEPARTMENT OF HEALTH AND HUMAN SERVICES. *National Survey of Worksite Health Promotion Activities: A Summary.* U.S. Department of Health and Human Services, Public Health Service, Office of Disease Prevention and Health Promotion, 1987c.

U.S. DEPARTMENT OF HEALTH AND HUMAN SERVICES. *Review of the Research on the Effects of Health Warning Labels. A Report to the United States Congress.* U.S. Department of Health and Human Services, June 1987d.

U.S. DEPARTMENT OF HEALTH AND HUMAN SERVICES. *Smoking, Tobacco, and Health Fact Book.* U.S. Department of Health and Human Services, Public Health Service, Centers for Disease Control, Center for Health Promotion and Education, Office on Smoking and Health. DHHS Publication No. (CDC) 87-8397, 1987e.

U.S. DEPARTMENT OF HEALTH AND HUMAN SERVICES. *The Health Consequences of Smoking: Nicotine Addiction. A Report of the Surgeon General, 1988.* U.S. Department of Health and Human Services, Public Health Service, Centers for Disease Control, Center for Health Promotion and Education, Office on Smoking and Health. DHHS Publication No. (CDC) 88-8406, 1988.

U.S. DEPARTMENT OF HEALTH, EDUCATION, AND WELFARE. *The Health Consequences of Smoking.* U.S. Department of Health, Education, and Welfare, Public Health Service, Health Services and Mental Health Administration. DHEW Publication No. (HSM) 73-8704, 1973.

U.S. DEPARTMENT OF HEALTH, EDUCATION, AND WELFARE. *The Health Consequences of Smoking, 1977–1978.* U.S. Department of Health, Education, and Welfare, Public Health Service, Office of the Assistant Secretary for Health, Office on Smoking and Health. DHEW Publication No. (PHS) 79-50065, 1978.

U.S. DEPARTMENT OF HEALTH, EDUCATION, AND WELFARE. *Smoking and Health. A Report of the Surgeon General.* U.S. Department of Health, Education, and Welfare, Public Health Service, Office of the Assistant Secretary for Health, Office on Smoking and Health. DHEW Publication No. (PHS) 79-50066, 1979.

U.S. OFFICE OF TECHNOLOGY ASSESSMENT. *Passive Smoking in the Workplace: Selected Issues.* U.S. Office of Technology Assessment, May 1986.

U.S. PUBLIC HEALTH SERVICE. *Smoking and Health. Report of the Advisory Committee to the Surgeon General of the Public Health Service.* U.S. Department of Health, Education, and Welfare, Public Health Service, Center for Disease Control. PHS Publication No. 1103, 1964.

U.S. SENATE. Senate Report No. 91-566. *U.S. Code Congressional and Administrative News* 2:2652–2680, April 1, 1970.

U.S.A. V. LIGGETT ET AL. 76 Civ. 811 (S.D.N.Y. 1981).

U.S.A. V. R.J. REYNOLDS TOBACCO CO., 1980–81, *Trade Cas. (CCH)* 63,847 (S.D.N.Y. 1981).

UNITED STATES V. 354 BULK CARTONS TRIM REDUCING-AID CIGARETTES, 178 F. Supp. 847 (D.N.J. 1959).

UNITED STATES V. 46 CARTONS, MORE OR LESS, CONTAINING FAIRFAX CIGARETTES, 113 F. Supp. 336 (D.N.J. 1953).

UTAH. Cigarette and Tobacco Tax Codification. House Bill No. 138, 1986.

UTAH. Cigarettes and tobacco—Advertising restrictions. *Utah Code Ann.* 76-10 102 (1978).

UTAH. House Bill No. 35. Increasing the Cigarette Excise Tax. 1987 Legislative Session, 1987.

UTAH HOUSE OF REPRESENTATIVES. An Act to Prohibit Smokeless Tobacco. House Bill 154, 1986 General Session.

UZYCH, L. Teen tobacco laws. Unpublished manuscript, 1987.

VETERANS ADMINISTRATION. VA announces plans for smoke-free hospitals. Press release. December 22, 1988.

VILNIUS, D. Rocky Mountain States take aim at tobacco. *Chronic Disease Notes and Reports* 1(2):9, December 1988.

WAGNER, S. *Cigarette Country: Tobacco in American History and Politics.* New York: Praeger Publishers, 1971a.

WAGNER, S. *The Federal Trade Commission.* New York: Praeger Publishers, 1971b.

WALKER, R.B. Medical aspects of tobacco smoking and the anti-tobacco movement in Britain in the nineteenth century. *Medical History* 24:391–402, 1980.

WALSH, D.C., GORDON, N.P. Legal approaches to smoking deterence. *Annual Review of Public Health* 7:127–149, 1986.

WALSH, D.C., MCDOUGALL, V. Current policies regarding smoking in the workplace. *American Journal of Industrial Medicine* 13:181–190, 1988.

WARNER, K.E. The effects of the anti-smoking campaign on cigarette consumption. *American Journal of Public Health* 67(7):645–650, July 1977.

WARNER, K.E. Possible increases in the underreporting of cigarette consumption. *Journal of the American Statistical Association* 73(362):314–318, June 1978.

WARNER, K.E. Clearing the airwaves: The cigarette ad ban revisited. *Policy Analysis* 5(4):435–450, Fall 1979.

WARNER, K.E. Cigarette smoking in the 1970's: The impact of the antismoking campaign on consumption. *Science* 211(4483):729–731, February 13, 1981.

WARNER, K.E. Cigarette excise taxation and interstate smuggling: An assessment of recent activity. *National Tax Journal* 35(4):483–490, December 1982.

WARNER, K.E. Cigarette advertising and media coverage of smoking and health. *New England Journal of Medicine* 312:384–388, February 7, 1985.

WARNER, K.E. Smoking and health implications of a change in the Federal cigarette excise tax. *Journal of the American Medical Association* 255(8):1028–1032, February 28, 1986a.

WARNER, K.E. *Selling Smoke: Cigarette Advertising and Public Health.* Washington, D.C.: American Public Health Association, October 1986b.

WARNER, K.E. Selling health: A media campaign against tobacco. *Journal of Public Health Policy* 7(4):434–439 Winter 1986c.

WARNER, K.E. The tobacco subsidy: Does it matter? *Journal of the National Cancer Institute* 80(2):81–83, March 16, 1988.

WARNER, K.E. Effects of the antismoking campaign: An update. *American Journal of Public Health* 79(2):144–151, February 1989.

WARNER, K.E., ERNSTER, V.L., HOLBROOK, J.H., LEWIT, E.M., PERTSCHUK, M., STEINFELD, J.L., TYE, J.B., WHELAN, E.M. Promotion of tobacco products: Issues and policy options. *Journal of Health Politics, Policy and Law* 11(3):367–392, Fall 1986a.

WARNER, K., ERNSTER, V.L., HOLBROOK, J.H., LEWIT, E.M., PERTSCHUK, M., STEINFELD, J.L., WHELAN, E.M. Public policy on smoking and health: Toward a smoke-free generation by the year 2000. A statement of a working group to the Subcommittee on Smoking of the American Heart Association. *Circulation* 73(2):381A–395A, February 1986b.

WARNER, K.E., GOLDENHAR, L.M. The cigarette advertising broadcast ban and magazine coverage of smoking and health. *Journal of Public Health Policy*, in press.

WARNER, K.E., MURT, H.A. Economic incentives for health. *Annual Review of Public Health* 5:107–133, 1984.

WASHINGTON POST. Smoking ban takes effect in California. *Washington Post*, January 3, 1988, p. A19.

WASILEWSKI, C. Auto insurance marketing—1986. *Best's Review (Property/Casualty)* 88(5):30–32, 122–124, September 1987a.

WASILEWSKI, C. Property insurance marketing—1986. *Best's Review (Property/Casualty)* 88(7):32–36, 119–120, November 1987b.

WATERSON M.J. *Advertising and Cigarette Consumption*. London: Advertising Association, December 1982.

WEIL, G. Testimony at the Hearings on Advertising of Tobacco Products before the Subcommittee on Health and the Environment of the Committee on Energy and Commerce, House of Representatives, 99th Congress, 2d Session, Serial No. 99-167, July 18, August 1, 1986.

WEINMAN, S.J., Actuarial Manager, Hanover Insurance Company. Personal communications to Chris Pashos, Institute for the Study of Smoking Behavior and Policy, John F. Kennedy School of Government, Harvard University, Cambridge, Massachusetts, May 1988.

WHELAN, E.M. *A Smoking Gun: How the Tobacco Industry Gets Away With Murder*. Philadelphia: George F. Stickley, 1984.

WHELAN, E.M., SHERIDAN, M.J., MEISTER, K.A., MOSHER, B.A. Analysis of coverage of tobacco hazards in women's magazines. *Journal of Public Health Policy* 2(1):28–35, March 1981.

WHITE, L. A total ban on cigarette advertising: Is it constitutional? *ACSH News and Views* 5(4):1, 4–7, September–October 1984.

WHITE, L. A license to lie. *ACSH News and Views* 9–10, May–June 1987.

WHITE, L., WHELAN, E.M. How well do American magazines cover the health hazards of smoking? The 1986 survey. *ACSH News and Views* 7(3):1, 7–11, May–June 1986.

WHITESIDE, T. *Selling Death: Cigarette Advertising and Public Health*. New York: Liveright, 1971.

WILSON, D.S. Cigars and pipe tobacco to get warning labels. *New York Times*, October 19, 1988a.

WILSON, D.S. Two ballot issues raise question: Is smoking becoming taboo? *New York Times*, October 25, 1988b.

WORLD HEALTH ORGANIZATION. *Smoking and Its Effects on Health, Report of a WHO Expert Committee*. Technical Report Series 568. Geneva: World Health Organization, 1975.

WORLD HEALTH ORGANIZATION. Comparative health legislation: Legislative action to combat smoking. *International Digest of Health Legislation* 27(3):491–706, 1976.

WORLD HEALTH ORGANIZATION. *Controlling the Smoking Epidemic. Report of the WHO Expert Committee on Smoking Control*. WHO Technical Report Series 636. Geneva: World Health Organizaition, 1979.

WORLD HEALTH ORGANIZATION. *Primary Prevention of Coronary Heart Disease. Report on a WHO Meeting*. EURO Reports and Studies 98. Copenhagen: World Health Organization, 1985.

WORLD HEALTH ORGANIZATION. *Smokeless Tobacco Control. Report of the WHO Study Group*. Geneva: World Health Organization, in press.

YENCKEL, J.T. Smoke: In the air and on the ground. *Washington Post*, June 5, 1988, p. E1, E13.

YOUNG, F.E. Testimony at the Hearing on the Health Consequences of Smoking: Nicotine Addiction, before the Subcommittee on Health and the Environment, Committee on Energy and Commerce, U.S. House of Representatives, 100th Congress, 2d Session, Serial No. 100-168, July 29, 1988, pp. 15–19.

YOUNG, T. The demand for cigarettes: Alternative specifications of Fujii's model. *Applied Economics* 15(2):203–211, April 1983.

ZAMRAZIL, K. Health promotion or regulation compliance. Smoking polices in Texas hospitals. *Texas Hospitals* 40(1):23–26, June 1984.

ZERNER, C. Graphic propositions: The efficacy of imagery and the impotence of warnings in cigarette advertising. *Tobacco Products Litigation Reporter* 1(10):4.71–4.85, November 1986.

CHAPTER 8

CHANGES IN THE SMOKING-AND-HEALTH ENVIRONMENT: BEHAVIORAL AND HEALTH CONSEQUENCES

CONTENTS

Introduction

As the preceding chapters have documented, concern about the hazards of smoking during the past 25 years has been associated with development and dissemination of scientific knowledge and with a wide variety of private and public sector activities intended to reduce the disease burden of smoking. Collectively, these efforts have been labeled "the antismoking campaign" (Warner 1977, 1989). This Chapter reports on research concerning the effects of the campaign and accompanying knowledge and attitudinal changes on cigarette consumption and its mortality toll. Whereas previous chapters have examined trends in smoking behavior and its health consequences, the research reviewed in this Chapter analyzes how these trends compare with those that would have been expected in the absence of changes in the smoking-and-health environment.

Prior to reviewing the evidence, the next section presents a brief discussion of what the term "antismoking campaign" is intended to connote throughout the Chapter.

The Antismoking Campaign

Activities directed at discouraging the use of tobacco products were reviewed in Chapters 6 and 7. While some of these activities have been developed explicitly as campaigns against smoking, such as efforts of the major voluntary societies, there has been no single, longstanding, organized, national campaign to reduce smoking and its associated disease burden. The widespread perception of the existence of a national "campaign" reflects the large number of antismoking activities, their shared goals of smoking prevention and cessation, and their persistence throughout the past 25 years. Smoking cessation and prevention activities predated the first Surgeon General's Report, but 1964 marked the beginning of the first period of sustained, substantial, and expanding antismoking activity. Hence "the antismoking campaign" is typically dated from publication of the first Report. Important developments related to smoking and health from 1964 through 1988 are presented in the Appendix to this Chapter.

Throughout this Chapter, the term "antismoking campaign" is used in a broader context as a convenient designation for the collectivity of these activities and for the changing social norms that have accompanied them (see Chapter 4). In essence, it serves as a shorthand expression covering smoking-and-health knowledge, concern, and reaction, the entirety of changes in the social environment spawned by scientific and social interest in the hazards of smoking. This includes the conduct of the tobacco industry in response to concerns about those hazards. Thus, for example, manufacturers' promotion of low-tar and -nicotine cigarettes in the 1970s is both a response to public concerns about smoking and a contributor to smoking behavior and its health consequences. Research on the behavioral and health implications of the campaign therefore examines the net effects of "pro" and "anti"-smoking information and activities.

Scholars have addressed the effects of both specific seminal events of the antismoking campaign and the consequences of the campaign in its entirety. Among the seminal events analyzed by researchers are publication and media coverage of the first Surgeon General's Report, the Fairness Doctrine broadcast media antismoking public service announcements of 1967–70, the ensuing ban on broadcast advertising of cigarettes, and the spread of nonsmokers' rights legislation in the 1970s and 1980s, all discussed in the preceding chapter. The pattern of one significant influence on cigarette consumption—excise taxation—has also been considered part of the antismoking campaign: a steady pattern of increases in State taxes in the 8 years following release of the first Surgeon General's Report might be construed as a campaign response, at least in part (Warner 1981b). Analysis of the role of excise taxation in the antismoking campaign, reviewed below, has treated taxation as both a component of the campaign and an independent phenomenon (Warner 1977, 1981a, 1989).

Research reviewed in this Chapter focuses on campaign effects since 1964, with one important exception: the shift from unfiltered to filtered cigarettes in the 1950s following the first widespread public concern about a link between smoking and lung cancer, and cigarette manufacturers' development and marketing of new filter-tipped products.

Behavioral Effects of the Campaign

In terms of health implications, the most significant behavior changes associated with the antismoking campaign likely relate to the most basic measures of smoking: prevalence and per capita cigarette consumption. Following examination of the evidence pertaining to impact of the campaign on these variables, this Section briefly reviews two other behavioral measures relating to smokers' choice of cigarette type: shifts toward filtered cigarettes and low-tar and -nicotine brands.

Smoking Prevalence

The most common index of changes in smoking behavior is smoking prevalence. Trends in prevalence by a variety of socioeconomic and demographic characteristics were reviewed in Chapter 5. Analytical studies relating prevalence trends to antismoking activities are relatively few in number, although the literature on cigarette excise taxation and the broadcast media advertising ban includes studies that have relied on survey-based prevalence data; these were reviewed in Chapter 7 (e.g., Lewit, Coate, Grossman 1981; Lewit and Coate 1982).

Evidence pertaining to the effects of the antismoking campaign on smoking in various age–sex cohorts was examined in a previous Surgeon General's Report (US DHEW 1979). Since publication of that Report, two studies have analyzed the cohort prevalence effects of the antismoking campaign in its entirety (Warner and Murt 1982; Warner 1989). Findings from these studies are reviewed in this Section. Discussions of the strengths and limitations of cohort analyses have been presented previously by the Surgeon General (US DHHS 1980) and by other scientists (Harris 1983; Brown and Kessler 1988).

Among changes in the prevalence of smoking since 1964, some logically suggest significant response to the smoking-and-health message. The decreasing prevalence of smoking among both men and boys serves as the most obvious example. Other patterns often have been interpreted as reflecting little response to the message. The most notable example is the relatively steady trend in adult female smoking prevalence from

1964 through the late 1970s, followed by relatively modest decreases in the 1980s. A second example is the apparent increase in smoking by teenage girls through the mid-1970s. (See Chapter 5.)

Warner and Murt (1982) argued that the female prevalence data have been misinterpreted. Conceptually, they suggested, the appropriate question was how prevalence in a given year compared with the rate that would have been experienced without the campaign, and not simply how prevalence had changed over time. In the case of women, smoking prevalence had been rising rapidly since World War II, paralleling the diffusion pattern of smoking by men two to three decades earlier. Without the antismoking campaign, Warner and Murt argued, smoking prevalence would have been expected to have continued to increase as it had with men. As such, the stability of female smoking prevalence in the mid-1960s, at a level far below that attained by men, should be interpreted as a significant response to the antismoking campaign.

Warner and Murt (1982) and Warner (1989) developed estimates of prevalence without the campaign, a process they described as necessarily involving the use of numerous assumptions whose quantitative precision or qualitative appropriateness can be challenged. The authors tested the overall validity of their estimates by converting the annual cohort projections into estimates of annual aggregate cigarette consumption and then comparing these with estimates derived by Warner (1981a, 1989) in a methodologically distinct analysis of aggregate cigarette demand. The pattern generated by aggregating the subjective data was highly similar to that estimated through use of regression analysis with objective data on cigarette production and sales. Nevertheless, the nature and number of assumptions recommend that the analysis be interpreted in qualitative terms, as a demonstration that smoking prevalence has been influenced, apparently substantially, by the smoking-and-health message.

Tables 1 and 2 illustrate the authors' comparative perspective for men and women, respectively. Each cell in each table records smoking prevalence for the relevant birth cohort and the relevant year, in 5-year increments from 1965 through 1985, based on survey respondents' self-reports. These entries are called "reported" prevalence (R in the tables). (See Harris 1983 for discussion of retrospective self-report biases.) Each cell also provides an estimate of the smoking rate that might have been expected in the absence of the antismoking campaign ("expected" prevalence, E in the tables). The difference between the two figures for the specific birth cohort in a given year represents an estimate of the percentage points of smoking prevalence avoided by the campaign. Avoided prevalence includes both campaign-related quitting and noninitiation of smoking. The data are from Warner's (1989) updating of the authors' original study (Warner and Murt 1982). Both references describe the method of determining "expected" prevalence. The updated study presents annual data for both "reported" and "expected" prevalence for 1964 through 1985.

Table 1 indicates, for example, that in 1975, 53 percent of men born between 1941 and 1950 reported themselves to be smokers. However, had their smoking patterns not been influenced by the antismoking campaign, an estimated 64 percent of them would have been smoking in 1975. Without a response to the campaign, their smoking prevalence would have been 11 percentage points, or 21 percent, higher than it actually was. By 1985, the cohort's smoking prevalence had fallen 15 points to 38 per-

TABLE 1.—Smoking prevalence for males (percent), 1965–85, reported and expected in the absence of the antismoking campaign

Year	Birth cohort											
	1901–10		1911–20		1921–30		1931–40		1941–50		1951–60	
	R	E	R	E	R	E	R	E	R	E	R	E
1965	45	46	60	61	62	66	59	63	46	48	2	3
1970	39	42	53	56	55	64	53	64	58	62	18	21
1975	30	37	46	54	47	62	46	62	53	64	38	50
1980	18	32	30	49	41	58	44	58	44	63	42	64
1985	16	25	22	45	32	53	35	54	38	60	38	66
E–R, 1985	9		23		21		19		22		28	

NOTE: R, reported; E, expected; E–R, expected minus reported.
SOURCE: Warner (1989).

TABLE 2.—Smoking prevalence for females (percent), 1965–85, reported and expected in the absence of the antismoking campaign

	Birth cohort											
	1901–10		1911–20		1921–30		1931–40		1941–50		1951–60	
Year	R	E	R	E	R	E	R	E	R	E	R	E
1965	21	21	36	37	43	45	44	46	30	32	1	2
1970	18	19	33	36	40	48	43	48	41	46	13	15
1975	15	18	28	35	38	48	42	50	40	50	35	40
1980	15	16	26	33	31	47	35	51	34	52	32	50
1985	8	14	18	31	27	44	32	49	32	52	32	54
E–R, 1985	6		13		17		17		20		22	

NOTE: R, reported; E, expected; E–R, expected minus reported.
SOURCE: Warner (1989).

cent. Prevalence expected in the absence of the campaign would have fallen too, but only by 4 points (to 60 percent). Consequently, the gap between reported prevalence and that which would have been anticipated without the campaign had increased to 22 percentage points. Thus, Warner (1989) estimated that for men born between 1941 and 1950, smoking prevalence would have been 58 percent higher than it was in 1985 (the 22 percentage-point gap divided by reported prevalence of 38 percent), had the men's smoking not been influenced by smoking-and-health knowledge and social change.

Table 2 shows that for women born between 1921 and 1930, expected prevalence exceeded reported prevalence by 10 percentage points in 1975. Both measures fell through the mid-1980s, although reported prevalence decreased more than expected prevalence without the campaign, so that the gap between the two widened to 17 percentage points by 1985. In that year, according to the estimates, in the absence of the antismoking campaign, smoking prevalence in this cohort of women would have been 63 percent higher than it actually was (the 17 percentage-point gap divided by reported prevalence of 27 percent).

Figures 1 and 2 illustrate this perspective on the impact of the campaign on smoking prevalence by plotting annual figures for reported and expected prevalence, as well as pre-1964 prevalence estimates, for two other cohorts, one male and one female. In each case, the solid line plots actual reported prevalence and the dashed line plots the anticipated prevalence in the absence of the antismoking campaign. The gap between the two lines constitutes a measure of the impact of the campaign on smoking prevalence for these two birth cohorts.

The analysis indicates that all 12 of the age–sex birth cohorts experienced substantial quitting or noninitiation of smoking as a result of the antismoking campaign. By 1985, the estimated gap between actual (reported) prevalence and that anticipated without the campaign ranged from a low of 6 percentage points for the eldest female cohort to a high of 28 percentage points for the youngest males.

The percentage-point gap is larger for each male cohort than for the same-age female cohort. This is consistent with the common observation that the campaign has encouraged more men to quit than women. However, because the actual smoking prevalence of each birth cohort is smaller for women than for men, this standard observation misses an essential consideration: the ratios of percentage points of campaign-related quitters and noninitiators to the percentages of actual smokers are quite comparable for men and women. Thus, when the 1985 percentage-point gap (the last row in Tables 1 and 2) is divided by actual prevalence in that year, this measure of relative quit-and-nonstart rate indicates little difference between males and females.

The percentage-point gap in 1985 generally increases from the older to the younger birth cohorts, especially for the females. Warner and Murt observed that this might be expected because decisions concerning the initiation of smoking occurred after 1964 for many members of the two youngest cohorts and well before 1964 for the older cohorts. Decisions not to start smoking may be easier than decisions to quit.

The expected prevalence figures indicate that a majority of each of the four youngest male cohorts would have been expected to be smokers in 1985 without the campaign, including two-thirds of men born from 1951 through 1960. In fact, fewer than 40 per-

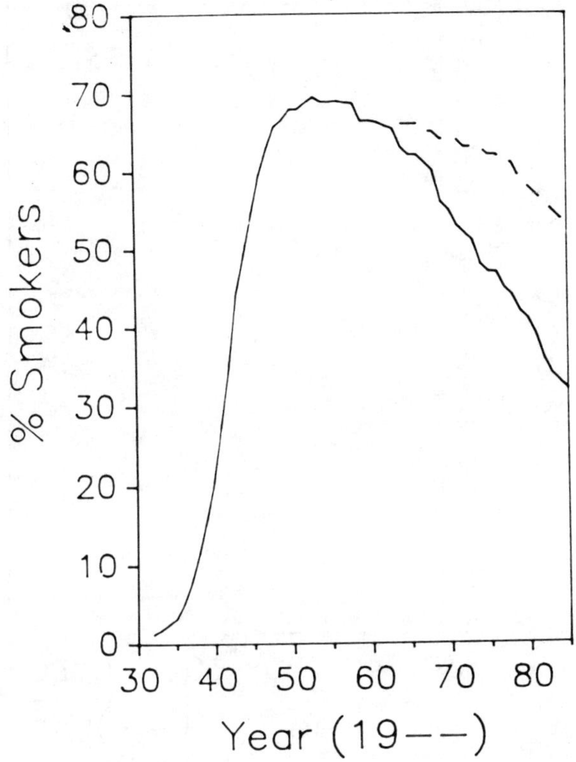

FIGURE 1.—Actual smoking prevalence history (solid line) and estimated prevalence for 1964–85 in the absence of the antismoking campaign (dashed line), 1921–30 male cohort

SOURCE: Warner (1989).

cent of each cohort reported themselves to be smokers that year. Similarly, without the campaign, smoking prevalence in the four youngest female cohorts would have been expected to include a majority or near majority of the women (44 percent for the 1921–30 birth cohort to 54 percent for the 1951–60 cohort). Yet each of these cohorts reported prevalence rates of either 27 percent (1921–30 cohort) or 32 percent (1931–60 cohorts).

Warner and Murt observed that the peak prevalence of the youngest cohort of males (born 1951–60), which fell short of 50 percent, made this cohort the first group of men born during the century never to have included a majority who were smokers. Supportive of the large gap found between this cohort's reported prevalence and the estimate of prevalence without the campaign are data on the peak prevalence of each of the older cohorts, reported by Harris (1983) and presented in Table 3. In the space of a single 10-year period, peak prevalence fell 16 percentage points, from 58 to 42 percent (for the 1941–50 and 1951–60 birth cohorts, respectively). In the span covered by three 10-year birth cohorts, the maximum percentage of men smoking fell by almost 30 percent-

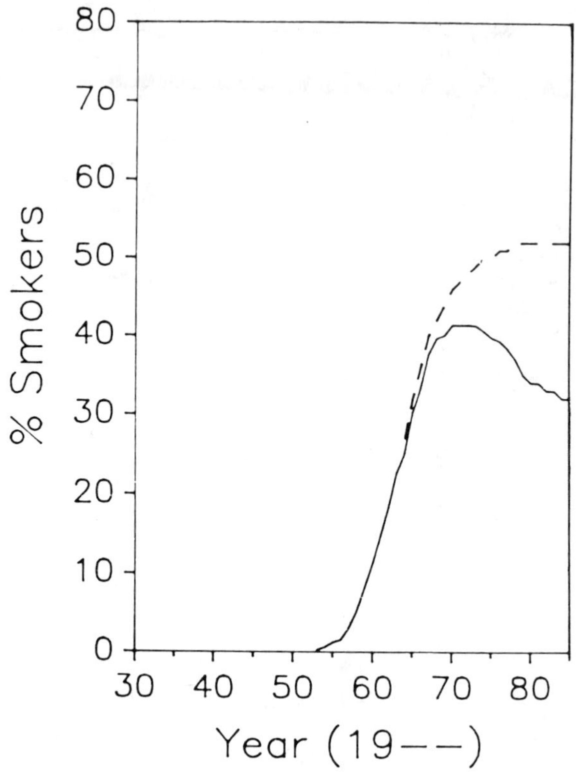

FIGURE 2.—Actual smoking prevalence history (solid line) and estimated prevalence for 1964–85 in the absence of the antismoking campaign (dashed line), 1941–50 female cohort

SOURCE: Warner (1989).

age points (from 70 percent for the 1921–30 cohort). Preliminary data from the 1987 National Health Interview Survey (NHIS), combined with other NHIS data from the 1980s, suggest that the peak prevalence for the cohort of males born between 1961 and 1970 may represent a further decrease of as much as 12 or 13 percentage points, to a rate of 29 to 30 percent.

The rates attained by the 1911–30 cohorts suggest that the expected peak prevalence figures for males in Table 1 may be conservative. This perception is reinforced by recognition that the 1921–30 cohort achieved its peak rate of smoking the year of the first major public concern about smoking and cancer, and that succeeding cohorts reached peak smoking age during other periods of concern about the health consequences of smoking.

In this context, had women's smoking patterns eventually mirrored those of men approximately three decades earlier, the expected prevalence figures in Table 2 would have to be considerably larger than they are. As such, the gaps between reported and

TABLE 3.—Peak smoking prevalence, males born 1901–60

Birth year	Year of peak prevalence	Prevalence (percentage)
1901–10	1938	62
1911–20	1947	71
1921–30	1953	70
1931–40	1962	61
1941–50	1969	58
1951–60	1980	42

SOURCE: Harris (1983); NHIS 1983.

expected prevalence for women may be conservative measures of the impact of the antismoking campaign on women's smoking prevalence.

Warner (1989) multiplied the reported and expected prevalence estimates for 1985 by cohort-specific population estimates to generate estimates of the 1985 population of smokers with and without the antismoking campaign. Including the cohort born 1961–70, and adjusting population estimates to reflect the differential mortality of smokers, Warner estimated that in 1985 there were 56 million American smokers born between 1901 and 1970. In the absence of the campaign, he estimated that there would have been 91 million smokers.

Not considered in Warner and Murt's analyses is change in the consumption of other tobacco products. Throughout much of the century, while the prevalence of cigarette smoking was first rising and then falling, the use of other smoking tobaccos and smokeless tobacco products was diminishing. From the mid-1970s into the present decade, decreases in the prevalence of smoking by boys occurred at the same time that the prevalence of smokeless tobacco use by boys was rising (Connolly et al. 1986). (See Chapter 5.) The significance of this most recent inverse correlation has not been established, but it implies that the prevalence of tobacco use by boys may not have decreased as much as data on cigarette smoking might suggest.

Per Capita Cigarette Consumption

While smoking prevalence is likely the best single measure of smoking behavior, a second measure has been employed frequently as an index of a society's smoking exposure: adult per capita cigarette consumption, typically defined as total cigarette consumption divided by the population over 17 years of age. One advantage of this measure is that it is derived from objective data. Aggregate consumption is calculated on the basis of cigarette production, tax, and sales data, adjusted for inventories (US DHEW 1979). (See Chapter 5.) Adult population estimates are from census data. Both sources are considered quite reliable. By contrast, self-reported cigarette consumption is subject to inaccuracies due to underreporting (Warner 1978) and "digit bias," the tendency to report daily consumption in terms of the number of cigarettes in the packs selected by smokers or in other round numbers (e.g., 10 and 30; see Chapter 5) (Kozlowski 1986).

Per capita consumption has the additional advantage of being a conservative measure of downward trends in smoking behavior, one thus unlikely to exaggerate the extent of change, because it does not take account of other smoking behavior changes that might increase one's estimation of response to the antismoking campaign. For example, smokers' switching to low-yield cigarettes could increase per capita consumption, because of the tendency to compensate for reduced nicotine yield per cigarette (US DHHS 1981, 1988; Gerstein and Levison 1982). As such, by itself, the market shift toward low-tar and -nicotine cigarettes may have introduced a tendency toward increases in per capita consumption that does not necessarily reflect any greater societal exposure to tobacco (Walker and Brin 1988). Thus, estimation of campaign response based on the pattern of per capita consumption may understate the extent of true response.

This advantage of the measure also points out its chief limitation: it masks changes in the composition and individual behavior of the smoking population. Per capita consumption offers no insight into variations in the sex, age, income, or education distribution of smokers; it fails to distinguish a change in the number of smokers from a change in the number of cigarettes the average smoker consumes; and, as just discussed, it ignores several other potentially important changes in smoking behavior, such as smokers' switching to low-yield cigarettes or reducing the amount of each cigarette smoked.

The analytical perspective involved in the per capita consumption studies is identical to that employed in the preceding cohort analysis: the objective remains to estimate smoking patterns that would have been expected without the antismoking campaign and then to compare them with realized patterns. The methodological approach is quite different, however, as has been the focal point of most of the relevant studies. Specifically, several authors have estimated impacts of the campaign in econometric analyses in which data on adult per capita cigarette consumption (the dependent variable) were regressed on data on a series of independent variables, including dummy variables and other measures intended to reflect years of prominent antismoking activity. Regression coefficient estimates in these studies indicate whether the years of special antismoking activity were associated with statistically significant decreases in per capita cigarette consumption, and if so, to what extent.

Effects in Years of Major Smoking-and-Health Events

Interest in major developments affecting the demand for cigarettes has emphasized changes in per capita cigarette consumption in and after the years in which they occurred. The developments studied have included the first widespread public discussion about the link between smoking and cancer in the United States in 1953 and 1954; publication of the first report of the British Royal College of Physicians on smoking and health in 1962 (Royal College of Physicians 1962); publication of the first Surgeon General's Report in 1964 (US PHS 1964); airing of the Fairness Doctrine antismoking messages on U.S. television and radio from 1967 through 1970; broadcast ad bans in several countries; and the spread of nonsmokers' rights laws in the United States beginning in the mid-1970s. Figure 3 indicates how decreases in adult per capita consumption in the United States corresponded to the timing of the major U.S. smoking-and-health events.

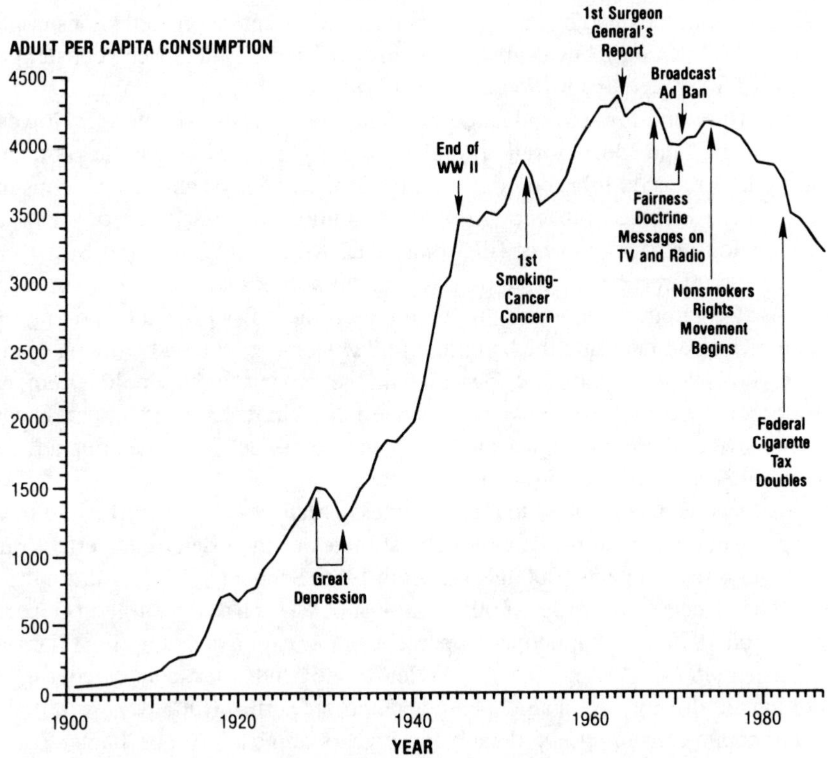

FIGURE 3.—Adult per capita cigarette consumption and major smoking-and-health events

SOURCE: Adapted from Warner (1985a).

Although there are exceptions (e.g., Fujii 1980), studies of individual "shocks to the system," such as publication of the first Surgeon General's Report, are quite consistent in their finding that cigarette consumption exhibited statistically significant decreases during these years, with the estimated magnitude ranging from about 3 to 8 percent of per capita consumption in the year of the event (Bishop and Yoo 1985; McGuinness and Cowling 1975; Radfar 1985; Witt and Pass 1983; Hamilton 1972; Atkinson and Skegg 1973, 1974; Atkinson and Townsend 1977; Peto 1974; Russell 1973; Ippolito, Murphy, Sant 1979; Doron 1979; Schneider, Klein, Murphy 1981; Warner 1977, 1981a, 1989). Many authors of these studies have concluded that these effects were transitory—that is, consumption rapidly returned to its previous baseline (e.g., Atkinson and Skegg 1973, 1974; Atkinson and Townsend 1977; Warner 1977, 1981a; Witt and Pass 1983)—but others believe that some of the shocks caused permanent shifts downward in the demand for cigarettes (e.g., Ippolito, Murphy, Sant 1979).

Considering antismoking activities after the 1964 Report and the Fairness Doctrine ads (discussed in Chapter 7), Doron (1979) concluded that antismoking publicity depressed per capita consumption by approximately 900 cigarettes in 1970. Schneider, Klein, and Murphy (1981) analyzed the effects of three antismoking events together and concluded that they had had a modest collective impact on cigarette consumption (decreasing it 8.3 percent), but a substantial impact on per capita tobacco consumption (a decrease of 39 percent from 1964 through 1978), because they encouraged smokers to switch to filter and low-tar and -nicotine cigarettes (discussed below). However, Schneider, Klein, and Murphy failed to account for changes in cigarette production technology that reduced tobacco consumption independent of changes in consumer demand. These included tobacco sheet reconstitution, increased use of stems and scraps, and addition of nontobacco filler materials. (See also Walker and Brin 1988.)

Considerable interest has focused on government policies with respect to broadcast advertising of cigarettes, encompassing both the Fairness Doctrine antismoking messages in the United States and the banning of television and radio advertising of cigarettes in several Western countries. Research on the impacts of these policies emerged soon after they were adopted. Analysis has reemerged in recent years in part because of the relevance of these experiences to the contemporary debate on banning advertising and promotion of tobacco products (Chapter 7).

Most analysts have concluded that the Fairness Doctrine ads were effective in discouraging cigarette consumption, although estimates of their deterrence effect range from relatively small impacts (Baltagi and Levin 1986; Schneider, Klein, Murphy 1981; Fujii 1980) to effects on the order of other major shocks, such as the Surgeon General's Report (Doron 1979), to as much as 14 percent of per capita consumption (Hamilton 1972; Warner 1977, 1981a, 1989). At least one study has concluded that the antismoking ads did not have an independent deterrence effect (Ippolito, Murphy, Sant 1979). Per capita consumption fell each of the years of the ads. (See Chapter 7.)

Because objective consumption data are not specific to groups of consumers, no analysis based on these data has investigated campaign effects on children and teenagers. The only econometric analysis to examine teenagers' consumption response to the Fairness Doctrine ads relied on survey-based prevalence data (Lewit, Coate, Grossman 1981). That study concluded that the messages produced a 5.2-percent decrease in teen smoking during their first year, but their novelty, and hence effectiveness, diminished by the second year.

With broadcast ad bans having been adopted in several Western countries, analysts have studied the effect of this major antismoking event in a variety of countries. While assessments of the impact of the U.S. broadcast ad ban effective in 1971 were reviewed briefly in Chapter 7, it is useful to reiterate those findings and supplement them with the conclusions of authors who have studied bans in other countries.

The U.S. broadcast ban on cigarette ads is the event for which there is least agreement in the literature about consumption implications. As discussed in Chapter 7, some analysts have concluded that the U.S. ban was counterproductive, actually contributing to increased cigarette consumption. Hamilton (1972) predicated this judgment on his evaluation of the relative effectiveness of pro- and antismoking advertisements. He estimated that prosmoking advertising increased per capita consumption by 95 cigarettes per year, while the Fairness Doctrine ads decreased it by 531. Consequently, prohibiting cigarette advertising, which also eliminated the need for broadcasters to donate time to the smoking-and-health cause, resulted in a net gain in cigarette sales. Schneider, Klein, and Murphy (1981) also concluded that the ban increased consumption, but primarily because it reduced a major cost of business for the tobacco companies—broadcast advertising—which, according to these authors, did not affect the aggregate level of consumption. They argued that decreased cost permitted price reductions,which, other things being equal, would increase consumption.

Other analysts have found no support for this position (Baltagi and Levin 1986). One of its premises was disproven soon after the ban, namely that cigarette advertising expenditures would fall sharply and remain, if not permanently lower, at least substantially lower for a long time, thus permitting the price of cigarettes to fall. Advertising expenditures did decrease in 1971, immediately following the broadcast ad ban, but they increased in succeeding years such that real expenditures (i.e., controlling for inflation) exceeded pre-ban levels by the mid-1970s (Federal Trade Commission 1988). Real cigarette price actually increased in the first 2 years of the ban period, although real manufacturers' wholesale prices declined during those years (excise taxes accounting for the increase).

Several analysts have concluded that broadcast bans have decreased consumption, albeit typically quite modestly (Bishop and Yoo 1985; Peto 1974). A common assessment, particularly in studies of the British broadcast ad ban, has been that the consumption impact of the ban trailed off, with consumption returning to baseline within 2 to 5 years (McLeod 1986; Witt and Pass 1983; Atkinson and Skegg 1974). As noted in Chapter 7, however, none of these analyses was designed to assess the long-run social influence of entire generations not being exposed to broadcast advertising of cigarettes (Warner 1979).

Many observers believe that the seminal smoking-and-health event in the United States in the past 15 years has been the growth of the nonsmokers' rights movement, reflected in passage of State and local laws and private business policies restricting smoking in public places and workplaces. Laws and policies and their effects were reviewed in the preceding chapter and, in greater depth, in the 1986 Surgeon General's Report (US DHHS 1986) and other recent publications (Bureau of National Affairs 1986, 1987).

As noted in the last chapter, to date few statistical studies using objective consumption data have examined the relationship between smoking restriction policies and per capita consumption. Three econometric analyses found a significant inverse relationship between restrictions and consumption, but none concluded that the relationship was causal. In one study, an index of the growth of State-level smoking restriction laws correlated strongly with the decline in adult per capita consumption after 1973 (Figure 3), but the author concluded that "This correlation seems unlikely to reflect causation. Rather, both declining consumption and growth in legislation probably reflect a prevailing nonsmoking ethos and the conversion of modified knowledge and attitudes into behavioral change" (Warner 1981a).

In the second econometric study, the author found a significant reduction in smoking associated with laws categorized as restrictive, but no significant reduction associated with less restrictive laws. The study could not determine, however, whether passage of restrictive laws preceded or followed decreases in consumption (Lewit 1988). In the third study, the authors concluded that the significant correlation between passage of laws and reduced cigarette demand likely reflected reverse causality; that is, that cigarette demand has a significant negative effect on the probability of passing a clean indoor air law (Chaloupka and Saffer 1988).

Aggregate Effects

While numerous econometric studies have contributed to understanding the impact of major individual smoking-and-health events, regression analysis has also been used by Warner (1977, 1981a, 1989) to estimate changes in per capita consumption associated with changes in the smoking-and-health environment over the entire period since 1964. In the two more recent studies, to estimate what consumption would have been in any given year without the antismoking campaign, Warner added the values of the relevant antismoking variables in the regression, multiplied by their corresponding coefficients, to the year's actual per capita consumption. (With the previous year's consumption included among the independent variables as a measure of the addiction effect, an antismoking effect was also carried forward into future years and was included in the analysis.) The resulting estimates of per capita consumption in the absence of the campaign were then compared with the realized levels of consumption to measure the aggregate impact of the campaign in the year in question.

Figure 4 presents the results of the most recent analysis (Warner 1989). The solid line in the Figure tracks actual adult per capita cigarette consumption from 1932 through 1987. (The regression covered the post-World War II period, 1947 through 1987.) The dashed and dotted lines are two estimated patterns that consumption would have followed from 1964 through 1987 had the demand for cigarettes never been influenced by the development and dissemination of scientific knowledge on the hazards of smoking and the associated social and policy developments.

The distinction between the two estimated lines lies in how price changes are treated. The dotted line results from the assumption that the pattern of price changes was itself a function of legislators' reactions to the emerging evidence on smoking and health (Warner 1981a,b). In particular, the real price of cigarettes rose every year from 1964 through 1972 and again from 1981 through 1987. The intervening period of real price decreases has been attributed to reduction in new State excise tax increases due to concern about interstate cigarette smuggling, the result of tax-based price differentials between low- and high-tax States (Advisory Council on Intergovernmental Relations 1985; Warner 1982). The resumption of real tax increases in 1981 may reflect reduced concern about smuggling, as a consequence of the diminishing real value of interstate tax differences during the preceding decade. (See Chapter 7.) To reflect the assumption that this pattern of price changes was a function of the antismoking campaign, the dotted line in Figure 4 treats price as if it had been constant (in real terms) in the years after 1963. This permits an assessment of the effects on consumption of price fluctuations possibly resulting from the campaign.

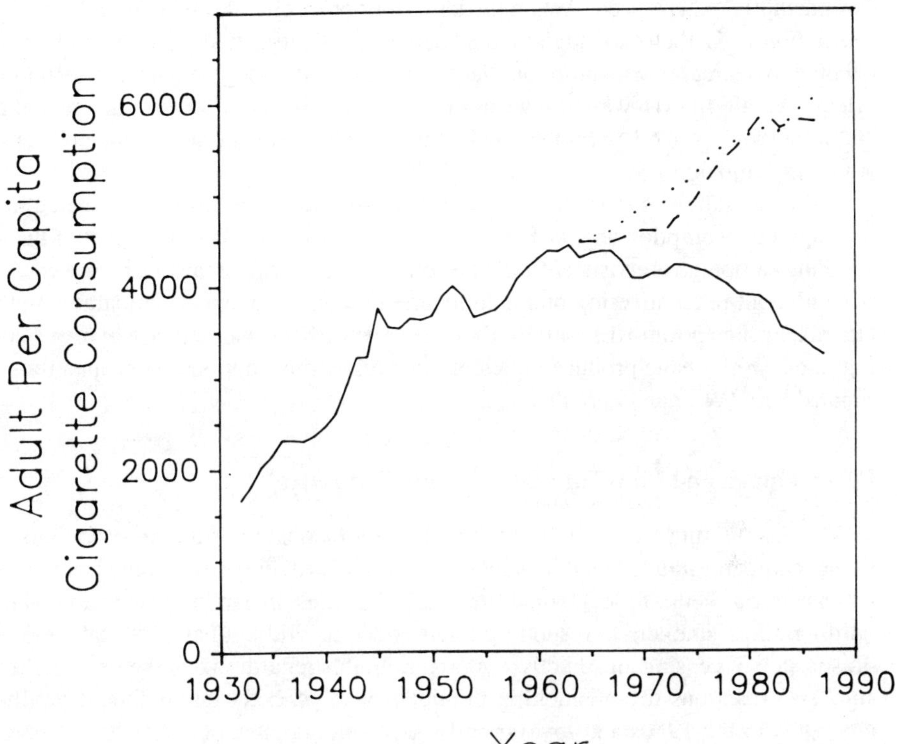

FIGURE 4.—Comparison of actual per capita cigarette consumption (solid line) with estimated consumption in the absence of the antismoking campaign (dashed line = actual cigarette prices; dotted line = real price held constant)

SOURCE: Warner (1989).

The dashed line treats the pattern of realized prices as independent of the antismoking campaign; actual experienced prices are reflected in the dashed line. Warner interpreted the gap between the solid line (actual consumption) and dashed line (estimated consumption, actual prices) as a measure of the " 'pure' publicity effect" of the campaign, whereas the gap between the dashed line and dotted line (estimated consumption, constant prices) measured the impact on consumption of changing prices. To the extent that the latter was attributable to smoking-and-health concerns of legislators, Warner considered it a measure of price-related campaign-induced changes in consumption.

While the precise pattern of estimated per capita consumption without the antismoking campaign depends on the treatment of price change, each of the estimated lines indicates a generally increasing pattern of consumption over time, in contrast to the pattern actually experienced. According to the analysis, in 1987, without the antismoking campaign, and treating price changes as independent of the campaign (i.e., the dashed line in Figure 4), per capita consumption would have been 79 percent greater than the level actually experienced. When the pattern of price changes is removed (the dotted line in Figure 4), the estimate rises to 89 percent, indicating that price fluctuations contributed to decreased consumption, but to a much smaller degree than did the publicity effect. An alternative way to interpret the 1987 figures is to observe that actual consumption was from 53 to 56 percent of the expected level in the absence of the antismoking campaign.

Two observations support the magnitude of the campaign impact estimated in this per capita consumption analysis. First, the finding of a substantial impact of the antismoking campaign is consistent with the cohort analysis of prevalence reviewed above. Second, continued diffusion of smoking among women to levels comparable to those attained by men prior to the mid-1960s, combined with the maintenance of men's smoking rates, would have produced rates of per capita consumption higher than those estimated here (Warner 1977).

Filter-Tipped and Low-Tar and -Nicotine Cigarettes

Whereas quitting smoking or avoiding initiation constitutes the most obvious reaction to campaign-related health or social concerns, switching to cigarettes perceived as less hazardous better reflects some smokers' responses, in part because actions short of quitting allow smokers to respond to their concerns without having to take the more drastic step of ceasing an addictive behavior. In this regard, two of the best markers of smokers' reactions to antismoking publicity have been the rapid spread of filtered cigarettes in the 1950s and low-tar and -nicotine cigarettes in the 1970s (Schneider, Klein, Murphy 1981).

While evidence linking cigarette smoking with cancer dates back at least to the 1930s, the period of sustained, intensive scientific investigation began in the late 1940s and early 1950s. (See Chapters 1 and 2.) A few popular publications transmitted the new scientific findings to the lay public soon thereafter, including *Reader's Digest* (Riis 1950; Norr 1952; Lieb 1953; Miller and Monahan 1954) and *Consumer Reports* (1953, 1954, 1955). At the same time, cigarette manufacturers were developing and marketing new filtered cigarettes. Cigarette filters were advertised as a technology to remove the harmful elements of smoke (Calfee 1986; Davis 1987; Tye 1986; Warner 1985b; Whelan 1984).

As the data in Chapter 5 indicate, the shift to filtered cigarettes at this time was swift. While filtered cigarettes had been available since the 1930s, they composed only 1 percent of the market in 1952. By 1954 the proportion of filtered cigarettes had increased to 9 percent. The filter-tip market share rose by at least 9 percentage points each of the next 3 years, reaching 38 percent in 1957. Three years later, the filtered cigarette became the dominant product on the market. This first widespread public concern about smoking and health was also associated with a 2-year decline in adult per capita cigarette consumption in 1953 and 1954 (Figure 3).

Two decades later, in the mid-1970s, the rapid shift toward low-tar and -nicotine cigarettes represented a second major change in consumers' choice of cigarette product. In the late 1960s, low-tar and -nicotine cigarettes (defined as cigarettes yielding 15 mg tar or less, as measured by the Federal Trade Commission) constituted from 2 to 3 percent of the cigarette market. In the early 1970s, cigarette manufacturers initiated an advertising campaign for low-tar and -nicotine cigarettes, which resulted in 50 percent of advertising dollars being dedicated to these products by 1977 (Schneider, Klein, Murphy 1981; Federal Trade Commission 1988). Many of the ads made health claims for the products, most implicitly (Altman et al., in press; Davis 1987; Tye 1986; Warner 1985b).

From 1970 through 1974, the market share of low-yield cigarettes increased from 4 to 9 percent. Three years later, with 50 percent of all cigarette ads devoted to the low-yield products, market share had increased to 23 percent. By the end of the decade, the market share exceeded 40 percent, and it hit 56 percent in 1981. Thereafter, the percentage backed off a few points, but the low-tar and -nicotine cigarette remained the principal product on the market (Federal Trade Commission 1988).

Surveys in the 1970s found that large proportions of the smoking public believed that some cigarettes posed little or no health risk (Federal Trade Commission 1981). (See Chapter 4.) As such, many smokers may have perceived low-tar and -nicotine cigarettes as an alternative to quitting smoking that would not compromise health. Some analysts have concluded that the shift to low-tar and -nicotine cigarettes, and before it to filter-tipped cigarettes, was the smoking public's principal behavioral response to concerns about the health hazards of smoking (Schneider, Klein, Murphy 1981).

Health Consequences of the Campaign

Given the health consequences of smoking, described in Chapters 2 and 3, the behavioral impact of the antismoking campaign implies that the campaign has had significant effects on the health of the American public. These health effects may be quite varied, reflecting the number and variety of behavioral changes, ranging from outright smoking cessation to shifts to low-tar and -nicotine cigarettes. In addition to reductions in the amount of smoking-related mortality, the mix of smoking-related deaths may have been altered by campaign responses, as a result of changes in the nature of the product and its disease-producing properties. (See Chapters 2 and 3 and US DHHS 1981.) Similarly, patterns of morbidity and disability may have been affected.

While smoking-related deaths have been averted as a result of people's responses to the antismoking campaign (as discussed below), it is also possible that some additional deaths have occurred because of campaign response. The latter could result, for example, if industry advertising, responding to smokers' health concerns, prompted smokers who otherwise would have quit smoking to switch to low-yield cigarettes. There is a clear consensus that among the principal factors motivating the growth of filtered cigarettes and the shift toward brands lower in tar and nicotine yield were concerns about the health effects of smoking—on the part of consumers, the Federal Trade Commission (which decided in 1967 to publish standardized tar and nicotine measurements), and the cigarette manufacturers in response (US DHHS 1981, 1988; Gerstein and Levison 1982; Schneider, Klein, Murphy 1981; Miles 1982). As noted above, analysts have concluded that, at the time of the shifts to filtered and low-yield cigarettes, cigarette advertising stressed the new products' health "advantages," with the apparent intent of allaying consumer fears and thereby discouraging quitting of smoking (Calfee 1986; Davis 1987; Tye 1986; Warner 1985b; Whelan 1984; Altman et al., in press).

A number of factors complicate assessment of the net health consequences of reduced-yield cigarettes. These include the unknown health effects of additives in low-yield cigarettes and the tendency toward nicotine regulation, both discussed in detail in previous reports of the Surgeon General (US DHHS 1981, 1988); the possibility that many low-yield-cigarette smokers would have quit smoking in the absence of the availability of lower yield products; and the possibility that the availability of low-tar and -nicotine brands may account in part for the increase in smoking by teenage girls and young women in the 1970s (Harris 1980). To date, the net health effects of the introduction and consumer acceptance of filtered and low-yield cigarettes have not been determined. Furthermore, no formal analysis has attempted to assess how much of the switch to lower yield products constitutes response to the antismoking campaign.

Only one measure of health impact of the campaign has been evaluated quantitatively: aggregate mortality associated with changes in smoking prevalence. The concluding section of this Chapter reviews the relevant findings.

Mortality Postponed by Campaign-Related Decreases in Smoking Prevalence

While the net health effects of filter and low-tar and -nicotine cigarettes have not been determined, Warner (1989) has estimated the mortality postponed as a result of campaign-induced decisions of smokers to quit and of nonsmokers not to start smoking. Updating an earlier analysis (Warner and Murt 1983), Warner applied epidemiologic data on age–sex-specific mortality rates of smokers, former smokers, and never smokers to the cohort-specific changes in smoking prevalence summarized above in Tables 1 and 2. The reduced mortality rates of former smokers (compared with continuing smokers) were multiplied by the estimated number of campaign-induced quitters and noninitiators (i.e., people influenced by the campaign not to start smoking) in each cohort and in each year from 1964 through 1985. This procedure generated estimates of the number of additional smoking-related deaths that would have occurred had the antismoking campaign not encouraged quitting and noninitiation. (See Chapter 3 for discussion of smoking-related deaths.) The analysis also produced estimates of life–years saved. These represent the life expectancy gained by campaign-induced quitters and noninitiators who avoided or postponed premature smoking-related deaths.

Given the need to make several assumptions to perform the study, Warner subjected his findings to four sensitivity analyses. He altered each of four variables' assumed values in a conservative direction to determine whether the specific values selected for the base case fundamentally affected the qualitative findings of the study. While the sensitivity analyses reduced the estimates of deaths postponed by the campaign, the author concluded that none reduced them sufficiently to alter the essential qualitative finding: from 1964 through 1985, hundreds of thousands of smoking-related premature deaths were delayed or avoided as a result of campaign-induced decisions to quit smoking or not to start.

Table 4 presents estimates of deaths postponed for each of the 12 age–sex cohorts identified in Tables 1 and 2, from 1964 through 1985. For Americans born after 1900, the total number of deaths postponed as a result of campaign response was estimated as 789,200. The distribution between men and women and across birth cohorts is seen in the individual cells of Table 4.

TABLE 4.—Deaths postponed by campaign-related smoking cessation and noninitiation, 1964–85 (in thousands)

Birth year	Males	Females	Total
1901–10	103.6	16.7	120.3
1911–20	182.0	46.0	228.0
1921–30	182.7	59.6	242.3
1931–40	83.2	22.7	105.9
1941–50	44.0	15.5	59.5
1951–60	29.0	4.2	33.2
Total	624.5	164.7	789.2

SOURCE: Warner (1989).

According to the estimates in Table 4, nearly four times as many men as women realized additional years. In part this reflects the greater consumption impact of the campaign on men, as well as their higher mortality rates. However, Warner's analysis utilized male smoker mortality ratios from an insurance study (Cowell and Hirst 1980) and adopted as a conservative assumption an estimate that women's excess smoker mortality ratios were half those of men. New data from the American Cancer Society's survey, analyzed in Chapter 3, demonstrate that women's excess smoker mortality ratios are closer to two-thirds those of men. Consequently, the data in Table 4 likely underestimate the number of women's deaths postponed relative to those of men.

Warner also estimated the number of life–years saved as a result of campaign-related smoking cessation and noninitiation. In total, the 12 cohorts gained 16.3 million additional life–years. The average number of life–years saved per death postponed was 20.6.

Figure 5 plots the cumulative number of smoking-related deaths estimated to have occurred within the 12 cohorts between 1964 and 1985 and the study's estimate of the number that would have occurred without the antismoking campaign. By 1985, when the cumulative number of postponed deaths was approaching 800,000, the number of smoking-related deaths during the period had totaled 5.7 million. Thus, life-savings attributable to the campaign equaled 12 percent of actual plus avoided smoking-related mortality. In Warner and Murt's earlier study, campaign-related life-savings through 1978 equaled 5 percent of actual plus avoided smoking-related mortality (Warner and Murt 1983). The increase reflects greater numbers of quitters and the health benefits of the passage of time, as former smokers' excess (smoking-related) mortality risks fall as years of smoking increase. Comparing the two analyses, one sees that almost three-

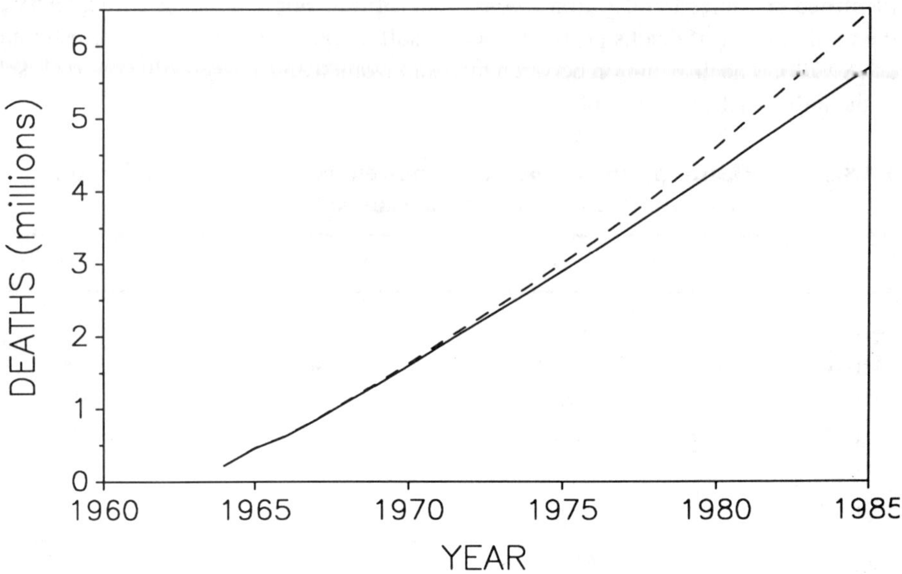

FIGURE 5.—Comparison of estimated cumulative smoking-related deaths (solid line) with estimate of the number that would have occurred without the antismoking campaign (dashed line), 1964–85

SOURCE: Unpublished data from study reported by Warner (1989).

quarters of the postponement of deaths occurred in the most recent 7 years of the 22 years studied. In particular, 112,400 deaths—14 percent of the total—were postponed in 1985 alone (Warner 1989).

For the youngest cohorts in the study, low overall death rates translated into relatively few deaths postponed through 1985. Given the substantial impact of the campaign on the smoking patterns of these cohorts, however, major life-saving accomplishments of antismoking efforts mounted to date will be realized two to three decades hence, when these cohorts reach the age at which smoking-related illnesses begin to take their greatest toll. Similarly, recent campaign-related quitting in the middle-aged cohorts will translate into large numbers of smoking-related deaths postponed or avoided in future years, as these recent quitters experience reduced smoking-related mortality rates. Thus, the health benefits of the antismoking campaign will continue to expand, both in absolute terms and as a percentage of the total potential burden of smoking-related mortality. This is illustrated by Warner's (1989) estimate that campaign-induced quitting and noninitiation through 1985 will result in the postponement or avoidance of an additional 2.1 million smoking-related deaths between 1986 and the year 2000.

The finding that men have realized a much greater collective health benefit from their responses to the antismoking campaign than have women reflects the fact that more men than women quit or did not initiate smoking as a result of the campaign, as well as the assumed lower smoker mortality ratios and death rates of women. As women's smoking patterns have approached those of men in recent years (see Chapter 5), the disparity between male and female smoker mortality ratios has diminished. (See Chapter 3.) Particularly in the younger cohorts, if women respond to the relatively new emphasis on the health consequences of their smoking (US DHHS 1980), the male–female differential for postponed deaths would be expected to decrease in the future (Warner and Murt 1983; Warner 1989).

The authors of these studies acknowledged that their estimate of deaths postponed as a result of the antismoking campaign was an incomplete measure of the health consequences of the campaign (Warner and Murt 1983; Warner 1989). As noted above, the net health effects of the switch to filtered and low-yield cigarettes have not been established, and no formal analysis has assessed the impact of campaign-related reductions in smoking prevalence on smoking-related morbidity and disability. Nevertheless, Warner and Murt concluded that the estimated life-savings associated with responses to the campaign constitute a major public health accomplishment. They cautioned, however, that the magnitude of the remaining burden of smoking "places the impressive successes of the antismoking campaign in context" (Warner 1989).

Conclusions

1. All birth cohorts born between 1901 and 1960 experienced reductions in the prevalence of smoking relative to the rates that would have been expected in the absence of the antismoking campaign. By 1985, the gap between actual (reported) prevalence and that which would have been expected ranged from 6 percentage points for the eldest female cohort to 28 percentage points for the youngest male cohort.
2. In 1985, an estimated 56 million Americans 15 to 84 years of age were smokers. In the absence of the antismoking campaign, an estimated 91 million would have been smokers.
3. Adult per capita cigarette consumption has fallen 3 to 8 percent in years of major smoking-and-health events, such as publication of the first Surgeon General's Report on smoking and health in 1964. Per capita consumption fell each of the years the Fairness Doctrine antismoking messages were presented on television and radio (1967–70).
4. By 1987, adult per capita cigarette consumption would have exceeded its actual level by an estimated 79 to 89 percent had the antismoking campaign never occurred.
5. One of the most substantial behavioral responses to concerns about smoking and health has been the shift toward filtered cigarettes in the 1950s and low-tar and low-nicotine cigarettes in the 1970s. The net health impact of these product changes is unknown.
6. As a result of the antismoking campaign, an estimated 789,000 deaths were postponed during the period 1964 through 1985, 112,000 in 1985 alone. The average life expectancy gained per postponed death was 21 years.
7. The avoidance of smoking-related mortality associated with the antismoking campaign will represent a growing percentage of smoking-related mortality over time,

as the principal beneficiaries of the campaign, younger men and women, reach the ages at which smoking-related disease is most common. Campaign-induced quitting and noninitiation through 1985 will result in the postponement or avoidance of an estimated 2.1 million smoking related deaths between 1986 and the year 2000.

Appendix

Selected Developments Related to Smoking and Health, 1964–88

1964

- *Smoking and Health: Report of the Advisory Committee to the Surgeon General*, the first major U.S. report on smoking and health, is published. Concludes that cigarette smoking is a cause of lung cancer in men and a suspected cause in women. Identifies many other causal relationships and smoking–disease associations. Calls for "appropriate remedial action."

- National Interagency Council on Smoking and Health, the first national antismoking coalition, is formed.

- National Association of Broadcasters (NAB) amends its television advertising code to discourage portrayal of cigarette smoking as a behavior worthy of imitation by youngsters.

- Cigarette manufacturers establish voluntary Cigarette Advertising Code for television and radio.

- Federal Trade Commission (FTC) announces proposed Trade Regulation Rule on Cigarette Labeling and Advertising.

- National Center for Health Statistics begins collecting information on smoking as part of the National Health Interview Survey. Collected periodically thereafter.

- American Medical Association (AMA) officially calls smoking "a serious health hazard."

- Public Health Service (PHS) and Indian Hospitals discontinue distributing free cigarettes. The Department of Defense and the Veterans Administration soon do the same in their medical installations.

- State Mutual Life Assurance Company becomes the first company to offer life insurance to nonsmokers at discounted rates.

1965

- Congress passes the Federal Cigarette Labeling and Advertising Act, requiring health warning on all cigarette packages: "Caution: Cigarette Smoking May be Hazardous to Your Health."

- PHS establishes the National Clearinghouse for Smoking and Health.

1966

- Health warning label appears on all cigarette packages.
- Congress enacts the Fair Packaging and Labeling Act to require fair, nondeceptive packaging and labeling. Tobacco and tobacco products are excluded.

1967

- Report of the Surgeon General concludes smoking is the principal cause of lung cancer.
- Federal Communications Commission (FCC) rules that the Fairness Doctrine applies to cigarette advertising. Stations broadcasting cigarette commercials must donate air time to antismoking messages.
- PHS, American Cancer Society (ACS), American Lung Association (ALA) (then known as the National Tuberculosis Association), and American Heart Association (AHA) launch public service advertising campaigns against smoking.
- FTC releases the first report on tar and nicotine yield in cigarette brands.
- National Institutes of Health initiates research planning for developing "less hazardous" cigarettes.
- First World Conference on Smoking and Health is held in New York City.

1968

- Action on Smoking and Health is formed to serve as a legal action arm for the antismoking community.
- National Clearinghouse for Smoking and Health produces the first Government antismoking poster.
- CBS airs "National Smoking Test" during prime time.

1969

- NAB endorses phasing out of cigarette ads on television and radio.
- ACS sponsors a quit-smoking series on PBS.
- ALA introduces its first smoking cessation materials.

1970

- Congress enacts the Public Health Cigarette Smoking Act of 1969 (passed in 1970), banning cigarette advertising on television and radio and requiring a stronger health warning on cigarette packages: "Warning: The Surgeon General Has Determined that Cigarette Smoking is Dangerous to Your Health."

- Due to the new statutory prohibition on broadcast advertising, the voluntary Cigarette Advertising Code is disbanded.

- Due to the broadcast ban, the FCC rules that the Fairness Doctrine no longer will apply to cigarette advertising (effective 1971).

- First National Conference on Smoking and Health is held in San Diego.

- World Health Organization takes a public position against cigarette smoking.

- Congress enacts the Controlled Substances Act. Tobacco is excluded from jurisdiction.

1971

- Surgeon General proposes a Government ban on smoking in public places.

- Cigarette advertising ends on radio and television. Fairness Doctrine antismoking messages also end.

- Cigarette manufacturers' voluntary agreement to list tar and nicotine yield in all advertising becomes effective.

- Six major cigarette companies agree voluntarily to include health warnings in all printed advertising.

- The FTC announces intent to proceed against cigarette companies for false and deceptive advertising.

- Second World Conference on Smoking and Health is held in London.

- Interstate Commerce Commission implements rules to restrict smoking to rear seats (not to exceed 20 percent of capacity) on interstate buses.

1972

- First Report of the Surgeon General to identify involuntary smoking as a health risk.

- Under a consent order with the FTC, six major cigarette companies agree to include a "clear and conspicuous" health warning in all cigarette advertisements.

- Congress enacts the Consumer Product Safety Act. Tobacco and tobacco products are excluded from jurisdiction.

- Supreme Court upholds congressional action banning cigarette commercials from television and radio.

- Department of Health, Education, and Welfare issues policy directive to establish no-smoking rules in departmental conference rooms, cafeterias, and certain work areas.

- ALA sponsors first State-level "no-smoking day" in Oklahoma.

1973

- Congress enacts Little Cigar Act of 1973, banning little cigar ads from television and radio.

- Civil Aeronautics Board requires no-smoking sections on all commercial airline flights.

- General Services Administration issues guidelines on smoking in Federal buildings.

- Arizona becomes the first State to restrict smoking in a number of public places and the first to do so explicitly because environmental tobacco smoke exposure is a public health hazard.

1974

- Connecticut passes the first State law to apply smoking restrictions to restaurants.

- ACS, ALA, and AHA cosponsor no-smoking day in Minnesota.

1975

- Cigarettes are discontinued in K-rations and C-rations provided to soldiers and sailors.

- Third World Conference on Smoking and Health is held in New York City. Conferees call for a unified worldwide campaign against smoking.

- Minnesota passes landmark comprehensive statewide clean indoor air law.

1976

- Interstate Commerce Commission modifies interstate bus rules to permit smoking in 30 percent of seats.

- Interstate Commerce Commission prohibits smoking in railroad dining cars and requires separate smoking and nonsmoking passenger cars.

- Congress amends the Federal Hazardous Substances Act to exclude tobacco and tobacco products from jurisdiction.

- Congress enacts the Toxic Substances Control Act. Tobacco and tobacco products are excluded from jurisdiction.

- ACS appoints National Commission on Smoking and Public Policy to hold hearings on major policy. Report issued in 1978.

1977

- Secretary of Health, Education, and Welfare establishes Task Force on Smoking and Health.

- ACS sponsors the first national "Great American Smokeout."

- Doctors Ought to Care is formed to provide a focal point for physicians' antismoking advocacy, especially through counteradvertising.

1978

- Secretary of Health, Education, and Welfare announces major Government initiative against smoking. Calls smoking "Public Health Enemy Number One."

- National Clearinghouse for Smoking and Health is renamed Office on Smoking and Health and transferred from Atlanta to Washington, DC. Given expanded function to coordinate Federal smoking and health activities.

- AMA releases "Tobacco and Health," summarizing findings of a tobacco research program that included 15 million dollars in financial support from the tobacco industry. Concluded that smoking is harmful to health.

- Utah enacts the first State law banning tobacco advertisements on any billboard, streetcar sign, streetcar, or bus.

1979

- Fifteenth Anniversary Report of the Surgeon General is issued. Most comprehensive review of smoking and health ever published.

- National Institute of Education survey shows that girls are smoking more than boys.

- Fourth World Conference on Smoking and Health is held in Stockholm.

- Minneapolis and St. Paul become the first cities to ban the distribution of free cigarette samples.

1980

- Report of the Surgeon General highlights health consequences of smoking to women.
- PHS announces Health Objectives for the Nation, which include a goal to reduce smoking to below 25 percent among adults by 1990.
- The FTC begins testing cigarettes for carbon monoxide yields.

1981

- Report of the Surgeon General focuses on "The Changing Cigarette." Concludes no cigarette or level of consumption is safe.
- The FTC concludes existing cigarette warning label is no longer effective. Recommends rotational warning label system.
- National Conference on Smoking or Health is held in New York City, sponsored by ACS. Leads to formation of Coalition on Smoking OR Health. (See 1982.)

1982

- Report of the Surgeon General focuses exclusively on smoking and cancer.
- Congress temporarily doubles the Federal excise tax on cigarettes to 16 cents per pack, to be in effect January 1, 1983, to October 1, 1985. First increase since 1951.
- Congress enacts No Net Cost Tobacco Program Act of 1982 to reduce taxpayers' costs for the tobacco price support program.
- ACS, ALA, and AHA form a tripartite Coalition on Smoking OR Health, primarily to coordinate Federal legislative activities related to smoking control.
- National Cancer Institute reorganizes its smoking research program, as the Smoking, Tobacco and Cancer Program, to focus on smoking behavior research and interventions.

1983

- Report of the Surgeon General focuses exclusively on smoking and cardiovascular disease.

- Fifth World Conference on Smoking and Health is held in Winnipeg.
- National Institute on Drug Abuse declares smoking to be the Nation's "most widespread form of drug dependency."
- *New York State Journal of Medicine* publishes the first U.S. medical journal all-tobacco edition focusing on health and social issues.
- San Francisco passes law to include smoking restrictions in private workplaces.

1984

- Report of the Surgeon General focuses exclusively on smoking and chronic obstructive lung disease.
- Congress enacts the Comprehensive Smoking Education Act, requiring rotational health warnings on cigarette packages and advertisements:

  "SURGEON GENERAL'S WARNING: Smoking Causes Lung Cancer, Heart Disease, Emphysema, and May Complicate Pregnancy."

  "SURGEON GENERAL'S WARNING: Quitting Smoking Now Greatly Reduces Serious Risks to Your Health."

  "SURGEON GENERAL'S WARNING: Smoking by Pregnant Women May Result in Fetal Injury, Premature Birth, and Low Birth Weight."

  "SURGEON GENERAL'S WARNING: Cigarette Smoke Contains Carbon Monoxide."

- Federal Interagency Committee on Smoking and Health, an advisory committee chaired by the Surgeon General, is established.
- Food and Drug Administration approves nicotine polacrilex gum as a "new drug."
- Congress enacts the Cigarette Safety Act of 1984, requiring research and a report on "fire-safe" cigarettes.
- Tobacco Products Liability Project is formed to support efforts to bring product liability suits against cigarette manufacturers as a public health strategy.
- Surgeon General announces his goal of a smoke-free society by the Year 2000.

1985

- Report of the Surgeon General covers smoking and occupational exposures.

- AMA calls for a ban on all tobacco advertising and promotion, consistent with similar calls by ALA, ACS, AHA, and numerous other health and medical organizations.

- Office on Smoking and Health initiates a national educational campaign regarding smoking during pregnancy.

- National Heart, Lung, and Blood Institute establishes a Smoking Education Program.

- ALA produces a television series, "Freedom from Smoking® in 20 Days."

- Minnesota enacts the first State legislation to earmark a portion of the State cigarette excise tax to support antismoking programs.

- STAT (Stop Teenage Addiction to Tobacco) is formed to focus on teenage tobacco use.

- Maine becomes the first State to adopt a law protecting supporters of worksite smoking policies against discrimination.

1986

- Report of the Surgeon General focuses exclusively on the health consequences of involuntary smoking.

- Special Report of the Surgeon General documents the health consequences of using smokeless tobacco.

- Congress enacts the Comprehensive Smokeless Tobacco Health Education Act of 1986. Requires rotation of three health warnings on smokeless tobacco packages and advertisements and bans smokeless tobacco advertising on broadcast media.

- Congress extends permanently the 16 cents per pack Federal excise tax on cigarettes.

- Congress enacts the Tobacco Program Improvement Act of 1986, further revising the price support program.

- Department of Health and Human Services releases the first biennial National Status Report to Congress on Smoking and Health.

- Department of Defense launches extensive antismoking education campaign for the military and other Department of Defense employees.

- Americans for Nonsmokers' Rights becomes National. Originally formed as California GASP (Group Against Smoking Pollution) in 1976.

- Minnesota enacts the first State law to ban free distribution of smokeless tobacco samples.

- Congress imposes a Federal excise tax on smokeless tobacco products.

1987

- General Services Administration implements regulations to prohibit smoking in Federal buildings, except in designated areas.

- Department of Health and Human Services (DHHS) establishes a smoke-free environment in its facilities, affecting 120,000 DHHS employees nationwide.

- Food and Drug Administration determines "Masterpiece Tobac" (chewing gum containing tobacco) to be an "adulterated food" subject to its jurisdiction, and "Favor" (a "smokeless cigarette" not containing tobacco leaf) to be a "drug" subject to its jurisdiction. Both products withdrawn from the market.

- Sixth World Conference on Smoking and Health is held in Tokyo.

- ACS, ALA, and AHA launch a joint project, "Tobacco-Free America."

- Minnesota Sports Commission votes to ban tobacco advertising in the Metrodome Sports Stadium effective 1992, the first such action in the United States.

- Minnesota passes a law requiring all hospitals in the State to ban smoking by 1990.

1988

- Report of the Surgeon General concentrates exclusively on nicotine addiction.

- Congressionally mandated smoking ban takes effect on domestic airline flights scheduled for 2 hours or less. Northwest Airlines voluntarily bans smoking on all fights in North America.

- ALA sponsors the first annual "Non-Dependence Day."

- In *Cipollone* v. *Liggett Group, Inc.*, plaintiff wins the first jury verdict against a tobacco company in a smoking and disease case.

- New York City clean indoor air ordinance takes effect, banning or severely limiting smoking in a wide variety of public places. Applies to over 7 million people, almost 3 percent of the U.S. population.

- New York Metropolitan Transit Authority (NYMTA) bans smoking on Long Island Railroad and Metro North Commuter Rail and trains, affecting 452,000 daily riders. Action prompted by a law Congress passed in 1987 to withhold Federal transportation funds to NYMTA unless it banned smoking.

- California implements statewide law banning smoking on all intrastate airplane, train, and bus trips.

- California suit against manufacturers and retailers of cigars, pipe tobacco, and roll-your-own cigarette tobacco seeks compliance with State law requiring labeling of consumer products containing carcinogens or reproductive toxins. Cigar Association of America indicates that most cigars sold in the United States will carry a warning label.

- R.J. Reynolds test markets Premier, a "new cigarette prototype" that the company calls "the cleaner smoke." Health organizations petition FDA to regulate the product as a drug or medical device.

- California voters pass referendum raising State cigarette excise tax by 25 cents per pack, the largest cigarette excise tax increase in U.S. history. Revenues earmarked for public health purposes.

References

ADVISORY COMMISSION ON INTERGOVERNMENTAL RELATIONS. *Cigarette Tax Evasion: A Second Look.* Washington, D.C.: Advisory Commission on Intergovernmental Relations, March 1985.

ALTMAN, D.G., SLATER, M.D., ALBRIGHT, C.L., MACCOBY, N. How an unhealthy product is sold: Cigarette advertising in magazines (1960–1985). *Journal of Communication* 37(4):95–106, Autumn 1987.

ATKINSON, A.B., SKEGG, J.L. Anti-smoking publicity and the demand for tobacco in the U.K. *Manchester School of Economics and Social Studies* 41(3):265–282, September 1973.

ATKINSON, A.B., SKEGG, J.L. Control of smoking and price of cigarettes—A comment. *British Journal of Preventive and Social Medicine* 28(1):45–48, February 1974.

ATKINSON, A.B., TOWNSEND, J.L. Economic aspects of reduced smoking. *Lancet* 2(8036): 492–495, September 3, 1977.

BALTAGI, B.H., LEVIN, D. Estimating dynamic demand for cigarettes using panel data: The effects of bootlegging, taxation, and advertising reconsidered. *Review of Economics and Statistics* 68:148–155, 1986.

BISHOP, J.A., YOO, J.H. "Health scare," excise taxes and advertising ban in the cigarette demand and supply. *Southern Economic Journal* 52(2):402–411, October 1985.

BROWN, C.C., KESSLER, L.G. Projections of lung cancer mortality in the United States: 1985–2025. *Journal of the National Cancer Institute* 80(1):43–51, March 2, 1988.

BUREAU OF NATIONAL AFFAIRS. *Where There's Smoke: Problems and Policies Concerning Smoking in the Workplace.* Washington, D.C.: Bureau of National Affairs, 1986.

BUREAU OF NATIONAL AFFAIRS. *Where There's Smoke: Problems and Policies Concerning Smoking in the Workplace*, Second Edition. Washington, D.C.: Bureau of National Affairs, 1987.

CALFEE, J.E. *Cigarette Advertising, Health Information and Regulation Before 1970.* Bureau of Economics, Federal Trade Commission, May 20, 1986.

CHALOUPKA, F., SAFFER, H. The demand for cigarettes and restrictions on smoking in the workplace. Working paper. New York: National Bureau of Economic Research, July 1988.

CONNOLLY, G.N., WINN, D.M., HECHT, S.S., HENNINGFIELD, J.E., WALKER, B. JR., HOFFMANN, D. The reemergence of smokeless tobacco. *New England Journal of Medicine* 314(16):1020–1027, April 17, 1986.

CONSUMER REPORTS. Cigarettes, the industry and its advertising: How harmful are they? *Consumer Reports* 18:58–74, February 1953.

CONSUMER REPORTS. Cigarette smoking and lung cancer. *Consumer Reports* 19:54–92, February 1954.

CONSUMER REPORTS. Cigarettes. *Consumer Reports* 20:56–73, February 1955.

COWELL, M.J., HIRST, B.L. Mortality differences between smokers and non-smokers. *Transactions of the Society of Actuaries* 32:185–213, 1980.

DAVIS, R.M. Current trends in cigarette advertising and marketing. *New England Journal of Medicine* 316:725–732, March 19, 1987.

DORON, G. *The Smoking Paradox: Public Regulation in the Cigarette Industry.* Cambridge, Massachusetts: Abt Books, 1979.

FEDERAL TRADE COMMISSION. *Federal Trade Commission Staff Report on the Cigarette Advertising Investigation.* Federal Trade Commission, May 1981.

FEDERAL TRADE COMMISSION. *Report to Congress Pursuant to the Federal Cigarette Labeling and Advertising Act.* Federal Trade Commission, February 1988.

FUJII, E.T. The demand for cigarettes: Further empirical evidence and its implications for public policy. *Applied Economics* 12:479–489, 1980.

GERSTEIN, D.R., LEVISON, P.K. (eds.) *Reduced Tar and Nicotine Cigarettes: Smoking Behavior and Health.* Washington, D.C.: National Academy Press, 1982.

HAMILTON, J.L. The demand for cigarettes: Advertising, the health scare, and the cigarette advertising ban. *Review of Economics and Statistics* 54:401–411, November 1972.

HARRIS, J.E. Public policy issues in the promotion of less hazardous cigarettes. In: Gori, G.B., Bock, F.G. (eds.) *Banbury Report. A Safe Cigarette?* Cold Spring Harbor, New York: Cold Spring Harbor Laboratory, March 12, 1980, pp. 333–340.

HARRIS, J.E. Cigarette smoking among successive birth cohorts of men and women in the United States during 1900–80. *Journal of the National Cancer Institute* 71(3):473–479, September 1983.

IPPOLITO, R.A., MURPHY, R.D., SANT, D. *Staff Report on Consumer Responses to Cigarette Health Information.* Bureau of Economics, Federal Trade Commission, August 1979.

KOZLOWSKI, L.T. Pack size, reported smoking rates, and public health. *American Journal of Public Health* 76(11):1337–1338, November 1986.

LEWIT, E.M. *Clean Indoor Air Laws and Male/Female Smoking Differences. Final Report of Program Activities.* Grant No. DA03641-02. Newark, New Jersey: University of Medicine and Dentistry of New Jersey, 1988.

LEWIT, E.M., COATE, D. The potential for using excise taxes to reduce smoking. *Journal of Health Economics* 1(2):121–145, 1982.

LEWIT, E.M., COATE, D., GROSSMAN, M. The effects of government regulation on teenage smoking. *Journal of Law and Economics* 24:545–569, December 1981.

LIEB, C.W. Can the poisons in cigarettes be avoided? *Reader's Digest* 63:45–47, December 1953.

MCGUINNESS, T., COWLING, K. Advertising and the aggregate demand for cigarettes. *European Economic Review* 6:311–328, 1975.

MCLEOD, P.B. Advertising bans, tobacco and cigarette consumption. *Economic Letters* 20:391–396, 1986.

MILES, R.H. *Coffin Nails and Corporate Strategies.* Englewood Cliffs, New Jersey: Prentice-Hall, 1982.

MILLER, L.M., MONAHAN, J. The facts behind the cigarette controversy. In: *Reports to Consumers on American Cigarettes.* Pleasantville, New York: Reader's Digest Association, 1954, pp. 3–8.

NORR, R. Cancer by the carton. *Reader's Digest*, December 1952, pp. 7–8.

PETO, J. Price and consumption of cigarettes: A case for intervention? *British Journal of Preventive and Social Medicine* 28:241–245, 1974.

RADFAR, M. The effect of advertising on total consumption of cigarettes in the U.K. *European Economic Review* 29(2):225–231, November 1985.

RIIS, R.W. How harmful are cigarettes? *Reader's Digest*, January 1950, pp. 1–11.

ROYAL COLLEGE OF PHYSICIANS. *Smoking and Health. Summary and Report of the Royal College of Physicians of London on Smoking in Relation to Cancer of the Lung and Other Diseases.* New York: Pitman Publishing Company, 1962.

RUSSELL, M.A.H. Changes in cigarette price and consumption by men in Britain, 1946–71: A preliminary analysis. *British Journal of Preventive and Social Medicine* 27(1):1–7, February 1973.

SCHNEIDER, L., KLEIN, B., MURPHY, K.M. Governmental regulation of cigarette health information. *Journal of Law and Economics* 24:575–612, December 1981.

TYE, J.B. *Sixty Years of Deception: An Analysis and Compilation of Cigarette Ads in Time Magazine, 1925 to 1985*, Volume 1. Palo Alto, California: Health Advocacy Center, 1986.

U.S. DEPARTMENT OF HEALTH AND HUMAN SERVICES. *The Health Consequences of Smoking for Women. A Report of the Surgeon General.* U.S. Department of Health and Human Services, Public Health Service, Office of the Assistant Secretary for Health, Office on Smoking and Health, 1980.

U.S. DEPARTMENT OF HEALTH AND HUMAN SERVICES. *The Health Consequences of Smoking. The Changing Cigarette: A Report of the Surgeon General.* U.S. Department of Health and Human Services, Public Health Service, Office of the Assistant Secretary for Health, Office on Smoking and Health. DHHS Publication No. (PHS) 81-50156, 1981.

U.S. DEPARTMENT OF HEALTH AND HUMAN SERVICES. *The Health Consequences of Involuntary Smoking. A Report of the Surgeon General.* U.S. Department of Health and Human Services, Public Health Service, Centers for Disease Control. DHHS Publication No. (CDC) 87-8398, 1986.

U.S. DEPARTMENT OF HEALTH AND HUMAN SERVICES. *The Health Consequences of Smoking: Nicotine Addiction. A Report of the Surgeon General, 1988.* U.S. Department of Health and Human Services, Public Health Service, Centers for Disease Control, Center for Health Promotion and Education, Office on Smoking and Health. DHHS Publication No. (CDC) 88-8406, 1988.

U.S. DEPARTMENT OF HEALTH, EDUCATION, AND WELFARE. *Smoking and Health. A Report of the Surgeon General.* U.S. Department of Health, Education, and Welfare, Public Health Service, Office of the Assistant Secretary for Health, Office on Smoking and Health. DHEW Publication No. (PHS) 79-50066, 1979.

U.S. PUBLIC HEALTH SERVICE. *Smoking and Health. Report of the Advisory Committee to the Surgeon General of the Public Health Service.* U.S. Department of Health, Education, and Welfare, Public Health Service, Center for Disease Control. PHS Publication No. 1103, 1964.

WALKER, W.J., BRIN, B.N. U.S. lung cancer mortality and declining cigarette tobacco consumption. *Journal of Clinical Epidemiology* 41(2):179–185, 1988.

WARNER, K.E. The effects of the anti-smoking campaign on cigarette consumption. *American Journal of Public Health* 67(7):645–650, July 1977.

WARNER, K.E. Possible increases in the underreporting of cigarette consumption. *Journal of the American Statistical Association* 73(362):314–318, June 1978.

WARNER, K.E. Clearing the airwaves: The cigarette ad ban revisited. *Policy Analysis* 5(4): 435–450, Fall 1979.

WARNER, K.E. Cigarette smoking in the 1970's: The impact of the antismoking campaign on consumption. *Science* 211(4483):729–731, February 13, 1981a.

WARNER, K.E. State legislation on smoking and health: A comparison of two policies. *Policy Sciences* 13:139–152, 1981b.

WARNER, K.E. Cigarette excise taxation and interstate smuggling: An assessment of recent activity. *National Tax Journal* 35(4):483–490, December 1982.

WARNER, K.E. Cigarette advertising and media coverage of smoking and health. *New England Journal of Medicine* 312:384–388, February 7, 1985a.

WARNER, K.E. Tobacco industry response to public health concern: A content analysis of cigarette ads. *Health Education Quarterly* 12(2):115–127, Summer 1985b.

WARNER, K.E. Effects of the antismoking campaign: An update. *American Journal of Public Health* 79(2):144–151, February 1989.

WARNER, K.E., MURT, H.A. Impact of the antismoking campaign on smoking prevalence: A cohort analysis. *Journal of Public Health Policy* 3(4):374–390, December 1982.

WARNER, K.E., MURT, H.A. Premature deaths avoided by the antismoking campaign. *American Journal of Public Health* 73(6):672–677, June 1983.

WHELAN, E.M. *A Smoking Gun: How the Tobacco Industry Gets Away With Murder.* Philadelphia: George F. Stickley, 1984.

WITT, S.F., PASS, C.L. Forecasting cigarette consumption: The causal model approach. *International Journal of Social Economics* 10(3):18–33, 1983.

GLOSSARY

AAFP	American Academy of Family Physicians
AAP	American Academy of Pediatrics
AARC	American Association for Respiratory Care
AC	advisory committee
ACCP	American College of Chest Physicians
ACHE	American College of Healthcare Executives
ACS	American Cancer Society
ADAMHA	Alcohol, Drug Abuse, and Mental Health Administration
AHA	American Heart Association
ALA	American Lung Association
AMA	American Medical Association
ANR	Americans for Nonsmokers' Rights
AR	attributable risk
ASH	Action on Smoking and Health
ASHA	American School Health Association
AUTS	Adult Use of Tobacco Survey
BATF	Bureau of Alcohol, Tobacco, and Firearms
BART	Bay Area Rapid Transit
BC/BS	Blue Cross–Blue Shield
BIOSEP	Biofeedback Smoking Education Project
BRFS	Behavioral Risk Factor Surveillance System
CAB	Civil Aeronautics Board
CC	Consensus Conference
CDC	Centers for Disease Control
CHD	coronary heart disease
CIS	Cancer Information Service
CNR	Californians for Nonsmokers' Rights
CNS	central nervous system
CO	carbon monoxide
COHb	carboxyhemoglobin
COLD	chronic obstructive lung disease
COPD	chronic obstructive pulmonary disease
CPS	Current Population Survey
CPS-I	Cancer Prevention Study I
CPS-II	Cancer Prevention Study II
CPSA	Consumer Product Safety Act

CPSC	Consumer Product Safety Commission
CVD	cardiovascular disease
DBP	diastolic blood pressure
DHHS	Department of Health and Human Services
DOC	Doctors Ought to Care
DOD	Department of Defense
EPA	Environmental Protection Agency
ETS	environmental tobacco smoke
FAA	Federal Aviation Administration
FCC	Federal Communications Commission
FDA	Food and Drug Administration
FEV_1	1-sec forced expiratory volume
FFDCA	Federal Food, Drug, and Cosmetic Act
FHSA	Federal Hazardous Substance Labeling Act
FTC	Federal Trade Commission
FTE	full-time equivalents
GASO	Great American Smokeout
GASP	Group Against Smoking Pollution
GSA	General Services Administration
HCN	hydrogen cyanide
HDL	high density lipoprotein
HES	Health Examination Survey
HHANES	Hispanic Health and Nutrition Examination Survey
HIAA	Health Insurance Association of America
HMO	health maintenance organization
HRSA	Health Resources and Services Administration
IAC	Interagency Committee
ICC	Interstate Commerce Commission
ICD-9	International Classification of Diseases, Ninth Revision
ICD-7	International Classification of Diseases, Seventh Revision
IPPB	Intermittent Positive Pressure Breathing Trial
IQ	I Quit
JCAHO	Joint Commission on Accreditation of Healthcare Organizations
LFL	"Live for Life"
LIRR	Long Island Railroad
MBTA	Massachusetts Bay Transportation Authority
MRFIT	Multiple Risk Factor Intervention Trial
MS	mainstream smoke
NAB	N′-nitrosoanabasine
NAIC	National Association of Insurance Commissioners
NASHS	National Adolescent Student Health Survey
NAT	N′-nitrosoanatabine
NCHS	National Center for Health Statistics
NCI	National Cancer Institute
NCSH	National Clearinghouse for Smoking and Health

NDN	National Diffusion Network
NHANES	National Health and Nutrition Examination Survey
NHES	National Health Examination Survey
NHIS	National Health Interview Survey
NHLBI	National Heart, Lung, and Blood Institute
NICHD	National Institute of Child Health and Human Development
NIDA	National Institute on Drug Abuse
NIH	National Institutes of Health
NNK	4-(methylnitrosoamino)-1-(3-pyridyl)-1-butanone
NNN	N′-nitrosonornicotine
NNS	National Natality Survey
NRC	National Research Council
NSBA	National School Boards Association
NSDA	National Survey on Drug Abuse
NSFG	National Survey of Family Growth
OASH	Office of the Assistant Secretary for Health
OCC	Office of Cancer Communications
OSH	Office on Smoking and Health
OSHA	Occupational Safety and Health Administration
OTA	Office of Technology Assessment
PAH	polynuclear aromatic hydrocarbon
PHS	Public Health Service
ppb	parts per billion
PSAs	public service announcements
RJR	R.J. Reynolds Tobacco Company
SCN^-	thiocyanate
SEP	Smoking Education Program
SES	socioeconomic status
SHCP	School Health Curriculum Project
SHD	State Health Department
SS	sidestream smoke
ST	smokeless tobacco
STAT	Stop Teenage Addiction to Tobacco
STCP	Smoking, Tobacco, and Cancer Program
TEFRA	Tax Equity and Fiscal Responsibility Act
TPLP	Tobacco Products Liability Project
TSG	Technical Study Group
TSNA	tobacco-specific N-nitrosamine
USDA	U.S. Department of Agriculture
USP	U.S. Pharmacopeia
VA	Veterans Administration
WHO	World Health Organization

INDEX

☆U.S.G.P.O. 1989 623-880/10288